# Selective Partial Ablation
# of the Frontal Cortex

# Selective Partial Ablation of the Frontal Cortex

## A Correlative Study of its Effects on Human Psychotic Subjects

BY

THE COLUMBIA-GREYSTONE ASSOCIATES

FRED A. METTLER, M.D., Ph.D.

EDITOR

PAUL B. HOEBER, INC.

MEDICAL BOOK DEPARTMENT OF HARPER & BROTHERS

SELECTIVE PARTIAL ABLATION OF THE FRONTAL CORTEX

## DEDICATION

The authors take pleasure in dedicating this volume to the nurses, attendants, and other personnel who were also true collaborators with us in this cooperative study. Your care and labor provided the greatest guarantee of safety for the patients and your enthusiasm was a constant source of stimulation to the authors.

# ACKNOWLEDGMENTS

The present constitutes the official group report of the first Columbia-Greystone Project conducted at the New Jersey State Hospital at Greystone Park, Dr. Marcus A. Curry, Medical Superintendent and Chief Executive Officer, under the auspices of the Department of Neurology of the College of Physicians and Surgeons, Columbia University, Dr. Edwin G. Zabriskie, Acting Executive Officer.

Financial assistance is acknowledged from the Myra Salzer Gift Fund, The Rockefeller Foundation, the Department of Neurology of the College of Physicians and Surgeons, the Pool-Heath Fund, several anonymous donors, the State of New Jersey and the United States Public Health Service under grant MH 118 to Columbia University, Dr. Fred A. Mettler, responsible investigator. The cooperation of several facilities of the Veterans Administration, particularly that at Lyons, New Jersey, of the Department of Mental Hygiene of the State of New York, of Montefiore Hospital, of Bellevue Hospital, of the Department of Zoology of the University of Indiana, and several other institutions and agencies in the use of apparatus and the help of their personnel is also gratefully acknowledged.

# LIST OF CONTRIBUTORS

BEECHLEY, ROBERT M., M.A.
  Psychologist, Northern New Jersey Mental Hygiene Clinic, The New Jersey State
  Hospital at Greystone Park, New Jersey.

CARPENTER, MALCOLM B., M.D.
  Fellow, Department of Neurology, College of Physicians and Surgeons, Columbia University, New York.

CLAUSEN, JOHS, M.A.
  Fellow, Psychiatric Institute, Columbia University, New York.

* COLLINS, LAURENCE M., M.D.
  Clinical Director, The New Jersey State Hospital at Greystone Park, New Jersey.

*† COTTON, HENRY A., JR., M.D.
  Former Deputy Commissioner for Mental Hygiene and Hospitals, State of New Jersey.

COWEN, DAVID, M.D.
  Assistant Professor of Neuropathology, College of Physicians and Surgeons, Columbia University, New York.

* CRANDELL, ARCHIE, M.D.
  Assistant Medical Superintendent, The New Jersey State Hospital at Greystone Park, New Jersey.

* CURRY, MARCUS A., M.D.
  Medical Superintendent and Chief Executive Officer of The New Jersey State Hospital at Greystone Park, New Jersey.

EMMEL, ELSIE, A.B., M.T.
  Clinical Laboratory, The New Jersey State Hospital at Greystone Park, New Jersey.

FEIRING, EMMANUEL, M.D.
  Associate Neurosurgeon, Beth Israel Hospital, New York. Consultant in Neurosurgery, New Jersey State Hospital at Greystone Park, New Jersey.

FRANKEL, EMIL
  Director, Division of Statistics and Research, New Jersey State Department of Institutions and Agencies, Trenton, New Jersey.

* GAMBILL, PERRY J., M.D.
  Senior Resident Physician, in charge of Ear, Nose and Throat Department, The New Jersey State Hospital at Greystone Park, New Jersey.

GARRISON, MORTIMER, JR., PH.D.
  Senior Research Scientist (Psychology), Psychiatric Institute, Columbia University, New York.

GASOREK, KATHRYN ALBERT, A.M.
  Psychologist, Psychiatric Institute, Columbia University, New York.

GASS, H. HARVEY, M.D.
  Resident, Neuropsychiatric Service, Montefiore Hospital, New York.

GRIMMELMANN, IHLER, M.A.
  Psychologic Intern, Psychiatric Institute, Columbia University, New York.

* Member of the Committee on Publication.
† Deceased.

HAMWI, VIOLET, A.B.
Psychologic Intern, Psychiatric Institute, Columbia University, New York.

* HEATH, ROBERT G., M.D.
Professor of Psychiatry and Neurology, the Tulane University of Louisiana; formerly Instructor in Neurology, College of Physicians and Surgeons, Columbia University, New York.

HOLSOPPLE, JAMES Q., PH.D.
Chief Clinical Psychologist, Veterans Administration Branch 2, New York.

KESSLER, EDWARD, M.D.
Senior Resident Physician, The New Jersey State Hospital at Greystone Park, New Jersey.

KING, HENRY EUGENE, PH.D.
Senior Research Scientist (Psychology), Psychiatric Institute, Columbia University, New York.

KING, WILBUR RICHARD, PH.D.
Psychologist, Psychiatric Institute, Columbia University, New York.

KIRK, VIRGINIA, PH.D.
Psychologist, Vanderbilt School of Medicine, Nashville, Tennessee.

KLINE, NATHAN S., M.D.
Executive Secretary, Research Committee, Veterans Administration Hospital, Lyons, New Jersey; Department of Neurology, College of Physicians and Surgeons, Columbia University, New York.

* LANDIS, CARNEY, PH.D., D.SC., M.D. (HON.)
Professor of Psychology, Columbia University; Principal Research Psychologist, Psychiatric Institute, Columbia University, New York.

LEAVENS, MILAM E., M.D.
St. Luke's Hospital, Chicago; formerly Baylor University School of Medicine, Houston, Texas.

LONGLEY, WILLIAM H., JR., M.D.
Senior Resident Physician, The New Jersey State Hospital at Greystone Park, New Jersey.

* MELVIN, DANIEL G., M.D.
Senior Resident Physician, The New Jersey State Hospital at Greystone Park, New Jersey.

* METTLER, FRED A., A.M., M.D., PH.D.
Associate Professor of Anatomy, College of Physicians and Surgeons, Columbia University, New York.

* POOL, J. LAWRENCE, M.D.
Director of the Service of Neurological Surgery, Neurological Institute, Presbyterian Hospital; Professor of Neurological Surgery, Columbia University, New York.

RAPPORT, ESTELLE, M.A.
Psychological Assistant, Rockland State Hospital, Orangeburg, New York.

RASHKIS, SHIRLEY REIDER, PH.D.
Research Assistant, Psychiatric Institute, Columbia University, New York.

ROTHFIELD, LAWRENCE, A.B.
New York University College of Medicine, New York.

RUST, RALPH M., PH.D.
Clinical Psychologist, Department of Health, Yale University, New Haven, Connecticut; formerly Research Assistant, Psychiatric Institute, Columbia University, New York.

* SAGERT, CARL M., M.D.
Senior Resident Physician and Pathologist, The New Jersey State Hospital at Greystone Park, New Jersey.

    * Member of the Committee on Publication.

SHEPPERD, LEWIS A., M.D.
Fellow in Otolaryngology, College of Physicians and Surgeons, Columbia University, New York.

STAUFFER, ANNE KENNARD, PH.D.
Research Assistant, Psychiatric Institute, Columbia University, New York.

VERNON, LEONARD J., M.D.
Anesthesiologist-in-Chief, John Gaston Hospital, Memphis, Tennessee; Acting Head Department of Anesthesiology of the University of Tennessee, College of Medicine; Consultant Anesthesiologist, St. Joseph Hospital, Memphis, Tennessee.

WEBER, JOHN J., M.D.
Research Assistant, Department of Neurology and the Psychoanalytic Clinic for Training and Research, College of Physicians and Surgeons, Columbia University, New York.

* WOLF, ABNER, M.D.
Associate Professor of Neuropathology, College of Physicians and Surgeons, Columbia University, New York.

YOUNG, KATHLEEN MARY, PH.D.
Junior Technician, Psychiatric Institute, Columbia University, New York.

* ZIGARELLI, JOSEPH F., M.D.
Senior Resident Physician, The New Jersey State Hospital at Greystone Park, New Jersey.

* ZUBIN, JOSEPH, PH.D.
Assistant Professor in Psychology, Columbia University; Associate Research Psychologist, Psychiatric Institute, Columbia University, New York.

* Member of the Committee on Publication.

# PREFACE

This book is a cooperative report of a truly cooperative endeavor. Our study derives not only from cooperation between several institutions, but also reflects the combined efforts of a large number of workers representing many disciplines. We were attempting to discover whether technically improved and less drastic neurosurgical approaches to the therapy of the mentally ill would yield results as satisfactory as, or better than, those obtained by lobotomy. More importantly, we endeavored to elucidate the mechanism by which any improvement occurs. Therefore we attempted to gather, in addition to the critical psychiatric data, as complete information as possible upon any reported or suspected function of different parts of the frontal cortex. We made use of the facilities and technics of clinic and laboratory.

In this report we present a detailed account of our study of the 48 patients in our series—24 of whom were operated upon and 24 in a control group. In Chapter I we described the process by which the patients were selected, and present a complete outline of the project. The details of the surgical procedures used are described and illustrated in Chapter IV. Chapter V is devoted to the cytoarchitecture of the brain which had to be studied afresh.

In Section II the reader will find a complete report of the medical survey of these patients, including the laboratory studies, the results of audiometric and vestibular studies, the testing of the visual apparatus, the roentgenologic determination of gastrointestinal motility, the contribution of electroencephalography, etc.

Section III, the largest portion of the book, contains a detailed report of the psychologic investigations, which were as exhaustive as we could make them within the limitations of time and the cooperative ability of our patients. In assembling an adequate battery of psychologic tests for our purposes, entirely new tests were devised which it is hoped have led to certain valid conclusions concerning the possible influence, or lack of such, of specific areas of the frontal lobe on behavior and mental life as well as brief observations on the nature of the changes produced by prefrontal lobotomy. This section includes a separate chapter devoted to follow-up tests one year after operation.

Section IV is devoted to the psychiatric, neurologic, and pathologic investigations, and in Section V we offer three separate summaries of our findings in the fields of anatomy and physiology, psychology, and psychiatry. In these summaries we attempt to point up what we feel has been learned from this exploratory research, both in terms of tentative conclusions and also by delineating areas and directions for future work which our studies have revealed.

While we feel that much has been accomplished by this project, much more remains to be done. We now see more clearly, and have attempted to set down, many of the hurdles which must be overcome before we understand the functions of various parts of the brain. We were occasionally frustrated in our efforts to follow certain lines of investigation, both by practical inability to apply known technics and also by the non-existence of technics for certain studies. These are among the areas requiring immediate study.

Perhaps the most significant implication of our work is the evidence it offers of both the productivity of cooperative research and the feasibility of such multidiscipline cooperation in peacetime. Our experience indicates that the type of integration exemplified in this report not only increases the scope and value of the cooperative result but also enriches the work of each member of the team.

Our patients were institutionalized people originally diagnosed as incurable cases of dementia praecox, manic-depressive psychosis, and involutional psychosis. Our evidence indicates, as summed up in Table 5, page 25, that a considerably higher proportion of those who received topectomy were improved and parolable from institutional care than might otherwise have been anticipated. Indeed, no patient was admitted to this group who had shown any improvement when treated by any of the alternative forms of therapy. Therefor our project, in addition to gratifying our desire for scientific information, has also served to restore several persons to community life who would otherwise have remained institutionalized. Follow-up studies for these people are reported here and are being continued.

# CONTENTS

# CONTENTS

## SECTION IV. PSYCHIATRY—NEUROLOGY—PATHOLOGY

## SECTION V. SUMMARY

**SECTION I**

# Introduction

*Chapter 1*

# Nature of the Project

FRED A. METTLER AND MARCUS A. CURRY

---

THE productive nature of cooperative research has never been better demonstrated than during the last war and the accomplishments of the Committee on Medical Research have been well explained in the second series publication of "Science in World War II" entitled "Advances in Military Medicine" (Andrus et al., '48) which, as Waldemar Kaempffert points out in his review, emphasizes the necessity for the continuance of at least some cooperative research in times of peace.

The present research was planned and executed as an application of modern cooperative methods to a specific psychiatric problem. As a coordinated attack upon problems in the field of neurology and psychiatry it was unique in method and magnitude but study of the succeeding pages will indicate many ways in which such an investigation could and should be improved. Indeed it is one of the purposes of the present communication to place on record such methodologic mistakes as we feel we have made, for in a study as costly in effort and money as this has been, mere repetition would be an extremely unenlightened enterprise. A considerable number of individual problems which do not require a large cooperative team for investigation have been turned up by the present study. Thus, far from stifling individual research, cooperative researches should have the effect of turning up many problems of a nature specifically susceptible to inquiry by the individual investigator.

In this chapter we are concerned with an explanation of the "climate of opinion" surrounding the development of the problem investigated, the formulation of the immediate problem, the background of the project, and an account of the manner in which it was carried out. In the course of dealing with these topics, data necessary to have in hand in order to understand more than one of the succeeding chapters will be immediately presented to avoid the necessity for repetition.

## DEVELOPMENT OF THE GENERAL PROBLEM

It should be clearly understood that this study was an outgrowth of the increasing use of surgical procedures for the treatment of psychiatric conditions. What we were primarily interested in was information as to whether less drastic and technically improved neurosurgical approaches would produce results as satisfactory or perhaps even better than those obtained by lobotomy. Secondarily, we hoped to elucidate the mechanism by which improvement occurs, when it does occur. Finally, we felt that no incidental bit of information should be allowed to slip by unnoticed if it were at all possible to detect it by any method at our disposal.

In order to understand why it was felt desirable to improve upon the neurosurgical methods of the treatment of psychiatric conditions, the general reader must realize that such operations had become relatively common at the time this study was begun. The circumstances underlying the growth of "psychosurgery," as it has been called, were somewhat as follows: During the past half-century the growth of medical specialism brought about a practical divorce between the various disciplines dealing with disorders of the neural system. We are not concerned in this place with an estimate of the desirability or undesirability of this process but only with an estimation of the position (in 1946) of "psychosurgery."

Once the more obvious aspects of psychotherapy had been explored, progress in the treatment of psychotics gradually decelerated. What might have happened is irrelevant in view of the introduction of shock therapy and surgical techniques. It is axiomatic that fixed lines of reasoning in medicine do not spontaneously alter their cyclical movement. When change occurs it is usually of a tangential type and is the result of the external impingement of a definitely profitable concept: one has but to consider the influence of the development of the vacuum tube upon all of medical technology.

At the end of the second decade of the present century there were two major courses which might be pursued in the treatment of malignant psychoses—psychotherapy and/or removal from society. Psychotherapy was costly, both in time and money, and produced good results in only a small number of the least serious cases. In the thirties, two additional though not entirely new therapeutic procedures attracted wide attention—convulsive therapy and "psychosurgery." If the rationale of convulsive therapy (Sakel, '35) was obscure it had the practical advantage that it often proved useful in treating temporary psychiatric episodes. Today shock therapy is increasingly utilized and additional investigation will undoubtedly reveal why it is often useful.

The original rationale for the use of surgical procedures for the relief of psychoses has been reviewed by Freeman and Watts ('42) who have also explained the events which occurred in this field in the thirties. Their book should be consulted for the details. In general, one may say that operation upon the human being was the natural outgrowth of intensive experimental work done on the cerebral cortex during the last quarter of the nineteenth century. The first operation was done by a Swiss, Gottlieb Burckhardt (1836-1907), who had written a work (Burckhardt, 1875) attempting to explain the pathophysiology of neural disorders. In 1882 he became Director of the Insane Asylum in Préfargier and soon instituted cortical removals (Burckhardt, 1890-'91). It was not until 1936 that any cerebral operations were done in this country for psychiatric conditions. Freeman and Watts (Freeman, '37) were the first operators and, although some few patients were operated upon by several others, their series of 80 was, with one exception, by far the largest series of operations done by April, 1941. The exception was a series of 73 patients operated upon by Schrader. The subsequent text will show that it was significant that Schrader's mortality rate at a state psychiatric institution—State Hospital No. 4, at Farmington, Missouri—was lower than that reported by other surgeons and his rate of improvement in chronic schizophrenics (52 percent) not very much lower than the total number of good results (63 percent) in the mixed series of Freeman and Watts.

At the time of entry of the United States into World War II relatively few laymen had heard of lobotomy or leucotomy, as the current "psychosurgical" operations were called, and these operations gave little indication of changing psychiatric treatment and management markedly for a long while to come. Morris Fishbein ('41), speaking in the capacity of editor of the Journal of the American Medical Association, approached frontal lobotomy in August 1941, with the bivalent caution characteristic of an undetermined trend, "No doctor can yet assert that this is or is not a truly worthwhile procedure. The ultimate decision must await the production of more scientific evidence." Shock therapy, meanwhile, made definite strides. It had not only been adopted by nearly all progressive state institutions but many private practitioners were using it, often under circumstances of potential danger.

Subsequent developments illustrated another characteristic feature of medical history, namely that profound changes in practice and theory are often brought about by influences outside the profession itself. This can be illustrated by calling attention to the important role played by public sentiment in accelerating changes in the care of medically discharged veterans of the late war. With the discharge of the first of what evidently was soon to become a large number of psychiatrically disabled veterans, the public became actively concerned about their rapid rehabilitation. By August 26, 1943, many relatives and guardians of patients who had failed to improve with shock therapy, began to demand more rapid and drastic treatment and on this day the Veterans Administration found it advisable to issue a communication concerning "prefrontal lobotomy." This was directed to all neuropsychiatric facilities and indicated that provision for the operation was then being prepared within the facilities by consultant neurosurgeons, working upon a fee basis, and by staff members who were to be sent for special training. Operation was to be authorized after presentation of the case to the Medical Director (Chas. M. Griffith), in Washington, and the receipt of approval from the Central Office. Cases to be selected were to be those "in which apprehension, anxiety, and depression are present, also cases with compulsions and obsessions, with marked emotional tension," and in which all other forms of therapy, including shock therapy, had failed. (A tabular presentation of the symptomatology present in the cases studied in our own series appears on p. 409.)

This communication also pointed out that special postoperative care of the patient was required to prevent "strangulation by excessive amounts of unswallowed food." Until the reorganization of the Veterans Administration in 1945 (again in response to public pressure for improved medical care) few suitable arrangements had been made for the performance of any significant number of such operations.

On April 8, 1946, applications for "prefrontal lobotomy," as it was called in circular No. 83 of that date, were ordered to be submitted for approval to the appropriate Branch office for the consideration of the Consultant in neuropsychiatry who was to see the patient wherever possible. In Technical Bulletin 10A-30 (March 28, 1947), rescinding circular 83, the operation to be done was designated as "prefrontal leukotomy" and the Branch chief in neurosurgery and the Branch chief in neuropsychiatry were authorized to delegate responsibility, for the selection of patients for the operation, to a "leukotomy committee" in any VA hospital or center; such committee to consist, when possible, of the consultant in neurosurgery, the consultant in neuropsychiatry, the chief of the service concerned, and the clinical psychologist. At this time it was said that criteria for the selection of patients were in the process of being developed.

In the meanwhile the public had begun to inquire why more radical therapy was not being employed among the chronic populations of civilian mental hospitals. We have already mentioned Schrader's early work in this field in Missouri. By March, 1947, over 2,000 lobotomies had been done in the United States, including a series of 200 at the Boston Psychopathic Hospital. Of this number over 1,725 were done since 1941. It is obvious that neurosurgery was being increasingly employed in the psychoses and this trend continued while the present study was in progress.

No one reading the present monograph is likely to be in need of reminder that the rationale for lobotomy or leucotomy still required clarification in 1947. Indeed, TB 10A-30 explicitly recognized the necessity for further attention to the development of criteria for the selection of cases and it is quite certain that little or nothing published up to that date provided any real objective evidence of what effects were produced by such operations. This is scarcely surprising since the operations were performed by blind procedures and it is difficult to compare the various elements in the data collected prior to that date.

Under favorable circumstances the mortality rate at the end of 1946, by blind operation, was about 4 percent but it was not uncommon for the death rate to reach 10, 15, or even 20 percent in some unpublicized groups of cases, even when operations were performed by neurosurgeons of unquestionable competence. Such experience indicates that, regardless of psychiatric condition, the "psychosurgical" patient is, for a specific critical period, primarily a neurosurgical patient and his pre- and postoperative management must rest securely in the hands of a competent and adequate staff trained in neurosurgical techniques.

From the point of view of management there is still another factor worth emphasizing, which suggests that the patient should have the benefit of skilled and continued neurosurgical care—the occurrence of convulsions in about 4 percent of the patients surviving operation. In any series of patients subjected to psychosurgery, by methods commonly in use in 1947, it might be anticipated that 4 percent would not survive the operation, an additional 4 percent would develop convulsions, and an additional 42 percent would show no very decided improvement.

### FORMULATION OF THE PARTICULAR PROBLEM

As commonly performed, up to 1947, the technique of frontal lobotomy was an empirical procedure. While all surgeons performing the operation were constantly attempting to probe as deeply as possible into the circumstances surrounding whatever changes were produced in their patients, little systematic information which did not appear in Freeman and Watts' original edition, was brought forward at the time the present investigation was begun. It is obvious that a systematic study of the effect of frontal lobotomy was long overdue and, in discussing this matter with members of the Veterans Administration prior to the issuance of TB 10A-30, Mettler suggested the advisability of collecting such data—an idea which must have occurred to even the casual observer. The implementation of such a program was, however, retarded by fiscal difficulties existent at the time and it is apparent that such a study, extensive, laborious, and exhaustive though it must have been, to be of any real significance, could only have served as a preliminary step until such time as the operative approach could be better controlled.

In practice the usual, initial, and often satisfactory lobotomy was theoretically carried out through a plane which ventrally lies just rostral to the temporal pole and dorsally cuts the junction of Brodmann's area 8 and 6. (Freeman and Watts, '47). If such a cut completely disconnected all cortex rostral to it, areas 10 and 46 would be disconnected together with most of Brodmann's areas 9, 11, 47, 32, and a slight amount of areas 8 and 45. Such total disconnection was uncommon, the usual incision of that time, despite its ventral origin, sparing most of the basal radiations (and thus areas 11, 47, and perhaps 32). That more or less other cortex was also spared is very probable since, while the occasional patient was well oriented, serious degradation occasionally followed complete transection carried out far rostral to the usual plane. Lobotomy at planes caudal to that noted above, was done in patients who failed to show improvement or in those having relapses. The plane then chosen, theoretically cut the caudal part of area 6 dorsally and its rostral part ventrally. Since, however, variation is of the essence in anatomy, from a practical point of view it is inconceivable that these cerebral incisions, based upon planes determined by cranial landmarks, as the lobotomy incision must be, would always fall at a particular place. The degree of expected variation as determined by Mettler and Rowland ('48) from measurements made on cadavers is of such a nature that one can hope to find the incision passing through some part of the pars triangularis of the inferior frontal gyrus in not much more than half the number of cases. In about a quarter of the number of cases the incision enters through area 44 or its borders. Rarely

TABLE 1.   POINT OF CEREBRUM EXPOSED IN THE LIVING HUMAN BEING BY EMPLOYING THE MEASUREMENTS OF FREEMAN AND WATTS FOR THE LATERAL TRANSCRANIAL APPROACH

| Case no. | Distance to lateral fissure | Distance to central fissure | Location of Point |
|---|---|---|---|
| 5 | 1.8 | 1.4 | Dorsocaudal quadrant of pars opercularis |
| 11 | 2.2 | 2.7 | Dorsorostral quadrant of pars opercularis |
| 20 | 2.4 | 2.8 | Dorsorostral corner of pars opercularis |
| 23 | 1.4 | 2.7 | Dorsocaudal part of pars triangularis |
| 28 | 2.3 | 2.6 | Dorsorostral quadrant of pars opercularis |
| 46 | 2.1 | 1.9 | Dorsorostral quadrant of pars opercularis |
| Range | 1.4–2.4 | 1.4–2.8 | |

it enters the middle frontal gyrus. While postmortem distortion accounts for a certain amount of the variation noted above the most fertile source of error lies in the difficulty encountered in locating the part of the coronal suture to be perforated (Rowland and Mettler, '48). This is, of course, harder to find in the living patient, especially if old, than in the cadaver. While the number of surgical cases in which we have been able to turn down a bone flap after marking the brain through a lobotomy burr-hole is small, it is apparent that variation is not entirely artifactual. The measurements in 6 living patients in whom the coronal suture was absolutely defined* are given in table 1.

Even in patients in whom the operation is done at a particular plane, the amount of disconnected cortex varies. Finally, even if one assumes that the same areas were always disconnected it would still be rationally desirable to determine the critical parts of this disconnected cortex.

We are thus brought to a concern beyond that of merely studying the effects of frontal lobotomy. Lobotomy requires analysis into its constituent elements in order to extricate desirable from undesirable effects and pertinent regions from those in which removal or disconnection contributes nothing to the possible therapeutic value of the operation. Could we find, for example, that only one cortical area need be removed to achieve a particular result, an essentially uncertain operation could be reduced to proper surgical technique and its unnecessary damage eliminated. It is possible that careful study might

* The measurements given here for the living are uninfluenced by shift in the brain after opening the skull case for a simple lobotomy. The brain may or may not shift its position after a large flap is turned down. It may not change its position even after much handling and turning of the head. Positional changes are most marked with alterations in circulatory flow or fluid balance. The largest shift we have so far observed was about 1 cm.

disclose areas of differential therapeutic value or even reveal the mechanism by which improvement is brought about. If this mechanism were accessible by medical rather than surgical means the highest possible degree of success might be said to have been achieved.

### BACKGROUND OF THE COLUMBIA-GREYSTONE STUDY

During the period from 1942-1944, the connections and functions of the primate frontal cortex were under restudy. These studies allowed the construction of a thalamocortical map (Mettler, '47) in which the various areas of Brodmann could be correlated with particular parts of the thalamic nuclei. This map offered little support for the then current belief that the medial thalamic nucleus projects to both rostral cortex and hypothalamus, a belief which figured prominently in current explanations for the manner in which frontal lobotomy was believed to exert a beneficial effect. It was our hope that these studies, and others of Freeman and Watts ('47) published together with them (see also Mettler, '47a), might prove of use in studying the effects of lobotomy as well as motor function in general. A previous study (Mettler, '44) had already indicated that while removals of most individual granular cortical areas exerted little if any effect upon the behavior of simians, removal of area 9 alone produced a definite change in the direction of increased spontaneous activity (an observation previously made by Richter and Hines, '38) while removal of all granular frontal cortex results in over-reactivity. More recently a number of writers, particularly Halstead ('47), have touched upon a phenomenon, designated as "stimulus bound," resembling over-reactivity; this phenomenon is similarly seen after frontal lobe lesion in the human being. Again, a heightened immediate reaction to noxious stimulation has been described after lobotomy (Chapman, Rose, and Solomon, '48). The fact that the portion of the medial nucleus which most frequently shows retrograde change in the human being after lobotomy is that which projects to area 9 suggested that functional changes due to disconnection of area 9 might be the critical factor in lobotomy regardless of whatever other changes might result from disconnection of additional areas. (There is here no implication that severance of the thalamocortical fibers is responsible for such improvement but merely that the thalamic degeneration is a means of determining what cortical area is really disconnected.)

At this time Dr. James Lawrence Pool occupied the position of Research Assistant in the Department of Neurology and Dr. Robert G. Heath, that of Tilney Fellow. Both were interested in the analysis of frontal lobe function and a conservative operative procedure (middle of superior frontal gyrus) was worked out which was tried by Dr. Pool on one of his private patients, Dr. Heath doing the psychiatric study of the case. Surprisingly enough (since there was no *a priori* reason to suppose that Brodmann's simian area 9 is identical either in structure or function with his area 9 in man) the results of this operation were encouraging (a second such patient also improved but in two others the results were equivocal).

About this time (the early fall of 1946) Mettler was giving a series of lectures under the auspices of the New Jersey Neuropsychiatric Association and this opportunity was taken to see whether a sufficiently large series of suitable patients might be available to continue the study of the results of such an operation.* A rather sizeable number of requests appeared for consideration. Naturally enough these requests came from the State of New Jersey and most came from the area taken care of by the New Jersey State Hospital at Greystone Park. In expressing his opinion of the matter in connection with one such patient, Dr. Curry stated that he was in accord with the psychosurgical approach and would be agreeable to having the relatives of the patient in question arrange for her transfer for operation. The patient, Mrs. S., was a schizophrenic and, at the time of the correspondence concerning her, Dr. Heath expressed some doubt as to the advisability of operation in this condition.

* By vote of the group on December 1, 1947, the operative procedure involved in such localized cortical ablation has been named topectomy, from τόπος and ἐκτομή.

Moreover, it was felt that if several patients from Greystone were to be available it might be more satisfactory to operate on the premises rather than to put the relatives to the difficulties of transferring such patients from the jurisdiction of one state to another.

On January 23, 1947, Dr. Curry wrote Dr. Mettler, in part, as follows: "this is to advise that I have taken this matter up with my Chief Surgeon (Dr. Collins) and the Director of Nurses (Miss Clark) and we very definitely feel that this procedure is another advancement in the treatment of mental disease and, accordingly, we shall be very glad to make our operating room available and to furnish scrub nurses during the operation."

It now became apparent, as might have been anticipated, that the patients concerning whom requests might be received were not necessarily those who were most likely to be benefited by a cortical operation. On the other hand, it was clear to Superintendent Curry that the relatives of very many suitable patients would request such operation if they knew it were possible to obtain such a service free of charge.

In spite of the improvement of the patients initially operated upon in New York (three of these underwent operation at the Neurological Institute and one at Doctors Hospital) several disturbing features presented themselves. It was feared that variation in the psychiatric condition of the patients studied would deprive any data collected of much of their significance. Moreover, even though the operative procedure used was based upon apparently valid experimental data and had, in part, proved useful, it might well be that the human frontal cortex contained regions of much greater significance than 9 and that these regions would never be discovered if the operation were not varied. Again, our ultimate goal was not to perform an operation but to find out why such an operation had a beneficial effect. This could not be done unless the patients were studied just as completely as it was possible for us to do so. Such a program must, of necessity, be a *tour de force.* To set up the requisite machinery for such a study without trying to collect data which might answer some of the outstanding questions about the frontal lobe would be a very wasteful enterprise. Finally, no cortical operation is ever quite comparable to another. Let us assume that area 9 had been removed from our patients initially operated upon (in point of fact the operations only approximately involved that area): Could we then assume that similarly favorable results could be obtained from every area 9 removal? Certainly not, since it was more than possible that the improvement might have been the result of the inadvertent dysfunction of some other region, either by severing its projections or interfering with its blood supply. If that were the case it might well be that an area 9 operation might prove to be essentially irrelevant.

The conclusions to be drawn from these considerations were obvious—nothing short of a complete study of the frontal cortex, area by area, could answer the problems before us. Moreover, as was subsequently pointed out by Dr. Cotton, in order to exclude a "total push" effect from the test procedures themselves, it would be necessary to include in the study a group of patients not undergoing operation who would be just as thoroughly studied and kept in precisely the same environment as those who were to be operated upon. A study such as this required a plan of attack surpassing anything heretofore attempted in the field of psychiatry. It presented problems in financing, personnel, supply, synchronization, and planning of no mean magnitude. To disentangle some of these problems a general conference was held at Greystone Park on February 1. Present at this conference were Drs. Collins, Cotton, Crandell, Curry, Heath, McMurray, Mettler, and Pool and Senator Abel. The results of the conference were summarized in a directive issued by Dr. Cotton on February 3 and in a preliminary plan drawn up by Dr. Mettler on February 4. The following is abstracted from these:

"Statement of Problem: An elucidation of the factors involved in leucotomy with a view toward employing a more discriminating and less drastic operation which will give a wider range of more selective functional results.

"Methods of study: . . . In order to evaluate the necessity or desirability of removing" various frontal areas "and with a view toward preserving those which need not be disconnected, selected areas . . . will be removed from a series of patients." (Preliminary plan.)

"the removal of a small portion of cortex . . . This operation should be much safer than the present practice" which carries "the risk of cutting aberrant blood vessels and otherwise causing severe damage to the brain."

On February 7, the project was approved by Edwin Garvin Zabriskie, Acting Executive Officer of the Department of Neurology, and an application for funds was signed on February 17 by Dean Willard C. Rappleye of the College of Physicians and Surgeons. On February 28, the New Jersey State Board of Control gave its approval.

The preliminary plan outlined a tentative method of procedure and, on March 10, the project was declared in operation and a definite protocol was drawn up. Approxi-

TABLE 2.  ROSTER OF PERSONNEL NOT LISTED ON PAGES vii–ix

ATTENDANTS AT GREYSTONE

Elsworth Bopp

George Bopp

Mrs. Frank Connelly

Mrs. Josephine Delaine

Mrs. Elizabeth Harple

John Hurta

Michael Lane

Abe Levy

Clifford Maines

Walter Peters (from Jefferson Medical College)

Ruth Coombs Tennyson

Mrs. Ruth Versen

JUNIOR TECHNICIANS AT COLUMBIA

Gloria Oliver

Irene Bookspan Sacks

LABORATORY TECHNICIANS AT GREYSTONE

Eleanor Coulter

Mary Jo Hatch

Dolores Pisapia

Ward C. Slawson

ROENTGENOLOGY TECHNICIANS AT GREYSTONE

Mrs. F. Mars

Rose Zaluk

SECRETARIES AT COLUMBIA

Frances Daniels

Irma Horst

Diana Leslie

Mary Marquette

Audrey Moore

William Schubring

Regina Unger

SECRETARIES AT GREYSTONE

Mary L. Byrnes

Mildred Herroder

SECRETARY AT GREYSTONE AND COLUMBIA

Dorothy Logan

SENIOR TECHNICIANS AT COLUMBIA

Mrs. G. Lubinsky

Mrs. C. Schogoleff

OCCUPATIONAL THERAPIST AT GREYSTONE

Mrs. Corinna Hegarty

EDITORIAL ASSISTANT

Mabel Kerr (College of Physicians and Surgeons, Columbia University)

ILLUSTRATOR

Mrs. Theresa Summers, Department of Neurology, College of Physicians and Surgeons

PHOTOGRAPHER

Peter Huber, *Department of Neurology, College of Physicians and Surgeons*

PHARMACIST (GREYSTONE)

Mr. Philip Roberts

NURSING STAFF (GREYSTONE)

| | |
|---|---|
| Betty Bacher | Kristine Jensen |
| Rose Campo | Frances Koonz |
| Adeline Collins | Morese Miller |
| Ann Eickhorn | Dorothy Minker |
| Edith Staats Emery | Jean Olson |
| Marion Evans | Dorothy Ramsey |
| Shirley Farley | Emma Robotkay |
| Mrs. Vivien Haliburton | Alice Rohr |
| Irene Hermandez | Edna Romoski |
| Helen Herschell | Alice Smith |
| Ruth Holley | Emma Sobers |

Margaret Swearingen

DIETITIAN (GREYSTONE)

Florence Pond

OPERATING ROOM STAFF (GREYSTONE)

| | |
|---|---|
| Joan Bolitho | Mrs. Lorraine Ewing |
| Marie Brinkman | Jeanne Leyhan |

Mrs. Gladys Paulos

RESEARCH ASSISTANT (NEUROLOGY, COLUMBIA)

Mrs. H. Edey (*New York University, College of Medicine*)

SUPERVISORS (GREYSTONE)

| | |
|---|---|
| Mrs. Virginia Callahan | Mrs. Jeannette Muller |
| Mrs. Dora Maxwell | Elsie Slobuski |

Alice Wilson

DIRECTOR OF NURSING (GREYSTONE)

Dorothy E. Clark

ANESTHETIST

D. Jeanne Richardson, M.D., *Department of Anesthesia, Bellevue Hospital*

SOMATOTYPE GROUP

Wm. H. Sheldon, Ph.D., M.D., *Research Associate, Department of Medicine, College of Physicians and Surgeons, Columbia University*

C. Wesley Dupertius, Ph.D., *Research Associate, Department of Medicine, College of Physicians and Surgeons, Columbia University*

SEX BEHAVIOR GROUP

Wardell Pomeroy, Ph.D., *Department of Zoology, Indiana University, Bloomington, Indiana*

Alfred C. Kinsey, Sc.D., *Watermann Research Professor of Zoology, University of Indiana, Bloomington, Indiana*

CONSULTANT ON VESTIBULAR FUNCTION

Edmund Fowler, Jr., M.D., *Professor of Otolaryngology, College of Physicians and Surgeons, Columbia University*

ASSISTANT SUPERINTENDENT, THE NEW JERSEY STATE HOSPITAL AT GREYSTONE PARK

George B. McMurray, M.D.

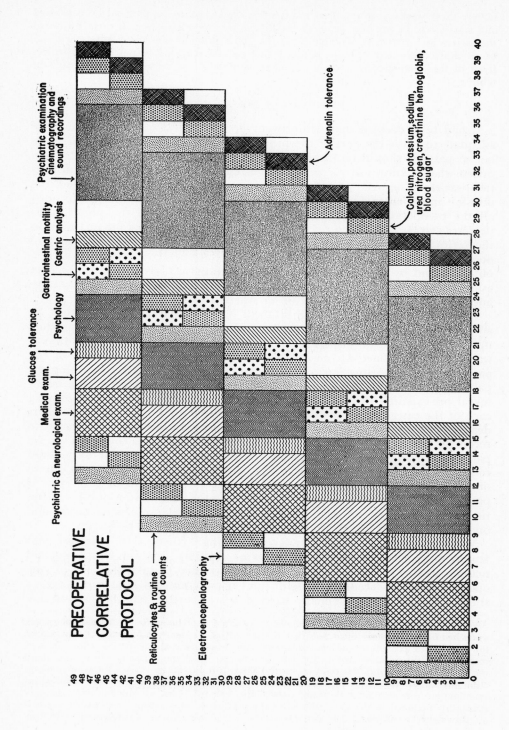

PREOPERATIVE CORRELATIVE PROTOCOL

Psychiatric & neurological exam.

Medical exam.

Glucose tolerance

Psychology

Gastric analysis

Gastrointestinal motility

Psychiatric examination cinematography and sound recordings

Reticulocytes & routine blood counts

Electroencephalography

Adrenalin tolerance

Calcium, potassium, sodium, urea nitrogen, creatinine hemoglobin, blood sugar mately three weeks were required to assemble the necessary supplementary personnel and start work. In practice many of the difficulties envisioned seemed to take care of themselves as we went along, thanks to the good common sense and indefatigability of all those concerned with the project. The collaborating personnel is listed in the front of this monograph, a roster of the remainder of the personnel is presented in table 2.

## EXECUTION OF THE PROJECT

It had been decided that while twenty-four bilateral operations would be adequate to cover the part of the brain under investigation, twice that number of patients should be included in the study. The extra 24 patients comprised what is known in succeeding pages as the "control" group. No distinction was made between any of the 48 patients prior to operation. Indeed, the decision in which group an individual patient belonged was not made until all the preoperative studies were complete. On March 10 the preoperative protocol (fig. 1) was drawn up, and by March 25 the patients for inclusion in the series had been selected (fig. 2 shows the distribution of controls and operatees by age and sex). By April 3 the special operative permits had been obtained and by April 5 the patients had been transferred to ward 17A set aside in the Clinic Building at Greystone Park. Preoperative study, in accordance with the schedule, was begun on April 7.

**Protocol.** In drawing up the protocol it was our intention to gather, in addition to the critical psychiatric data, as complete information as possible upon any reported or suspected function of the frontal lobe. In addition it was necessary to have a complete estimate of the medical condition of the patient (the age, sex, marital condition, and other general data concerning the patients is shown in table 3) and certain precautionary data which might reveal pre-existing intracranial disease or anomaly. The reasons for studying each of the categories of data selected will appear upon reading the chapters dealing with those categories. In drawing up the protocol we were forced to reconcile ourselves to the deletion of certain studies. The condition of the patients prevented us from carrying out studies of basal metabolism, fluid intake and output, caloric requirements, and urinary secretion. It was one of our purposes to see what could be done with the problem of that type of patient who might be expected to spend the rest of his life in a public institution. Under such circumstances behavior is likely to be somewhat casual and one is forced to do without some data.

We also had to reconcile ourselves to doing without skin resistance and temperature measurements and studies of capillary flow for which we had neither apparatus nor personnel. We did not care to take the risk of preoperative pneumoencephalograms or lumbar puncture, and thus had to forego studies of the hematoencephalic barrier. It was further felt that it was pos-

---

FIG. 1. This diagram shows the manner in which the preoperative work-up of the cases was scheduled and clearly illustrates that the pattern of temporal dispersion is a function of the number of procedures and patients when the work load of the testing teams is kept constant. Patient numbers are on the left (no case 43); days from start of testing are along the abscissa. The schedule for the various disciplines is indicated by various forms of shading; clear blocks, electroencephalography. Included in the time allotted to the neurological examination were vestibular tests and tests of thermal, two-point, vibrational, and gustatory sensibility. Included in the time allotted to the psychiatric examination were gastrointestinal motility rechecks and visual field determinations. The above protocol was followed by routine skull roentgenologic examination.

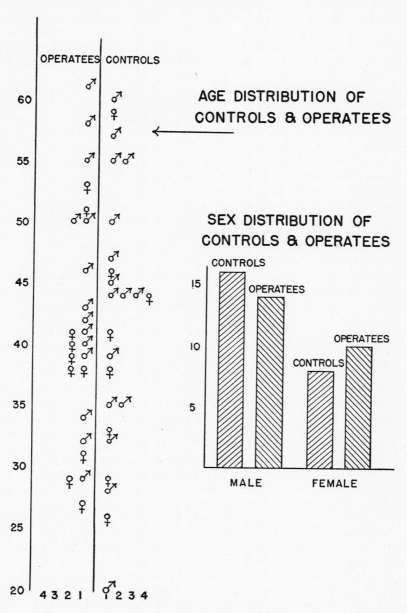

Fig. 2. Distribution of controls and operatees by age and sex.

sible to carry the gathering of data into a realm where the law of diminishing returns would become operative and we thus ruled out myographic study and direct electrical recordings from the cortex at operation. The latter procedure would have unduly prolonged an already lengthy operation and complicated the surgical set-up; therefore, although excellent apparatus and expert personnel were available for such work, it was left out of the protocol. Finally, the number of investigative procedures which could be performed was limited by the maximum number of postoperative examinations which were consistent with the welfare of the patients.

It was not expected that the protocol would be rigidly followed but examination of the data subsequently presented indicates that, in actual practice, its gathering proceeded with surprisingly few hiatuses. While undue crowding of a program such as this is certainly to be avoided it is probably advisable to arrange schedules of this type so that the work of any given team flows along in a fairly uninterrupted manner. In no case should an unscheduled break in activity be allowed to develop. Alternative critical personnel should be immediately available for all teams as replacements in case of illness and also to supply help if an incorrect estimate of the work load has been made.

**Selection of Patients for the Group.** The selection of the patients is further discussed on p. 21. It was our original desire to work with patients of as nearly the same kind as possible. While it was theoretically possible to draw against other institutions in New Jersey, the population at Greystone (5,700) is so extensive that there seemed to be no reason for going outside that hospital. While it is improbable that anyone of experience would expect to be able to discover 50 identical cases from among even so large a number as 5,700 (even when these are already largely selected because of geographic and economic factors) the degree of divergence we ultimately found in our group was surprising and seriously complicated the interpretation of the subsequent data. It must not be supposed that such variation is peculiar to our series. Many, if not most, psychiatric studies are conducted upon groups less homogeneous than ours but the factor of variation is consciously or unconsciously minimized or ignored. This seems to us to be a peculiarly blind procedure which leads not only the reader but the investigator himself into confusion. At first we thought there was something radically wrong with our method of selection (some ways in which it can be improved are subsequently indicated) but we soon found that we had uncovered an unexpected error in the clinical method. Once the members of a selected group are brought together, at the same time and place, and simultaneously examined under identical conditions very surprising differences emerge which might not have been apparent under other circumstances. It must be emphasized that the factor of difference is thrown into relief in this way as by no other. If one examines a particular patient in January and another in February, one's criteria have already had time to undergo a subtle evolution; moreover, one cannot go from the one patient to another and make an immediate comparison. It will be one of the purposes of chapter 25 to emphasize the differences brought out under such conditions. Spatial and temporal juxtaposition therefore reduce the illusion of uniformity. Moreover, patients exhibit highly labile kinetic variations, the degree of which is only perceptible by a method of study such as that here employed. The condition of psychotic patients is especially unstable and not a few of ours changed perceptibly during preoperative study (see also p. 22) and several original diagnoses required revision as the patients' patterns of

TABLE 3.  BASIC DATA FOR THE 48 PATIENTS IN THE PROJECT
(There is no number 43)
(For cytoarchitectonic maps see Chapter 5 and with regard to apparent discrepancies in succeeding chapters, concerning removals of various areas see p. 78)

| No. of patient | Age | Sex | Marital condition | I.Q. | Occupation | Final preoperative diagnosis | Operative removal |
|---|---|---|---|---|---|---|---|
| 1[k] | 35707 55 | M. | Single | 119 | Electrician | Sch. Cat. | Control |
| 2 | 38803 46 | M. | Married | 107 | Blueprint sketcher | Sch. Heb. | 8, 6$^b$, 9$^b$ (leucot.$^a$) |
| 3[k] | 38077 61 | M. | Married | 125 | Accountant | Inv. Mixed | 9$^b$, 6$^b$ |
| 4[i,k] | 47130 55 | M. | Single | 92 | Porter | Ob. Incip. Schiz.$^f$ | 46 |
| 5[h,k] | 44574 35 | M. | Married | 83 | Welder | Sch. Heb. | Control (leucot.) |
| 6[a] | 45650 32 | M. | Single | 92 | Shipping clerk | Sch. Heb. | 8$^b$, 6$^d$, (6$^e$) |
| 7[i,k] | 41443 40 | M. | Married | 93 | Machinist | Sch. Par. | 8, 9$^b$, 10$^b$ |
| 8[a,k] | 43486 29 | M. | Single | 90 | Cook | Psych. (?), Incip. Sch.$^f$ | 10$^b$, 46$^b$, 9$^b$,8$^b$ |
| 9[k] | 38170 44 | M. | Single | 113 | Baker | Sch. Par. | Control |
| 10 | 26023 44 | M. | Single | 76 | Driver | Schiz. Heb. | Control |
| 11[i,k] | 41610 44 | M. | Married | 91 | Laborer | Schiz. Par. | Control (leucot.$^a$) |
| 12 | 44893 57 | M. | Married | 109 | Upholsterer | Schiz. Par. | Control |
| 13[a,i,k] | 44060 43 | M. | Married | 96 | Waiter | Schiz. Par. | 9$^b$, 10$^b$, 45, 46 |
| 14 | 37249 47 | M. | Married | 119 | Physician | Schiz. Heb. | Control |
| 15[i,k] | 33491 55 | M. | Widowed | 81 | Laborer | Schiz. Heb. | Control |
| 16 | 35143 50 | M. | Single | 83 | Clerk | Sch. Heb. (?) Org. Psych. | Control |
| 17 | 28282 60 | M. | Married | 104 | Salesman | Schiz. Heb.$^f$ | Control |
| 18 | 42228 39 | M. | Divorced | 127 | Research physicist | Schiz. Heb. | 11$^b$ |
| 19 | 37380 50 | M. | Married | 102 | Candymaker | Schiz. (?) MDD$^f$ | 45$^b$ |
| 20[h,i,k] | 40370 28 | M. | Single | 55 | Farmer | Schiz. Heb. | Control (leucot.$^a$) |
| 21[i,k] | 26619 42 | M. | Single | 104 | Butcher | MDD | 10 |
| 22[a,i,k] | 47390 50 | M. | Married | 101 | Weaver | Schiz. Par. or In. P. | 9, 10, 46 |
| 23 | 45947 39 | M. | Divorced | 117 | Letter carrier | Schiz. Heb.$^f$ | Control (leucot$^a$) |
| 24 | 29624 41 | M. | Single | 67 | Baker | Schiz. Cat. | 6$^d$ (6$^e$) |
| 25[i,k] | 45317 58 | M. | Married | 95 | Mailer | Inv. D.+Pos. Org. Br. Dis. | 8, 9, 46, 10$^b$ |
| 26 | 43551 35 | M. | Divorced | 89 | Laborer | Schiz. Heb. | Control |
| 27[k] | 43105 34 | M. | Single | 84 | None | Schiz. Heb. | 10$^b$, 9$^b$, 8$^b$, 6$^b$ |
| 28 | 43840 27 | M. | Single | 57 | Laborer | Schiz. Heb. | Control (leucot.$^a$) |
| 29 | 44891 20 | M. | Single | 89 | None | Schiz. Cat. | Control |
| 30 | 26777 45 | M. | Separated | 74 | Laborer | Schiz. Heb. | Control |
| 31 | 45743 51 | F. | Married | 96 | Domestic | Inv. Par. | 9 |
| 32 | 39651 41 | F. | Married | 131 | Secretary | MDM | 8$^b$, 9, 10$^b$ |
| 33[k] | 46102 27 | F. | Single | 94 | Mill worker | Schiz. Heb.$^f$ | 10$^b$, 46$^b$, 45, 44$^b$ |
| 34[i,k] | 46307 33 | F. | Single | 121 | Shop steward | Schiz. Par. | Control |
| 35 | 47227 59 | F. | Divorced | 111 | Dressmaker | Schiz. Par.$^f$ | Control |
| 36[k] | 44784 53 | F. | Separated | 93 | Houseworker | Inv. Par.$^f$ | 10, 11, 45, 46, 47$^l$ |
| 37 | 43992 38 | F. | Married | 76 | None | Schiz. Heb. | Control |
| 38[a,i,k] | 45216 38 | F. | ? | 106 | Bookkeeper | MDM | 6, 8, 9, 10$^e$ |
| 39[i,k] | 42886 44 | F. | Widowed | 101 | Clerical work | Schiz. Heb.$^f$ | Control |

TABLE 3. BASIC DATA FOR THE 48 PATIENTS IN THE PROJECT—*Continued*

| No. of patient | Age | Sex | Marital condition | I.Q. | Occupation | Final preoperative diagnosis | Operative removal |
|---|---|---|---|---|---|---|---|
| 40[g] | 43788 | 29 | F. | Single | 91 | Salesgirl | Schiz. Par. | 24[b] (ventricle) |
| 41 | 32936 | 46 | F. | Married | ? | Waitress | Schiz. Heb. | Control |
| 42[g,i,k] | 44878 | 40 | F. | Married | 113 | Salesgirl | MDM—Schiz. | 11 |
| 44 | 41144 | 38 | F. | Married | ? | Bookkeeper | Schiz. Heb. | 47[bl] (leucot.[a]) |
| 45 | 40705 | 41 | F. | Married | ? | Farmwork | Schiz. Heb. | Control |
| 46 | 45052 | 29 | F. | Single | ? | Telephone operator | Schiz. Heb. | Control (leucot.[a]) |
| 47 | 40202 | 31 | F. | Single | 74 | Sewer | Schiz. Heb. | 44 |
| 48 | 39338 | 26 | F. | Single | 67 | Worked for NYA | Schiz. Heb. | Control |
| 49[i,k] | 27718 | 39 | F. | Single | 111 | None | Schiz. Par. | 10, 11[b], 46[b] |

? Unable to determine.
[a] Done five months after original operation or visit to surgery.
[b] Part only.
[c] Unilateral verification done five months after original operation.
[d] Incomplete original removal (caudally).
[e] Venous ligation.
[f] See chapter 25 for elaboration of diagnosis and changes made after visit to surgery.
[g] Convulsions following topectomy.
[h] Convulsions following lobotomy.
[i] Out of hospital on July 1, 1948. On Oct. 18, 1948, 2 topectomies, cases 7, 8, in this group had been returned to the institution but 2 others (19, 27) had been discharged. All controls in this group were still out; of the leucotomies, case 20 had been returned. There were no new discharges among the controls or leucotomies.
[k] Considered to have shown temporary or permanent improvement.
[l] Area 47 appears to be indistinguishable from area 10

behavior became clearer. As we came to know our patients better we realized that uniformity was an unobtainable goal, but we now feel that we have perfected a technique for drawing closer to that goal than that employed when we began this work. The important points here are: (1) that our group was not uniform, (2) that this lack in uniformity complicates the interpretation of the results, (3) that this failing is not peculiar to our work, (4) that methods to circumvent the difficulty have yet to be devised, (5) that our method of study enables one to perceive variations which would otherwise be missed, and (6) that we feel, as a result of the present study, we have been able to devise criteria and methods which will enable us to draw even closer to the theoretical ideal.

Some idea of the difficulty of obtaining a "homogeneous" group can be obtained from the results of a later survey made at Greystone and based upon the following criteria: absence of obvious mental disease in the blood relatives, absence of obvious medical complications, completion of at least the eighth grade of an American school, the existence of some sort of stable supportive social situation to which the patient might return, existence of the illness without remission for at least two years, and limitation of chronological age to a ten-year span as follows: schizophrenics and psychoneurotics, 25 to 35; manic depressive and involutionals to 45 to 55. The initial survey detected only 54 hebephrenic, 16 catatonic, 3 paranoid, 4 manic depressive, and 16 involutional patients who offered promise of meeting these criteria. The preliminary psychiatric review reduced the eligible cases to 20 hebephrenic, 10 catatonic, and 10 involutional cases. Further investigation reduced the eligibles still farther. It is evident that very strenuous efforts must be used and a hospital population larger than 6,000 to obtain

48 psychiatric patients who are relatively uniform with regard to more than one or two variable factors.

Having encountered and perceived the factor of variation we decided to turn it to good account and we found that it enabled us to try to fit our operations to the needs of the case. This was the final determining factor (medical condition being the primary factor) in selecting the patients for

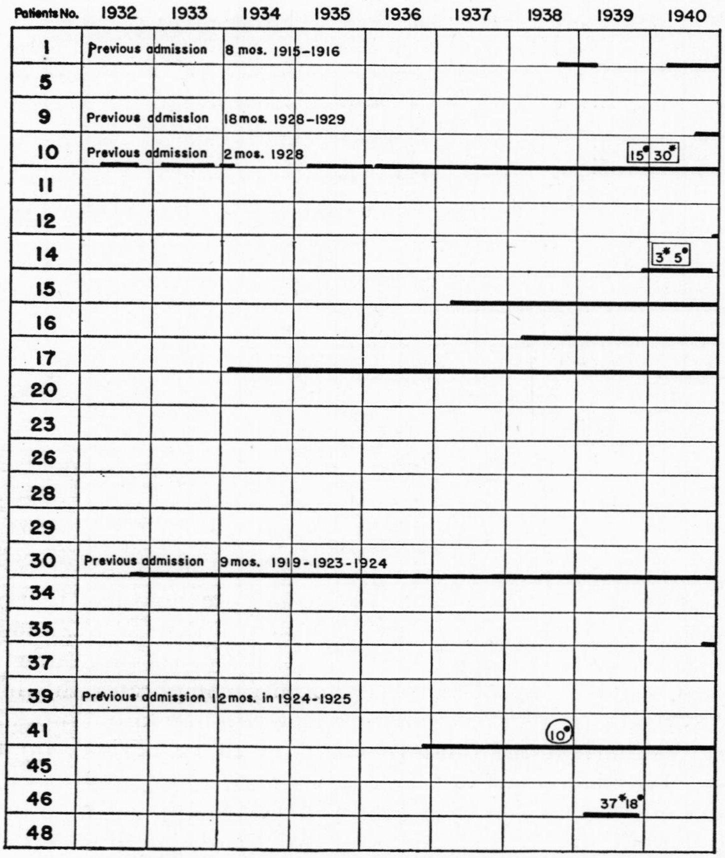

| Patients No. | 1932 | 1933 | 1934 | 1935 | 1936 | 1937 | 1938 | 1939 | 1940 |
|---|---|---|---|---|---|---|---|---|---|
| 1 | Previous admission | 8 mos. 1915-1916 | | | | | | | |
| 5 | | | | | | | | | |
| 9 | Previous admission | 18 mos. 1928-1929 | | | | | | | |
| 10 | Previous admission | 2 mos. 1928 | | | | | | 15° 30° | |
| 11 | | | | | | | | | |
| 12 | | | | | | | | | |
| 14 | | | | | | | | 3* 5° | |
| 15 | | | | | | | | | |
| 16 | | | | | | | | | |
| 17 | | | | | | | | | |
| 20 | | | | | | | | | |
| 23 | | | | | | | | | |
| 26 | | | | | | | | | |
| 28 | | | | | | | | | |
| 29 | | | | | | | | | |
| 30 | Previous admission | 9 mos. 1919-1923-1924 | | | | | | | |
| 34 | | | | | | | | | |
| 35 | | | | | | | | | |
| 37 | | | | | | | | | |
| 39 | Previous admission | 12 mos. in 1924-1925 | | | | | | | |
| 41 | | | | | | | 10° | | |
| 45 | | | | | | | | | |
| 46 | | | | | | | | 37* 18° | |
| 48 | | | | | | | | | |

**CONTROLS**

FIG. 3.  Control group. Periods of institutionalization and the nature and effectiveness of therapy. Simple arabic number—electroshock treatments. Arabic number with asterisk—insulin treatments; arabic number followed by black circle—metrazol treatments. Where these numbers appear without a box or circle around them the treatments were considered

operation. The reader's attention is called to the fact that, independently of postoperative data, the present constitutes a very comprehensive study of many previously ignored aspects of a population sample from a public psychiatric institution.

It is unnecessary to say that no patient was included in the study who had not already undergone every known, accepted form of therapy which seemed to offer any promise. The length of time each of the patients had been under institutional observation and treatment, and the past record of convulsive and coma therapy are shown in figures 3 and 4. Perusal of them will disclose further variables which should be eliminated in subsequent work of this type. The basic data in figures 3 and 4 are compared in table 4.

**Independence of Studies.** In setting up the project the factor of preconception was protected against by arranging independent categories allocated to separate teams, the members of each of which had no free access to

| 1941 | 1942 | 1943 | 1944 | 1945 | 1946 | Mos. institu-tionalized | Metrazol treatment | Shock treatment | Insulin treatment |
|---|---|---|---|---|---|---|---|---|---|
| [8] | | | | | | 101 | | 8 | |
| | | | | 31* 10 | [31* 11] | 21 | | 21 | 62 |
| 3? | (9)(9)? | 6 | 3? | | | 61 | | 21? | 9 |
| [10] | | | | | | 153 | 15 | 10 | 30 |
| | | | 16* 13 | 8* 6 | [27* 29] | 26 | | 48 | 51 |
| | | | | | | 25 | | | |
| | | | | | | 80 | 5 | | 3 |
| | | | | | | 121 | | | |
| | | | | | | 109 | | | |
| | | | | | | 183 | | | |
| | | (19* 14) | (12*)(23* 18) | | | 30 | | 32 | 54 |
| | | [28*] | | | | 33 | | | 28 |
| | | | 17* 12 | [68* 36] | | 30 | | 48 | 85 |
| | | | 30* 3 | [18]+ | | 28 | | 21+ | 30 |
| | | | | 14+ (86* 20) | | 25 | 20 | 14+ | 86 |
| | | | | | | 192 | | | |
| | | | | | (10) | 13 | | 10 | |
| | | | | | | 17 | | | |
| | | | (38/32*) | | | 34 | | 38 | 32 |
| | 14/29* | | (41* 33) | | | 59 | | 47 | 70 |
| | | | | | | 126 | 10 | | |
| | | 14/31* | [72* 20] | | | 53 | | 34 | 103 |
| | | | | | | 33 | 18 | | 37 |
| | | | | | | 69 | | | |

FIG. 3—*Continued*

effectual; where they are encircled the treatments exerted less than the desired effect; where they are boxed treatment was ineffectual. Where a number is followed by a question mark it is believed additional unrecorded treatments were given. Where a number is followed by a plus mark it is known that additional treatments were given but their exact number is unknown.

the data gathered by the others. It was thus impossible for an unconscious preconception to be carried beyond any given team and the teams were so set up that the data of one (or more) served as an automatic check on that of others.

**Preoperative Data Collected.** Upon removal to the study ward, each patient received a Wassermann recheck, medical examination, complete psychiatric recheck, and neurological examination (three independent examiners), and roentgenogram of the frontal sinuses and skull were made. All patients

| Patient No. | 1932 | 1933 | 1934 | 1935 | 1936 | 1937 | 1938 | 1939 | 1940 | 1941 | 1942 | 1943 | 1944 | 1945 | 1946 | Mos. institutionalized | Metrazol treatment | Shock treatment | Insulin treatment |
|---|---|---|---|---|---|---|---|---|---|---|---|---|---|---|---|---|---|---|---|
| 2 | | | | | | | | | | | | | | | | 77 | | | |
| 3 | | | | | | | | | 14* 19* | | | | | | 23 | 82 | 19 | | 14 |
| 4 | | | | | | | | | | | | | | | | 9 | | 23 | |
| 6 | | | | | | | | | | 48* 4* | | | | | 66* 26 | 25 | 14 | 26 | 114 |
| 7 | | | | | | | | | | | 12 15 | 22* 8 | * 20 | 39* 6 | 17 | 23 | | 43 | 35 |
| 8 | | | | | | | | | | | | | | 47* 6 | 9* 20 | 29 | | 33 | 39 |
| 13 | | | | | | | | | | | | | 35* 12 | | | 21 | | 36 | 56 |
| 18 | | | | | | | | | | | | | | | | 47 | | 12 | 35 |
| 19 | | | | | | | | | 17* | | | | | | | 76 | | | 17 |
| 21 | | | | | | | | | | | | | 11* | | | 102 | | | |
| 22 | | | | | | | 28* | | | | | | | | | 12 | | | 11 |
| 24 | | | | | | | | | | | | | | | | 153 | 28 | | |
| 25 | | | | | | | | | | | | | | 21 | | 17 | | 21 | |
| 27 | | | | | | | | | | | | | | | 53* 13 + | 39 | | 13+ | 53 |
| 31 | | | | | | | | | | 28* 15 | | | | 12 | 5? 5? | 22 | | 15 | 28 |
| 32 | | | | | | 22* | | | | | | | 20 42* | | 14 | 50 | 22 | 34 | 42 |
| 33 | | | | | | | | | | | | | | | | 22 | | 22? | |
| 36 | | | | | | | | | | | | | | | | 15 | | 9 | 9 |
| 38 | | | | | | | | | | | | 9* 9 | | 31* | 38* | 26 | | 1 | 41 |
| 40 | | | | | | | | | | | | | | | | 29 | | | |
| 42 | Previous admission 6 mos. 1928-9 | | | | | | | | | | | | | | | 67 | | | |
| 44 | | | | | | | | | | | | 37* 28 + 6 | | | | 61 | +6 | 28 | 37 |
| 47 | | | | | | | | | | | 41* 20 + 12 | | | | | 64 | +12 | 20 | 41 |
| 49 | Previous admission 1 year 1929-30 | | | | | | | | | | | | | | | 165 | | | |

Previous admission 5 mos. 1926-7 (Patient 21)

were typed for blood group. Special laboratory tests included three red, white, differential and reticulocyte counts, three hemoglobin, blood sugar, urea, creatinine, calcium, sodium and potassium analyses, a glucose tolerance test, and gastric analyses. Special clinical studies included adrenalin tolerance, color vision (Ishihara) and visual field determination by the tangent screen method, audiogram and examination of the vestibular system, roentgenologic determination of gastrointestinal motility, voice recording, cinematographic study, and electroencephalography. Psychologic study included a full battery of tests, some specially developed for this project. These tests are described in section III. Throughout the work it was evident that there is considerable room for further progress in instrumentation, the development of more rapid laboratory techniques, and the improvement of psychometric testing methods. Except in the latter field no progress was made in these matters.

TABLE 4. COMPARISON OF CONTROL CASES AND OPERATEES.
HOSPITALIZATION AND THERAPY*

| | Months institutionalized to 1947 | Number of cases receiving | | |
| --- | --- | --- | --- | --- |
| | | Metrazol treatment | Electroshock | Insulin |
| Controls | 1622 (67) | 5 (13) | 13 (27) | 14 (48) |
| Operatees | 1232 (51) | 6 (16) | 15 (22) | 15 (38) |

* Figures in parentheses indicate average period of institutionalization per patient and average number of treatments per patient receiving particular treatments.

**Selection of Patients for Operation.** Once the preoperative data were in hand the group was divided into 24 control patients and 24 considered appropriate for operation. The manner in which this was done was as follows:

Two lists were drawn up in each of which the patients on one were matched against those on the other according to psychologic characteristics. The matchings were as follows (patients finally operated upon in boldface type): 1-3, 2-12, 4-28, 5-6, 7-17, **8-29**, 9-14, 10-30, 11-19, 13-21, 15-22, 16-25, 18-23, 20-24, 26-27, **31-36**, **32-35**, **33-44**, **34-38**, 37-47, 39-42, 40-49, 41-45, 46-48 (alternative matches 37-33, 48-47, 35-31, 46-44). The judgment as to which one of the pair of matched patients was to be operated upon was made on the basis of medicosurgical and prognostic considerations, evidence of spontaneous improvement, and temporary unwillingness on the part of the patient to be operated upon. As the laboratory and medical findings became available it was obvious that surgery was inadvisable in certain patients and these had to be placed in the list of patients not selected for operation. Patients so excluded and the reasons for excluding them were: 12, low erythrocyte count;

FIG. 4. Operatees. Periods of institutionalization and nature and effectiveness of therapy. Simple arabic number—electroshock treatments. Arabic number with asterisk—insulin treatments; arabic number followed by black circle—metrazol treatments. Where these numbers appear without a box or circle around them the treatments were considered effectual; where they are encircled the treatments exerted less than the desired effect; where they are boxed treatment was ineffectual. Where a number is followed by a question mark it is believed additional unrecorded treatments were given. Where a number is followed by a plus mark it is known that additional treatments were given but their exact number is unknown.

15, pneumonia; 17, duodenal ulcer; 26, leucocytic inversion; 34, duodenal ulcer; 35, arteriosclerotic heart disease; 37, shock risk; 39, low erythrocyte count; 41, edema; 46, doubtful Wassermann reaction.

It was a principle of the investigation that no patient would be operated upon unless both the relatives and guardian gave their consent and the patient himself wished to have the operation. If any doubt was expressed, even though the patient was patently incompetent at the time, such patient was excluded from the operative list. Patients excluded for reasons of this type were 9, 29, and 30.

Although all the patients in the group had been selected because they had been adjudged unimprovable by other means, it was felt that if a patient exhibited evidence of improvement (howsoever illusory this might ultimately prove to be) during the preliminary study period of forty days it would be inadvisable to operate. Not only is one dealing here with the question of physician-patient relationship but such a policy protected the operative data to a marked extent from the inclusion of patients whose improvement might be unrelated to the actual operative procedure. Patients so excluded were numbers 1, 34, and 39 (34 and 39 already excluded, see above).

In the remaining cases in which the psychologic pairing was allowed to stand, judgment as to which of the pair of patients should be operated upon was based upon prognostic considerations. Eight matched pairs were broken, viz. 9-14, 10-30, 13-21, 31-36, 33-44, 40-49, 41-45, and 46-48 because of prognostic considerations. These patients occupied the following order in the prognostic listing—good, 13, 21, 31, 36, 40; poor, 9, 14, 30, 49; bad, 33, 44; nil, 10, 41, 45, 46, 48. Patients 9 and 30 were not operated upon for the reasons noted above. Patient 14 was considered to have organic brain damage and consequently was rejected. As matters turned out the postoperative results coincided with the prognosis in exactly half the patients operated upon in this group and it is therefore doubtful whether anything was gained by breaking the psychologic matchings. Certainly this tended to render interpretation of the psychologic data more difficult. It is realized that in any list such as the original the matchings are at most only approximate and can only serve as a guide for ultimate arrangement (for reasons mentioned above), but the initial matching enabled us to determine that the ideal preliminary group in a study such as this should be approximately four times the size of the definitive group. Circumstances which render operation inadvisable must always be expected to arise which will complicate the process of matching, and previously studied replacements should be available from outside the working group. In the present study it was impossible to handle a group any larger than forty-eight. Since the preoperative studies were of a comprehensive nature the load on the clinical and x-ray laboratories alone was extremely heavy. Had the number of cases been larger it would also have been necessary to expand the psychometric staff in such a way that more than one person might have had to administer some particular tests which would have introduced undesirable inequivalence in the raw data.

At the end of the four-month postoperative period the control patients adjudged improved were those numbered 1, 9, 15, 34, 39. Of these 5 patients, 3 (1, 34, and 39) had been detected in the preoperative study period. Patient 15 had been so ill of pneumonia that we had not formed any judgment as to his preoperative psychiatric trend and had already excluded him from the operative list. Patient 9 showed rapid deterioration in the postoperative period and had to be put on shock therapy in order to keep him self-sustaining. Despite the fact that shock therapy had previously proved to be inadequate really to change this patient's condition for any length of time, the improvement he did show was related in this case to that procedure.

**Complicating Factors Anticipated in the Surgical Procedure.** Since our primary concern was to determine whether removal of one or more cortical areas would produce psychiatric improvement, our next problem was to work out an operative protocol which would enable us to differentiate between the true effect of removal of areas and spurious effects which might follow removal of one area but really be due to the interference of function of another (either because of vascular or conducting factors). There are eleven Brodmann areas rostral to area 4 (which no one has considered so far to be implicated in lobotomy). Two of these (24 and 32) might best be removed together. We therefore had ten primary operative removals to do, viz.: 6, 8, 9, 10, 11, 24, and 32, 44, 45, 46, and also 47. From the point of view of conduction, if the effects of removal of an area such as 9 were due to interruption of fibers of passage from 10, then such effects should appear when 10 was removed by itself, and so on. Vascular factors would not, however, be automatically controlled by such a selection. Removal of area 45 might conceivably interfere with the blood supply of area 46 and part of 9. Removal of 45, 46, and 9 was therefore planned to see if it produced the same result as removal of 45 alone. Removal of 9, 8, and 46 was similarly planned to control removal of 46 and of 9, while removal of 9, 10, and 46 was planned to control removal of 46, of 10, and of 9. These three additional removals increased the protocol to thirteen operations.

It is obvious that cortical removals must of necessity interrupt the venous drainage and our series was therefore increased to fourteen, by including one operation in which no cortex was removed but only the venous drainage to the superior sagittal sinus ligated.

Until the specimen is sectioned and perhaps not even then, it is, of course, impossible to know exactly what area is removed from a brain if that area is not electrically excitable or does not display characteristic action currents. Mettler ('44, see p. 107) has further emphasized the lack of necessary correlation between a removed piece of cortex and the dysfunctional regions of the cortex. Any operative protocol such as the above, in order to be meaningful, must be drawn up in such a way as to give adequate results no matter what the arrangement of cortical areas may be. One cannot become dependent on the accuracy of the Brodmann or any other extant map, but any such map can be used as an arbitrary means of subdividing the frontal lobe. The investigator can then use it in his search for responsible foci, but he must allow for errors in judgment in locating the regions whatever they are. He must further take into consideration the possibility that the frontal lobe may have been subdivided far beyond its functional units and, finally, he needs to control the element of mere mass. In the three combined removals already noted, possible errors in judgment in locating areas 44, 45, 46, 9, and 10 had been adequately controlled but we still needed to control removal of areas 8 and 6. Combined removals of 8, 9, and 11 and 6 and 8 were therefore added to our list as well as repetitions of the single removals of 9 and 10 and 11. Three mass factor operations were added without regard to areas, viz. the removals of the superior, middle, or inferior frontal gyri alone, as far back as area 4.

Mettler ('44) has pointed out that aggregate removals of a number of areas, which when removed alone give but minimal similar effects, may result in a significant physiologic effect and that this phenomenon is not a mere function of mass but depends upon exceeding the law of physiologic safety. In order to compare the aggregate effects of elements in the rostral and caudal halves of frontal cortex rostral to area 6, we therefore scheduled a removal in one case of areas 10, 11, 45, 46, and 47 in order to compare the results with those following already scheduled removal of areas 8 and 9. To further control a possible error in judgment of the rostral border of the latter operation, combined removal of 8, 9, and 10 was scheduled.

Each Brodmann area (other than areas 32 and 24) was therefore to be removed more than once. The number of times individual areas appeared in the protocol of specific removals (either partial or total) is as follows: 6 (4), 8 (8), 9 (10), 10 (6), 11 (3), 24 and 32 (1), 44 (2), 45 (4), 46 (7), 47 (2). In addition each of the three frontal gyri was to be removed separately and a rostrodorsal venous ligation was scheduled.

**Selection of Operation for Individual Patients.** The operative protocol thus drawn up represented twenty areal operations,* seventeen of which differed in some respect from one another (three of the twenty were duplicates), three gyrectomies, and one venous ligation. *A priori* there was no reason to suppose that any of these operations other than those involving areas 6 and 44 would result in effects more deleterious than might theoretically be expected after conventional lobotomy, but our cadaver measurements suggested that area 44 was commonly damaged in that operation. In drastic lobotomy, moreover, area 6 can scarcely escape damage. However, to be on the safe side, 2 of the 4 patients chosen for operation involving area 6 were ones in which conventional lobotomy would not have been employed but rather the more drastic posterior cut encroaching upon area 6. One of the two remaining patients so operated upon had only partial removal of area 6. In the other, in whom all of area 6 was ablated, catatonia with periods of universal tremor was present and it will be recalled that removal of area 6 is not infrequently used in treating tremor. Removal of area 44 was done in a patient whose most distressing symptom was continuous babbling and that area was also involved in the inferior frontal gyrus removal which was performed on a patient who had gradually grown mute.

Operations (see chapter 4) were begun on May 15. Each patient in the operative series was accompanied to the operating room by a patient of compatible blood in the control series. Both were anesthetized with sodium pentothal and 500 cc. of blood was withdrawn from the control (to balance blood loss in the patient upon whom operation was performed) whenever conditions allowed. The control was then returned to the wards. The nature of the operation was recorded photographically, by diagram, and by description. The precise nature of the operation was known only to the surgeon and anatomist who made the records and the records were not made available to the remainder of the group until after the patients had been re-examined by the general staff at Greystone with respect to suitability for parole (i.e. not until after the three-month postoperative check-up). (For method of handling the specimens obtained at operation see chapter 5.)

When the patients reached the ward a record of the pulse, blood pressure, respiration, and temperature was made hourly during the waking period and

* See footnote on p. 8.

the laboratory procedures were reinstituted as soon as valid data were available. The same tests were performed on the patients subjected to operation and the controls. All other significant studies were resumed as soon as possible and repeated in three months.

**Comparison between Topectomy and Lobotomy.** At the end of the three-month postoperative study (which required an additional month) the progress notes were collected from the senior psychiatrist (Dr. Heath) and all patients were remanded to the regular Greystone Staff for evaluation without

TABLE 5. EVALUATION OF PATIENTS IN PROJECT BY GREYSTONE STAFF ON SEPTEMBER 25, 1947

| Improved and parolable[a] | | | Improved but not parolable | | Unimproved | | |
|---|---|---|---|---|---|---|---|
| Operated—20 | | Control—5 | Operated—1 | Control—0 | Operated—3 | Control—19 | |
| 3 | 27 | 1 | 2 | | 6[d] | 5[h] | 28 |
| 4 | 31 | 9[g] | | | 24 | 10 | 29 |
| 7 | 32 | 15 | | | 44 | 11 | 30 |
| 8[b] | 33 | 34 | | | | 12 | 35 |
| 13[c] | 36 | 39 | | | | 14 | 37 |
| 18 | 38[d] | | | | | 16 | 41 |
| 19 | 40[e] | | | | | 17 | 45 |
| 21 | 42[f] | | | | | 20[d] | 46 |
| 22[d] | 47 | | | | | 23 | 48 |
| 25 | 49 | | | | | 26 | |

[a] For further course of these patients see chapter 25.

[b] Convulsions postoperatively and on Sept. 4, 11, 21, Oct. 4, 1947, and approximately every two weeks since, if not controlled by medication. Reoperated Oct. 20, 1948. Some convulsions after reoperation.

[c] Convulsions on Mar. 3 and Apr. 20, 1948.

[d] One postoperative convulsion in immediate postoperative period.

[e] Convulsions on Dec. 13, 1947, Jan. 16, and Feb. 10, 1948.

[f] Convulsions on Jan. 23 and Apr. 15, 1948.

[g] Decline in postoperative period. Convulsive therapy in July for two treatments. Improvement dating from this period. Relapse and readmission to hospital in February, 1948.

[h] Postoperative convulsion and convulsive bout on Nov. 2, 1947.

any data from the study groups, with the request that the patients be evaluated according to routine criteria. The results were as shown in table 5. (It should be pointed out that the Greystone Staff had no knowledge of our intention to perform a second operation upon patients who were not improved and that judgments were therefore uninfluenced by such a consideration.)

We were now faced with three significant questions: (1) Would operatees who were not improved by the procedures we employed have been improved if we had ablated different areas or done a lobotomy? (2) What would the test procedures we employed have shown if we had done lobotomies instead of topectomies? (3) What would have been the course of the control patients had they not been introduced into the study group?

1. Unless operation is a nonspecific procedure or unless neighborhood effects complicate removals of small areas such as 44, 45, 46, or 47, one would hardly anticipate improvement from these operations. Some of the unimproved operatees might therefore have been expected to have been improved by different or more extensive topectomies. There were, however, certain patients, such

as 44, in whom no topectomy might have been beneficial. In order to determine whether such patients would have been benefited by lobotomy we now
decided to perform lobotomies on 2 of the 4 operatees who had shown little
or no improvement. The patients chosen as most likely to benefit from this
procedure were 2 and 44.

2. In order to arrive at an opinion as to what our test procedures would
have disclosed if we had employed lobotomy *instead* of topectomy, 6 unimproved control patients were selected for this operation. These patients' numbers were 5, 11, 20, 23, 28, 46. Their further course is described in chapter 25.

3. The question as to the probable course of the control patients had they
not been included in the study group is considered in chapter 2 and need
not be elaborated here beyond pointing out that no prognosis is infallible
and at least one definite value of the "total-push" technique is the exposure of
erroneous diagnosis and the correction of prognoses. Such inaccuracies should
become apparent in a relatively short period and the 4 patients who began to
show improvement in the preliminary testing period probably represent errors
in judgment of this type.

**Interpretation of Temporal References in This Monograph.**  All references to temporal relations in this study are computed from the day of the
visit to the surgery. This day is referred to as "O" in control patients and
"Day of Operation" in the operatees. Periods prior to this are designated by
minus symbols and periods after it by plus.

**Methodology.**  Considerable difficulty was experienced, throughout the
project, in maintaining satisfying scientific criteria. The reason for this is,
of course, that clinical investigations rarely satisfy criteria which can be met
in the laboratory. There is a widespread tendency among laboratory investigators, who observe this, to discount much clinical investigative work
despite the fact that the urgency of clinical problems demands definite action.
Clinical investigators who attempt to create an illusion of scientific certainty
are themselves responsible for some of this distrust.

In the present research we were constantly forced to deal with data of varying degrees of objective validity and the reader will do well to recognize this
at the outset. A certain amount of confusion between data of different types
has been avoided by the method of subsequent presentation in which essentially different approaches are allocated separate chapters. In attempting
to correlate these data our conclusions fall into distinctly different categories
of certainty and, in order to avoid creating a false sense of security, an attempt
is made throughout, and in the final chapter, to distinguish between these
categories and to indicate what we believe to be reasonably certain, what we
consider probable, and what still seems to be very doubtful. There should be
no serious objection to such a method of presentation but it is obvious that
the caution we have urged upon the reader should be maintained by him in
applying our conclusions to his practice.

# Chapter 2

# Prognostic Expectations of the Patients Under Ordinary Institutional Care

## HENRY A. COTTON, JR., AND EMIL FRANKEL

THE 48 patients in the series, including both the controls and operatees, were originally classified as follows (for final preoperative diagnosis, see table 3, page 17):

| | |
|---|---|
| Dementia praecox | 39 |
| Manic-depressive psychosis | 4 |
| Involutional psychosis | 5 |

The average stay in the hospital for these patients was four years. During this time, they were subjected to the usual forms of treatment, including the various types of shock therapy (where indicated), occupational therapy, recreational activities, and general institutional care. However, it must be conceded that they had received very little psychotherapy. Group psychotherapy has been

TABLE 6. ADMISSIONS TO, AND DISCHARGES ALIVE FROM THE NEW JERSEY STATE HOSPITALS FOR THE DIAGNOSTIC CATEGORIES INDICATED

| Diagnosis | Number of admissions | Number of discharges | Rate of discharges alive per 100 admissions |
|---|---|---|---|
| Involutional | 602 | 427 | 70.9 |
| Manic-depressive | 1232 | 1041 | 84.5 |
| Dementia praecox | 1972 | 1181 | 59.9 |
| Total specified psychoses | 3806 | 2649 | 71.7 |

started too recently for it to have had any effect on this series of patients and individual therapy is practically impossible with a relatively small staff of trained psychiatrists. While it is realized that psychotherapy is probably the most important method of treatment which psychiatry has to offer, it is a generally accepted fact that many psychotics fail to show a favorable response even under ideal conditions, such as are provided by the small psychiatric units attached to medical schools and research centers.

In order to make an objective evaluation of the effects of topectomy on this group of patients, one must consider what the chances for recovery or improvement would have been if this treatment had not been carried out.

In table 6 are given the number of patients admitted and the number of living patients discharged for the various diagnostic groups as well as the rate of discharges per one hundred admissions in each category for the New Jersey State hospitals during the period 1944 through 1946.

In table 7 is shown the length of stay of members of the above group of

TABLE 7. LENGTH OF TIME SPENT IN HOSPITALS, PRIOR TO DISCHARGE, BY THE PATIENTS SHOWN IN TABLE 6

| Diagnosis | Duration of hospital life of first admissions before discharge | | |
|---|---|---|---|
| | Under 6 months | 6–11 months | 1 year and over |
| Involutional................... | 73.1% | 16.6% | 10.3% |
| Manic-depressive............... | 77.7 | 11.9 | 10.4 |
| Dementia praecox.............. | 54.2 | 19.3 | 26.5 |

patients in the hospital prior to discharge. It will be noted that by far the largest percentage of patients were discharged in the first six months after admission.

While it might be argued that patients of the above group have not been followed long enough to draw any final conclusions, there seems to be little likelihood on the basis of past experience of any increased discharge rate. On the other hand, it is quite possible that some of these patients now in the community may return to an institution at a later date.

A relatively long-term study has been carried out on a combined group of 500 patients, including both those having dementia praecox and manic-depressive psychoses, who were committed to New Jersey State mental hospitals for the first time in 1930 and followed for an eight-year period thereafter. Table 8 was

TABLE 8. WHEREABOUTS OF 500 COMMITTED MANIC-DEPRESSIVE AND DEMENTIA PRAECOX PATIENTS DISCHARGED FROM MENTAL HOSPITALS IN 1930

| After | Percent | | |
|---|---|---|---|
| | Released | In hospital | Died |
| One year.............. | 51.5 | 41.7 | 6.8 |
| Two years............. | 55.4 | 36.0 | 8.6 |
| Three years............ | 60.1 | 29.9 | 10.0 |
| Four years............. | 60.6 | 29.1 | 10.3 |
| Five years............. | 60.2 | 28.8 | 11.0 |
| Six years.............. | 60.2 | 28.1 | 11.7 |
| Seven years............ | 61.4 | 26.5 | 12.1 |
| Eight years............ | 62.1 | 25.5 | 12.4 |

based on the whereabouts of each individual patient at the end of each twelve-month period after his own admission, noting the status at that time without regard to the intervening happenings in the life of that patient which might include return or readmission for a short temporary period.

Table 8 and figure 5 indicate that by far the greater number of patients who are discharged leave the hospital during the first two years and after that time there is very little expectancy of further improvement or recovery.

While it is true that these patients were admitted for the first time before shock therapy was started in New Jersey mental hospitals, unfinished studies on later series of patients indicate that even with shock therapy the opportunities for improvement or recovery are negligible after the first two years.

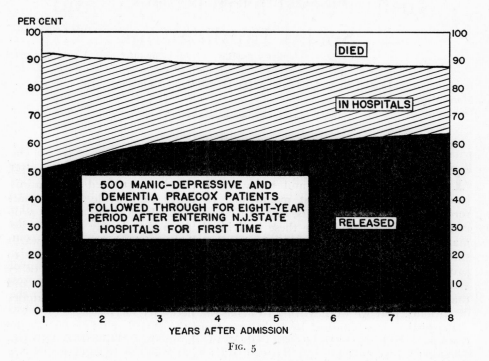

FIG. 5

A survey of the literature indicates that in the case of dementia praecox the majority of patients who are going to show improvement or recovery do so within the first year and that the percentage diminishes during the second year, following which time there is very little expectancy of further change.

In the case of the manic-depressive and involutional psychoses, one finds reports of patients who have shown improvement or recovery after longer periods of time, but here again changes are most apt to occur during the first two years of the patient's stay in the hospital and the opportunity for recovery or improvement after that time lessens considerably.

Bearing these facts in mind, it can be assumed with reasonable certainty that any improvement shown in the series of patients treated surgically was due to the topectomy operation.

# Chapter 3

# Institutional Management and Social Implications

MARCUS A. CURRY AND HENRY A. COTTON, JR.

## INSTITUTIONAL MANAGEMENT

THE development of a program of this type in a large mental hospital, critically overcrowded and badly understaffed, constituted an administrative problem of the first magnitude. In order to provide an adequate number of nurses, attendants, and other institutional personnel for the project, it was necessary to take these individuals from the already badly undermanned wards in other parts of the hospital. It was felt that separate wards should be provided for all patients involved in the project, and in order to provide these it was necessary to increase the existing overcrowding in other areas. It was only because we felt that this project was so worthwhile, and that it offered certain possibilities which would be helpful to a large number of patients, that we were willing to make the necessary sacrifices.

Permission was obtained by Dr. Curry from the Board of Managers of the Greystone Park State Hospital to embark on the project. Dr. Cotton, in turn, obtained authorization from the Commissioner of the Department of Institutions and Agencies and the New Jersey State Board of Control.

A good deal of over-all planning was required in advance to set the program in operation. Time schedules were made up designating definite dates for completion of the various steps involved. Regular schedules were established for the performance of the large number of diagnostic tests and other procedures to which the patients were subjected prior to operation. Frequent meetings were held of all those concerned in order that every phase of the program might be clearly understood. A number of circulars were issued at frequent intervals for the guidance of the professional staffs. As a result of this planning, the examinations were conducted in an orderly manner, and there was no delay or confusion.

Particular emphasis was placed on the provision of adequate clerical personnel, filing space, and office equipment for handling the numerous records of preoperative and postoperative examinations. All records connected with the program were handled separately from those for the remainder of the institution.

All personnel working with patients in the project was carefully selected and indoctrinated as to the purpose of the program. Only those individuals who evidenced definite interest in being associated with such a program were actually assigned to duties with it. Orientation for personnel included a complete explanation of the operative procedures, what results might reasonably be expected or anticipated, and instruction as to how the patients were to be handled, particularly with regard to information to be given to patients and relatives. It was emphasized that in no case were relatives' hopes to be raised unduly. A conservative attitude was followed by all concerned in order to avoid sensationalism or undue optimism. The number of physicians, nurses, attendants, and other personnel assigned to the project was sufficient to insure that the patients were adequately cared for and observed at all times. This provided much more adequate care and intensive observation than is ordinarily found in a large mental hospital. Nursing personnel maintained its own schedules of the various examinations, operations, and other activities, so that there were no delays in having the patients report at the appointed places on time.

The use of separate wards made it possible for all patients in both the operatee and control groups to be relatively isolated from the general patient population. A program of recreational and occupational activities was established to insure that the patients were reasonably occupied during such time as they were not undergoing examinations and treatments. It must be admitted that this problem was again more intensive than that which is ordinarily in operation in the remainder of the institution. This segregation made it possible to insure uniform personal care of the patients and uniform sanitary and hygienic conditions particularly with regard to bathing, diets, and the like.

The operating room and such of its staff as were necessary were regularly assigned to the project on scheduled days with the result that the operations proceeded in an orderly manner without necessity for changing the schedule. Such other facilities, including x-ray and laboratory, were made available on a regular basis, although this resulted in considerable interference with the normal activities in the hospital.

When patients were selected for surgery, a letter was written to the responsible relative outlining the nature of the procedure and enclosing a permission slip for operation. No operations were performed unless the slip was signed. In cases of doubt, the relatives were asked to visit the hospital so that the procedure could be explained to them in more detail. No patient was subjected to surgery without not only the written permission but also the active cooperation of the responsible relatives. The operative procedure was also formulated carefully to each patient in order to reduce misunderstanding and possible antagonism to a minimum. As a result of careful planning along this line, the patients were extremely cooperative.

As the Greystone Park State Hospital was already operating on a limited budget, special arrangements were made with the Department of Institutions and Agencies to make available the minimal additional funds necessary for the purchase of the additional supplies required. This made it possible to complete the project without delays.

It should be emphasized that the resources of the Greystone Park State Hospital in terms of personnel, finances, and equipment would have been inadequate to have carried out a project of this type without the assistance received from the College of Physicians and Surgeons. Only the close association and cooperation between the representatives of the two institutions which prevailed throughout made it possible to carry on the project so successfully.

The time which was devoted to preliminary planning and meetings between the two groups bore fruit in efficient operation of the various activities later on.

## SOCIAL IMPLICATIONS

In recent years many advances have been made in the treatment of psychotic patients. The use of the various forms of shock therapy in conjunction with psychotherapy, particularly in group form, together with narcosynthesis, recreational and occupational therapy and their adjuncts, have made it possible for a sizable number of patients suffering from functional psychoses to return to community life. In spite of all that has been accomplished, there still remains an appreciable number of these patients who either do not respond adequately to the forms of treatment enumerated, or who, after a brief period of improvement, relapse and become long-term institutional charges. Since many of these patients enter the institution while they are still relatively young and may be expected to live until they are in their sixties or seventies, this constitutes a source of increasing overcrowding. For these reasons alone, it is very desirable to develop new forms of treatment. The restoration of additional patients to the point where they can adjust in community life is also extremely desirable from a socioeconomic standpoint.

It is quite true that favorable outcome with the more accepted forms of treatment depends on such factors as the pre-psychotic personality, heredity, and, in the case of schizophrenics, the amount of affective elements in the psychotic picture. One should not assume, however, that even if these factors appear adverse, that there are not types of treatment which can be developed to operate successfully in spite of them.

During recent years, there has been increasing interest in psychiatry on the part of the public. This is partly owing to publicity given to nervous and mental illness attendant to selective service and military neuropsychiatry, and also to the efforts of national organizations such as the Committee for Mental Hygiene. The moving picture, popular literature, and the radio have all been giving more attention to the subject of mental illness, again increasing public interest, even though such portrayals have often been melodramatic and inaccurate. Publicity given to the Freeman-Watts operation has resulted in many inquiries from relatives regarding the possibilities of neurosurgery. In some instances the relatives have removed patients from the Greystone Park State Hospital in order to have operative procedures, such as lobotomy, carried out elsewhere.

For these reasons, it appeared to be desirable to take a series of patients in whom the usual forms of treatment had been relatively ineffective and subject them to neurosurgery. The operation of topectomy, as developed by the Columbia group, appeared to have certain advantages over the more commonly used Freeman-Watts technique.

The neurosurgical program has already been very favorably received in terms of public relations. The reaction of relatives has been almost uniformly favorable. There has been general appreciation of the fact that an effort was being made to do something for patients who otherwise, presumably, would have very little expectancy of ever leaving the institution. This appreciation has been extended to the surrounding communities. However, care has been taken to avoid sensational publicity. No false hopes have been offered, and efforts have been made to present the operative procedure in as objective a manner as possible.

The question of follow-up of patients who have improved sufficiently as the result of operation to be returned to community life has received careful consideration. These patients have come up against the same problems as those discharged following other forms of treatment. Many of them have had difficulty in finding employment, not because they were incapable of it, but because of the stigma which, in spite of all our efforts, is still attached to those who have been treated in a mental hospital. In other instances, families and friends have been reluctant to accept the patients back to their homes and social circles. Hospital social workers assigned to follow up the patients have made every effort to overcome these factors. Wherever possible, relatives and friends are interviewed prior to the patient's release and an effort made to formulate the patient's problems to them and to prepare a more favorable home and community environment. Families and friends have been urged to treat these patients with sympathetic understanding, and to render more active assistance in bringing about successful community adjustments than has been the case in the past.

From an over-all standpoint, the project has several possible implications. In the first place, a relatively new avenue of approach has been opened up for patients who were formerly considered to be on a long-term basis after failure to show adequate improvement with the commonly accepted forms of treatment. Even under ideal conditions in research institutions many patients fail to respond satisfactorily to psychotherapy and the various forms of shock treatment. The possibility, and so far it is only a possibility, has been raised for making a real reduction in the number of long-term patients suffering from functional psychoses in the mental hospitals in the State. Just how great this reduction will prove to be and what effect it may have on the mental hospital building program in the future, it is impossible to state at the present time, but certainly the implications are far-reaching.

It should be emphasized that topectomy, if used at all, should not be resorted to until after the possibilities of other forms of treatment have been exhausted. Also, when patients are subjected to neurosurgery, full use should be made of psychotherapy and its various adjuncts.

Finally, a program of this type marks another step in the long road toward bringing the mentally ill into the same category as patients suffering from medical and surgical conditions. It should help the efforts of psychiatrists to get the public to regard mental patients as individuals suffering from treatable disorders, rather than as candidates for custodial care.

# Chapter 4

# Surgical Procedure

J. LAWRENCE POOL, LAURENCE M. COLLINS,
EDWARD KESSLER, LEONARD J. VERNON, AND
EMANUEL FEIRING

---

## INTRODUCTION

IN A SERIES of 23 psychotic patients, segments from different parts of both frontal lobes of the brain were symmetrically excised in the effort to induce desirable alterations in behavior without detriment to intellectual or emotional capacity.* In 20 of the 23 cases an effort was made to confine these segmental removals as nearly as possible to cytoarchitectonic areas according to Brodmann's map (fig. 55) of the human cerebral cortex or to combinations of these areas. As explained in the footnote on p. 8 the surgical procedure has been called "topectomy." In 3 cases bilateral "gyrectomy" rather than topectomy was carried out; that is, removal of the superior frontal gyri in one case (27), of the middle frontal gyri in another (8), and of the inferior frontal gyri in a third (33). In an additional case (38), making a total of 24 patients upon whom intracranial surgery was performed, the procedure was confined to ligation of the superior cerebral (corticodural) veins of both frontal lobes, no incision into the brain having been made.

It is clearly recognized that only a rough approximation to the boundaries of Brodmann's areas can be arrived at by gross inspection of the brain. For the sake of convenience (as explained on p. 53), however, cortical removals will hereinafter be described in terms of Brodmann's areas. In estimating the sites

* In discussing the surgical aspects of topectomy at a symposium on "Problems of the Human Frontal Lobe" held at the New York Academy of Medicine in March 1948 (under the auspices of the Columbia-Greystone Associates; sponsored by the New York Society of Neurosurgery), an invited guest, Dr. Jacques LeBeau of Paris, France made the following remarks: "In March 1947 Dr. J. Lawrence Pool suggested to me the bilateral removal of areas 9 and 10 of Brodmann in connection with the treatment of some mental disorders and intractable pain. This was performed on 15 patients with my associates Drs. Feld and Rosier from April, 1947, to February, 1948, in the clinic of the late Professor Clovis Vincent.

*General Conclusions:* The patients are much less anxious than before operation, without a marked change in their so-called "personality," and they are much more "themselves" than after prefrontal leucotomy. The operation has made agitated patients much quieter and socially educable. No postoperative fits were observed to date. Cases with intractable pain were relieved of their discomfort, but when asked about pain described it as before operation. As to the function of the frontal lobe in regard to mental disorders and intractable pain, it already seems as if the cortex in the region of the junction of areas 9 and 10 had a special importance, although a word of caution must be insisted upon: the follow-up of our patients is definitely not long enough to feel confident of their future."

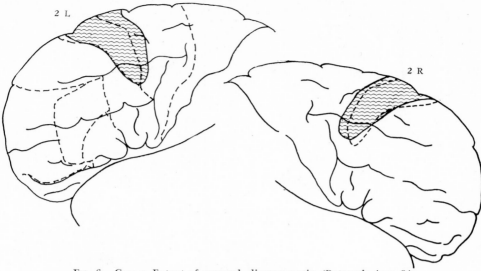

FIG. 6.   Case 2. Extent of removal, diagrammatic. (Protocol: Area 8.)

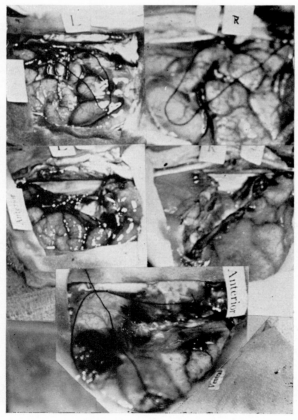

FIG. 7.   Case 2. Photographs. *Upper left:* Left frontal lobe. Thread indicates site for excision. *Lower left:* Left frontal lobe showing actual excision. Semilunar white space below *L* is falx. *Upper right:* Right frontal lobe. Thread indicates site for excision. *Lower right:* Right frontal lobe showing actual excision. White space below *R2* is falx. *Lowest photograph* (approximately 1.5× magnification shown in lower right photograph): Site of excision on right at operation five months later. Diagonal thread marks plane of coronal suture.

Note: The photographs of the ensuing cases are not always of the same degree of magnification, although an effort was made to keep them so.

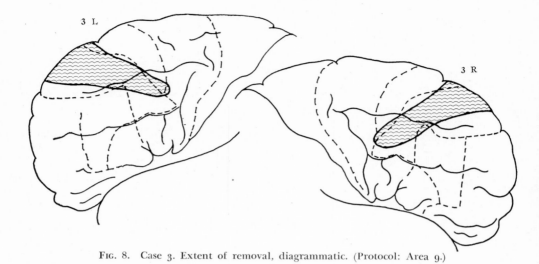

Fig. 8.  Case 3. Extent of removal, diagrammatic. (Protocol: Area 9.)

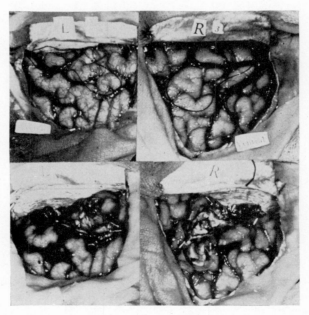

Fig. 9.  Case 3. Photographs. *Upper left:* Left frontal lobe. Thread indicates site for excision. *Lower left:* Left frontal lobe showing actual excision. *Upper right:* Right frontal lobe. Thread indicates site for excision. *Lower right:* Right frontal lobe showing actual excision. Beneath black traction suture on the dura is the falx.

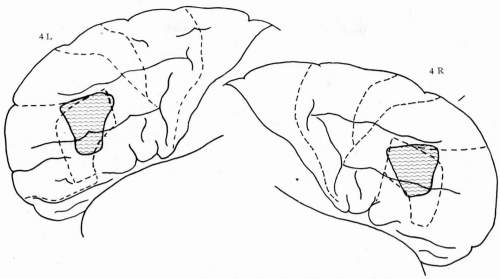

FIG. 10. Case 4. Extent of removal, diagrammatic. (Protocol: Area 46.)

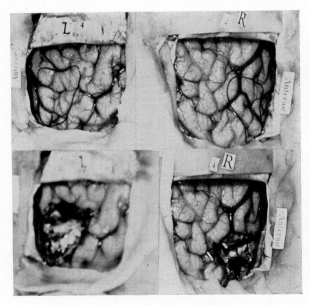

FIG. 11. Case 4. Photographs. *Upper left:* Left frontal lobe. Thread indicates site for excision. *Lower left:* Left frontal lobe showing actual excision. *Upper right:* Right frontal lobe. Thread indicates site for excision. *Lower right:* Right frontal lobe showing actual excision.

Note: In comparing this figure with figure 10 it must be realized that while diagrams can be made to a constant projection it is not always possible to photograph the brain from the same angle, thus the perspectives of diagrams and photographs necessarily often differ.

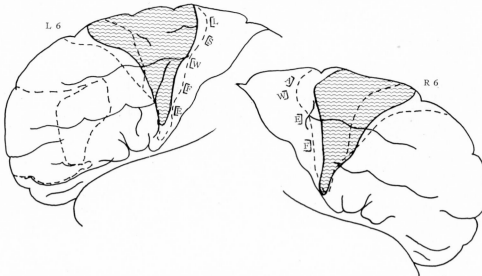

FIG. 12. Case 6. Extent of removal, diagrammatic. (Protocol: Areas 6 and 8.)

Lettering indicates observed contralateral motor effects upon electrical stimulation of the cortex as follows: Left (L 6): *L*=leg; *S*=shoulder; *W*=wrist; *F*=flexion of fingers; *E*=extension of second finger. Right (R 6): *A*=arm; *W*=wrist; *E*=contraction (extensor) of fingers; *F*=face. (The rostral or anterior margin of each paper label marks the rostral extent of excitable motor cortex.)

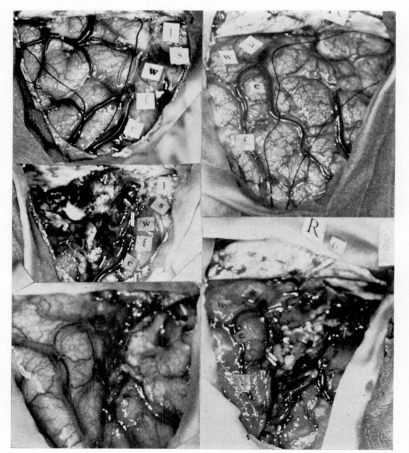

FIG. 13. Case 6. Photographs. *Upper left:* Left frontal lobe. Thread indicates site for excision. *Middle left:* Left frontal lobe showing actual excision. White space at upper left is falx. *Upper right:* Right frontal lobe. Thread indicates site for excision. *Lower right:* Right frontal lobe showing actual excision. *Lower left* photograph shows site of excision (on right) upon re-exploration five months later.

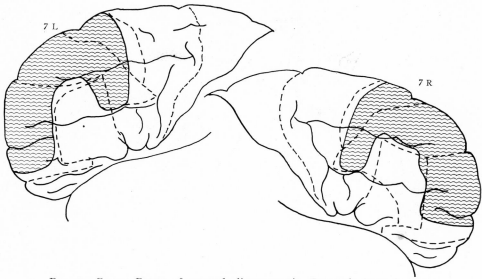

FIG. 14. Case 7. Extent of removal, diagrammatic. (Protocol: Areas 8, 9, 10.)

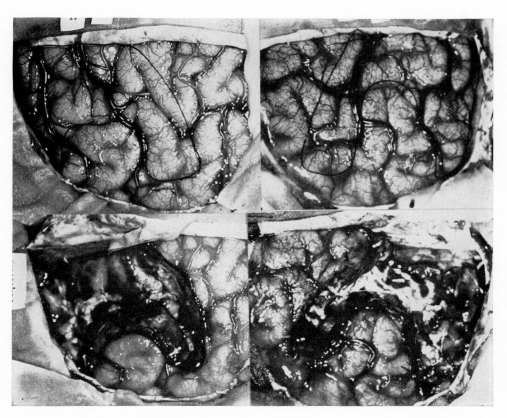

FIG. 15. Case 7. Photographs. *Upper left:* Left frontal lobe. Thread indicates site for excision. *Lower left:* Left frontal lobe showing actual excision. *Upper right:* Right frontal lobe. Thread indicates site for excision. *Lower right:* Right frontal lobe showing actual excision.

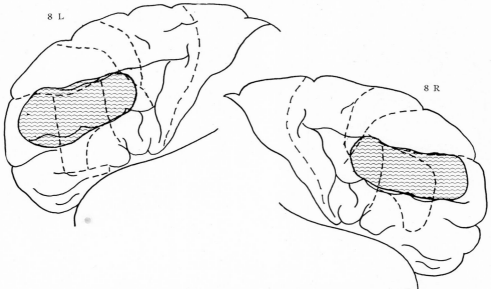

FIG. 16. Case 8. Extent of removal, diagrammatic. (Protocol: Middle frontal gyri.)

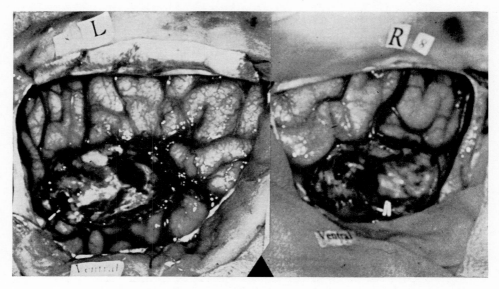

FIG. 17. Case 8. Photographs. *Left:* Left frontal lobe showing actual excision. *Right:* Right frontal lobe showing actual excision.

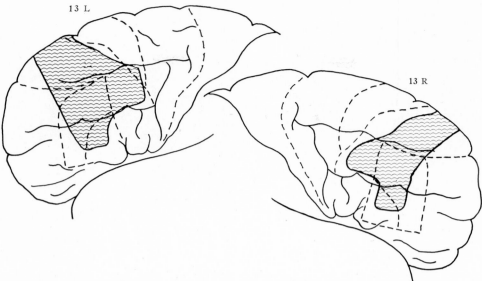

FIG. 18. Case 13. Extent of removal, diagrammatic. (Protocol: Areas 9, 45, 46.)

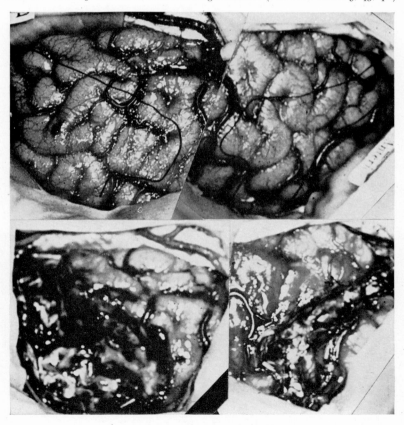

FIG. 19. Case 13. Photographs. *Upper left:* Left frontal lobe. Thread indicates site for excision. *Lower left:* Left frontal lobe showing actual excision. *Upper right:* Right frontal lobe. Thread indicates site for excision. *Lower right:* Right frontal lobe showing actual excision.

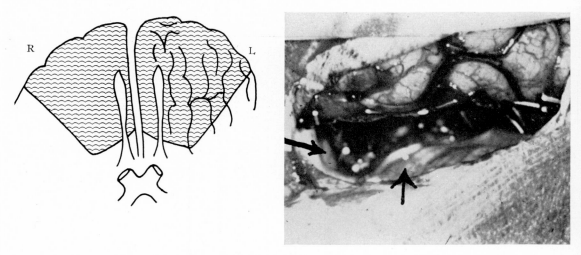

FIG. 20. Cases 18 and 42. *Left:* Extent of removal, diagrammatic. (Protocol: Area 11 for both cases.) *Right:* Photograph indicates operative field (left side) after excision of orbital gyri. Arrow at bottom points to floor of anterior fossa; arrow at left points to rostroventral aspect of falx.

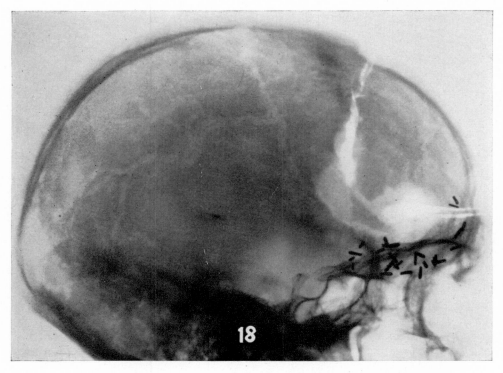

FIG. 21. Case 18. Postoperative x-ray indicating extent of excision as outlined by silver clips. (X-rays of case 42 were similar to this.)

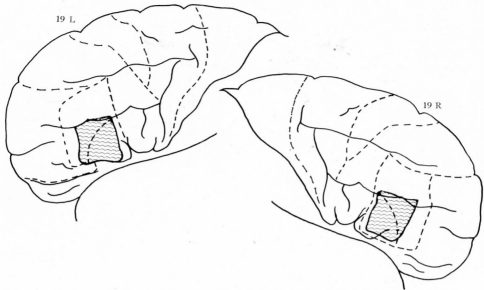

FIG. 22. Case 19. Extent of removal, diagrammatic. (Protocol: Area 45.)

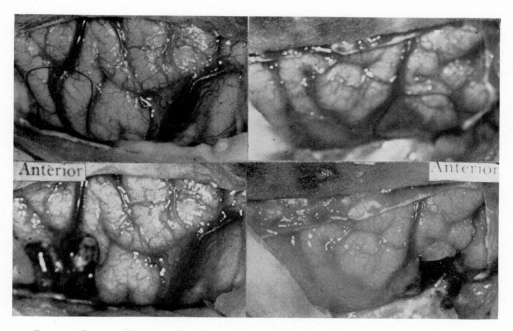

FIG. 23. Case 19. Photographs. *Upper left:* Left frontal lobe. Thread indicates site for excision. *Lower left:* Left frontal lobe showing actual excision. *Upper right:* Right frontal lobe. Thread indicates site for excision. *Lower right:* Right frontal lobe showing actual excision.

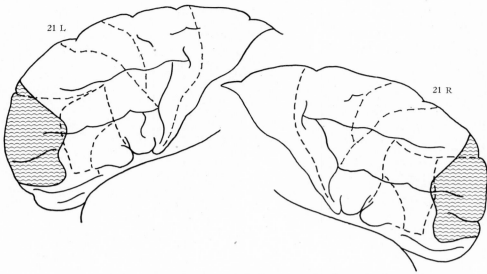

Fig. 24.  Case 21. Extent of removal, diagrammatic. (Protocol: Area 10.)

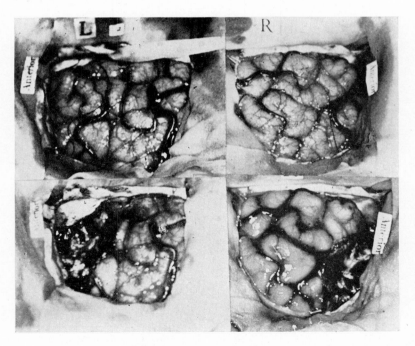

Fig. 25.  Case 21. Photographs. *Upper left:* Left frontal lobe. Thread indicates site for excision. *Lower left:* Left frontal lobe showing actual excision. *Upper right:* Right frontal lobe. Thread indicates site for excision. *Lower right:* Right frontal lobe showing actual excision.

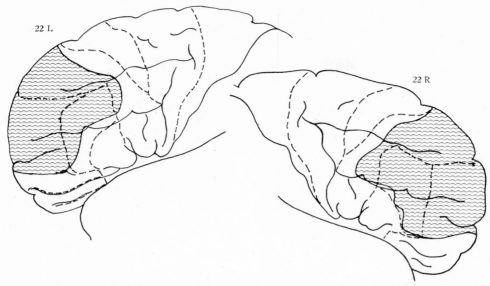

Fig. 26.　Case 22. Extent of removal, diagrammatic. (Protocol: Areas 9, 10, 46.)

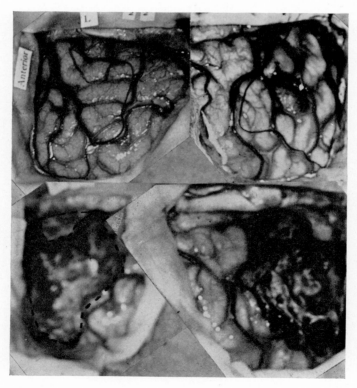

Fig. 27.　Case 22. Photographs. *Upper left:* Left frontal lobe. Thread indicates site for excision. *Lower left:* Left frontal lobe showing actual excision. *Upper right:* Right frontal lobe. Thread indicates site for excision. *Lower right:* Right frontal lobe showing actual excision.

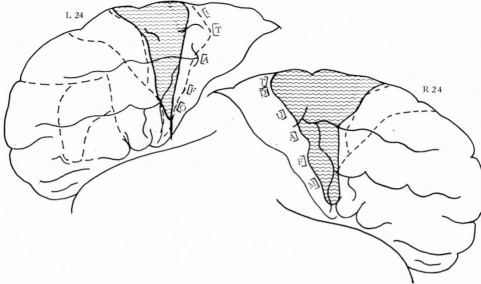

FIG. 28.   Case 24. Extent of removal, diagrammatic. (Protocol: Area 6.) Lettering indicates observed contralateral motor effects upon electrical stimulation of the cortex as follows: Left (L 24): *t*=toes; *T*=thigh; *A*=arm; *F*=face; *O*=orbicularis oculi. Right (R 24): *T*=toes; *D*=thigh; *U*=ulnar deviation of wrist; *A*=arm; *F*=face; *M*=mouth.

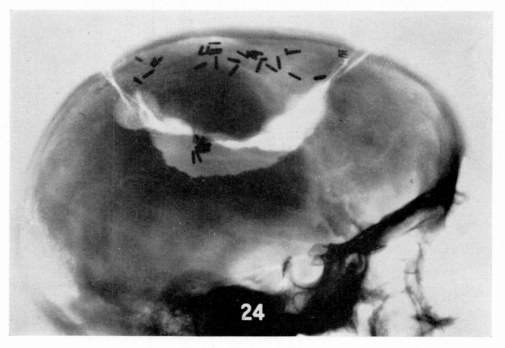

FIG. 29.   Case 24. Postoperative x-ray. Group of silver clips occupying central portion of bone flaps indicates sites of cortical excisions. (Clips near extreme margins of bone flaps are placed on edges of dural flaps.)

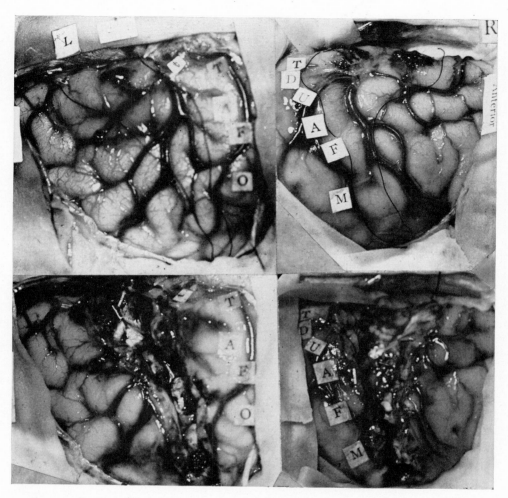

FIG. 30.   Case 24. Photographs. *Upper left:* Left frontal lobe. Thread indicates site for excision. *Lower left:* Left frontal lobe showing actual excision. *Upper right:* Right frontal lobe. Thread indicates site for excision. *Lower right:* Right frontal lobe showing actual excision.

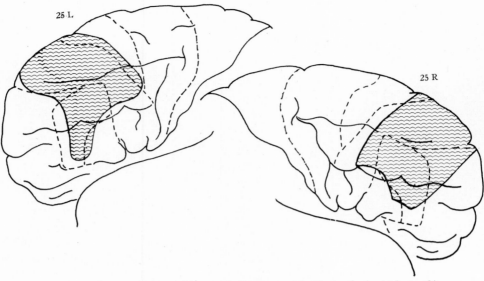

FIG. 31. Case 25. Extent of removal, diagrammatic. (Protocol: Areas 8, 9, 46.)

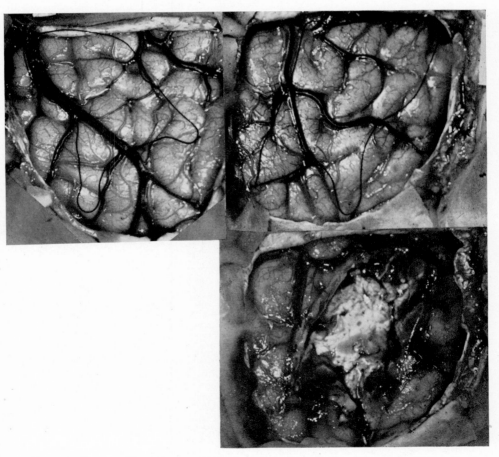

FIG. 32. Case 25. Photographs. *Upper left:* Left frontal lobe. Thread indicates site for excision. *Lower left:* (Photograph missing). *Upper right:* Right frontal lobe. Thread indicates site for excision. *Lower right:* Right frontal lobe showing actual excision.

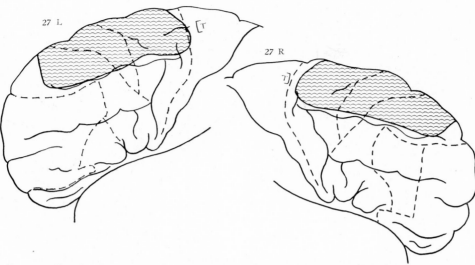

FIG. 33. Case 27. Extent of removal diagrammatic. (Protocol: Superior frontal gyri.) (*T:* indicates movements of contralateral toes on electrical stimulation.)

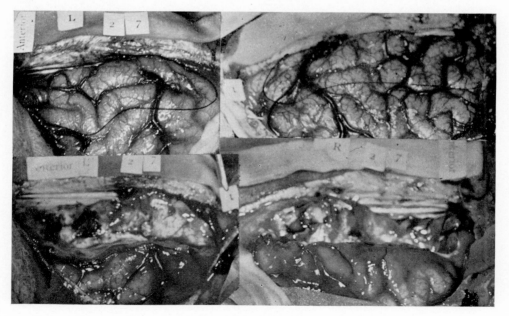

FIG. 34. Case 27. Photographs. *Upper left:* Left frontal lobe. Thread indicates site for excision. *Lower left:* Left frontal lobe showing actual excision. *Upper right:* Right frontal lobe. Thread indicates site for excision. *Lower right:* Right frontal lobe showing actual excision.

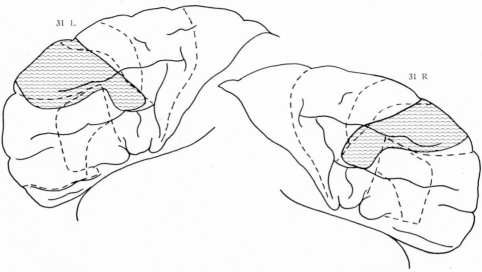

FIG. 35. Case 31. Extent of removal, diagrammatic. (Protocol: Area 9.)

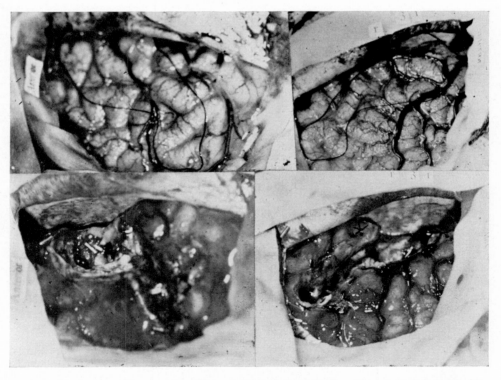

FIG. 36. Case 31. Photographs. *Upper left:* Left frontal lobe. Thread indicates site for excision. *Lower left:* Left frontal lobe showing actual excision. *Upper right:* Right frontal lobe. Thread indicates site for excision. *Lower right:* Right frontal lobe showing actual excision. Note exposure of falx after each excision.

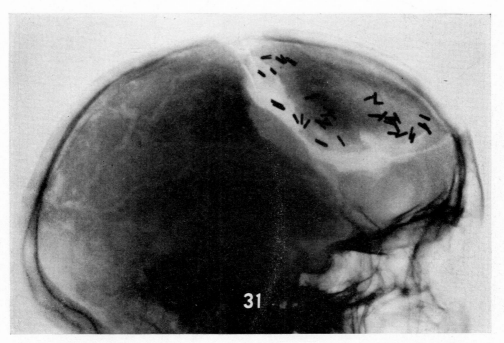

FIG. 37.   Case 31. Postoperative x-ray. Ventrally situated clusters of silver clips indicate site of cortical removal. (Dorsocaudal clips are placed on dura.)

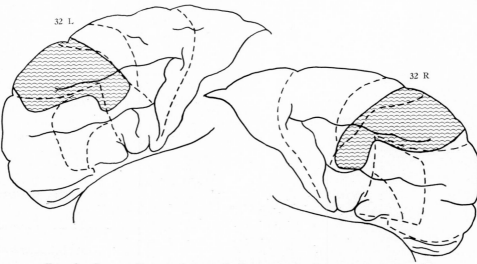

FIG. 38.   Case 32. Extent of removal, diagrammatic. (Protocol: Areas 8 and 9.)

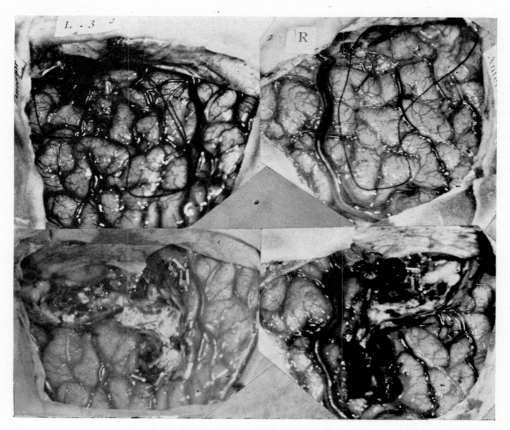

FIG. 39.   Case 32. Photographs. *Upper left:* Left frontal lobe. Thread indicates site for excision. *Lower left:* Left frontal lobe showing actual excision. *Upper right:* Right frontal lobe. Thread indicates site for excision. *Lower right:* Right frontal lobe showing actual excision. Note exposure of falx after excisions.

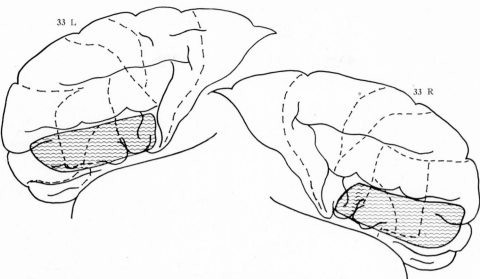

FIG. 40.  Case 33. Extent of removal, diagrammatic. (Protocol: Inferior frontal gyri.)

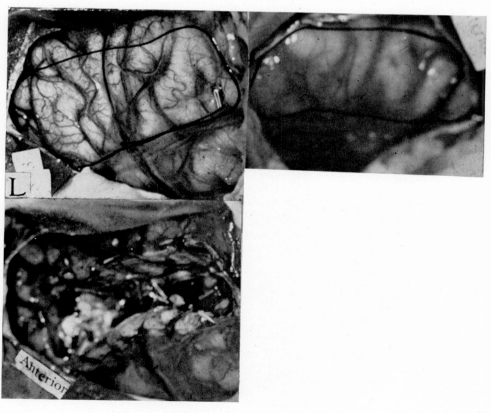

FIG. 41.  Case 33. Photographs. *Upper left:* Left frontal lobe. Thread indicates site for excision. The sylvian fissure lies immediately below and parallel to the lowermost part of the black thread. *Lower left:* Left frontal lobe showing actual excision. *Upper right:* Right frontal lobe. Thread indicates site for excision. *Lower right:* (Photograph missing).

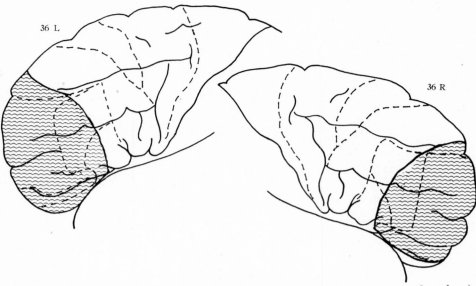

FIG. 42.   Case 36. Extent of removal, diagrammatic. (Protocol: Areas 10, 11, 45, 46, and 47.)

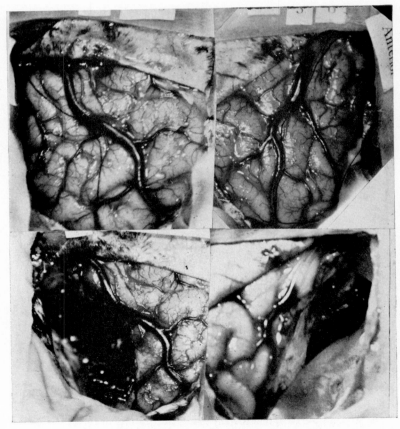

FIG. 43.   Case 36. Photographs. *Upper left:* Left frontal lobe. Thread indicates site for excision. *Lower left:* Left frontal lobe showing actual excision. *Upper right:* Right frontal lobe. Thread indicates site for excision. *Lower right:* Right frontal lobe showing actual excision.

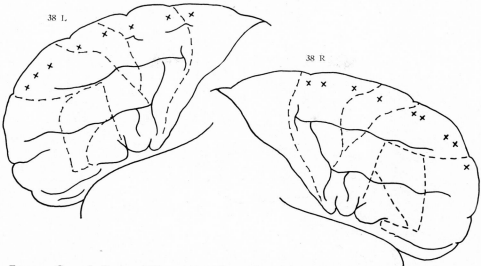

FIG. 44. Case 38. Crosses indicate approximate site of superior cerebral veins divided after ligation with silver clips. (No excision of cortical tissue.)

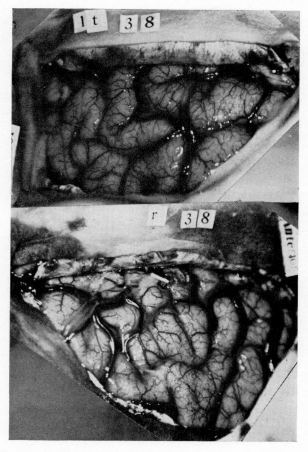

FIG. 45. Case 38. Photographs. *Upper:* Left frontal lobe before venous ligation. *Lower:* Right frontal lobe after ligation of superior cerebral veins.

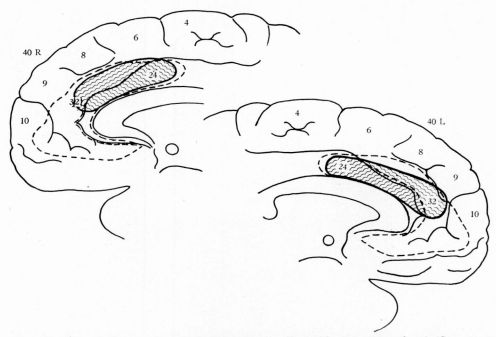

FIG. 46. Case 40. Extent of removal, diagrammatic. (Protocol: Areas 24 and 32.) (Case 42. [Protocol: Area 11]: see diagram and x-ray for case 18 [figs. 21 and 22].)

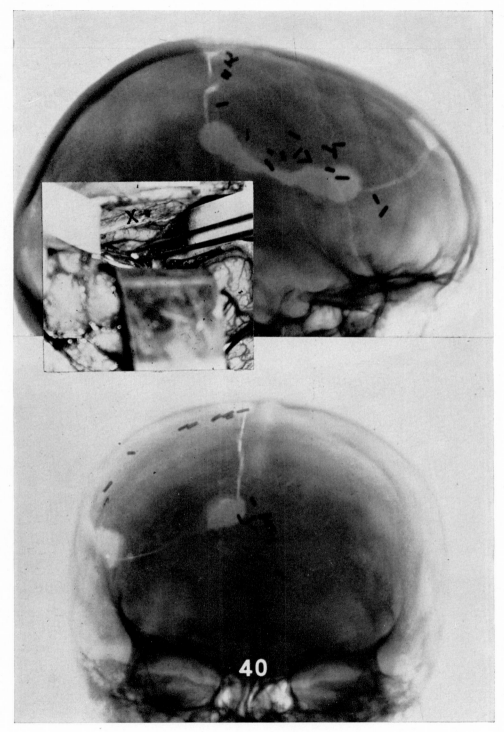

Fig. 47.   Case 40. Postoperative anteroposterior and lateral x-rays showing position of right frontal bone flap. The deeply situated silver clips close to the midline indicate the approximate extent of cortical removal. Insert (photograph) shows operative approach to cingular gyri. Right frontal lobe is being retracted. Falx (X) is shown and part of the medial surface of the left frontal lobe beneath it. The small white area between forceps tips is the corpus callosum.

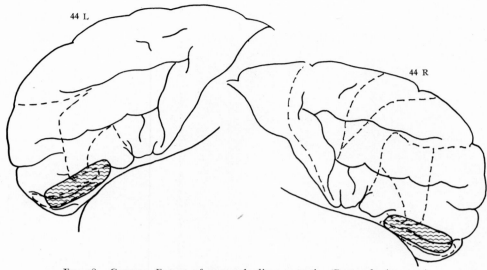

FIG. 48. Case 44. Extent of removal, diagrammatic. (Protocol: Area 47.)

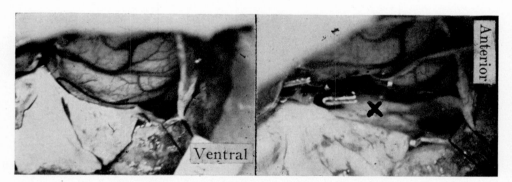

FIG. 49. Case 44. Photographs. *Left:* Thread in place along base of right frontal lobe, ventrolaterally. *Right:* Site of excision. The floor of the anterior fossa (X) is visible at the bottom of the photograph.

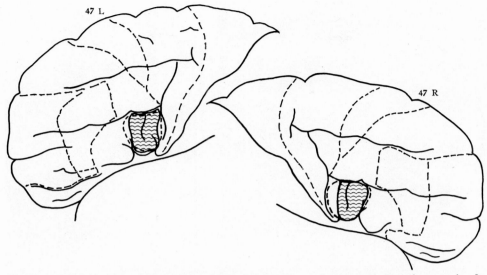

FIG. 50.   Case 47. Extent of removal, diagrammatic. (Protocol: Area 44.) For photograph of cortical removal in this case see figure 67, facing page 77.

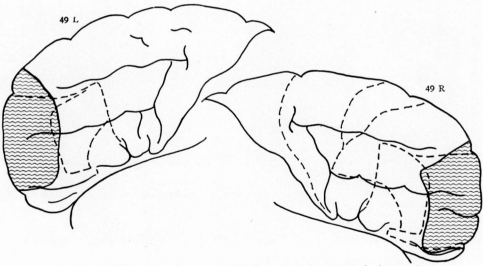

FIG. 51.   Case 49. Extent of removal, diagrammatic. (Protocol: Area 10.)

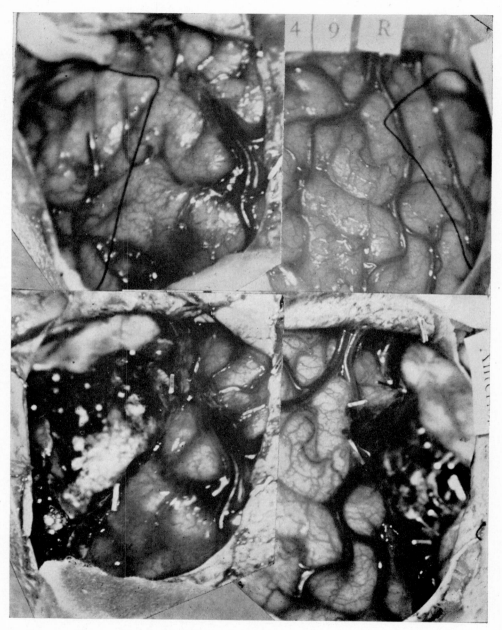

FIG. 52.  Case 49. Photographs. *Upper left:* Left frontal lobe. Thread indicates site for excision. *Lower left:* Left frontal lobe showing actual excision. *Upper right:* Right frontal lobe. Thread indicates site for excision. *Lower right:* Right frontal lobe showing actual excision. Note falx exposed by each excision.

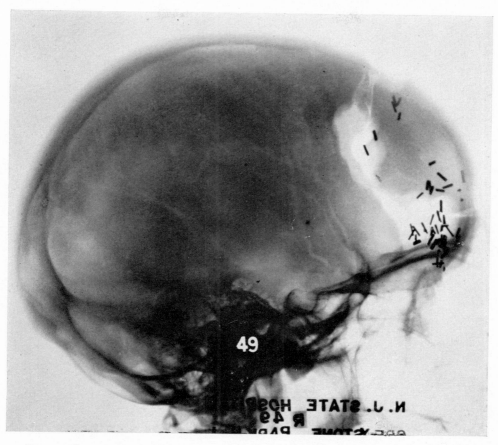

Fig. 53. Case 49. Postoperative x-ray. Large rostroventral cluster of silver clips indicates approximate extent of cortical removal. (The small group of dorsocaudally situated clips is on the dura.)

for cortical excision, fundamental cortical landmarks serving as reference points depended on the site of the exposure and included the sylvian fissures, the central and precentral sulci, the superior and inferior frontal sulci, the pars triangularis and pars opercularis, the corpus callosum, the orbital gyri, the olfactory tracts and optic nerves, and the gyri of the insula. Other useful reference points included the coronal and temporal sutures, the sphenoid ridge, the floor of the anterior fossa, and the falx cerebri. Electrical stimulation of the excitable motor cortex served as an additional localizing aid in 3 cases: 6, 24, and 27.

After exposure of the cortex, the proposed site of each excision was checked in every case by the neurosurgeon and the anatomist, with the aid of enlarged charts and photographs prepared from Mettler ('42, figs. 64, 78, 80, 82, 84, and 333). A photograph of the exposed cortex was then made, after which a black silk thread was laid along the boundaries of the area to be removed and a second photograph taken with this thread in place. A third photograph was taken after each cortical ablation had been completed. When enlarged to actual size, these photographs were used to prepare figures 6-53. In addition, diagrams and measurements of each cortical ablation were made during the course of each operation, while the weight of each specimen of freshly excised cortex was recorded directly upon its removal. These weights appear in table 9 together with an *estimation* of the total weight of tissue removed, computed according to the volume of the cavity in the brain created by the removal. (Since it was usually not feasible to excise the entire specimen completely in one block, gentle suction with a small suction tip was employed to complete the removal.)

Anteroposterior and lateral x-ray films of the skull taken three to six weeks after each operation served to corroborate the estimated site and extent of the cortical extirpations, outlined by silver brain clips. From the above data each cortical resection could be charted with reasonable accuracy, as illustrated in figures 6-53.

### SURGICAL PROCEDURE IN INITIAL GROUP OF OPERATIONS

**Consent for Operation.** The consent of the family or the next of kin was obtained for each operation. An order for surgery was also given by the Medical Superintendent and Chief Executive Officer, and Clinical Director and Chief Surgeon of the New Jersey State Hospital at Greystone Park. No patient, even though irrational, was operated upon who objected.

**Preoperative Preparation.** The battery of tests described in chapter 1 having been completed, the day before operation a final physical examination was carried out, the blood cross-matched with a compatible donor, an enema ordered, and the patient's entire head shaved. Nothing was allowed by mouth during the eight hours prior to operation. One hour before operation, morphine sulfate (8 to 10 mg.) and atropine (0.4 mg.) were given by hypodermic. On arrival in the anteroom, the patient's pharynx and larynx were cocainized (in all but 4 patients) with an atomizer containing a 5 percent solution of cocaine. A saline infusion was then started and used as a vehicle for the administration of 3 percent sodium pentothal. Curare (Squibb's "Intocostrin") was administered (intravenously) in 17 of the 24 cases, the dosage ranging from 20 to 60 units (see table 10).

**Anesthesia and Treatment during Operative Procedure.** Anesthesia was induced with sodium pentothal administered intravenously, followed by oral intratracheal intubation, after which the scalp was infiltrated with 70 to 100 cc. of 1 percent procaine hydrochloride solution (without epinephrine).

TABLE 9. WEIGHTS OF SPECIMENS IN GRAMS

| Case No. | Areas removed | Side of removal | Actual weight of fresh tissue removed | Estimated weight according to volume of cerebral cavity [a] | Estimated weight of brain tissue removed by suction | Estimated total weight (both sides) |
|---|---|---|---|---|---|---|
| 2 | 8, 6[b], 9[b] (8[c]) | Left | 5.8 | 9.3 | 3.5 | |
| | | Right | 7.1 | 8.1 | 1.0 | 17.4 |
| 3 | 9[b], 6[b] | Left | 6.3 | | | |
| | | Right | 6.4 | | | |
| 4 | 46 | Left | 5.8 | 10.8 | 5.0 | |
| | | Right | 4.8 | 10.0 | 5.2 | 20.8 |
| 6 | 8[b], 6[d] (6[c]) | Left | 9.6 | 13.7 | 4.1 | |
| | | Right | 16.3 | 11.2 | | 24.9 |
| 7 | 8, 9[b], 10[b] | Left | 25.5 | 30.0 | 4.5 | |
| | | Right | 20.0 | 34.0 | 6.0 | 64.0 |
| 8 | 8[b], 9[b], 10[b], 46[b] (MFG) | Left | 7.8 | 17.0 | 9.2 | |
| | | Right | 8.7 | 13.0 | 4.3 | 30.0 |
| 13 | 9[b], 10[b], 45, 46 | Left | 13.5 | 15.1 | 1.6 | |
| | | Right | 14.0 | 16.5 | 2.5 | 31.6 |
| 18 | 11[b] | Left | 4.2 | 12.0 | 7.8 | |
| | | Right | 4.3 | 14.0 | 9.7 | 26.0 |
| 19 | 45[b] | Left | 1.8 | 7.5 | 5.7 | |
| | | Right | 1.8 | 4.3 | 2.5 | 11.8 |
| 21 | 10 | Left | 8.2 | 16.1 | 7.9 | |
| | | Right | 5.2 | 9.3 | 4.1 | 25.4 |
| 22 | 9, 10, 46 | Left | 23.1 | 24.7 | 1.6 | |
| | | Right | 19.5 | 24.7 | 5.2 | 49.4 |
| 24 | 6[d] (6[c]) | Left | 7.6 | 12.8 | 5.2 | |
| | | Right | 10.8 | 18.4 | 7.6 | 31.2 |
| 25 | 8, 9, 46, 10[b] | Left | 11.3 | 20.9 | 9.6 | |
| | | Right | 14.1 | 17.5 | 3.4 | 38.4 |
| 27 | 6[b], 8[b], 9[b], 10[b] SFG | Left | 16.9 | 24.8 | 7.9 | |
| | | Right | 17.8 | 30.2 | 12.4 | 55.0 |
| 31 | 9 | Left | 13.0 | 20.0 | 7.0 | |
| | | Right | 10.7 | 13.1 | 2.4 | 33.1 |
| 32 | 8[b], 9, 10[b] | Left | 12.5 | 12.7 | 0.2 | |
| | | Right | 17.0 | 17.1 | 0.1 | 29.8 |
| 33 | 44[b], 45, 46[b], 10[b] IFG | Left | 12.9 | 14.5 | 1.4 | |
| | | Right | 7.0 | 15.1 | 8.1 | 29.6 |
| 36 | 10, 11, 45, 46, 47 | Left | 23.8 | 36.9 | 13.1 | |
| | | Right | 29.0 | 36.6 | 5.6 | 73.5 |
| 38 | 6, 8, 9, 10[e] | | | | | |
| 40 | 24[b] | Left | Not weighed | 7.0 | .... | |
| | | Right | | 7.2 | | 14.2 |
| 42 | 11 | Left | 4.9 | 12.5 | 7.6 | |
| | | Right | 5.0 | 14.5 | 9.5 | 27.0 |
| 44 | 10[b] (47) | Left | 2.5 | 5.7 | 2.2 | |
| | | Right | 2.0 | 5.5 | 3.5 | 11.2 |
| 47 | 44 (44[c]) | Left | 3.0 | 8.2 | 5.2 | |
| | | Right | 3.6 | .... | .... | |
| 49 | 10, 11[b], 46[b] | Left | 9.0 | 17.1 | 8.1 | |
| | | Right | 10.0 | 25.0 | 15.0 | 42.1 |

[a] Measurements in centimeters are given in chapter 5.   [b] Part only.
[c] Unilateral verification done five months after original operation.
[d] Incomplete original removal caudally.   [e] Venous ligation only.

TABLE 10. OPERATING ROOM DATA FOR TOPECTOMY CASES

| Case No. | Duration surgery Hrs. | Duration surgery Min. | Dose curare in units | Gm. pent. for intubation | Gm. pent. total | Fluid therapy in cc Glucose | Fluid therapy in cc Plasma | Recovery reflex in O.R. |
|---|---|---|---|---|---|---|---|---|
| 2 | 4 | 30 | — | .7 | 1.1 | 1400 | 500 | Extubated self |
| 3 * | 6 | 5 | — | .6 | 2.3 | 2000 | 500 | Present; awake |
| 4 | 4 | 50 | — | .8 | 1.6 | 1400 | 500 | Present |
| 6 | 5 | 10 | 40 | .33 | 1.5+ | 1800 | 250 | Present |
| 7 | 7 | 20 | 40 | ? | 2.5+ | 2200 | 500 | Present; moaning |
| 8 | 5 | 40 | — | .6 | 2.3 | 2000 | 500 | Present; awake |
| 13 | 6 | 20 | — | .8 | 2.8 | 1000 | 500 | Present |
| 18 | 5 | 30 | — | 1.1 | 2.5 | 1300 | 500 | Present; moaning |
| 19 | 4 | 30 | 40 | .5 | 1.7 | 1800 | 250 | Present |
| 21 | 5 | 10 | — | .6 | 2.6 | 1000 | 500 | Present |
| 22 * | 5 | 30 | — | .8 | 2.3 | 1800 | 500 | Present |
| 24 * | 8 | 15 | 60 | 1.0 | 2.5+ | 2000 | 500 | Absent |
| 25 | 5 | 20 | 40 | .5 | 1.2 | 1300 | 250 | Present; open eyes |
| 27 * | 5 | 30 | 60 | .7 | 2.6 | 1500 | 250 | Absent |
| 31 | 5 | 0 | 20 | .4 | 1.0 | 1600 | 250 | Present; talking |
| 32 | 6 | 15 | 20 | .23 | 1.7 | 2000 | 250 | Climbed to stretcher |
| 33 * | 6 | 30 | 20 | .5 | .94 | 1800 | 250 | Present; eyes open |
| 36 | 5 | 35 | 20 | .23 | 1.0 | 1400 | 250 | Present; talking |
| 38 | 4 | 40 | 20 | .5 | 1.5 | 2000 | 250 | Present |
| 40 | 4 | 55 | 60 | .5+ | 1.0+ | 2200 | 250 | Present |
| 42 | 5 | 20 | 40 | .6 | 1.75 | 1800 | 250 | Present; talking |
| 44 | 5 | 25 | 20 | .23 | 1.5 | 1500 | 250 | Present; open eyes |
| 47 | 4 | 45 | 20 | .4 | 1.3 | 1600 | 250 | Present |
| 49 | 6 | 25 | 40 | .3 | 1.2 | 2000 | 250 | Climbed to stretcher |

* Transfusions (whole blood): case 3, 200 cc.; case 22 and case 27, 500 cc.; case 24, 600 cc.; case 33, 800 cc.

Following intubation a semiclosed absorption to-and-fro system was set up and a 75-25 mixture of nitrous oxide-oxygen delivered for twenty minutes or more. The system was then changed to a closed one and the bag filled with the same mixture. This mixture was rebreathed for approximately fifteen minutes after which the bag was emptied and refilled with the same mixture again. During the fifteen-minute rebreathing periods 400 cc. of oxygen per minute flowed continuously. At no time was cyanosis noted and at no time following the occasional short apnea during induction were respirations depressed or inadequate.

Secretions during these long procedures were frequently excessive and required repeated suctioning. Increasing the dose of atropine premedication from 0.4 to 0.6 mg. did not solve the problem, nor did repeating the drug intravenously within two to three hours of premedication time. Stimulation of the trachea during passage of the suction catheter inevitably produced the familiar "bucking" phenomenon. Surgery was usually halted until the "bucking" disappeared and additional pentothal was seldom needed after removal of the tracheal irritant. Thorough suctioning before removal of the endotracheal tube at the conclusion of surgery consistently yielded large quantities of thick secretions.

Glucose in distilled water, normal saline, and plasma were given liberally and routinely, and 5 patients also received a transfusion of whole blood (table 10). Clinically, none of the patients showed any evidence of traumatic or hemorrhagic shock during operation. In only one patient did the blood pressure fall to a level of 85/60 and that patient had arrived in the operating room with a blood pressure of 95/60. This patient did not develop the clinical picture of shock and the blood pressure responded favorably to transfusion therapy. The blood pressure in the other patients showed only insignificant alterations, remaining approximately at the preoperative level in each case.

During operation the pulse rate remained fairly constant in the majority of patients, but in patients 2, 19, 21, 25, 27, 31, 33, and 44 a decrease in rate followed removal of cortex from one or the other frontal lobe. The most marked change (96 per min. to 72 per min.) occurred in patient 25. The depth of anesthesia was not altered and canisters were not changed at the time of these observations. The pulse never slowed abruptly as in patients with altered vagal reflexes, but presented a gradual transition to a slower rate, which was usually maintained to the end of anesthesia. A similar phenomenon has been observed in the course of prefrontal lobotomy operations.

Variations in rate and depth of respiration were not unusual and were not associated with the cortical excisions.

The amount of pentothal needed to maintain these patients varied depending upon the size of the patient, the duration of operation, and whether or not curare was used as an aid to intubation. When curare was not used, the maximum dose for any one patient was a 2.8 gm. and the minimum 1.1 gm.; the average dose for this group was 2.17 gm. In the curare group the maximum dose was 2.6 gm. and the minimum 0.94 gm., the average dose being 1.57 gm. The duration of anesthesia in the shortest operation was four and one-half hours and in the longest eight and one-quarter hours (table 10).

The recovery of the patients following discontinuance of anesthesia was prompt in all but 2 cases. In one of these (case 24) there was lapse into preoperative catatonic stupor. The other patient (case 6) had a generalized convulsion during operation lasting fifteen seconds following electrical stimulation of his cerebral cortex. It is questionable whether or not the convulsion effected the delayed recovery from anesthesia. Immediately after operation, 2 patients transferred themselves unaided onto the stretchers, and 3 spoke coherently before leaving the operating room, while 1 patient extubated himself and the rest of the group had recovered sufficiently to make the insertion of an oral airway unnecessary.

The postoperative follow-up of these cases is reported in the section contributed by the medical clinical investigators.


### DETAILS OF OPERATIVE PROCEDURE

**Position of the Patient.** Each operation was performed with the patient lying on his back, the head being elevated 30 to 45 degrees from the horizontal. For subfrontal exposures the head was dropped into a slightly dependent position once the bone flap had been elevated. This facilitated the operative approach by allowing the brain to fall away from the floor of the anterior fossa. For relatively low, ventrally placed craniotomies, the drapes were so arranged that the head could be turned to either side; otherwise it was never necessary to readjust the position of the head.

**Instrument Table.** Instruments were arranged before each operation, ready for immediate use, on a large instrument table wheeled into place so that it straddled the operating table. (Additional space for the anesthetist and for inspection of the patient during cortical stimulation could be provided were the height of the table made adjustable.)

**Preparation of Scalp.** Immediately before operation the scalp was thoroughly cleansed with green soap and water, and then with ether, before being painted with tincture of iodine, and finally washed with 70 percent alcohol. The site of the proposed incision was then outlined with methylene blue and infiltrated with 1 percent procaine hydrochloride.

**Draping.** The operative field was first draped with sterile rubber sheeting over which appropriately sized double-thickness drapes were laid.

**Operative Approaches.** For most of these operations a generous bilateral exposure of cortex was required, for which a coronal scalp incision was used, crossing the midline close to or caudal to the coronal suture and then curving forward so that the scalp could be reflected anteriorly as far as the supraorbital ridge.

The bone flaps were made in the usual fashion by making holes with a Hudson drill and sawing between them with a Gigli saw. Each bone flap hinged on the temporal muscle. In most cases the medial margin of each bone flap was placed as close to the midline as possible, leaving a narrow bridge of bone about 1 cm. in width over the superior longitudinal sinus. In 8 cases this procedure was varied, a single saw-cut being made medially along the course of the longitudinal sinus, thus creating a bivalve type of flap. Well-beveled edges allowed such bivalved flaps to be seated firmly upon closure.

The rostral margins of the bone flaps were in general placed as far forward as the extent of the frontal sinuses permitted, while the caudal margins were planned according to the region of cortex to be exposed. After reflecting each flap, a small amount of bone was usually removed ventrally with rongeurs.

For comparatively small flaps, situated above the upper limit of the temporal muscles, an H-shaped scalp incision was made (2 cases), the bar of the "H" being directly over, and parallel to, the superior longitudinal sinus. In this type of flap the scalp was not dissected from the periosteum.

Limited exposures for the removal of small areas (such as area 44) confined to the lower gyri of the frontal lobes were readily accomplished by turning moderately small flaps, one on either side, through separate curved incisions. In case 40 a single flap on the right side sufficed to expose the desired portion of the medial surface of each frontal lobe down to the corpus callosum.

**Placement of Bone Flaps.** Variations in the placement of bone flaps for adequate exposure of the various segments of the frontal lobes under discussion may be summarized as follows:

*Brodmann's Areas 4 and 6.* Medially the rostral margin of the bone flap may be begun halfway between the supraorbital ridge and the bregma, while the caudal limb follows a line drawn through the external auditory meatus perpendicular to Reid's base line (Mettler, '42, p. 120, fig. 84).

*Area 8.* An "H" type of flap was used (see above), the rostral margin being halfway between the supraorbital ridge and the bregma, while the caudal margin begins an equal distance caudal to the bregma.

*Area 9.* Exposure of the full extent of this area requires a flap extending from the supraorbital ridge to a point 1.5 cm. caudal to the bregma, and thence ventrally almost to the sylvian point.

*Area 10.* Essentially the same as for area 9, though not necessarily as far caudally.

*Area 11.* For excision of the orbital gyri of each frontal lobe, each flap must be placed as far rostrally as possible, as if for a bilateral pituitary approach, since the olfactory tracts and optic nerves must be visualized.

*Areas 45 and 46.* Although more ventrally placed, otherwise essentially the same as for area 9, since a wide exposure of cortical landmarks is necessary in order to identify the approximate site of areas 45 or 46.

*Areas 44 and 47.* Separate, relatively small, ventrally placed bifrontal flaps may be used. Area 44 lies close to the angle formed by the junction of the coronal and squamous sutures, so that the bone flap should be centered over this junction. For area 47 (a part of area 10) a similar flap may be made, but should be extended farther rostrally.

*Areas 24 and 32.* For an approach to areas 24 and 32 a large unilateral, rostrally placed flap seems sufficient. By retracting the presenting cerebral hemisphere laterally from the falx, the medial surface of each frontal lobe can be exposed down to the corpus callosum as far caudally as area 4.

*Combined Removals.* To remove more than one of Brodmann's areas in a given case, each bone flap must be modified according to the suggestions just outlined so that each exposure is adequate.

*Frontal Gyri.* Flaps should be situated close to the midline for removal of the superior frontal gyri; ventrally and rostrally for removal of the inferior frontal gyri; and in an intermediate position for removal of the middle frontal gyri.

**Identification of Cortical Segments.** *Area 4.* Most of area 4 lies between the central and precentral sulci, with its broadest extent at the dorsal aspect of the precentral gyrus whence it extends medially as indicated on Brodmann's map (fig. 55). The rostral margin, irregular in outline, usually disappears ventrally into the depths of the central fissure. For identification of area 4 by gross inspection alone it is obviously necessary to identify the central and sylvian fissures. It is advisable to identify the precentral sulcus also. While exact delimitation of area 4 is difficult if not impossible, its boundaries may be determined approximately by means of electrical stimulation. (In this series no elaborate effort was made to identify 4s, nor the caudal boundary of area 4.)

Although area 4 was not excised its rostral extent was delimited by electrical stimulation in order to determine the caudal border of area 6.

*Area 6.* The caudal border of Brodmann's area 6 lies immediately rostral to area 4 (fig. 55), while area 6 occupies the bulk of the ventral portion of the precentral gyrus and thence extends rostrally in a somewhat curved fashion, encroaching upon the caudal portion of the middle frontal gyrus, and to a greater extent upon the caudal portion of the superior frontal gyrus. In outlining the approximate extent of area 6, it is therefore important to identify the central, the precentral, and the superior and inferior frontal sulci. In our cases, as a safeguard against trauma to area 4, the actual removal of area 6 along its caudal border followed a line 2 mm. or more rostral to the rostral extent of excitable motor cortex (cases 6 and 24).

*Area 8.* Area 8 is roughly a comma-shaped segment cutting obliquely across the superior frontal gyrus immediately rostral to area 6, terminating ventrally in the caudal portion of the middle frontal gyrus, rostral to the precentral sulcus.

*Area 9.* The ventrorostral margin of area 9 roughly bisects horizontally the superior half of the middle frontal gyrus and then swings almost at a right angle, in a ventral direction, to follow a line continuous with the rostral boundary of area 44. The ventrocaudal margin of area 9, approximately 1 cm. in length, is marked by the ventral border of the middle frontal sulcus close to its junction with the precentral sulcus. Thence, the caudal margin of area 9 runs in a medial or dorsal direction, crossing the middle frontal gyrus obliquely until it reaches the superior frontal sulcus, whence it turns sharply in a rostral direction. Thus the key points in locating the approximate extent of area 9 are the superior and inferior frontal sulci and the precentral sulci. With an adequate exposure these structures are not difficult to identify.

*Area 10.* Area 10 is roughly a rectangular segment of cortex comprising the rostral third of the frontal lobe. Its dorsal or medial margin roughly bisects the rostral third of the middle frontal gyrus, while its ventral margin parallels the base of the inferior frontal gyrus.

Note: Excisions of area 6, 8, 9, and 10 also included the cortex on the medial surface of each frontal lobe believed to represent these areas.

*Area 44.* Area 44 can be readily identified as the pars opercularis of the inferior frontal gyrus. It lies immediately in front of the lowermost portion of the precentral sulcus, and occupies the caudal third of the inferior frontal gyrus. Thus area 44 is bounded dorsally by the inferior frontal sulcus, ventrally by the sylvian fissure, caudally by the precentral sulcus, and rostrally by area 45 (pars triangularis). Removal of area 44 exposes the underlying gyri breves of the island of Reil. In case 47, hemostasis of area 44 was accomplished with silver clips exclusively.

*Areas 45 and 46.* Between areas 10, 9, and 44 there lies a roughly rectangular zone of cortex. Its ventrocaudal portion, representing area 45, is comprised for the most part of the pars triangularis, which can be readily identified. The remainder of the rectangle comprises area 46, the approximate boundaries of which can be identified by criteria used to identify the areas bordering upon it (see above).

*Area 47.* Area 47 is apparently represented by a rather thin strip of cortex along the base of the inferior frontal gyrus, and extends caudally to the sylvian fissure.

*Area 11.* Area 11 comprises the bulk of the four orbital gyri. Medially, it extends somewhat caudal to the full extent of the medial orbital gyrus. During the exposure of area 11 the olfactory tracts and optic nerves are brought into view, as well as the anterior cerebral arteries.

*Area 24.* As can be seen from Brodmann's map, area 24 occupies most of the rostral portion of the gyrus cinguli. By carrying the operative exposure down to the corpus callosum along its rostral half, there is no difficulty in identifying the appropriate gyri, except for that portion of the cortex lying ventral to the genu of the corpus callosum, where (case 40) the removal of area 24 (and 32) was not pursued.

*Frontal Gyri.* Little difficulty is incurred in locating the extent of the superior, middle, and inferior frontal gyri, provided the exposure is adequate. Before removing the superior frontal gyrus, the rostral extent of the excitable motor cortex should be determined by electrical stimulation (case 27), so that area 4 may be preserved. In the case of the middle and inferior frontal gyri, identification of the precentral sulcus clearly indicates the caudal boundaries of the excision.

*Technique of Electrical Stimulation.* During electrical stimulation of the motor cortex, the patient was maintained under light nitrous-oxide-oxygen anesthesia. A Rahm stimulator and bipolar electrodes were used, at a frequency of 60 cycles per second. The effects of successive stimuli were tested, applied at intervals separated by at least one minute, beginning at a current strength of 0.8 volt applied to the dorso-caudal aspect of the central gyrus close to the central fissure. The voltage was then increased by 0.2 volt with each successive stimulus (unless a response was elicited) to a maximum of 2.5 volts, and the duration of each stimulus (unless a response was observed) was twelve to fifteen seconds. Successive points were stimulated in similar fashion, each point being 2 to 3 mm. rostral to the previous site of stimulation. Cortical sites yielding a response were appropriately marked with small paper labels.

The electrodes were now applied to the cortex 1.5 cm. rostral to the labeled points, and the voltage doubled. The cortex was then stimulated at successive points in a caudal direction, until a response was again observed. The point at which this response occurred, even though the voltage had been doubled, usually corresponded closely with the previously labeled point, marking part of the rostral extent of area 4. This whole procedure was then repeated successively at more ventrally situated portions of the precentral gyrus.

**Technique of Cortical Excision.** All patients in this series were operated upon with only one assistant. (With two assistants the operating time for a topectomy has been reduced to less than three hours.)

Prior to excision of cortical tissue, hemostasis of the surface veins, and then the arteries, was first carried out, along the line of the proposed incision marked with black thread, by means of silver clips and fine silk ligatures passed beneath the vessels on a one-half-inch curved needle. (One or two of the deeper vessels in the parasagittal sulci were sometimes missed and had to be secured during or after removal of the block of tissue.) The cortex was then incised perpendicular to its surface, with a no. 11 scalpel blade to the depth of 1.9 cm., and undercut with a curved dissector so that it could be removed as one block. It was often necessary, however, to complete removal and to smooth the edges of the cortical cavity, after the excision, with gentle suction. In a few instances the bulk of the removal was accomplished with suction, as in the removal of areas 44, 11, and 24 where difficulty of access and the proximity of important blood vessels made block removal undesirable. Each excision was carried down to the depths of the gray matter but no farther. The margins of the wound were then made smooth and even, to the depth of the gray matter, all around each cavity by means of a small-bore suction tip. Hemostasis was completed with silver clips and the application of oxidized cellulose ("Hemopak," Johnson and Johnson). In only rare instances was light application of the electrocautery used. The patient was then made to "buck" or cough by the anesthetist to make certain that hemostasis was satisfactory. Five cc. penicillin solution (1000 units per cc.) were now inserted in each wound and watertight closure of the dura accomplished with black silk sutures. The bone flap was replaced, the periosteum sutured, and the scalp approximated with a layer of galeal and superficial sutures. When subaponeurotic drains were used, they were removed twenty-four hours later. Normal saline solution at a temperature of 99° to 104° F. was used liberally during each operation to irrigate each wound and the exposed surfaces of the brain. The measurements of the extent of the cerebral cavities following cortical excision are given in pp. 64-77, and the weights of tissue removed, in table 9, p. 36.

With regard to the three operations (cases 6, 24, and 27) in which electrical stimulation was used to outline the approximate rostral extent of the excitable motor cortex on the lateral convexity of the brain, it is believed that the caudal margin of each cortical excision included cortex within a few millimeters of area 4, so that presumably a considerable portion of 4's adjacent to these cortical excisions was either extirpated or traumatized. Finally, in cases 6 and 24 (see below), when electrical stimulation of the motor cortex was carried out at a second unilateral operation five months later, under similar conditions of anesthesia and operative technique, it was observed that the rostral extent of the excitable motor cortex had apparently become shifted to a more caudal plane. This shift was probably due to loss of viable neurones immediately caudal to the line of the first cortical excision, as indicated in figure 66.

### POSTOPERATIVE NOTES

Several patients had begun to recover consciousness as they were being moved off the operating-room table, although some required longer intervals to regain consciousness (table 10, p. 37). Postoperatively, fluids were administered by vein (and in a few cases by gastric tube) until nourishment could be taken by mouth, and each patient was given 30,000 units of penicillin every three hours intramuscularly for five days as a precaution against postoperative pneumonia. Three patients required aspiration of serosanguineous fluid from beneath their scalp wounds.

In this series of twenty-four successive bilateral operations, carried out from May 26 to June 6, 1947, there were no fatalities, no wound infections, and no cases of postoperative pneumonia. Signs of delayed postoperative shock were promptly and effectively treated by transfusion. One patient (40) postoperatively had a small amount of blood in the cerebrospinal fluid as judged clinically and confirmed by spinal puncture. This had cleared by the tenth postoperative day, and may well have been occasioned by a small opening inadvertently made in the medial wall of the left lateral ventricle during removal of part of the cingulate gyrus. The incidence of transitory postoperative motor weakness, incontinence, and of convulsive seizures are among the subjects discussed in pp. 430-452.

### Prefrontal Lobotomy (8 cases)

From October 27 through November 3, 1947, approximately five months after the first series of twenty-four operations had been completed, 8 patients were subjected to bilateral prefrontal lobotomy. Six of these patients were selected from the control group, and 2 (2 and 44) from the group previously operated upon. In case 2, area 8, and in case 44 the ventral portion of area 10 (? area 47) had previously been bilaterally removed.

The preoperative preparation, the technique of anesthesia, and the position of the patient on the operating table were similar to those used for the initial group of operations.

**Operative Technique.** With the patient in position for operation the site selected for lobotomy was marked on each side of the head so as to correspond as closely as possible to the operative site described by Freeman and Watts ('42); that is, in the coronal suture 6 cm. above the zygoma, perpendicular to a point 3 cm. caudal to the lateral margin of the orbit. This point was marked with a drop of methylene blue injected beneath the pericranium with a hypodermic needle. A coronal scalp flap was then reflected anteriorly as far as the supraorbital ridge, and a trephine opening made through the coronal suture bilaterally at the sites previously marked with methylene blue.

In each case a small incision was next made through the dura, in the center of the trephine opening (on the right side only), and a silver brain clip placed on the underlying cerebral cortex as a marker. A bone flap was then reflected to expose the right frontal lobe around the marker indicating the site of the lobotomy incision. Observations, photographs, and measurements were then made indicating the precise location of the proposed lobotomy incision with respect to its position on the surface of the cortex. (The results of these determinations are described on p. 7.) Color photographs of the exposed cortex were taken before and after lobotomy.

Prefrontal lobotomy was accomplished through a small cortical incision at the selected site, by means of a small spatula swept through the white matter to within 1.5 cm. of the falx cerebri medially, and 1.0 to 1.5 cm. of the floor of the anterior fossa at its junction with the sphenoid ridge, in a plane parallel to the coronal suture line, immediately rostral to the anterior extent of the lateral ventricle. The depth of each incision through the white matter and the position of the anterior extent of each lateral ventricle were previously determined by exploration with a brain needle. A biopsy of the cortex rostral to each right-sided lobotomy incision was then taken (without resort to the electrocautery). In cases 2 and 44 the biopsy included part of the scar resulting from the operative removal five months previously. Finally, the depths of the lobotomy incisions were outlined with silver brain clips to facilitate postoperative x-ray studies. Hemostasis being complete, each wound was closed in layers with interrupted silk sutures.

On the left side in each of these cases, the trephine opening at the designated point in the coronal suture was enlarged with rongeurs, along the coronal suture line, in a ventral and dorsal direction to facilitate the lobotomy. Five cc. penicillin solution (1000 units per 1 cc.) were instilled into each cerebral wound before closure.

**Observations.** *Cortical Scars.* In cases 2 and 44 cortical scars were found representing the removal, five months previously, of areas 8 and 47 respectively. The scars were lightly adherent to the overlying dura, which was quite easily peeled away, and were smooth, glistening, quite sharply demarcated, and somewhat concave. They appeared to be appropriately situated as regards the intended cortical removals. Small venous channels on the surface of each scar oozed slightly after separation of the dura. The cortex immediately adjacent to each scar appeared slightly yellowish and softened for a distance of about 0.5 cm. Otherwise the surrounding surface of the brain looked grossly normal.

*Vascular Changes Following Lobotomy.* In 4 cases, immediately following prefrontal lobotomy on the right side, it seemed that the larger cortical arteries exposed by the craniotomy flap diminished in caliber while the surface of the exposed cortex became paler. These observations were confirmed by subsequent study of the color photographs taken immediately before and after lobotomy, which in each case was always completed on the right side before being done on the left.

**Postoperative Course.** Postoperative convalescence, from the surgical point of view, proceeded smoothly in all but 2 cases. In case 5 the patient failed to respond well, stiffness of the neck developed, and spinal puncture on the second postoperative day revealed blood-tinged cerebrospinal fluid. On the third day after lobotomy the condition of this patient was further complicated by four convulsive seizures, beginning in the right upper extremity, so that he was taken to the operating room where exploration of each wound, under local anesthesia, revealed no evidence of hemorrhage on either side but cerebral edema on the left. Following this exploratory procedure the patient improved steadily so that five days later he was alert, able to speak and move all his extremities.

Patient 2 removed his dressing and clawed at his wound before the sutures had been removed. As a result, a low-grade wound infection with osteomyelitis developed, despite local and systemic administration of pencillin and sulfadiazine, necessitating another operation for the removal of necrotic bone and infected granulation tissue. Following this procedure wound healing was satisfactory.

## REOPERATION (UNILATERAL)

Approximately five months after the first operation reoperation was undertaken in two patients (patient 6—right side, October 27, 1947; patient 24—left side, October 28, 1947.

**Anesthesia.** Sufficient anesthesia was induced by sodium pentothal (intravenously) to pass an intratracheal tube, after spraying the pharynx with 1 percent pantocaine hydrochloride. The scalp was then infiltrated with approximately 80 cc. 1 percent procaine. Thereafter light inhalation anesthesia was maintained with nitrous-oxide-oxygen.

**Operation Procedure.** Re-elevation of the previous craniotomy flap on one side only (see protocols below) was rendered somewhat difficult owing to adhesions between the bone flap and the dura. Adhesions between the dura and the underlying cortex were also encountered, at the site of the previous cortical resections. Electrical stimulation of the excitable motor cortex was then carried out in each case, using a special grid (see below).

At the conclusion of stimulation, the rostral limits of excitable motor cortex were marked by a black thread. Shallow incisions were then made on the cortex (with the point of a no. 11 scalpel blade) approximately 2 mm. rostral to the thread. Photographs were now taken, the grid removed, and another photograph taken. As described in chapter 4, resection of cortex was then carried out from a line just caudal to the scalpel marks rostrally, to include the caudal border of the previously made cortical excision. These resections extended to a depth of approximately 2.0 cm. and were further deepened by about 1.5 cm. to serve as unilateral lobotomy. After hemostasis, the wounds were closed in the usual fashion and 5 cc. penicillin solution (1000 units per cc.) inserted beneath the dura.

It should be noted that prior to stimulation in case 24 it was necessary to apply the electrocautery lightly at several points along the margin of the cortical scar. In case 6 the cautery was not applied to the cortex. Small wisps of oxidized cellulose were applied over one or two bleeding points from the cortical scars in both cases. In case 6, the inner surface of the dura was lightly adherent only to the rostral aspect of the cortical scar. The scar itself was well circumscribed and its surface slightly concave.

In case 24 the cortical scar extended caudal to the limits of the previous excision, and was diffusely and densely adherent to the overlying dura. The extensive pathologic change in the cortex in case 24 may be attributed to the long duration of the first operation, and possibly also to the fact that there was extensive exposure of the cortex to the heat of photographic lights. Finally, it should be observed that during the first operation in this case some subarachnoid extravasation of blood had occurred on the left side.

**Apparatus for Cortical Stimulation:**  a Rahm stimulator, calibrated as to voltage output only and supplied by 110 volt AC. Bipolar electrodes 2.0 mm. apart were used for stimulation. The stimulator was controlled by Dr. Harry Grundfest. Electrical contact was made by means of a foot switch controlled by the surgeon.

To facilitate charting the excitable motor cortex a grid was laid over the exposed cortex prior to stimulation. The grid was made of black silk thread woven into squares approximately 1.5 cm.×1.5 cm., the horizontal threads of the grid being placed, as nearly as possible, parallel to the midline. The squares were designated by sterilized, numbered, paper tickets. A diagram was now made indicating the relationship of cortical landmarks to the squares of the grid. Each square was arbitrarily divided into points 2.5 mm. apart, to which stimulation was confined. Abscissae and ordinates were designated as "ventral" and "rostral" respectively. The extreme dorsocaudal point of each square chosen for stimulation was referred to as "ventral-zero; rostral-zero," while the extreme ventrorostral point was designated as "ventral-7.5 mm.; rostral-7.5 mm."; etc. These points could thus be readily plotted on the prepared diagram for future reference.

**Technique of Cortical Stimulation.**  The duration of each stimulus was exactly fifteen seconds unless a muscle response was first obtained, whereupon stimulation was always terminated at once. An interval of at least sixty seconds was allowed between the termination of one stimulus and the beginning of the next. When a convulsion occurred, an interval of five minutes or more was allowed between stimuli.

In each square, stimulation was carried out successively from a dorsocaudal point, in a rostral direction, at 2.5-mm. intervals, whereupon the adjacent portion of the square 2.5 mm. ventral to this zone was then investigated in like manner, and so on until the whole square had been tested. Each point was initially stimulated with a low voltage, and if no response was observed, the same point was again repeatedly stimulated with progressively increased voltages within reasonable limits until it became apparent that no observable response could be expected. After one whole square had thus been stimulated, the square immediately rostral to it was then studied in like manner. When tests in each row of squares had been completed, the subjacent row of squares was next studied in the same sequence, and so on.

Trained observers were posted so that movements of the four extremities and the face could be carefully watched and recorded during these tests.

**Photography.**  Photographs of the exposed cortex were taken, without moving or readjusting the camera, in the following sequence: (1) immediately after completing exposure of the cortex; (2) after laying the grid on the surface of the cortex; (3) after placing numbered tickets in the approximate squares of the grid; (4) after indicating with black thread (a) the rostral limits of cortex yielding observed muscle response upon electrical stimulation, (b) the line marked by scalpel cuts—approximately 2 mm. rostral to line (a), and (c) after cortical resection had been completed.

## CRITICISM

In reviewing the surgical aspects of this series of cases, certain criticisms as to technique became apparent.

First of all, while the electrocautery was used sparingly and with due caution for occlusion of superior cerebral veins prior to cortical excision, and occasionally for hemostasis during an excision, it should never have been used at all in close proximity to cortical tissue in this type of operative procedure.

Secondly, a subpial dissection technique should have probably been used within the margins of each ablation prior to cortical excision, to reduce the degree of circulatory changes in the adjacent cortex. Thus certain side effects, such as incontinence and motor weakness, due to dysfunction of adjacent cortex, and perhaps also the incidence of postoperative seizures might have been reduced. This improvement in technique has been used in subsequent topec-tomy cases of another series.

Thirdly, the alleged location of Brodmann's areas might have been more precisely determined, or the technique of cortical ablations been better stand-arized, had the extent of the excitable motor cortex been determined bi-laterally in each case, to serve as a point of departure in charting the areas to be excised. It must be said, however, that even had time permitted the universal application of this technique, the variability in cranial sizes and cerebral configurations from case to case would tend to vitiate the supposed accuracy of measuring distances rostral to the central fissure.

Fourthly, the technique of electrical excitation of the motor cortex as car-ried out in 3 of our cases (five operations) seems in retrospect unsatisfactory, although it was intended more as a check on cortical landmarks than as a formal investigation of cortical function. Even though our patients were lightly anesthetized during cortical stimulation, for this purpose it would have been better had the entire operative procedure been carried out under local anes-thesia alone. Another criticism is that an insufficient number of excitable motor points were determined in our cases.

In this series it was also unfortunate that some degree of subarachnoid bleeding occurred in 1 case, and that a small opening into a lateral ventricle was made in 2 cases (36 and 40).

When considered as a new approach to an uncharted problem, carried out in a hospital almost totally inexperienced in neurosurgical techniques, the thirty-six surgical procedures just described on the whole proceeded in a sur-prisingly satisfactory manner. The only fatality was that of patient 24 who succumbed thirteen days after a second operation, following aspiration of food. Since he had recovered sufficiently to sit up in a chair, his demise can hardly be regarded technically as "postoperative."

*Chapter 5*

# Cytoarchitecture

FRED A. METTLER

---

A S FAR as the present author is aware the attempt to define histologically the extent and location of specimens taken from the human frontal cortex of any considerable number of different individuals has not previously been made. It has been necessary therefore to elaborate a technique for this purpose as well as to carry it out.

## PROCEDURE

Preliminary studies have indicated the relative futility of attempting to determine the cytoarchitectural characteristics of pieces of cortex removed during routine neurosurgery and delivered to the laboratory through conventional channels. Anyone intending to expend any considerable effort, time, or funds in such an enterprise should be present at the operation and make careful photographs and sketches of (a) the site of operation, (b) the site to be excised, after delimiting this with a thread placed upon its surface (it might be useful to prepare sterilizable flexible patterns to help in placing the thread), and (c) the operative site before closure. The last step is important since it may provide an explanation for subsequently observed divergencies between individuals who have been subjected to presumably identical operations. The preincision photographs help evaluate the possibility of interference with surface vasculature, interference with which might also be responsible for the subsequent divergencies.

The tissue to be excised should be carefully marked to facilitate its later orientation in determining the subsequent plane of section, and should be immediately fixed. It may be considered advisable to weigh and sketch or photograph the specimen before fixation, but much time should not be lost in these enterprises. Weight is deceptive. It can be spuriously increased by the presence of blood clots in the sulci or an unusual amount of white matter.

Following fixation, it is wise to subject the specimen to a roentgenologic examination to make certain that no silver clips have been insinuated into its depths. All specimens should then be oriented according to the same plane of reference, embedded *in toto*, and cut serially.

It is obvious that the excision itself should be carried out in such a manner as to reduce the necessity for subsequent contact with the brain.

It may be considered advisable to measure the operative crater. Measurement of the operative site, like weighing the tissue removed, is subject to perceptible error since the operative crater tends to fall open or close up, especially if situated in a location where much sound tissue overhangs the crater. Estimates of the amount of tissue removed may be hazarded by using the volume of the crater expressed in cubic centimeters (1 cc. of brain weighs slightly less than 1 gm.), but these estimates are usually too high since some of the original crater is generally occupied by indentations of variable size.

In the present study the above procedures were followed excepting that in order to provide samples for histopathologic study it was necessary to cut these out of the specimen (usually from its center) before fixation. Comparison between the weights of tissue actually removed and weights estimated to have been removed (computed on the basis of measurement of the operative crater, as shown in table 9, chapter 4) indicates that spurious upgrading of the weight of the specimens and inaccuracies of volume, as determined by measurement, were negligible factors of error as contrasted with that produced by post-excisional manipulation of the operative site.

TABLE 11.   PERCENTILE RATIO OF MASS OF SPECIMENS ACTUALLY REMOVED TO TOTAL AMOUNT OF TISSUE ESTIMATED (BY MEASUREMENT OF THE OPERATIVE CRATER) TO HAVE BEEN REMOVED

| Case No. | Left | Right | Case No. | Left | Right |
|---|---|---|---|---|---|
| 2 | 62 | 88 | 24 | 59 * | 59 * |
| 4 | 54 * | 45 * | 25 | 54 * | 81 |
| 6 | 70 | 146 | 27 | 67 * | 59 * |
| 7 | 85 | 59 * | 31 | 65 * | 82 |
| 8 | 46 * | 67 | 32 | 97 | 100 |
| 13 | 89 | 85 | 33 | 42 * | 46 * |
| 18 | 42 * | 31 * | 36 | 65 * | 79 * |
| 19 | 24 * | 42 | 42 | 39 * | 34 * |
| 21 | 51 * | 56 | 44 | 44 | 36 |
| 22 | 94 | 79 * | 47 | 37 * | not determined |
|  |  |  | 49 | 53 * | 48 * |

* Specimens marked with an asterisk indicate discrepancies of more than 5 Gm. See also Table 9.

**Estimate of the Factor of Correspondence between Specimen Removed and Nonfunctional Area of Brain.**   As indicated in the preceding paragraph, the specimens removed rarely corresponded to the full extent of the operative crater. The approximate discrepancy (that is, making no allowance for upgrading of weight or inaccuracy of measurement) in the cases for which both weights and measurements are available is given in table 11.

It is obvious that at least one (6R) of these relationships is impossible and the ratios indicated in table 11 can only be regarded as approximations. What we are interested in, however, is information pointing to notable involvement of areas which we cannot expect to find in the specimens at hand. Examination of the ratios given in table 11 may be very deceptive in this respect. Where the specimen removed was very small, as in case 19 (1.8 gm.), it is apparent that the removal of an additional 5 or 6 gm. of tissue could easily have resulted from very minor cleaning up of the crater and could scarcely have notably extended the excision to other areas. If we discount extensions of the original ablation by 5 gm. or less we are left with 16 cases (those marked with an asterisk in table 11) in which appreciable discrepancy between the specimen and total ablated tissue may have existed.

Such a discrepancy need not indicate that the surgical excision exceeded the area intended for removal. Thus, in case 18 where it was intended to remove area 11, it was considered advisable, because of poor visibility, to remove *en bloc* only its rostral half, the remainder of the excision being completed by suction. If the specimen at our disposal includes nothing but area 11 (as happens to be the case) there would be no reason to suppose that the ablation exceeded its intended limits. For the completion of this analysis of the possibilities of excessive removals, as a result of postexcision clearing of the crater, the reader is referred to the description of the histologic specimens of individual cases.

The present writer has previously pointed out (Mettler, '44, p. 107) that there are still other reasons why the examination of a specimen removed at operation fails to give one an adequate conception of the total cortical area which may ultimately become nonfunctional. Examination of the specimen may show that the surface exhibits acute changes due either to undue exposure, the use of saline which was not isotonic or too warm, or to undue cautery play. The presence of such artefacts in the specimen should lead one to suspect their existence in cortex which was not removed. Some artefacts of such a nature were found in the following cases: 2R, 4RL, 7L, 8RL, 13RL, 18RL, 22RL, 25R, 31R, and 42R. It is apparent, in instances such as these, that evidence of acute pathologic or chemical changes must be disregarded unless these appear in cortex in the depths of the sulci.

Examination of the operative records and preoperative photographs of the operative sites disclosed instances in which neighboring vasculature might have been bilaterally interfered with in the following cases: 2 (to interfere with area 9), 3 (10), 4 (9, 10), 6 (9), 7 (46), 8 (9, 45), 31 (46), 32 (10), 33 (9, 45, 46 and walls of fossa lateralis), 49 (46).

Such interference might have been expected to result in an unusual leucocytic response. Possible leucocytic responses of this nature were observed in cases 6, 18, and 49.

**Summary.** Histologic examination cannot be expected to disclose the maximum extent of nonfunctional cortex. Whether it is of any use in telling whether particular parts of cortex were certainly removed we shall now make inquiry.

### Selection of Cytoarchitectonic Plan

Systematic studies upon the cytoarchitecture of the human frontal lobe as a whole are not numerous. Named in chronologic order, maps have been prepared by A. W. Campbell ('05) (see our fig. 54), C. and O. Vogt ('19), K. Brodmann ('25), C. v. Economo and G. N. Koskinas ('25), Cristoforo Jacob ('41), and Von Bonin ('44).

Most studies so far brought forward are complicated by at least one or two features disturbing to the investigator who seeks to identify the character of a *piece* of cortex taken from an otherwise intact brain. It is one thing to subdivide a given hemisphere into cubes and then decide if the histologic character of these differs. Under such circumstances the investigator knows when he begins, that his cubes come from necessarily different loci. It is quite another problem to sit down to specimens which all come from different hemispheres and which may or may not involve comparable loci. In the latter case the finding of transitional characteristics is of no great value. One can concern oneself only with notable similarity and definite difference.

Another common difficulty in identification of unknown samples is the tendency of previous investigators to cut their specimens from different loci

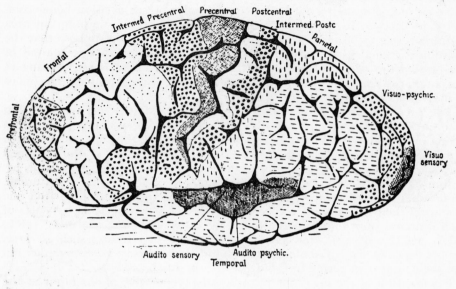

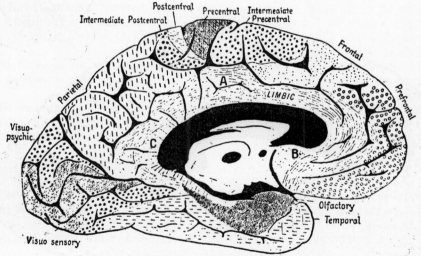

FIG. 54. Campbell's cytoarchitectural schemata.

in different planes. Here again it is one thing to examine selected sections all cut at right angles to the axis of a gyrus, but the person who sets out to determine what areas are or are not included in a given piece of tissue is obliged to cut the whole of it and if he is to do this without losing significant material he must cut the block *seriatim* and *in toto*. For this purpose he must choose a constant plane of reference and adhere to that plane in all his studies. In their recent atlas of "The Neocortex of Macaca Mulatta," Von

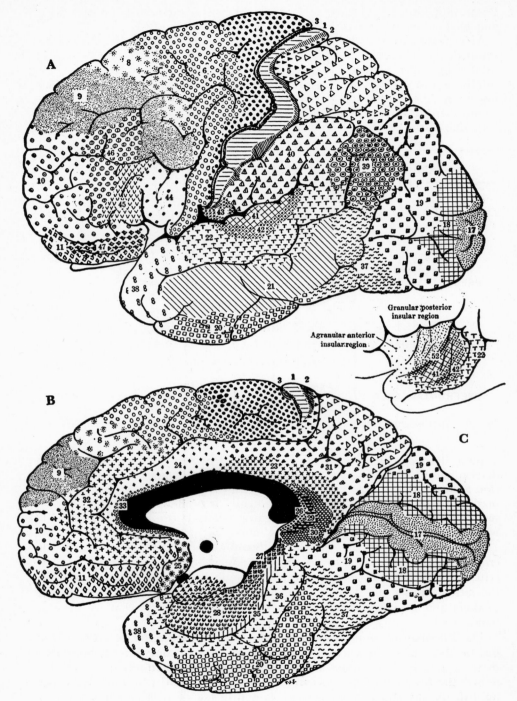

FIG. 55. Cytoarchitectural map of the human cortex according to Brodmann. *A*, lateral side; *B*, medial side; *C*, insular region.

Bonin and Bailey ('47) have very wisely taken this factor into consideration and have adhered to constant planes for each brain studied.

As a possible alternative to using one or another of the maps already developed, the suggestion has been advanced that one might employ a plan of subdivision of the cortex based upon the well-known cortical sectors (i.e. subdivision of the cortex upon the basis of the different thalamic nuclei playing upon different cortical parts), but the areas of cortex which receive projections from distinctly different thalamic masses are so large (Mettler, '47), that little which is discriminative can be obtained by the use of such

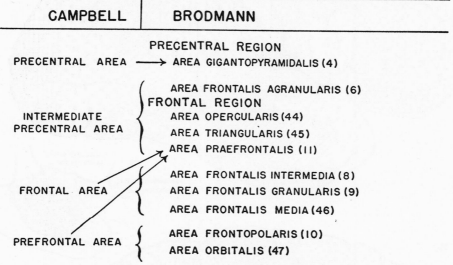

FIG. 56. Approximate equivalence between cytoarchitectural schemata of Campbell and Brodmann.

a plan. Besides, such an approach merely transfers the problems of the determination of function to a still more inaccessible locus, yields information about only one aspect of cortical function (its afferent systems), provides no data about the significance of variations in cortical structure within known sectors, and finally leaves the investigator without any means of knowing where he is when he works with cortex only.

One comes then to the necessity either of following as best he may the criteria established by one or another preceding author or of developing new criteria for himself. Since Bailey and Von Bonin have already embarked upon the latter venture the development of more satisfactory criteria may be left to them and we may presently see what can be done with what we have at hand.

The cytoarchitectonic plan one employs for identification of cortex need not be the same as is selected for operative protocol but it is obvious that there is a certain advantage in using the same scheme throughout. In this respect the Brodmann map possesses some virtue. Although Brodmann did not publish the descriptive matter to explain fully, or even clearly, his map for the human (some photomicrographs appear in his publication of 1908) it is one to which the criteria of Campbell or of Economo and Koskinas can easily

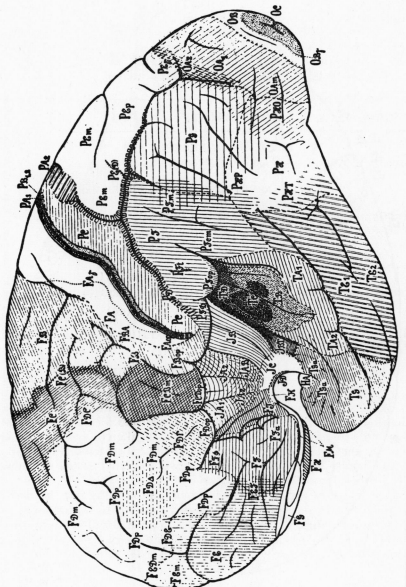

Fig. 57. Cytoarchitectural schema of Economo and Koskinas. Lateral surface.

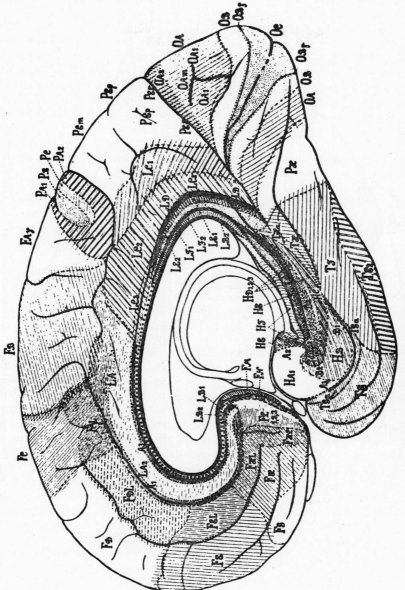

FIG. 58. Cytoarchitectural schema of Economo and Koskinas. Medial surface.

be applied as examination of figures 54 through 59 will show. These may be employed by anyone seeking to convert the data given in the present monograph to either the nomenclature of Campbell or that of Economo and Koskinas.

The characteristics described by Campbell for his areas are generally, if one makes allowance for the differences engendered by his use of a nomenclature for seven layers instead of six, the same as those given by Economo and Koskinas for comparable areas. It does not take long, however, to discover that while Campbell's areas are distinct from one another they are not homogeneous. When confronted with an unknown section from the frontal cortex it is a useful policy to determine first to which of the Campbell areas it belongs and then to search for further differentiating characteristics.

TABLE 12.   CAMPBELL'S CRITERIA FOR DISTINGUISHING BETWEEN PRINCIPAL
DIVISIONS OF FRONTAL CORTEX
(Terminology converted to Brodmann numbers and six-layer usage)

|  | 4 | 6, 44, 45 | 8, 9, 46 | 10, 47 |
|---|---|---|---|---|
| I | deep | ——— | ——— | ——— |
| II | poor | poor | notable | notable |
| III | large pyramids | large pyramids | small pyramids | very small pyramids |
| IV | indistinct | indistinct | distinct | cells small |
| V | Betz cells | moderate sized cells | small cells | very small cells |
| VI | ——— | ——— | ——— | ——— |

The criteria given in table 12 for distinguishing between the Campbell divisions are those of Campbell himself (terminology converted to Brodmann numbers and six-layer usage) and indicate that as one proceeds rostrally the development of the granular layers becomes more, and that of the pyramidal and ganglionic layers less, pronounced. In essence, Campbell has distinguished four degrees of such alteration as indicated above.

Certain it is that distinction between the agranular Brodmann areas, notably 4 (Economo and Koskinas' FA gamma) and 6 (Economo and Koskinas' FB) is accomplished with reasonable ease but there is no occasion to place with area 6 the opercular and triangular parts of the inferior frontal gyrus, that is Brodmann's 44 (Economo and Koskinas' FCB m) and 45 (Economo and Koskinas' FD gamma). Areas 44 and 45 have distinct granular characters which set them off from area 6, and there is, especially in 45, an interesting balance between the development of the granular layers on the one hand and the pyramidal and ganglionic on the other. Thus 45 has fairly large cells in the third and fifth layers as well as distinct granular development. If development of a cytoarchitectonic map were the writer's present concern I would be inclined to employ a different pattern for the intermediate third of the frontal lobe than that used by Campbell. Instead of lumping areas 6, 44, and 45 together in one category and 8, 9, and 46 in another it would seem more natural to consider area 6 as a distinct region, to place 44 with 8, and 45 and 46 with 9. This would introduce a certain additional amount of heterogeneity in 9, but Brodmann's 9 is the least homogeneous of his areas anyway.

The study of Economo and Koskinas has not been popular with investi-

gators of human material and this is not surprising since it is not easily available for use beside the microscope and not a little leisure is needed to
familiarize oneself with it. Economo and Koskinas carried the subdivision of
the cortex through simple qualitative differences into the realm of quantitative measurement. One must be prepared to sit down with photomicrographs
of one's own material, made at a constant factor of enlargement, and examine
them with calipers, crosslines, and counter before one can say that Economo
and Koskinas overextended their data. When this is done not only can most
of the Economo and Koskinas subdivisions be verified but additional nuances

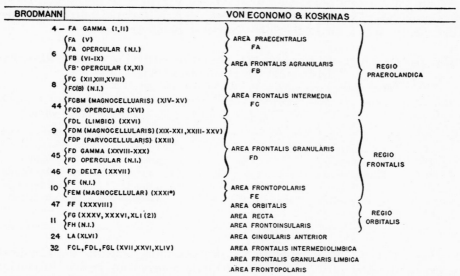

FIG. 59. Approximate equivalence between cytoarchitectural schemata of Brodmann and
of Economo and Koskinas. (Roman numerals refer to plates in Economo and Koskinas' Atlas.
N.I., not illustrated. *There is a discrepancy in the atlas figure and key diagram with
regard to this designation.)

of difference are likely to suggest themselves until one begins to take into
account the factors of individual variation. We may ask ourselves, moreover,
how useful such a laborious procedure is likely to be. Although the entire
atlas of Economo and Koskinas was reproduced for use in the present research
(these negatives are available in our laboratory for anyone who wishes to
make reproductions for his own use of one or another part of the difficultly
accessible atlas) and our own specimens photomicrographed for measured
comparison, it was felt, in the face of the variables already mentioned, that
it would contribute nothing to the ultimate utility of the data to reproduce
or describe this material here and we have restricted present textual description and determination to differences which were apparent upon inspection
without the use of measurement or counting. Since the tabulation (given in
figure 59) of equivalence between the areas of Brodmann and those of Economo and Koskinas includes the numbers of the illustrative plates in the
atlas of Economo and Koskinas and since this is our point of reference neither
has it been felt necessary to reproduce illustrative sections here.

In our present study we have accordingly employed the Brodmann map not only for surgical protocol but also in connection with the study of the histologic characteristics of the tissue removed. The histologic criteria used in identifying the Brodmann areas are those of Economo and Koskinas after appropriate conversion to the Brodmann plan.

Attention should be directed to another possible advantage of the Brodmann plan. None of the maps available for the human cortex provide us with a satisfactory anatomic substrate for function; too little of real value is known about the functions of this region. The only methods which have yielded suggestive information about the basic functions of subsidiary parts of the frontal cortex are those of ablation and stimulation (I have recently reviewed [Mettler, '48] the data so obtained) as carried out on experimental animals. Since the Brodmann plan has been a favorite among experimentalists, a fair degree of functional correlation has been worked out for that plan for the monkey. Measured by human standards, however, simian behavior is simple and stereotyped and transference to the human is not an easy matter. Moreover, one would not be justified in transferring, without further investigation, even these correlations to the Brodmann map for the human for there is no proved correspondence between areas bearing identical numbers in the Brodmann maps for the simian and human brains. Should we find physiologic evidence for some kind of equivalence we shall have opened the way for the clinical application of knowledge from the laboratory and provided a new significance for further experimental work. The trial of the Brodmann terminology and cytoarchitectonic plan in the present instance is, therefore, distinctly worth attempting and in no way interferes with the interpretation, in the light of any other of the cytoarchitectonic plans, of the data obtained.

### CRITERIA EMPLOYED FOR DISTINGUISHING THE BRODMANN AREAS

#### DORSOLATERAL AND DORSOMEDIAL CORTEX

**Area 4.** Because of its agranular nature and the presence of gigantopyramids in its ganglionic layer, cortex from this region is perhaps the easiest of the frontal areas to distinguish. Other than this it is the deepest of the frontal cortices. The external and internal granular layers are either absent or so poor in cells as to be difficult to distinguish (depending upon the thickness of the sections studied). Its outer layers are richer in cells than the inner and lack radial striation which may not extend beyond the polymorphic layer. Vertical division or layering is not very distinct and the ganglionic layer is not split.

**Area 6.** If one restricts area 4 to the description given in the preceding paragraph and insists on the presence of a distinct, continuous phalanx of gigantopyramids for its definition, there is no trouble about distinguishing between areas 6 and 4, even though the remaining characteristics of the two areas are much the same. Where the pyramids of the fifth layer of area 4 are small it is helpful to recall that radial striation is reasonably distinct in the caudal half of area 6. Distinction between area 6 and the Brodmann areas which impinge upon it rostrally is more difficult. Area 9, which is distinctly granular as described below, is probably the easiest to differentiate. Area 44 which is also somewhat granular, but usually designated as intermediate pyramidal in type, is somewhat more difficult to make out (see p. 62). The caudal part of area 8 may be very hard to distinguish from the rostral part of 6.

**Area 8.** This region is generally described as transitional between 9 and 6. This gives one the idea that it either maintains a constant appearance, intermediary between 6 and 9, or that its appearance gradually changes from the one type to the other. In my own experience neither statement is quite correct and I am inclined to look upon it as much closer to 6 in appearance than to 9. This also seems to be Von Bonin and Bailey's conclusion with regard to their simian area 8. (This is an interesting point for the location of Brodmann's simian area 8 does not appear to correspond at all to that of his area 8 for the human brain whereas that chosen by Von Bonin and Bailey does.) Although the appearance of 8 does change somewhat, as one progresses either forward or backward in a horizontal direction, the alteration upon passing into area 9 is much more abrupt than upon passing into 6. Indeed, the present writer would be at a total loss to fix upon characteristics which distinguish absolutely cortex from area 8 from that of area 6 if the cortex selected were taken from the region of transition between the two.

Area 8 is said to possess an underdeveloped granular layer and while this is true for its rostral part it should be emphasized that this granular characteristic is very difficult to distinguish caudally. All specimens I have seen from this caudal region have lacked the heavy concentration of cells in the external granular layer which one sees in area 9 and also its decided horizontal stratification. Area 8 is said to display less distinct radial striation than area 6. Though it is said that such radial striation can often be detected as far peripherally in area 6 as the external granular layer, this has not been my experience with regard to its most rostral part. Area 8 gives the impression of having somewhat smaller cells than 6, an impression which can be verified by measurement but which is often worthless during simple inspection. The separation of the cortex of area 8 from the underlying medullary substance is said to be less distinct than one sees in area 6, but this again is a valueless characteristic in junctional regions. For practical purposes then, area 8 is not hard to distinguish from 9, but it is very difficult to delimit from 6. Unless one can see what the histologic character of the cortex lying before or behind a given specimen is, it would be hard indeed to tell whether a bit of tissue from the back of 8 or front of 6 came from area 6 or area 8. It is worth emphasizing that the granular layers become progressively more pronounced as one proceeds rostroventrally, being most notable in the region of the olfactory bulbs.

**Area 9.** This area is very distinctly granular. The cells in the external granular layer are relatively abundant and it is distinctly laminated. While the area is not uniform in appearance throughout, these characteristics are preserved. As indicated above it can be distinguished from area 8 without too much difficulty. Its pyramidal layer is relatively narrow and in some loci contains large pyramids (in some parts of area 9 the pyramidal cells of the ganglionic and polymorphic layers are relatively smaller than those lying in layers more externally placed). Elsewhere the cells of the pyramidal layer may not be notable for size. With regard to distinguishing between it and neighboring areas, notably 10, 44, 45, and 46, the ensuing descriptions of these areas should be consulted. The most ventrocaudal part of area 9 (the ventral half of the caudal part of the middle frontal gyrus) is the so-called "area of agraphia" of Henschen-Broca.

**Area 10.** Area 10 resembles area 9 in general appearance but its cells are distinctly smaller. This is particularly true with regard to the pyramidal layer

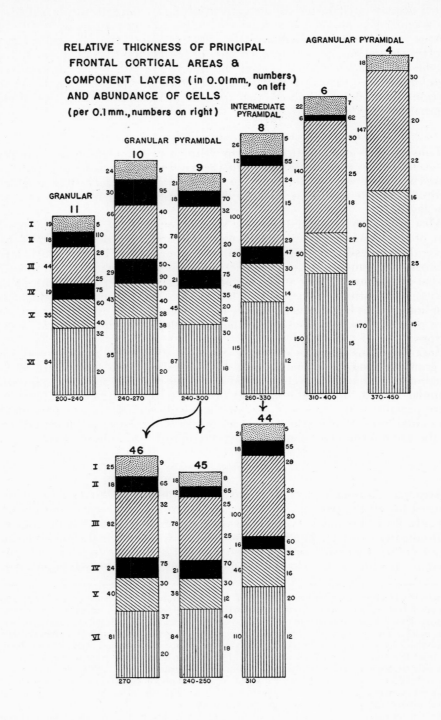

RELATIVE THICKNESS OF PRINCIPAL
FRONTAL CORTICAL AREAS &
COMPONENT LAYERS (in 0.01mm., numbers on left)
AND ABUNDANCE OF CELLS
(per 0.1mm., numbers on right)

which displays a characteristic atrophic appearance. Area 10 displays distinct horizontal layers and shows a degree of radial arrangement as well.

**Area 11.** Like 10 this region is distinctly granular. Its cells are small. It displays clearer horizontal laminae than 10. It is radially striated. As in area 10, the pyramidal layer is poor but the internal granular layer is relatively more pronounced than in area 10. The ganglionic and polymorphic layers are horizontally subdivided into cell-rich and cell-poor parts, in their external and internal halves respectively.

### MEDIAL CORTEX

Thus far it is obvious that one can distinguish with reasonable certainty between areas 4, 6, 8, 9, and 10, with the exception that a definite junction between areas 6 and 8 cannot be established with certainty. The cingulate cortex is characteristic in appearance. One notable feature is its lack of granular layers.

**Area 24.** Both granular layers are absent from area 24 though the upper part of the pyramidal layer is condensed and upon casual examination may create the impression of being an external granular layer. The molecular layer is broad, the ganglionic layer distinct and contains characteristic rod cells. Radial arrangment is poor at the summit of the gyrus and in the depth of the sulcus. It is distinct in the walls. The division between the pyramidal and ganglionic layers is indistinct. Area 24 is considered by many writers to be the most potent of the "suppressor" (in the "physiological neuronographic" sense) regions.

**Area 32.** This region is distinctly granular. Except for the narrowness of its granular layers it resembles area 9. The cells of the lower part of the ganglionic layer are relatively few and small but to either side of the internal granular layer a considerable number of large cells are to be seen. These are more prominent in the upper part of the ganglionic than lower part of the pyramidal layer. Von Bonin ('44, p. 80) thinks that area 32 is connected with all the physiologic neuronographically determined "suppressor" areas.

### VENTROLATERAL CORTEX

**Area 44.** Although it is far from clear that the term "Broca's area" should be used for all the pars opercularis of the inferior frontal gyrus and nothing but this, Economo and Koskinas so characterize the pars, which is the location of Brodmann's area 44. The facts are as follows: In his original communication Broca (1861) attempted only a very general localization (second and third frontal convolution) for motor aphasia. By 1896 Broca had overextended his

---

FIG. 60. Diagram of relative thickness of principal frontal cortical areas and their component layers (given in 0.01 mm., numbers to left of each block) computed at summit of gyri, and average number of cells per 0.1 mm. of each layer (numbers along right of each block). The appearance of several numbers by any given block indicates that the layer is subdivided and that its subdivisions contain the number of cells indicated. (These figures are from Economo and Koskinas and cannot be used for tissue from living humans.)

It will be observed that the transition from area 4 through 11 is in the direction of progressively thinner cortex and greater granular development. Areas 44 to 46 are profitably regarded as ventral parallels of this plan beginning with 44 which has much in common with 8 and progressing through 45 and 46 which resemble 9.

With regard to areas 44, 45, and 46 it will be observed that in the last the pyramidal layer is undivided, in area 45 it is double, and in 44 it is triple.

data (Broca and Maubrac, 1896) and indicated the caudal half of the pars opercularis (i.e. the caudal half of area 44) as the area which, when damaged, is provocative of motor aphasia.

The validity of Broca's ultimate dictum has, of course, frequently been questioned. Pierre Marie ('06), who felt that motor aphasia is invariably the result of the combination of anarthria with sensory aphasia, brought forward such devastating data against Broca's dictum that it is difficult to see how it survived. Bolton ('11) offered an interesting explanation for the failure of Broca's dictum to stand up under examination. Bolton postulated that a lesion in Broca's area (in the restricted sense) might or might not result in motor aphasia depending upon individual variation in the location and extent of the "educated psychomotor area." In recent years Broca's teaching has enjoyed a variable degree of acceptance with no outspoken active resistance. Surgeons have in general been unwilling to take the risk of encroaching upon the pars opercularis (Penfield and Rasmussen, '47) and it is still unclear whether the occurrence of aphasia, when lesions are found in this area, is due to cortical or subcortical damage (Mettler, '48a).

Area 44, like the transitional region between areas 6 and 8, shows only rudimentary granular characteristics and closely resembles such transitional cortex in other respects but differs from it by the presence of very large pyramidal cells in the lower part of the pyramidal layer. Von Bonin ('44, see p. 51 *et seq.*) has given a very circumstantial recent description of this region.

**Area 45.** Although distinctly granular, the horizontal demarcations of area 45 are less evident than in area 9. Area 45 exhibits large cells in the pyramidal layer and distinct radial striation. It is advisable to compare sections suspected to be from this region with known sections, from areas 9, 44, and 46. The large pyramids of the pyramidal layer of area 45 are not so close to the internal granular layer and do not form such a definite band as in area 44.

**Area 46.** This region has the same general character as area 9 but is not so distinctly laminated horizontally. Its molecular layer is said to be unusually broad but this may not be obvious. When seen it is a useful distinguishing characteristic. The external granular layer is somewhat poorer in cells than that in area 9. The pyramidal layer is relatively broader. In contrast to areas 9 and 45 the cells of this layer are smaller. The internal granular layer is unusually broad. The region is not sharply differentiated from its neighbors. In area 46 the cells in the pyramidal layer are much smaller than in some parts of area 9 and the cells in the granular layer relatively larger. In order to be certain that one is examining such material it is advisable to compare it with known cortex from area 9 and area 45.

**Area 47.** The present writer has not been able to distinguish, histologically, cortex taken from the location of Brodmann's area 47 from other specimens taken from the location of his area 10. Hans Kreht ('36), who has described a number of subsidiary fields in the inferior frontal gyrus, is evidently not of this opinion and some subsequent German writers have followed his plan, but my own feeling is that area 47 should probably be dropped from future maps of the region.

## RESULTS

For the convenience of the reader I reproduce herewith two charts (figs. 60, 61) that I have found useful in the practical identification of the material about to be described. It should be emphasized that these charts represent no

| Characteristic | 4 | 6 | 8 | 9 | 10 | 11 | 44 | 45 | 46 | 47 | 24 | 32 |
|---|---|---|---|---|---|---|---|---|---|---|---|---|
| Radial striation | | Notable | | | Notable | Distinct | Definite, narrow | Definite, narrow | | | Notable | |
| Type | Heterotypical | Heterotypical | Homotypical | Homotypical | Homotypical | Homotypical | Homotypical | Homotypical | | | Heterotyp. | Homotyp. |
| Cell prominence in layer III | ++++ | ++++ (Large pyramids) | ++ | +++ | | + | ++++ (Large pyramids) | ++++ | + | + | + | ++ |
| Cell prominence in layer V | ++++ (Giganto-pyramids) | ++++ | | +++ | | + | ++ | ++ | | | + | |
| Splitting of V | None. | | Double | Triple | | | Double | | None | Triple | Double | Double |
| Types — Agranular, pyramids | + | + | | | | | | | | | | |
| Types — Intermediate pyramids | | | + | | | | + | | | | | |
| Types — Granular, pyramids | | | | + | + | | | + | + | + | + (Special cells) | + |
| Types — Granular | | | | | | + | | | | | | |
| Granular pyr. modification — Relatively narrow III and large pyramids | | | | +* | | | | | | | | |
| Granular pyr. modification — Broad III and small pyramids | | | | | | | | | + | | | |
| Granular pyr. modification — Very narrow III and large pyramids | | | | | | | | + | | | | |

*True of only some parts of area 9, elsewhere pyramids are small

FIG. 61. Tabulation of distinguishing characteristics of frontal cortex, other than those shown in figure 60.

original findings and were, in the first instance, compiled from Economo and Koskinas' data. As in the previous descriptions I have seen fit to emphasize what I thought helpful and to drop what I considered confusing or useless.

Case 2.   Protocol: Area 8.   *Summary:* Asymmetrical removal of area 8 with infringement upon the right area 9 and bilateral infringement upon area 6.

*Operation.*   On May 28, 1947, both frontal lobes were exposed. On the left, a triangular piece of tissue weighing 5.8 gm. was removed at 10:52 a.m. and all samples were fixed by 10:58. On the right, a roughly quadrilateral block weighing 7.1 gm. was ablated at 11:45 a.m. and all samples were fixed by 11:52. So far as could be determined by comparison with the Brodmann map and measurement, the operative sites, after subsequent cleaning, were as follows:

Left: Area 8 and rostral part of 6. Ventrorostral edge, 4.5 cm.; caudal, 3 cm.; medial, 3.3 cm.; depth, 1.9 cm. Medial cortex removed to depth of 1.8 cm.

Right: Area 8. Ventrorostral edge, 4.7 cm.; caudal, 4.2 cm.; medial, 1.8 cm.; depth, 1.9 cm. Medial cortex removed to depth of 1.9 cm.

*Tentative Summary.*   The operative sites were grossly unsymmetrical, that on the left being almost twice as long, along the medial margin of the hemisphere (presumably at the expense of area 6), and not extending so far ventrally (presumably sparing the ventral part of area 8).

*Histologic Study.*   The cortex of the left specimen was fairly uniform in thickness throughout, as was its structure. It lacked the characteristic appearance of granular cortex and the decision required to be made was whether it was characteristic of area 8 or 6 (i.e. Economo and Koskinas' area frontalis intermedia or agranularis). The specimen at hand lacked the heavy concentration of cells in the external granular layer which one often finds in cortex taken from area 9 and also its more or less decided horizontal stratification, so that there is little reason to suppose that the specimen contained any area 9 cortex. Caudal sections might be from either area 8 or 6 as far as the present observer can determine. Sections from the rostral and caudal parts of the right specimen were markedly dissimilar. Those from the rostral edge of the right specimen were distinctly granular in character and there was evident encroachment upon area 9. The caudal sections looked like those from the left side.

*Summary.*   Area 8 and a variable amount of area 6 were removed bilaterally. Area 9 had been infringed upon on the right side. Area 6, if involved, was less damaged on the left than right.

*Reoperation.*   On October 29, 1947, the right cerebral scar was exposed and removed. The ventrorostral edge of the old scar measured 4 cm. (as against 4.7 cm. originally), the caudal edge measured 3 cm. (as against 4.2), and the medial edge of the hemisphere was discontinuous for a distance of 2.6 cm. (as against 1.8). It was 1.4 cm. deep (as against 1.9). The scar was now excised *en bloc* (the block weighed 17 gm.) at 11:23 a.m. through apparently sound cortex and all specimens were fixed by 11:32 a.m.

*Histologic Study of Operative Site.*   None of the now removed and supposedly sound cortex was normal. As one passed from definite scar tissue centrifugally several zones of disorganization were apparent. The first of these (about 5 mm. wide) was marked by disintegration of all layers except the sixth which was represented by some degenerated neurocytes and much gliosis. In the next zone (about 8 mm. wide) the outermost two layers were entirely acellular and vacuolated and the upper half of the pyramidal layer was also so affected. The remainder of the pyramidal layer contained some pyknotic disorganized neurocytes but the lower three layers were relatively normal in appearance except for a very slight amount of gliosis. The third zone (about 1 cm. wide) was characterized by a loss of cells in, and vacuolation of, the upper part of the pyramidal layer without notable disturbance either above or below this. Presumably zone 3 corresponds to retrograde degeneration of cells giving rise to short association fibers and the other two zones to damage of the supracortical capillary net. The specimen included cortex of the intermediate pyramidal type which had large pyramids in the third layer and presumably came from area 44.

**Case 3. Protocol:** Area 9. *Summary:* Removal of caudal part of 9 with invasion of area 6.

*Operation.* On May 15, 1947, both frontal lobes were exposed. On the right, an angular piece of tissue weighing 6.4 gm. was removed and on the left, a quadrilateral piece weighing 6.3 gm. was ablated.

*Tentative Summary.* So far as could be determined by comparison with the Brodmann map the operative sites were, on the right, most of area 9 and, on the left, only the part of area 9 in the superior frontal gyrus.

*Histologic Study.* The specimen presented a uniform histologic appearance in its rostral two-thirds. Caudal to this, its ventral edge developed a somewhat differently stratified structure. All sections were definitely granular in nature. The question raised by this specimen is whether it lies in area 9 or 10. The arrangement of cells in its rostral part coincides closely with the arrangement of Economo and Koskinas' area frontalis granularis. The caudal sections, however, contained not a few large pyramids in the lower part of the ganglionic layer suggesting that the ventrocaudal limit of the ablation may have impinged upon area 4. Forward projection of area 4 toward the middle frontal sulcus is known to occur as an individual variation in the macaque (Nañagas, '23) and perhaps the same circumstances occur in the human being. The cells in question in the present case did not, however, measure up to the full dimension of Betz cells and, since areas 9 and 6 (particularly the latter) often contain large cells in the ganglionic layer, their presence does not necessarily indicate transgression beyond area 6. Sections through the rostral part of the right specimen presented the appearance of area 9. Those through its caudal part were not so distinctly granular, suggesting infringement upon area 6.

*Summary.* The caudalmost part of area 9 appears to have been removed bilaterally. On the left, the ablation was apparently carried far enough caudally to pass into area 6. It may impinge upon area 4. On the right, the ablation did not go so far caudally but the specimens are consistent with the opinion that area 6 was invaded.

**Case 4. Protocol:** Area 46. *Summary:* Area 46 with infringement on left areas 9 and 45 and right area 10.

*Operation.* On May 19, 1947, both frontal lobes were exposed. On the left, a triangular piece of tissue weighing 5.8 gm. was removed at 11:25 a.m. and all samples were fixed by 11:35. On the right, a roughly square piece of tissue weighing 4.8 gm. was removed at 12:15. It is possible that this piece was rotated during transfer from the head so that its orientation may have been disturbed. The operative sites, after subsequent cleaning, so far as could be determined by comparison with the Brodmann map and measurement were as follows:

Left: Area 46. Rostral edge, 2.8 cm.; dorsal edge, 2.9 cm.; caudoventral edge, 3.9 cm.; ventral edge, 1 cm. Ablation, 1.9 cm. deep.

Right: Dorsal two-thirds of area 46. Rostral edge, 2.3 cm.; dorsal edge, 2.9 cm.; caudoventral, 2.1 cm.; ventral edge, 1 cm. Ablation, 1.6 cm. deep.

*Tentative Summary.* The ablation corresponded fairly closely to area 46.

*Histologic Study.* Sections from the rostral part of the left specimen had the character of area 9. As one progressed caudally the appearance rapidly changed to cortex characterized by a broad molecular layer and cell-poor external granular layer. The character of area 46 was maintained through the remainder of the specimen, though its caudal part exhibited a few large pyramids, characteristic of area 45. The right specimen began with cortex which seemed transitional between 10 and 46. One soon passed into cortex resembling area 46.

*Summary.* The specimen contained cortex of area 46 bilaterally. On the left, areas 9 and 45 were infringed upon and on the right area 10 may have been. Since the cortical crater was estimated to have been capable of holding about twice the mass of cortex as appeared in the specimen, one would assume that this presumptive extension was in the direction of areas 9 and 45 on the left and 10 on the right.

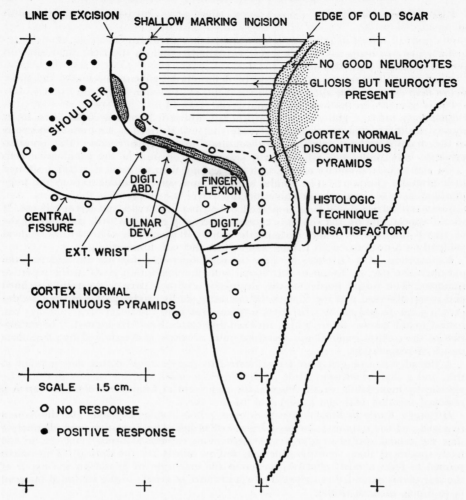

FIG. 62. Operative site of right hemisphere in case 6 at time of reoperation. Rostral to the right, caudal to the left. This figure shows the histologic condition of the cortex excised at the time of reoperation and also illustrates the responses obtained by electrical stimulation at that time. The shallow marking incision, within the excised block, was made just in front of the rostral border of excitable cortex. The zones of cell absence (stippled), gliosis in the presence of good cells (horizontals), normal cortex with discontinuous pyramids (white), and region of continuous pyramids (heavy shading) within the block excised at reoperation are indicated. The crosses mark distances of 1.5 cm.

Case 6.   Protocol: Areas 6 and 8.   *Summary:* Subtotal removal of areas 6 and 8.
   *Operation.*   On May 27, 1947, both frontal lobes were exposed. On the left, a triangular piece of tissue weighing 9.6 gm. was removed at 7:06 p.m. and all samples were fixed by 7:12. On the right, a roughly curved piece of tissue weighing 16.3 gm. was removed at 8:47 and all samples were fixed at 8:56. The operative sites, after subsequent cleaning, so far as could be determined by comparison with the Brodmann map and measurement, were as follows:
   Left: Dorsorostral part of area 6 and most of area 8 removed. Rostroventral edge, 5 cm.; caudal edge, 5 cm.; medial edge, 4 cm.; depth along medial side of hemisphere, 1.5 cm. The ventral third of area 6 and its caudal half were therefore missed.

Right: Rostroventral edge, 8 cm.; caudal edge, 7 cm.; medial edge, 3 cm.; depth along medial surface, 2.5 cm. The dorsocaudal part of area 6 was missed and the caudal part of area 9 in the middle frontal gyrus was evidently infringed upon.

*Tentative Summary.* The ablation was more complete on the right than left. On both sides area 8 was removed and some of area 6 was missed. On the left, the ventral third of area 6 was missed as well as part of the caudal edge of 6. On the right, the dorsocaudal part of 6 escaped ablation.

*Histologic Study.* Sections from the rostral part of the left specimen showed a rudimentary internal granular layer which was absent in caudal sections. The latter showed distinct radial striation. The former did not. Horizontal lamination was poor in the caudal sections, the pyramidal cells rather distinct in the general undistinguished cytologic background but no gigantopyramids were obvious in the ganglionic layer.

On the right the situation was the same except that the rostral sections showed little granular character except in the external layer. In the caudal sections the polymorphic layer was more distinct than on the left.

*Summary.* Areas 8 and 6 were represented in both the right and left specimens. It would appear that on the left the removal closely corresponded with the rostral part of area 8 but that on the right it fell somewhat short of this. The area 6 removal evidently was not carried far enough caudally to encroach upon area 4.

*Reoperation.* On October 27, 1947, the right operative scar was exposed and the old operative site was found to correspond with the description given in the tentative summary. The rostral border of the electrically excitable area was carefully defined and it was observed that the edge of the operative scar lay 2 cm. rostral to the shoulder area, 1.5 cm. rostral to the wrist area, 0.75 cm. rostral to the finger area, and 0.75 cm. rostral to the central fissure where no excitable cortex could be located. The estimation of the cortical removal was therefore quite accurate as determined by physiologic means at reoperation.

A thread was arranged 3 to 4 mm. rostral to the excitable cortex and parallel to this, and a shallow incision made in the cortex to mark the line of this thread. The electrically inexcitable cortex between the right central fissure and old scar was now removed together with the caudal part of the scar.

*Histologic Study of Second Area Removed.* The histologic character of the cortex removed and the responses obtained are shown in figure 62. It is interesting to observe that the caudal spread of gliosis was much more extensive dorsally (1.5 cm. in the fresh specimen) than ventrally where a shallow sulcus lay (no spread). This sulcus seemed to form a fairly effective barrier to the extension of gliosis. In the depth of the scar gliosis extended centripetally for a distance of 4 mm. in the sectioned material (5 to 6 mm. of fresh tissue).

**Case 7. Protocol:** Areas 8, 9, 10. *Summary:* Area 8 removal, subtotal removal of areas 9 and 10 and possible encroachment upon area 46.

*Operation.* On May 22, 1947, both frontal lobes were exposed and a semilunar piece of tissue weighing 17 gm. was removed from the left side of the brain at 11:42 a.m. All samples of tissue were fixed by 11:47. An additional piece weighing 8.5 gm. was delivered from the surgery while the first was being weighed. On the **right**, a piece of tissue having the shape of an inverted U and weighing 20 gm. was removed at 2:52 p.m. The operative sites, as far as could be determined after subsequent cleaning and by comparison with the Brodmann map and measurement, were as follows:

Left: Areas 8, 9, 10. Rostral dorsoventral diameter, 4.1 cm.; middle dorsoventral diameter, 3 cm.; caudal dorsoventral diameter, 4.3 cm.; caudorostral length, 5.5 cm. Intact segment (areas 45 and 46), dorsoventral diameter, 1.8 cm.; rostrocaudal diameter, 2.8 cm.

Right: Areas 8, 9, 10. Rostral dorsoventral diameter, 5 cm.; caudal dorsoventral diameter, 5.5 cm.; caudorostral length, 4.5 cm. Intact segment (areas 45 and 46), dorsoventral diameter, 3.2 cm.; rostrocaudal diameter, 2.5 cm.

*Tentative Summary.* In spite of some discrepancy in sizes and weights of the removals of the two sides, areas 8, 9, and 10 appeared to have been reasonably accurately removed from both sides.

*Histologic Study.* The rostral part of the left specimen was granular in character and distinctly laminated horizontally. Its cells were small and the third layer poorly developed. Farther caudally the granular nature of the cortex became more pronounced and then less so. The most caudal sections still showed a very poorly developed granular layer. Such sections exhibited little radial striation.

On the right, the most rostral sections resembled those on the left but their medial extent was more typically granular. The caudal sections were not definitely granular except in their lateral parts.

*Summary.* Cortex of areas 8, 9, and 10 was removed on both sides. Apparently the most ventral parts of the left areas 9 and 10 escaped inclusion in the specimen. According to the estimate of postexcisional additional removal, the right ablation was very notably extended. This extension was principally in the dorsoventral direction and either represented extension to include all of the ventral parts of areas 9 and 10 or encroachment upon area 46.

**Case 8.    Protocol:** Middle frontal gyrus.    *Summary:* Asymmetrical removal of middle frontal gyri, encroaching upon area 6 caudally and 10 rostrally.

*Operation.* On May 16, 1947, both frontal lobes were exposed. On the left, a quadrilateral piece of tissue weighing 7.8 gm. was removed and, on the right, a somewhat larger piece of approximately the same shape and weighing 8.7 gm. The operative sites, after subsequent cleaning and so far as could be determined by comparison with the Brodmann map and measurement, were as follows:

Left: Middle frontal gyrus removed as far back as but not encroaching upon areas 8 and 6. Medial aspect of brain spared, dorsal quarter of lateral surface of area 10, dorsal half of area 46, and ventral third of lateral surface of area 9. Dorsal edge, 4.5 cm.; rostral edge, 2.4 cm.; caudal edge, 2.5 cm.; ventral edge, 5.5 cm.

Right: As for left side; dorsal edge, 4.0 cm.; rostral edge, 1.8 cm.; caudal edge, 2.0 cm.; ventral edge, 4.5 cm.

*Tentative Summary.* Bilateral excision of middle frontal gyrus as far caudally as areas 8 and 6.

*Histologic Study.* On the left, the sections began in cortex which was evidently of type 10 and ended caudally in cortex of type 9.

On the right, the specimen began rostrally in cortex which had a better developed pyramidal layer than one would expect to find in area 10. The sections terminated caudally in agranular cortex which was distinctly radially striated medially but not laterally.

*Summary.* On the left, the ablation of the middle frontal gyrus invaded area 10 and proceeded caudally into area 9. There was no area 6 in the specimen. On the right, area 10 was not included in the rostral part of the specimen but its caudal part infringed upon areas 8 and 6. The left cortical crater was notably enlarged after excision and the right to some extent. Presumably the right enlargement extended into area 10 and the left into 6.

**Case 13.    Protocol:** Areas 9, 45, 46.    *Summary:* Removal of areas 45, 46, and subtotal removal of 9 with encroachment upon area 10.

*Operation.* On May 20, 1947, both frontal lobes were exposed. On the left, an L-shaped piece of tissue weighing 13.5 gm. was excised at 7:28 p.m. All specimens were fixed by 7:40 p.m. On the right, a triangular piece weighing 14 gm. was excised at 8:45 p.m. and all samples were fixed by 8:55 p.m. The operative sites, after subsequent cleaning, so far as could be determined by comparison with the Brodmann map and measurement, were as follows:

Left: The operative excision only approximated the borders of the areas specified in the protocol. Thus, the dorsal part of area 9 in the concavity of area 8 was avoided as was the ventrocaudal half of area 45. The dorsocaudal edge of area 10 was included in the ablation. The medial edge of the hemisphere was removed for a distance of 1.2 cm. The rostral edge of the ablation measured 6 cm. and its ventro-caudal border 2.8. The ablation was 1.2 cm. deep.

Right: On this side the ablation closely corresponded with the predetermined site, except that the dorsocaudal corner of area 10 was also ablated. The medial edge of the hemisphere was removed for a distance of 1.2 cm. The rostral edge of the ablation measured 5.8 cm. Its ventral edge followed the ventral edge of the pars triangularis and measured 1.6 cm., then moved up along the caudal edge of this for 1.1 cm. and directly caudal for 1.2 cm. The dorsocaudal edge measured 6 cm.

*Tentative Summary.* On the left, all of area 46, half of area 45, and half of area 9 appear to have been removed, together with a fragment of area 10. On the right, areas 46, 45, and 9 were removed, together with a fragment of area 10.

*Histologic Study.* On the left, the rostral sections presented an appearance consistent with area 9. Caudally, cortex with notable pyramids in the third layer was included.

On the right, the most rostral sections apparently came from area 10. The caudal sections had the appearance of area 9 medially and area 45 laterally.

*Summary.* The rostral part of area 9 was apparently removed bilaterally, the excision including a part of area 10 on the right. Caudally the last sections from both sides still exhibited cortex of type 45. The specimen apparently did not include all of the caudal part of area 9. There was no notable extension of the crater following excision of the specimen.

**Case 18. Protocol:** Area 11. *Summary:* Subtotal removal of area 11.

*Operation.* On May 21, 1947, both frontal lobes were exposed. On the right a quadrilateral piece of tissue weighing 4.3 gm. was removed at 4:15 p.m. All specimens were fixed at 4:22 p.m. On the left a similar piece weighing 4.2 gm. was removed at 5:20 p.m. The operative sites, after subsequent cleaning, so far as could be determined by comparison with the Brodmann map and by measurement, were as follows:

Right: Rostral three-quarters of area 11. Rostrocaudal diameter, 4.5 cm.; medio-lateral, 5.0 cm.; depth, 1 cm.

Left: Rostral three-quarters of area 11 sparing laterocaudal edge. Rostrocaudal diameter, 4.5 cm.; mediolateral, 4.5 cm.; depth, 1 cm.

*Tentative Summary.* Bilateral removal of rostral three-quarters of area 11.

*Histologic Study.* The appearance of the rostral sections from both sides was consistent with the belief that these samples had been taken from area 11. Caudal sections from the left showed less distinct subdivision of the ganglionic and poly-morphic layers than farther forward but were still of the same type.

*Summary.* All tissue in both specimens was of the sort found in area 11. In this case no attempt was made to remove all of area 11 *en bloc* because of the limited visibility of the area and danger of infringing upon the rostral vasculature of the brain. The sites of excision were therefore notably extended caudally by suction. There is no reason to believe that anything but area 11 was removed but the caudal quarter or third of this escaped removal.

**Case 19. Protocol:** Area 45. *Summary:* Area 45 with probable encroachment upon area 46.

*Operation.* On May 26, 1947, both frontal lobes were exposed and a small semi-circular piece of tissue weighing 1.8 gm. was removed from the left hemisphere at 11:07 a.m. All specimens were immediately fixed. A piece of the same size and weight was removed from the right hemisphere at 11:58 a.m. All specimens were fixed by 12:04 p.m. The operative sites, after subsequent cleaning, so far as could be determined by comparison with the Brodmann map and by measurement, were as follows:

Left: Area 45 and ventral third of area 46; horizontal diameter, 2.0 cm.; vertical, 2.5 cm.; depth, 1.5 cm.

Right: Area 45 and ventral third of area 46; horizontal diameter, 1.7 cm.; vertical diameter, 1.5 cm.; depth, 1.7 cm.

*Tentative Summary.* Bilateral ablation of area 45 and ventral third of area 46.

*Histologic Study.* Only the right specimen was available for histologic study, the left having been used in the search for pathologic changes. The piece was small and uniform in appearance. Its external granular layer contained very small cells but the internal granular layer was evident. Considerable numbers of large pyramidal cells were present in layer 3 and radial striation was marked.

*Summary.* Only the right cortical specimen was available. It presented a structure consistent with the belief that it was taken from area 45. Both craters were notably enlarged after excision. The extension was more marked in the vertical direction on the left than right, presumably at the expense of area 46.

**Case 21.** **Protocol:** Area 10. *Summary:* Area 10 with possible encroachment upon areas 45 and 46.

*Operation.* On May 20, 1947, both frontal lobes were exposed. On the right, a semicircular piece of tissue weighing 5.2 gm. was excised at 11:10 a.m. All specimens were fixed by 11:25 a.m. On the left, a roughly quadrilateral piece of tissue weighing 8.2 gm. was removed at 12:15 p.m. All specimens were fixed by 12:22 p.m. The right sample represented only the lateral half of the area ultimately removed since the medial aspect of the region was ablated by suction. As nearly as could be determined, by comparison with the Brodmann map and by measurement, the ablations were as follows:

Right: The ventral half of area 10 and of area 46 were removed together with some encroachment upon the rostral part of area 45. The dorsoventral diameter measured 1.3 cm. and the rostrocaudal 4.5 cm.

Left: Removal of area 10; dorsoventral diameter, 3.7 cm.; rostrocaudal, 2.7 cm.

*Tentative Summary.* The removals were grossly asymmetrical. On the left, the ablation corresponded well to area 10 but on the right only the ventral half of area 10 was removed and the excision included the ventral half of area 46 and encroached upon area 45.

*Histologic Study.* All specimens from both sides exhibited the abnormally wide granular layers and atrophic pyramidal layer which is seen in area 10.

*Summary.* Only area 10 appeared in the specimens. The ablation had been considerably extended by suction so that presumably not only all of 10 had been removed but there may have been some infringement upon areas 45 and 46 on the right.

**Case 22.** **Protocol:** Areas 9, 10, 46. *Summary:* Areas 9, 10, and 46.

*Operation.* On May 19, 1947, both frontal lobes were exposed. On the left, an incomplete quadrilateral of tissue weighing 23.1 gm. was removed at 7:25 p.m. All specimens were fixed at 7:40 p.m. On the right, a roughly triangular-shaped piece weighing 19.5 gm. was ablated at 8:13 p.m. All specimens were fixed by 8:22 p.m. After subsequent cleaning, the removals appeared to be, so far as could be determined by comparison with the Brodmann map and by measurement, as follows:

Left: The removal appeared to coincide fairly closely with areas 9, 10, and 46. The dorsoventral diameter measured 4.5 cm. and the rostrocaudal, 4.5 cm.; the depth of the excision was 1.5 cm.

Right: In spite of some differences in measurement the removal on the right appeared to be comparable to that on the left. The right measurements were: dorsoventral diameter, 5.3 cm.; rostrocaudal, 3.6.

*Tentative Summary.* Bilateral removal of areas 9, 10, 46.

*Histologic Study.* All sections were of the granular pyramidal type. Rostral sections through both specimens showed a relatively atrophic pyramidal layer. Caudal sections did not exhibit this characteristic and radial striation was less pronounced. There were, however, no very large pyramids in the third layer. Intermediate sections showed cortex, in their lateral edges, of a character consistent with area 46.

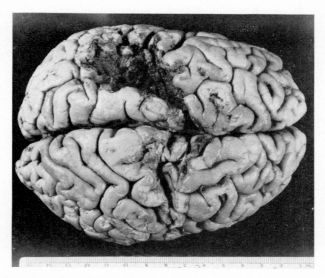

FIG. 63. Brain (norma dorsalis) of patient 24, who died twenty-two days after reoperation (left side). The lesion on the right represents the extent of the original operation. Metric scale below. (See also figure 66.)

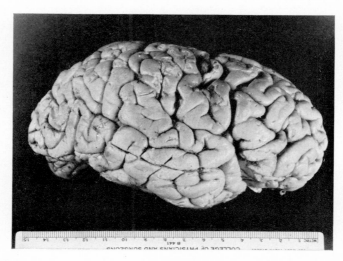

FIG. 64. Brain (norma lateralis dexter) of patient 24 showing ventrolateral extent of original operative lesion made one hundred and eighty days prior to decease. Metric scale below.

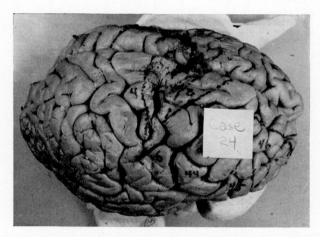

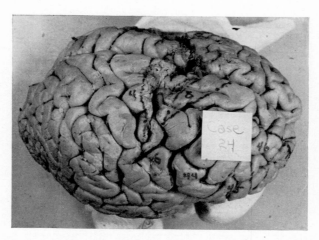

Fig. 65. Dorsolateral view of brain of patient 24 with assumed position of Brodmann areas marked in neutral red. Subsequent histologic study indicated that little if any area 6 remained at the location here bearing the numeral 6. This region was apparently area 9.

*Summary.* Areas 9, 10, and 46 were included bilaterally. There is no reason to suppose that these removals fell far short of or exceeded these areas.

**Case 24. Protocol:** Area 6. *Summary:* Subtotal removal of area 6.

*Operation.* On May 23, 1947, both frontal lobes were exposed. On the right, a triangular piece of tissue weighing 10.8 gm. was removed at 1:45 p.m. All specimens were fixed by 1:53 p.m. On the left, the tissue removed was somewhat fragmented and was delivered in two pieces which weighed 7.6 gm. in the aggregate. These were taken out at 3:45 p.m. and fixed by 3:53 p.m. So far as could be determined, by comparison with the Brodmann map and by measurement, the removals were as follows:

Right: Area 6, the operative bed measured 6.7 cm. dorsoventrally, along the medial margin it was 3 cm. wide, along its dorsoventral middle it measured 2 cm. rostrocaudally, and at its ventral extent was 1.3 cm. wide. The excision was 1.3 cm. deep

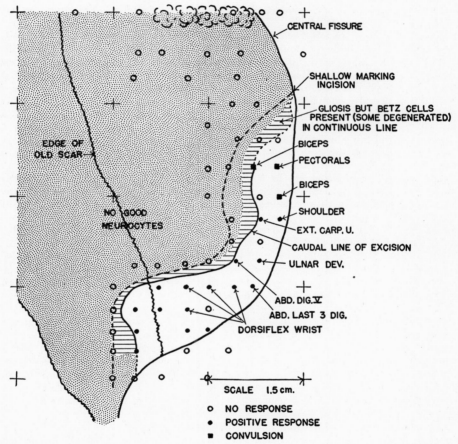

Fig. 66. Operative site of left hemisphere of case 24 (rostral to left, caudal to right) at time of reoperation to show degree of histologic alteration in caudal part of operative area. The edge of the old scar and the caudal line of the reoperative excision are indicated. The latter follows the line of excitable points (indicated here) as determined by electrical stimulation at the time of reoperation. The cortex was marked, before excision, by making a shallow incision just rostral to the line of excitable points. The stippled area contained no good neurocytes; the striated region contained gliosis but a few Betz cells, in apparently good condition, remained.

along the medial hemispheric margin, 1.5 cm. deep behind the middle frontal gyrus, and 0.8 cm. deep behind the pars opercularis.

Left: Rostral two-thirds of area 6, the operative bed measured 7.5 cm. dorsoventrally, along the medial margin it was 2.2 cm. wide, along its dorsoventral middle it measured 1.5 cm. rostrocaudally, and at its ventral extent was 0.8 cm. wide. The excision was 1.5 cm. deep along the medial hemispheric margin, 1.5 cm. deep behind the middle frontal gyrus, and 1.5 cm. deep behind the pars opercularis.

*Tentative Summary.* Right, area 6; left, rostral two-thirds of area 6.

*Histologic Study.* None of the sections of either specimen exhibited any internal granular layer except in their lateral edge where area 9 may have been infringed upon.

*Summary.* The cortex in the specimens at hand was of the type seen in area 6. Although both ablations were notably extended by suction, the right more than the left and to a larger size, there is no reason to suppose that the removals extended beyond area 6. Presumably, the left removal fell short of area 6. The other alternative would be that it coincided with 6 and the right exceeded it. This question was answered by reoperation.

*Reoperation.* On October 28 the left hemisphere was re-exposed and the caudal edge of the old excision was found to lie 3 cm. rostral to the central fissure dorsally. It lay 2.25 cm. rostral to the most rostral excitable part for the biceps and 1.5 cm. rostral to the most rostral electrically excitable point for the abductor of the little finger. In the ventral region, from which dorsiflexion of the wrist could be evoked, the old scar actually encroached upon the electrically excitable area and such movements could be evoked by stimulation of its bed (with minimal current strengths) as much as 7 mm. rostral to the caudal edge of the old excision. The inexcitable cortex between the old left scar and the central fissure was now removed. The rostral incision was carried through the floor of the old scar and the caudal just along the edge of most rostrally determined excitable points. The block weighed 28 gm.

*Postmortem Examination of the Brain.* This patient died of bronchopneumonia on November 19, 1947, and gross examination of the right side of the brain at that time was consistent with the belief that area 6 had been removed on that side (figs. 63-65).

*Histologic Study of Specimen Removed at Second Operation.* A thread was laid along the rostral border of the left electrically excitable cortex and a shallow incision made in the cortex just in front of and parallel to this border. The excision was then carried out along the actual border of the excitable area. The histologic appearance of the tissues removed and character of the responses obtained by stimulation at the time of the second operation are shown in figure 66.

**Case 25. Protocol:** Areas 8, 9, 46. *Summary:* Areas 8, 9, and 46 with infringement upon area 10 and possibly other areas.

*Operation.* On May 26, 1947, both frontal lobes were exposed. On the left an H-shaped piece of tissue weighing 11.3 gm. was removed at 6:55 p.m. All specimens were fixed by 7:05 p.m. On the right an H-shaped piece of tissue weighing 14.1 gm. was removed at 7:58 p.m. and all specimens were fixed by 8:07 p.m. After subsequent cleaning, so far as could be determined by comparison with the Brodmann map and by measurement, the removals were as follows:

Left: Areas 8, 9, 46. The distance of medial hemispheric margin excised was 2.5 cm., the rostroventral margin measured 6 cm., and the dorsocaudal 4 cm. The ventral rostrocaudal diameter was 3.1 cm. and the depth 1.6 cm.

Right: Area 8, 9, 46. The distance of medial hemispheric margin excised was 1.6 cm., the rostroventral margin measured 6 cm., and the dorsocaudal 5 cm. The ventral rostrocaudal diameter was 3 cm., and the depth 1.5 cm.

*Tentative Summary.* Bilateral ablation of areas 8, 9, 46.

*Histologic Study.* On the right, the rostral specimens were of a distinctly granular type. The most forward of the group appeared to be altering in the direction of the type of cortex seen in area 10. Caudally, the internal granular layer was very poorly developed and the ganglionic layer was double instead of triple. On the left, the rostral sections had the appearance of area 9 and caudally the internal granular layer was poorly developed. Intervening sections on both sides showed a structure consistent with area 46.

*Summary.* The specimens evidently included all of area 9 and at least parts of areas 46 and 8. On the right, area 10 was infringed upon. On both sides the operative site was enlarged after excision of the specimen, the left removal being finally notably longer in the rostrocaudal direction than the right. It is not clear in which directions the additional removals extended.

**Case 27. Protocol:** Superior frontal gyrus. *Summary:* Superior frontal gyri encroaching rostrally on area 10 and caudally on area 6.

*Operation.* On May 27, 1947, both frontal lobes were exposed. On the left, a long quadrilateral piece of tissue weighing 16.9 gm. was removed at 11:52 a.m. All specimens of tissue were fixed by 12:02 p.m. On the right, a similar piece weighing 17.8 gm. was excised at 1 p.m. There is no note to indicate exactly when all the parts of this piece were fixed. After subsequent cleaning of the operative site, as nearly as could be determined by comparison with the Brodmann map and by measurement, the removals were as follows:

Right: Superior frontal gyrus as far caudally as area 4 and rostrally as area 10, i.e. dorsal three-quarters of area 6, dorsal four-fifths of area 8, and dorsal four-fifths of area 9. Rostrocaudal measurement, 6 cm.; dorsoventral, 2.8 cm.; depth removed from medial surface, 1.8 cm.

Left: Superior frontal gyrus as far caudally as caudal part of area 6 and rostrally as area 10, i.e. dorsal three-quarters of area 6 sparing its most caudal part, dorsal four-fifths of areas 8 and 9. Rostrocaudal measurement, 5.2 cm.; dorsoventral, 2.8 cm.; depth removed from medial surface, 1.8 cm.

*Tentative Summary.* Bilateral removal of superior frontal gyri, i.e. most of areas 6, 8, and 9.

*Histologic Study.* Rostral sections through the right specimen had an appearance characteristic of area 10 and those through the caudal end were practically devoid of an internal granular layer. On the left, the most rostral sections had the appearance of type 9 cortex but the caudal sections exhibited a poorly developed internal granular layer.

*Summary.* The superior frontal gyri were removed—on the right, at least as far forward as area 10 and at least as far back as area 6. On the left, the excision fell short of these limits. Both removals were subsequently enlarged—the right more than the left. This enlargement must have occurred at the expense of area 6 or 10 or both.

**Case 31. Protocol:** Area 9. *Summary:* Area 9.

*Operation.* On May 29, 1947, both frontal lobes were exposed and an angular piece of tissue weighing 10.7 gm. was removed at 6:38 p.m. from the right side. All specimens were fixed by 6:48 p.m. On the left, a similarly shaped piece weighing 13 gm. was removed at 7:48 p.m. All specimens were fixed by 8:00 p.m. The operative sites, after further cleaning and as nearly as could be determined by comparison with the Brodmann map and by measurement, corresponded as follows:

Right: Area 9, dorsocaudal border, 4.5 cm.; medial margin of hemisphere removed, 2.5 cm.; rostroventral border, 6 cm.; depth of medial surface removed, 1.4 cm.

Left: Area 9, dorsocaudal border, 4.5 cm.; medial margin of hemisphere removed, 3.0 cm.; rostroventral border, 5.5 cm.; depth of medial surface removed, 1.8 cm.

*Tentative Summary.* Bilateral removal of area 9.

*Histologic Study.* All of the sections had an appearance which coincided with all criteria for type 9 cortex.

*Summary.* The tissue excised did not infringe upon anything but area 9. Both craters were extended following excision, the left particularly. There is no reason to suppose that the ultimate ablation trespassed upon other areas.

**Case 32. Protocol:** Areas 8, 9. *Summary:* Area 9 with infringement upon areas 8 and 10.

*Operation.* On June 6, 1947, both frontal lobes were exposed and, on the left, an angular piece of tissue weighing 12:5 gm. was removed at 11:45 a.m. All specimens were fixed at 11:49 a.m. On the right, a similarly shaped piece of tissue weighing 17 gm. was removed at 12:45 p.m. All specimens were fixed at 12:49 p.m. After subsequent cleaning, the operative site, as nearly as could be determined by comparison with the Brodmann map and by measurement, corresponded as follows:

Left: Areas 8, 9. Dorsocaudal margin, 4.1 cm.; medial margin of hemisphere removed, 3.3 cm. to a depth of 1.8 cm.; rostral part of ventral margin, 3.3 cm.; caudal part, 1.8 cm.; ventral drop, between, 1.8 cm.

Right: Areas 8, 9. Dorsocaudal margin, 5.0 cm.; medial margin of hemisphere removed, 2.8 cm. to a depth of 1.8 cm.; rostral part of ventral margin, 2.7 cm.; caudal part, 1.5 cm.; rostral drop, between, 2.5 cm.

*Tentative Summary.* Areas 8 and 9.

*Histologic Study.* On the left, the sections throughout had an appearance characteristic of area 9. On the right, the rostral sections appeared to be from area 10 and the caudal from 8.

*Summary.* There was little or no extension of the cortical wound following ablation of the specimens. On the left, the removal did not proceed beyond area 9. On the right, area 8 was included and area 10 infringed upon.

**Case 33. Protocol:** Inferior frontal gyrus. *Summary:* Inferior frontal gyri with encroachment rostrally upon area 10 and caudally upon area 44. Possible dysfunction in cortex of lateral cerebral fossa.

*Operation.* On May 30, 1947, both frontal lobes were exposed and on the left, a long quadrilateral piece of cortex weighing 12.9 gm. was removed at 12:20 p.m. All specimens were fixed by 12:28 p.m. On the right, a shorter piece of the same type and weighing 7 gm. was removed at 3:15 p.m. All specimens were fixed by 3:25 p.m. After subsequent cleaning, the operative sites appeared to correspond, as nearly as could be determined by comparison with the Brodmann chart and by measurement, as follows:

Left: Areas 44, 45, ventral half of 46, and caudal part of area 10. Dorsal margin, 6.3 cm.; ventral, 6.5 cm.; dorsoventral distance, 2.2 cm.; rostral depth, 1.9 cm.; caudal depth, 2.7 cm., exposing gyri breves and rostral part of transverse temporal gyrus of Heschl. At the depth of the exposure, the insulary rami of the middle cerebral vessels were visible. It was the author's impression that one of the branches of these vessels supplying the insulary aspect of the inferior frontal gyrus, or perhaps the insula itself, was ligated (see p. 449 concerning the neurological findings in this case).

Right: Areas 44, 45, and ventral half of 46. Dorsal margin, 5 cm.; ventral, 4.5 cm.; dorsoventral distance, 1.8 cm.; depth, 1.8 cm. throughout without exposure of insula.

*Tentative Summary.* Bilateral ablation of areas 44, 45, and half of 46. On the left, area 10 was involved and there probably was involvement of the cortex of the lateral cerebral fossa.

*Histologic Study.* The rostral sections of the left specimens were definitely granular with very small cells in the pyramidal layer. The caudal specimens, though still granular, exhibited the large cells in the lower part of the pyramidal layer which are found in area 44. On the right, the rostral sections resembled those from the left, the pyramidal layer being even less well developed than on that side. Caudal sections from the right were definitely granular but no large pyramids could be found in the lower part of the granular layer.

*Summary.* On the left the specimens began in area 10 and invaded area 44 caudally. On the right, the specimens seem to have reached farther rostrally (farther into area 10) but not so far caudally (not beyond area 45). There is no reason to believe that the operative site was subsequently extended on the right to involve area 44.

**Case 36.  Protocol:** Areas 10, 11, 45, 46, and 47.  *Summary:* Areas 10, 11, 45, 46, 47.*

*Operation.* On June 3, 1947, both frontal lobes were exposed and an angular piece of tissue weighing 23.8 gm. was removed from the left at 11:30 a.m. All specimens were fixed by 11:37 a.m. On the right, a piece of similar shape weighing 29 gm. was removed at 1:10 p.m. and all specimens were fixed by 1:15. After ablation the supraorbital defect tended to close up so that measurements were rather meaningless. So far as could be determined, by comparison with the Brodmann chart, the removals were as follows: areas 10, 11, 45, 46, and 47, ablation of orbital cortex as far back as optic foramina, ablation of lateral cortex of middle and inferior frontal gyri as far back as anterior ascending limb of lateral cerebral fissure.

*Tentative Summary.* Bilateral removal of areas 10, 11, 45, 46, and 47.

*Histologic Study.* All specimens from the left cortex were definitely granular. Rostral sections varied in appearance but most sections showed a very poor pyramidal layer. The appearance of the caudal sections was consistent with the belief that area 45 had been invaded. On the right, the rostral sections had the character of area 11 and the caudal sections showed scattered large pyramids, such as are seen in area 45.

*Summary.* The appearance of the specimens is consistent with the belief that areas 10, 11, 45, 46, and 47 were removed. Extension of the crater after excision of the specimens was appreciable but there is no reason to suppose that this exceeded the areas listed in the protocol.

**Case 40.  Protocol:** Areas 24, 32.  *Summary:* Subtotal removal of area 24.

*Operation.* On June 2, 1947, the right frontal lobe was exposed and a small specimen removed at 12:10 p.m. This was immediately fixed for enzyme studies. At 12:51 a further small piece was removed from the medial side of the left hemisphere without opening that side of the head. This piece apparently came from area 24. It was subdivided and fixed by 12:58. It was impossible for the author to visualize the sites of removal. These measured 3.9 by 1 cm. on the right, and 4.2 by 1.5 cm. on the left. Apparently the supracallosal parts of areas 24 and 32 were removed but not the parts below the callosum.

*Tentative Summary.* Bilateral removal of most of area 24 and the dorsal and caudal half of 32.

*Histologic Study.* Only a small specimen from the right side was available for cytoarchitectural study. This was typical mesocortex and, coming from the region from which it was taken, could have been nothing but area 24.

*Summary.* The ablation included at least part of area 24.

**Case 42.  Protocol:** Area 11.  *Summary:* Subtotal removal of area 11.

*Operation.* On May 29, 1947, both frontal lobes were exposed and an indeterminate fragment of rostral orbital cortex was removed at 10:52 a.m. This weighed 2 gm. and was divided and put in special fixatives by 11:02 a.m. A further piece from the caudal part of this surface was obtained at 11:05 a.m. It weighed 2.9 gm. and was fixed for cytoarchitectonic study by 11:08. Subsequently, a traumatized fragment weighing 1 gm. was obtained but discarded. At 12:30 p.m., a 5-gm. piece representing the rostral part of area 11 was obtained and put in formalin fixative at 12:35 p.m. An additional 2 gm. was subsequently obtained from this hemisphere at 12:40 p.m. and put in special fixatives by 12:45. After subsequent cleaning, the operative sites, as far as could be determined by comparison with the Brodmann map and by measurement, were as follows:

Left: Rostral three-fourths of area 11. Mediolateral measurement, 4.5 cm.; medial rostrocaudal distance, 4 cm.; lateral, 4.3 cm.

Right: Rostral three-quarters of area 11. Mediolateral measurement, 4.3 cm. (rostrally) and 2 cm. (caudally); medial rostrocaudal distance, 3.7 cm.; lateral, 4.5 cm.

*Tentative Summary.* Bilateral removal of rostral three-quarters of area 11.

* Area 47 seems to be indistinguishable from 10. See case 44.

*Histologic Study.* All sections were very prominently granular and showed the horizontal lamination of the ganglionic layer which is seen in cortex from area 11.

*Summary.* The specimens were derived from area 11. Although they represent only a portion of the cortex ultimately removed, there is no reason to believe that the ablation exceeded the projected removal of area 11, of which the rostral three-quarters were taken out.

**Case 44. Protocol:** Area 47. *Summary:* Subtotal removal area 10.

*Operation.* On June 4, 1947, both frontal lobes were exposed. On the left, a small piece of tissue was removed at 10:50 a.m. and a bit of it put in formalin at 10:53. On the right, another very small sample was obtained at 1:25 p.m. This was too small to divide for all fixatives so none was put aside for cytoarchitectonic study. At the time the tissues were removed the balance was temporarily out of adjustment and the weights were only estimated at 2.5 and 2.0 gm. respectively. Following subsequent cleaning, the site of ablation was considered, upon comparison with the Brodmann charts and by measurement, to be as follows:

Left: Area 47 and edges of adjacent areas 10 and 11. Rostrocaudal measurement, 3.8 cm.; dorsoventral, 1.0 cm.

Right: Area 47 and edges of adjacent areas 10 and 11. Rostrocaudal measurement, 3.7 cm.; dorsoventral, 1.0 cm.

*Tentative Summary.* Bilateral ablation of area 47.

*Histologic Study.* Only the left specimen was available for sectioning. It presented a character indistinguishable from that seen in area 10.

*Summary.* There is no way to tell whether the present specimens were removed from some part of area 10 or whether area 47 is a spurious locus which does not differ in any notable histologic manner from area 10.

*Reoperation.* On October 28, 1947, the right hemisphere was exposed and the operative scar was excised in a block in which the scar lay in its rostroventral part. A sample was also removed from the left side.

*Histologic Study of Operative Site.* The left sample had to be discarded because of buried silver clips. The right specimen exhibited the characteristics of area 11. The old scar was very shallow and its borders showed little neighborhood alteration.

**Case 47. Protocol:** Area 44. *Summary:* Area 44.

*Operation.* On May 28, 1947, both frontal lobes were exposed. On the left, a small quadrilateral piece of tissue weighing 3 gm. was obtained at 5:41 p.m. All specimens were fixed by 5:46. On the right, a similarly shaped piece of tissue weighing 3.6 gm. was removed at 7:50 p.m. All specimens, which did not include any for cytoarchitectural study, were fixed by 7:55 p.m. After subsequent cleaning, the sites of ablation were, as nearly as could be determined from comparison with the Brodmann maps and by measurement, as follows:

Left: Area 44. Caudal half removed *en bloc,* rostral half by suction. The record fails to list any measurement of the extent of the operated site on this side so a photograph (fig. 67) is presented herewith.

Right: Area 44. Dorsal edge, 2.0 cm.; ventral edge, 1.3 cm.; caudal edge, 2.3 cm.; rostral edge, 2.3 cm. Depths along these edges were respectively 2.0 cm., 1.0 cm., 1.9 cm., 1.1 cm.

*Tentative Summary.* Area 44.

*Histologic Study.* Only the left specimen was available for cytoarchitectural study. The character throughout was that of area 44 (see fig. 68). The specimen studied represented only the caudal half of the pars opercularis but figure 67 clearly indicates that the rostral half was also ablated.

*Summary.* Ablation of area 44.

**Case 49. Protocol:** Area 10. *Summary:* Area 10 with infringement upon areas 11 and 46.

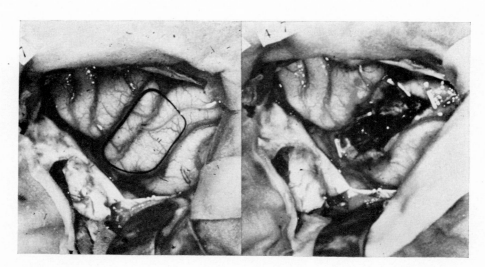

FIG. 67. Case 47. *Left,* Area to be removed (pars opercularis) outlined by thread. The caudal half (lower right) was removed *en bloc* (see fig. 68) and the remainder removed by suction. The final operative crater is shown in the right figure.

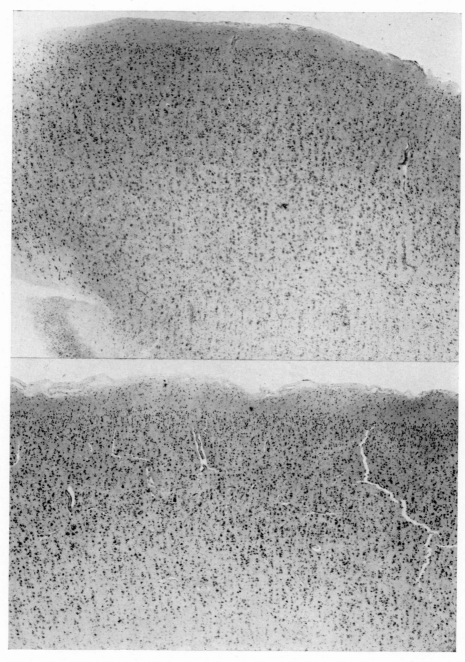

FIG. 68. Histologic appearance (x32) of left block removed from patient 47. The appearance of the rostral sections is shown above and the appearance of the caudal sections is shown below. The cortex is of intermediate pyramidal type and contains large pyramids in the third layer.

*Operation.* On June 5, 1947, both frontal lobes were exposed. On the right, a quadrilateral piece of tissue weighing 10 gm. was removed at 12:40 p.m. All specimens were fixed by 12:47 p.m. On the right, a similarly shaped piece of tissue weighing 9 gm. was removed at 2:10 p.m. All specimens were fixed by 2:16 p.m. After cleaning, the operative sites appeared to correspond, so far as could be determined by comparison with the Brodmann map and by measurement, as follows:

Right: Area 10, dorsal margin, 3.5 cm.; rostral margin, 4.6 cm.; caudal margin, 2.7 cm.; ventral margin, 4.0 cm.; depth, 2.2 cm.

Left: Areas 10 and 46, dorsal margin, 2.2 cm.; rostral margin, 4.5 cm.; caudal margin, 3.5 cm.; depth, 1.8 cm.; falx exposed over a distance of 1.5 cm.

*Tentative Summary.*   Bilateral removal of area 10, left removal of area 46.

*Histologic Study.*   On the right, the rostral sections had a character consistent with area 11 and the caudal that of area 10. On the left, the rostral sections apparently came from area 10 while the caudal resembled area 46.

*Summary.*   Bilateral removal of area 10, infringing upon the right upon area 11 and on the left upon area 46.


### DISCUSSION AND CONCLUSIONS

The Brodmann cytoarchitectural map of the human frontal cortex is of practical value for designation of the approximate area from which a specimen was taken. This statement is subject to the qualification that no distinguishing characteristics for area 47 were found, that the division between areas 8 and 6 is indefinite, that area 9 presents notable heterogeneity and that areas 45 and 46 resemble it. Subsidiary parts shown in the plans of Campbell, Brodmann, and of Economo and Koskinas all have a practical basis and the plans are mutually convertible.

The greatest difficulties in telling with certainty which cortical areas are nonfunctional, following ablation of a piece of cortex, are, in order of greatest seriousness, postexcisional manipulation of the crater, interruption of vessels to and from neighboring areas, probable individual differences in the arrangement of the cortical patterns, the growth of scar tissue in the floor of the crater, which scar tissue may interrupt projection fibers (to a depth of 5 to 6 mm. after twenty-one weeks) concerned with areas still in place, and changes due to exposure of the cortex, the use of saline, and the cautery. Study of the cortex adjacent to the site of a localized ablation shows that after five months the operative crater is reduced to about 75 percent of its original size and that the cortex bordering it is surrounded by three zones of disintegration. The first, about 5mm. wide, lacks all cell layers except the sixth. The second, about 8 mm. wide, lacks the first two layers and upper half of the third. The third zone, about 10 mm. wide, shows a loss of cells in the outer half of the third layer only. It is believed that the first two zones, totalling about 13 mm., reflect damage to the supracortical capillary net and that the third represents retrograde degeneration of cells sending association fibers to the ablated area. The first two zones are narrower or wider depending upon whether sulci do or do not lie close to the edge of the ablation.

In the present series of cases the correspondence with the plans of operations and the parts removed was good. Wherever an area was to have been removed it was generally removed at least in part. There was a distinct tendency for the operative removals to be somewhat larger than the protocols called for. What inaccuracies exist do not invalidate the possibility of allocating any effects noticed to the general region ablation of which was called for in the protocol. It would be a mistake to insist upon the absolute allocation of such noticed effects to ablation of the precise limits of particular areas as these are shown in the Brodmann charts.

While the actual operative removals were conducted upon a purely topographic basis, using the convolutional pattern and the Brodmann map as an arbitrary guide for the removal of cortex, it should be obvious that absolute coincidence with the Brodmann areas is not of critical importance in determining whether (1) removal of relatively restricted cortical areas produces therapeutically significant results in psychotics or whether (2) different parts of the frontal cortex mediate different functions (and if so what these are). Should it, however, prove (and whether or not it did is discussed in succeeding chapters) that function and alleged cytologic differences coincide, the method adopted was so arranged that such a correlation should not have entirely escaped unnoticed though, in the opinion of the present writer, the series was scarcely large enough to prove, beyond all shadow of doubt, the existence of such a correlation.

Table 3 summarizes, in rough form, the nature of the cortical ablations in individual cases but it is obvious, from the more precise descriptions given of individual cases in this chapter, that such a rough summary may be misleading. Furthermore it has been pointed out that even the best cytologic examinations of tissue removed do not ascertain the maximum extent of nonfunctional cortex. In the various other chapters of this book there are certain discrepancies between the manner in which different writers evaluate the nature of the ablations. Thus the fact that an area adjacent to the principal removal may have been infringed upon may be interpreted by one writer as evidence of its dysfunction. Another writer may discount such encroachment as inconsequential. Since the cytologic examination is but an approximation, at best, the editor has felt that forcing an arbitrary uniformity upon the various authors would result in imposing a false sense of exactitude upon the reader and such discrepancies have been allowed to stand. They are not, in themselves, of critical importance. It is probably better that the reader should be aware of their existence than that he should be given a false sense of security.

The reader may be interested to know that during the time the preceding material was in press Dr. Rowland and I conducted a quantitative study of the number of cells in the specimens discussed above. Imagine our surprise to discover that our schizophrenic patients' frontal lobes contained more cells than previous investigators have reported for normal humans! We believe the explanation for this inconsistency to be in the fact that our specimens were obtained from living humans whereas previous investigators have worked with postmortem material which evidently undergoes a variable degree of swelling. Reliable "normal" figures evidently have still to be obtained. The details of the quantitative studies noted above will be published shortly by Rowland and myself as a separate communication.

SECTION II

# Medical Survey

## Laboratory Findings
## and
## Special Tests

## Chapter 6

# General Medical Condition
# and Laboratory Findings

ROBERT G. HEATH, MALCOLM B. CARPENTER, H. HARVEY GASS,
AND JOHN J. WEBER

IN ADDITION to a survey of the general medical condition of the patients this section includes the results of several special tests performed before and after operation. For convenience and ready reference it will be subdivided into the following headings: (1) general medical condition of the patients, (2) glucose tolerance tests, (3) gastric acidity, (4) epinephrine tolerance studies, (5) blood pressure, and (6) fluctuations in weight.

### GENERAL MEDICAL CONDITION OF THE PATIENTS

Most of the patients were in good physical condition. The abnormalities found are listed in table 13.

Two patients (35 and 39) had clinical evidence of heart disease though neither gave a history of decompensation. Patient 39 had inactive rheumatic disease with mitral valve involvement. Patient 35, age 58 years, had generalized arteriosclerosis with evidence of aortic valvular disease.

During the radiologic survey, 2 patients (34 and 17) were found to have peptic ulcers. Both were asymptomatic. One patient (49) had mild chronic bronchitis.

During the workup, patient 15 developed a right lower lobe pneumonia and was excluded from preoperative testing for three weeks. Many of the patients repeatedly consulted the internist during the study with hypochondriacal complaints. A few of the patients, especially those with hypochondriacal symptoms, had been subjected to numerous operations. There was a high incidence of inguinal hernia in the males; 8 of the 30 had hernias, in 6 repair had been made.

Four patients were immediately excluded from operation for obvious medical reasons: the 2 with duodenal ulcers, the patient with lobar pneumonia, and the patient with generalized arteriosclerosis. During the course of the project several patients in both the control and the operatee group suffered minor injuries as a result of impulsive behavior. Two sustained fractures; patient 7 had a fracture of a proximal phalanx of the hand and patient 17, a Colles' fracture of the left forearm. Two others sustained lacerations of the hand by thrusting their fists through windows.

TABLE 13.  SUMMARY OF PHYSICAL EXAMINATIONS ON ALL PATIENTS*

| Number of Patient | Findings |
|---|---|
| 1 | Left indirect inguinal hernia |
| 3 | External hemorrhoids |
| 5 | Gross impairment of auditory function without organic aural disease |
| 4 | External hemorrhoids |
| 7 | Status postherniorrhaphy (right); right atrophic undescended testicle |
| 8 | Status postthoracotomy (right posterolateral) |
| 9 | Moderate thoracic scoliosis; cutaneous lipoma, anterior abdominal wall |
| 11 | Status postherniorrhaphy (right); recurrent right inguinal hernia (direct) |
| 12 | (a) Status postsuicidal attempt—scar left side neck anteriorly |
|  | (b) Status posttraumatic back injury with laminectomy 7–12 thoracic vertebrae (x-ray evidence of old compression fracture of lumbar I) |
|  | (c) Status postherniorrhaphy (left) |
|  | (d) Generalized hypoplasia of genitals |
| 13 | External hemorrhoids |
| 14 | Status postappendectomy |
| 15 | Chronic emphysema; left direct inguinal hernia |
| 16 | Status postlaparotomy (reason unknown, scar midline from umbilicus) |
| 17 | Status postherniorrhaphy (right); status postlaparotomy (reason unknown, right paramedian rectus scar) |
| 18 | Status postappendectomy; status postherniorrhaphy (right) |
| 19 | Traumatic ptosis left eye (secondary to burn) |
| 21 | Bilateral cryptorchidism with testicular atrophy |
| 23 | Status postappendectomy; perforated left tympanic membrane |
| 24 | (a) Status healed abdominal wounds (two) |
|  | (b) Urethritis (nonspecific) |
|  | (c) Atrophy intrinsic muscles of both hands |
| 28 | Left testicular hydrocele |
| 30 | Status postherniorrhaphy (right) |
| 32 | Status postcesarean section; hypoplasia of mammary glands (bilateral) |
| 34 | (a) Chronic cystic disease of breasts (bilateral) |
|  | (b) Duodenal ulcer (diagnosed on x-ray) |
|  | (c) Large keloid over sternum |
| 35 | (a) Status postoophorectomy (bilateral) |
|  | (b) Status postcholecystectomy |
|  | (c) Status postgastrojejunostomy |
|  | (d) Status postsuicidal attempt (scars cubital fossae bilaterally) |
|  | (e) Arteriosclerotic heart disease with mitral stenosis |
| 36 | Status postsalpingo-oophorectomy with hysterectomy |
| 38 | Rheumatic heart disease, inactive, with mitral involvement |
| 40 | Status postthyroidectomy |
| 44 | Status postappendectomy |
| 45 | Bilateral pterygii |
| 47 | Bilateral amputation of fourth toes |
| 49 | Status postthyroidectomy; chronic bronchitis |

* All physical examinations were performed at the beginning of the project, between April 9 and May 5, 1947. Only positive findings are summarized in this table. Patients 2, 6, 10, 20, 22, 25-27, 29, 31, 33, 37, 41, 42, 46, and 48 exhibited no abnormal findings.

## GLUCOSE TOLERANCE TESTS

### ALTERATIONS FOLLOWING ABLATION OF THE FRONTAL CORTEX

Glucose tolerance tests were performed on 24 psychotic patients, in 23 of whom one or a combination of Brodmann's areas were to be removed as treatment of the psychosis; in the twenty-fourth (patient 38) the superior cerebral veins of both frontal lobes were ligated. The same tests were performed on 24 control psychotics who underwent the same workup, but who were given only a general anesthetic without actual operation. On each subject, one preoperative (or preanesthesia) test was taken, and four tests were performed at three to five days, eight to ten days, twenty-eight to thirty-five days, and ninety to one hundred days, postoperatively.

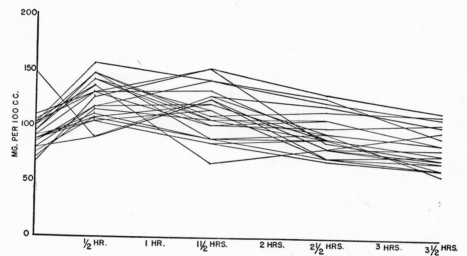

FIG. 69.   All preoperative glucose tolerance curves of operatees. There are no diabetic curves.

For each test, after a fasting specimen of blood was taken, the patient was given 1.75 gm. of glucose in water per kilogram of body weight. Venous blood specimens were then taken at intervals of one-half hour, one and one-half hours, two and one-half hours, and three and one-half hours.

The curves for the controls were essentially the same after anesthesia as before, but in some of the operatees there were marked changes. The nature of the change was in: (1) increased peak of the curve, (2) delayed fall in the curve, or (3) both.

Figure 69 shows all of the preoperative curves of patients subsequently operated upon. It is noted that all fell within normal range. In each patient in whom the curve was postoperatively altered the changes were essentially the same. On figure 70 the five curves of patient 13 are charted together to illustrate these changes.

Of particular interest was the finding that there was relatively little fluctuation in fasting sugars. The principal alteration was in the inability of the patients to tolerate sugar. This was temporary and had disappeared in all cases after one to two months. A graph (fig. 71) was made to show these particular characteristics. All fasting readings are charted on the lowest level, all one-half-hour readings on the next line above, all one and one-half-hour above this, and all three and one-half-hour readings above this.

Various graphs were made in order to determine if there was a correlation between the observed sugar tolerance curves and (1) weight of brain tissue removed, (2) degree

of clinical improvement, and (3) relationship to specific areas. The intake of carbohydrate during the postoperative period was considered to determine whether or not
some of the alterations might be a starvation phenomenon.

**Correlation between Weight of Removed Brain Tissue and Alterations in Toler-
ance Curve.** On figure 71 patients are lined up on the abscissa according to weight
of brain tissue removed,* the patients with smallest weight of brain removed being
on the left and those with the greatest amount removed on the right. It is apparent
that no relationship exists between the weight of brain removed and the alteration
in the glucose tolerance curve.

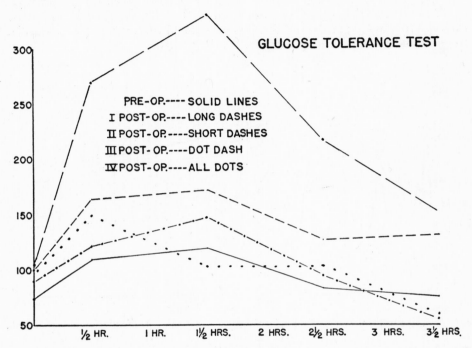

FIG. 70.   Preoperative and postoperative glucose tolerance curves on patient 13. (For time of
postoperative tests see text.)

**Correlation between Clinical Improvement and Alterations in Tolerance Curve.**
In order to make the correlation between the degree of clinical improvement and
alterations in the glucose tolerance curve all operatees were graded as to improvement
in social behavior. A rating was given preoperatively and another five months postoperatively, according to the following scale:

> 5=Most disturbed ward
> 4=Moderately disturbed ward
> 3=Best ward with ground parole
> 2=Home with supervision
> 1=Home and working, or capable of working.

The figure for improvement was arrived at by subtracting the postoperative from the
preoperative rating. In figure 72, this improvement figure was plotted against the sugar
tolerance curve (patients are lined up on the abscissa so that those with greatest

* As noted in chapters 3 and 4 the weight of brain removed was determined by weighing
the tissue carefully as soon as it was excised. In a few instances, when all the tissue could not
be excised because of difficulty in exposure, the weight of the tissue removed by gentle
suction was calculated from the volume of the resulting cavity.

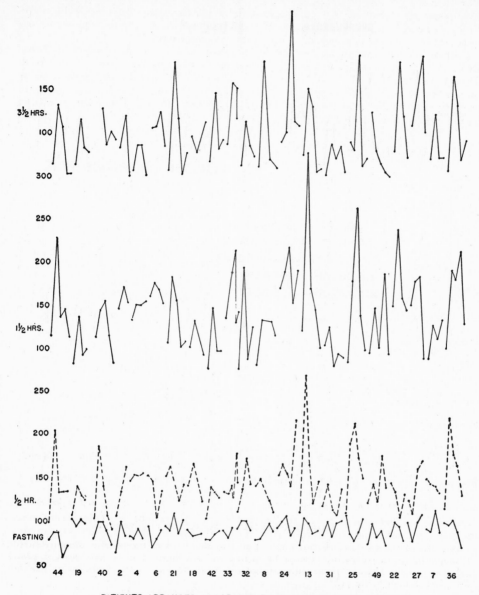

PATIENTS ARRANGED ACCORDING TO WEIGHT OF BRAIN REMOVED

FIG. 71. Glucose levels in patients upon whom operation was performed. In this chart the fasting sugars of each patient, taken at different times, are charted in one level, viz. the fasting levels before operation and three days, ten days, thirty days, and ninety days after operation are charted in the lowest level. Just above are the one-half-hour readings; first the preoperative, then the various postoperative values; above this are the one and one-half-hour readings, and at top are the three-hour readings.

On this chart patients are arranged on the abscissa according to the weight of the brain tissue removed.

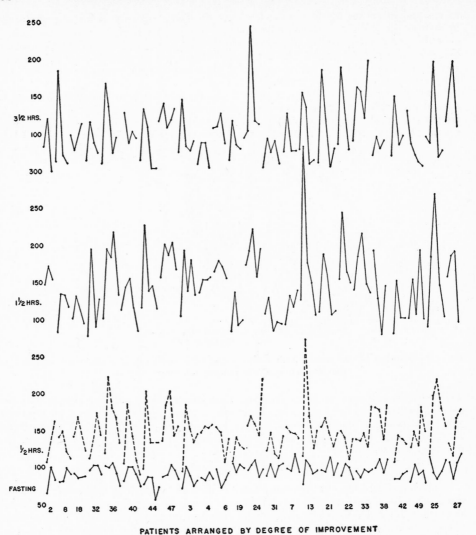

FIG. 72.   Relationship of clinical improvement to alteration in the glucose tolerance curves. Patients are arranged on the abscissa by degree of improvement; those with least improvement are on the left and those with greatest improvement are on the right. Sugar readings are plotted as in figure 71.

improvement are on the right, those with the least on the left). No correlation was found between the amount of clinical improvement and the altered sugar curves. Since the principal effects of the operation were in the affective sphere, the degree of alteration in affect at the time the various curves were taken was charted against the sugar curve. There was again no correlation. (These graphs are not included.)

**Relationship of Glucose Curve to Removal of Specific Areas.** Nineteen of the 24 patients operated upon showed an increase over the preoperative curve of at least 50 mg. per 100 cc. in one or more of the postoperative blood specimens. In 18 of these patients the rise was greatest on the first postoperative curve. One patient (24) failed to show a significant rise until the third postoperative curve was taken. He refused to eat and often regurgitated tube feedings. This late diabetic curve was attributed to malnutrition. Eight patients showed a rise of at least 100 mg. per 100 cc. of blood over the preoperative curve, and 2 patients showed a rise of over 150 mg. per 100 cc. over the preoperative curve. The 2 patients with a rise of greater than 150 mg. per 100 cc. were 25 and 13. For diagrams of areas supposedly removed in these cases figures 32 and 19 may be consulted.

Every patient in whom areas 9, 10, 24, 44, 45, and 47 were removed alone or as part of a combination of areas showed an increase of at least 50 mg. per 100 cc. In no patient in whom areas 6 and/or 8 were removed without infringement on more rostral areas was there a significant rise. There were 3 such patients (2, 6, and 24).

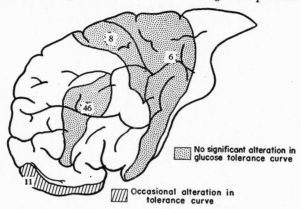

FIG. 73. Diagram of the frontal lobe showing the relationship of site of cortex removed to the alteration of the glucose tolerance curves.

Two patients had area 11 alone removed. One showed no significant change and the other showed an increase of 50 mg. per 100 cc. One patient had area 46 removed alone and failed to show a significant rise. In figure 73 the shaded parts indicate the areas of frontal cortex which when removed failed to produce a significant rise in the height of the curve.

ALTERATIONS FOLLOWING LOBOTOMY

Analyzing data from the lobotomy cases is difficult, since it is impossible to determine what has been cut. Of the 8 lobotomy cases, in 2 there was failure to show significant differences between the preoperative and postoperative curves. In the other 6 the changes were of the same nature as those seen in the topectomy cases, i.e. increased peak, delayed fall, or both. Here, too, these changes were temporary and disappeared in one month. Two patients who had previously had topectomy were included in this group. Patient 2, who earlier had area 8 and part of area 6 removed with no significant change in the sugar tolerance curve, after lobotomy showed an increase peak of 120 mg. per 100 cc. over the preoperative curve. Patient 44, who previously had area 47 removed with an increase of over 100 mg. per 100 cc., showed an equally great rise after lobotomy.

DISCUSSION

Changes in glucose metabolism have been reported associated with virtually every variety of encephalic abnormality. Hyperglycemia has been described clinically with concussion and skull fractures (Davidson and Allen, '25; Wooley, '36), brain tumors (Feinblatt, '23), encephalography (Bradley, '37), basal ganglia diseases and hypothalamic lesions (Morgan, Vonderahe, and

Malone, '37; Vonderahe, '37; Noltie, '38; Ingram and Barris, '36; Davis, L., '34). Experimentally, it has been reported when the intracranial pressure is raised in cats. Numerous references are available to indicate the extensive influence which peripheral (afferent) and autonomic impulses exert upon the level of blood sugar (Brooks, '31; Cannon, Shohl, and Wright, '11; Griffith, Lockwood, and Emery, '38; Bodo and Benaglia, '38; Noltie, '38; Brouha, Cannon, and Dill, '39; Davis, L., '34). The endocrine glands, particularly the adrenals, have often been implicated in such alterations of glucose levels (Donhoffer, and MacLeod, '32; Brobeck, Tepperman, and Long, '43; Cannon, Shohl, and Wright, '11; Griffith, Lockwood, and Emery, '38; Britton, '28; Lewis and Turcatti, '35). Emotional stimuli have long been recognized as capable of affecting blood sugar (Cannon, Shohl, and Wright, '11). In the direction of reducing blood sugar levels the reports available are as numerous and as widespread in their field of coverage. Encephalitis (Meakins, '40), experimental decerebration (Daniel and Maxim, '29), stimulation of afferent nerves (Brooks, '31), and Horsely-Clarke lesions of the hypothalamus (Barris and Ingram, '36; Davis, L., '34) have all been studied in this context. It is significant that most of the changes reported in association with cerebral stimulation or trauma have been transitory, and Peters and Van Slyke ('46) state that no definitely localized center for carbohydrate metabolism has been found higher than Bernard's center in the floor of the fourth ventricle, although higher levels of integration have long been sought, and there is evidence they do exist.

The present series illustrates once more the lability of carbohydrate balance and the degree to which it is subject to interference at the level of the telencephalon. For the first time, as far as we are aware, localized and discrete surgical removal of presumably normal frontal cortex has been shown to produce alterations in the amount of circulating glucose. These alterations were in the direction of increase of peak values and subsequent delayed fall and were transient, lasting not more than two months. The effect follows removal of rather widespread regions of frontal cortex, but only results when granular cortex is removed. These findings justify the assumption that the granular cortex of the frontal lobe exerts an influence on carbohydrate metabolism.

SUMMARY

1. Bilateral surgical ablations of discrete areas of frontal cortex were carried out on 23 psychotic patients.

2. Significant alterations in glucose tolerance curves, with higher peaks and general prolongation of the curves, were observed in 18 patients following operation.

3. These changes were transitory and did not appear after two months following operation.

4. Similar tests were performed on 8 lobotomy patients. Changes of the same type occurred in 6 of this series.

5. Attempts to correlate glucose values with nutrition, weight of brain removed, clinical course, or preoperative psychopathology were all unsuccessful. Removal of areas 9, 10, 24, 44, 45, and 47, either alone or in combination, always resulted in significant increase in the peak of the sugar tolerance curve, whereas removal of areas 6, 8, 11, and 46 consistently failed to produce a significant change.

6. It is concluded that the changes observed justify the assumption that the granular cortex of the frontal lobes exerts an influence in carbohydrate metabolism.

## EFFECTS OF TOPECTOMY AND PREFRONTAL LOBOTOMY UPON GASTRIC ACIDITY

It has been clearly established by many investigators that gastrointestinal function is subject to cerebral control. Alterations in gastric secretion and motility and the development of gastric mucosal hemorrhages and ulcers have been demonstrated both clinically and in the laboratory as a result of stimulation or destruction of various parts of the brain. Information regarding the role of the frontal lobes specifically in the control of gastric acidity is meager. Watts and Fulton ('34) noted that stimulation of premotor cortex caused increased gastric secretion. Mettler, Spindler, Mettler and Combs ('36) demonstrated erosions of the gastric mucosa following ablation of the frontal cortex in cats. In lobotomized patients a more prompt response of gastric secretion to histamine with a higher free hydrochloric acid content than in normal individuals was found by Petersen and Buchstein ('47). More recently Reed's ('48) observation of increased gastric secretion following prefrontal lobotomy suggests confirmation of this effect.

Topectomy and lobotomy as carried out in this project offer an opportunity for further confirmation of this tendency and continued investigation of the relationship between gastric acidity and the frontal lobes.

### METHOD OF INVESTIGATION

Two phases of gastric acidity were investigated, the gastric and the psychic or cephalic phase. The stimulus for the gastric phase was a test meal in the topectomy group and a histamine subcutaneous injection in the lobotomy group. The stimulus for the psychic phase was insulin (parasympathetic stimulation) in one series of tests and epinephrine (sympathetic stimulation) in a second series. The psychic phase was not studied in the lobotomy patients.

**Gastric Phase.** Gastric analysis was done preoperatively and postoperatively on the 24 patients operated upon in the topectomy series. Fourteen control patients were similarly studied under identical conditions as the operatees. Preoperative analyses were done on all patients about three weeks before the operative period and during the third postoperative week analyses were made on the control group as well as patients upon whom operations were performed. A test meal consisting of 60 cc. of a thin wheat gruel and not over 100 cc. of water was used, gavage feedings being employed where necessary. In each test a fractionated analysis was carried out over three consecutive days as follows: on each of these days, following a twelve-hour fast, the gastric contents were withdrawn after which the gruel meal was given. In addition to the fasting specimen only one other specimen was taken on any given day. On the first day this second specimen was withdrawn one-half hour following the test meal; on the second day, the second specimen was withdrawn one hour after the test meal; and on the third day it was taken two hours afterwards. An average of the three fasting specimens was used in evaluating the data.

In 8 patients who underwent bilateral prefrontal lobotomy a histamine (0.5 mg. histamine base) gastric analysis was done pre- and postoperatively, postoperative analyses being done during the second postoperative week. Single-day fractionated analyses were used with specimens taken at fifteen, thirty, forty-five, and sixty minutes following the histamine injection.

**Psychic Phase.** Insulin Rehfuss tests were performed on all patients in the topectomy series one month postoperatively. At the same time this test was carried out on 5 patients

TABLE 14. TABULATION OF MAXIMAL ACIDITIES IN TOPECTOMY PATIENTS AND CONTROLS IN THE GASTRIC PHASE OF SECRETION WITH A GRUEL MEAL STIMULUS

(Acidity is expressed in degrees)

| Patient No. | Areas removed | Maximal HCl | | Change | Maximal comb. Acid | | Change |
|---|---|---|---|---|---|---|---|
| | | Preop. | Postop. | | Preop. | Postop. | |
| **Operatees:** | | | | | | | |
| 2 | 8, 6[a] | 26 | 10 | −16 | 34 | 20 | −14 |
| 3 | 9, 6[a], 8[a], 45[a] | 29 | 0 | −29 | 28 | 11 | −17 |
| 4 | 46, 10[a] | 5 | 20 | +15 | 18 | 33 | +15 |
| 6 | 6, 8 | 18 | 6 | −13 | 13 | 7 | − 6 |
| 7 | 8, 9, 10, 46[a] | 44 | 32 | −12 | 16 | 13 | − 3 |
| 8 | 6[a], 8[a], 9[a], 10[a], 46[a] | 0 | 3 | + 3 | 6 | 7 | + 1 |
| 13 | 9, 45, 46, 10[a] | 25 | 14 | −11 | 8 | 14 | + 6 |
| 18 | 11 | 34 | 0 | −34 | 26 | 8 | −18 |
| 19 | 45 | 0 | 6 | + 6 | 20 | 17 | − 3 |
| 21 | 10 | 26 | 22 | − 4 | 23 | 13 | −10 |
| 22 | 9, 10, 46 | 39 | 17 | −22 | 15 | 13 | − 2 |
| 24 | 6 | 10 | 18 | + 8 | 26 | 46 | +20 |
| 25 | 8, 9, 46, 10[a] | 30 | 34 | + 4 | 20 | 22 | + 2 |
| 27 | 6[a], 8[a], 9[a], 10[a] | 13 | 20 | + 7 | 14 | 12 | − 2 |
| 31 | 9 | 10 | 0 | −10 | 15 | 12 | − 3 |
| 32 | 9, 8[a], 10[a] | 24 | 0 | −24 | 8 | 6 | − 2 |
| 33 | 45, 10[a], 44[a], 46[a,b] | 17 | 24 | + 7 | 8 | 16 | + 8 |
| 36 | 10, 11, 45, 46, 47 | 15 | 30 | +15 | 11 | 9 | − 2 |
| 38 | (6[a], 8[a], 9[a]) | 8 | 28 | +20 | — | 15 | — |
| 40 | 24 | 0 | 0 | 0 | 12 | 8 | − 4 |
| 42 | 11 | 24 | 44 | +20 | 14 | 12 | − 2 |
| 44 | 47 | 3 | 0 | − 3 | 11 | 10 | − 1 |
| 47 | 44 | 16 | 16 | 0 | 11 | 14 | + 4 |
| 49 | 10, 11[a], 46[a] | 0 | 12 | +12 | 19 | 12 | − 7 |
| **Controls:** | | | | | | | |
| 1 | | 12 | 5 | − 7 | 15 | 9 | − 6 |
| 5 | | 14 | 0 | −14 | 18 | 12 | − 6 |
| 9 | | 28 | 22 | − 6 | 22 | 19 | − 3 |
| 12 | | 8 | 3 | − 5 | 17 | 10 | − 7 |
| 14 | | 34 | 22 | −12 | 14 | 26 | +12 |
| 16 | | 27 | 21 | − 6 | 20 | 17 | − 3 |
| 17 | | 28 | 26 | − 2 | 24 | 14 | −10 |
| 20 | | 17 | 57 | +40 | 12 | 18 | + 6 |
| 30 | | 9 | 6 | − 3 | 12 | 10 | − 2 |
| 35 | | 0 | 0 | 0 | 10 | 9 | − 1 |
| 37 | | 20 | 20 | 0 | 10 | 9 | − 1 |
| 39 | | 50 | 44 | − 6 | 18 | 14 | − 4 |
| 41 | | 18 | 16 | − 2 | 26 | 8 | −18 |
| 45 | | 3 | 0 | − 3 | 11 | 10 | − 1 |

[a] Indicates partial removal of an area. Otherwise area removals are total or nearly so.

[b] In addition to areas indicated, the superior frontal gyrus was presumably destroyed or damaged by ligation of vessels to it.

Areas included within parentheses were presumably affected by ligation of vessels to them. No cortex removed.

not subjected to operation who are considered as controls for these postoperative values. For each test a fasting gastric specimen and a fasting blood sample for glucose level was taken after which 15 units of regular insulin was given intravenously. Thereafter blood samples for glucose were drawn one-half hour, one and one-half hours, two and one-half hours, and three and one-half hours later. Gastric specimens were obtained at half-hour intervals for three hours.

Epinephrine Rehfuss tests were performed on 21 topectomy patients about six weeks postoperatively. Five patients not subjected to operation and not participating in the insulin tests were used as controls. Gastric and blood samples were taken as in the insulin test except that blood specimens were drawn at half-hour intervals for two hours. One cc. of 1/1000 dilution of epinephrine by subcutaneous injection was used as a test dose.

Free, combined, and total acidity were determined on each specimen by titration with o.1N sodium hydroxide using Topfer's reagent, phenolphthalein, and/or 1 percent aqueous solution of alizarin sulfonate as indicators.

### RESULTS

Classification of the essential data is made solely on the basis of the maximal acidity (free and combined treated separately) obtained in a single analysis for each of the test stimuli used. For purposes of clarity and because no significant information was yielded therefrom, the factors of quantity of secretion, total acidity, and time at which peak acidity was reached have been omitted. Comparisons between pre- and postoperative maximal values in the gastric phase are made for each patient in the operatee and in the control series as well as for the lobotomy patients. In the cases of insulin and epinephrine Rehfuss tests, maximal acidity values are matched against a value obtained by averaging the maximal acidities of the appropriate control patients.

When the topectomy patients are considered as a unit with regard to their free acid changes in the gastric phase after operation (table 14), it would appear at first that a chance distribution of changes has occurred. Thus, out of 24 patients, 11 after operation showed an increase in acidity ranging from 3 to 20 degrees with an average increase of 10.6 degrees, whereas 11 others after operation showed a decrease in acidity ranging from 3 to 34 degrees with an average decrease of 16 degrees. Two patients showed no change. The magnitude of these changes is within the limits expected by daily normal variations in gastric acidity. This is true also of the magnitude of change within the control group in the preanesthesia and postanesthesia tests. However, judging from the control group, a chance distribution of change was not to be expected inasmuch as in that group only 1 patient out of 14 showed an increase in acid in the second test whereas 11 patients showed a decrease. Thus, the apparent even distribution of changes in acidity in both directions following topectomy, in actuality represents a weight in the direction of increased free acidity. The average increase of 40 degrees in the control group is of no significance since this value is based upon the change in only 1 patient. The tendency towards reduction in acid in the second test of the control patients perhaps reflects the increased tranquillity coming from greater care and attention during the prolonged testing and operative periods beyond that to which the subjects had been accustomed. In that sense this would be psychic effect, the changes indicated above following topectomy implying the absence of this effect.

In the lobotomy group 5 out of 8 patients showed an increase in free acid following operation (table 15). Three patients showed a decrease. The range of changes in each direction in these patients is compatible as is the average of these changes. The average increase and decrease is greater than corresponding values in the topectomy series. This may be the result of the use of the much stronger stimulus, histamine, in the lobotomy group.

This trend towards increased free acid in both topectomy and leucotomy groups, although slight, is credible in the light of the similar results in leucotomy patients noted by Petersen and Buchstein and by Reed. Analysis of the data on topectomy patients who showed increases in acidity following operation failed to reveal any dependence of this effect upon specific areas or regions of the frontal lobes. On the contrary, removal of area 9 seemed to be followed by a tendency towards decreased free acidity much more often than by increased free acidity. Although the greatest decrease in free acidity occurred in a patient who had area 11 alone removed, this was offset by increases occurring in other patients who had area 11 removed.

TABLE 15.  MAXIMAL ACIDITIES IN LOBOTOMY PATIENTS FOLLOWING
HISTAMINE STIMULATION
(Acidity is expressed in degrees)

| Patient No. | Lobotomy | | | Histamine | | |
| | Maximal HCl | | Change | Maximal comb. acid | | Change |
| | Preop. | Postop. | | Preop. | Postop. | |
|---|---|---|---|---|---|---|
| 2 | 79 | 85 | + 6 | 24 | 10 | −14 |
| 5 | 70 | 6 | −64 | 27 | 30 | + 3 |
| 11 | 65 | 47 | −18 | 15 | 60 | +45 |
| 20 | 31 | 76 | +45 | 32 | 94 | +62 |
| 23 | 53 | 56 | + 3 | 13 | 30 | +17 |
| 28 | 34 | 32 | − 2 | 14 | 59 | +45 |
| 44 | 0 | 32 | +32 | 7 | 28 | +21 |
| 46 | 43 | 67 | +24 | 25 | 18 | − 7 |

A number of patients in both the topectomy and the control groups failed to show any free acid following gruel test meals. Although the number of such patients increased considerably postoperatively in the topectomy group, this is probably without significance inasmuch as a comparable increase occurred in the control series.

In the control patients, with respect to changes in the maximal combined acid in the gastric phase, only 2 out of 14 showed an increase in the postanesthesia test whereas 12 showed a decrease (table 14). The ranges of change and the average changes were comparable in both directions and within the expected normal variation. In the topectomy series only 7 out of 24 patients showed an increase of combined acid postoperatively which varied from 1 to 20 degrees with an average increase of 8 degrees. Sixteen patients showed a decrease ranging from 1 to 18 degrees with an average decrease of 16 degrees. As with the free hydrochloric acid, attention focused on the topectomy series alone gives a false impression of the changes in the combined acid maximums. When compared to the expected variation as determined by the control group distribution, there is evident a weight in the direction of greater numbers of patients than expected showing an increase in combined acid postoperatively. This is offset to some extent, however, by the greater average of decreased maximal combined acid values in the topectomy group—16 as compared to 6 degrees for the controls. The removal of regions of the frontal lobes towards the pole, in particular areas 9, 10, and 11, moreover, seems to be followed by a tendency for combined acid to decrease.

A more definite trend is discernible in the changes of the maximal combined acidity values which followed lobotomy. Here, 6 patients out of 8 showed an increase in combined acidity postoperatively whereas only 2 showed a decrease. Moreover, 4 of these patients showed increases of considerably more than 14 degrees which was the greatest decrease that occurred. The average of the maximum combined acidity

TABLE 16. TABULATION OF MAXIMAL ACIDITIES IN THE PSYCHIC PHASE OF SECRETION AS INDICATED IN THE INSULIN REHFUSS TEST
(Acidity is expressed in degrees)

| Patient No. | Areas removed | Topectomy Minimal Blood Sugar mg. per 100 cc. | Maximal free HCl | Insulin Rehfuss Change from control maximum average | Maximal combined acid | Change from control maximum average |
|---|---|---|---|---|---|---|
| **Operatees:** | | | | | | |
| 2 | 8, 6ᵃ | 62 | 86 | +21 | 10 | −11 |
| 3 | 9, 6ᵃ, 8ᵃ, 45ᵃ | 44 | 14 | −51 | 18 | − 3 |
| 4 | 46, 10ᵃ | 60 | 86 | +21 | 12 | − 9 |
| 6 | 6, 8 | 56 | 48 | −17 | 10 | −11 |
| 7 | 8, 9, 10, 46ᵃ | 50 | 82 | +17 | 16 | − 5 |
| 8 | 6ᵃ, 8ᵃ, 9ᵃ, 10ᵃ, 46ᵃ | 50 | 40 | −25 | 14 | − 7 |
| 13 | 9, 45, 46, 10ᵃ | 41 | 64 | − 1 | 16 | − 5 |
| 18 | 11 | 39 | 0 | −65 | 6 | −15 |
| 19 | 45 | 48 | 72 | + 7 | 18 | − 3 |
| 21 | 10 | 60 | 58 | − 7 | 14 | − 7 |
| 22 | 9, 10, 46 | 47 | 96 | +31 | 8 | −13 |
| 24 | 6 | 52 | 58 | − 7 | 20 | − 1 |
| 25 | 8, 9, 46, 10ᵃ | 40 | 120 | +55 | 16 | − 5 |
| 27 | 6ᵃ, 8ᵃ, 9ᵃ, 10ᵃ | 60 | 42 | −23 | 24 | + 3 |
| 31 | 9 | 38 | 20 | −45 | 7 | −14 |
| 32 | 9, 8ᵃ, 10ᵃ | 38 | 41 | −24 | 12 | − 9 |
| 33 | 45, 10ᵃ, 44ᵃ, 46ᵃ,ᵇ | 42 | 36 | −29 | 19 | − 2 |
| 36 | 10, 11, 45, 46, 47 | 56 | 50 | −15 | 15 | − 6 |
| 38 | (6ᵃ, 8ᵃ, 9ᵃ) | 36 | 58 | − 7 | 10 | −11 |
| 40 | 24 | 42 | 0 | — | 13 | − 8 |
| 42 | 11 | 36 | 44 | −21 | 12 | − 9 |
| 44 | 47 | 36 | 28 | −37 | 39 | +18 |
| 47 | 44 | 40 | 40 | −25 | 20 | − 1 |
| 49 | 10, 11ᵃ, 46ᵃ | 38 | 90 | +25 | 11 | −10 |
| **Controls:** | | | | | | |
| 5 | | 60 | 80 | | 16 | |
| 16 | | 54 | 65 | | 18 | |
| 23 | | 50 | 36 | | 16 | |
| 30 | | 55 | 80 | | 44 | |
| 35 | | 48 | 0 | | 12 | |

Patient 35 is excluded in calculating the average maximum free acidity since he had achlorhydria. Patient 40 had achlorhydria consistently in all gastric analyses and is therefore not compared to the control maximum average.
ᵃ Indicates partial removal of an area. Otherwise area removals are total or nearly so.
ᵇ In addition to areas indicated, the superior frontal gyrus was presumably destroyed or damaged by ligation of vessels to it.
Areas included within parentheses were presumably affected by ligation of vessels to them. No cortex removed.

TABLE 17.  MAXIMAL ACIDITIES IN THE PSYCHIC PHASE OF SECRETION AS
INDICATED IN THE EPINEPHRINE REHFUSS TEST
(Acidity is expressed in degrees)

| Patient No. | Areas removed | Maximal blood sugar mg. per 100 cc. | Maximal free HCl | Change from control maximum average | Maximal Combined acid | Change from control maximum average |
|---|---|---|---|---|---|---|
| **Operatees:** | | | | | | |
| 2 | 8, 6$^a$ | 173 | 50 | +20 | 9 | − 4.8 |
| 3 | 9, 6$^a$, 8$^a$, 45$^a$ | 140 | 0 | −30 | 12 | − 1.8 |
| 4 | 46, 10$^a$ | 150 | 0 | −30 | 12 | − 1.8 |
| 6 | 6, 8 | 198 | 10 | −20 | 10 | − 3.8 |
| 7 | 8, 9, 10, 46$^a$ | 136 | 44 | +14 | 10 | − 3.8 |
| 8 | 6$^a$, 8$^a$, 9$^a$, 10$^a$, 46$^a$ | 146 | 0 | −30 | 12 | − 1.8 |
| 13 | 9, 45, 46, 10$^a$ | 146 | 66 | +36 | 8 | − 5.8 |
| 18 | 11 | 121 | 0 | −30 | 12 | − 1.8 |
| 19 | 45 | 155 | 19 | −11 | 16 | + 2.2 |
| 21 | 10 | 122 | 44 | +14 | 12 | − 1.8 |
| 22 | 9, 10, 46 | 139 | 58 | +28 | 8 | − 5.8 |
| 24 | 6 | 144 | 15 | −15 | 14 | + 0.2 |
| 25 | 8, 9, 46, 10$^a$ | 135 | 0 | −30 | 7 | − 6.8 |
| 27 | 6$^a$, 8$^a$, 9$^a$, 10$^a$ | 164 | 38 | + 8 | 14 | + 0.2 |
| 31 | 9 | 178 | 0 | −30 | 13 | − 0.8 |
| 32 | 9, 8$^a$, 10$^a$ | 113 | 0 | −30 | 4 | − 9.8 |
| 33 | 45, 10$^a$, 44$^a$, 46$^{a,b}$ | | | | | |
| 36 | 10, 11, 45, 46, 47 | 193 | 38 | + 8 | 32 | +18.2 |
| 38 | (6$^a$, 8$^a$, 9$^a$) | 204 | 28 | − 2 | 13 | − 0.8 |
| 40 | 24 | 167 | 0 | — | 13 | − 0.8 |
| 42 | 11 | 204 | 7 | −23 | 9 | − 4.8 |
| 44 | 47 | | | | | |
| 47 | 44 | | | | | |
| 49 | 10, 11$^a$, 46$^a$ | 182 | 48 | +18 | 12 | − 1.8 |
| **Controls:** | | | | | | |
| 1 | | 149 | 16 | | 9 | |
| 9 | | 204 | 44 | | 17 | |
| 12 | | 182 | 0 | | 12 | |
| 14 | | 163 | 56 | | 14 | |
| 39 | | 114 | 36 | | 17 | |

Patient 40 had achlorhydria consistently in all gastric analyses and is therefore not compared to the control maximum average.

$^a$ Indicates partial removal of an area. Otherwise area removals are total or nearly so.

$^b$ In addition to areas indicated, the superior frontal gyrus was presumably destroyed or damaged by ligation of vessels to it.

Areas included within parentheses were presumably affected by ligation of vessels to them. No cortex removed.

increases was 32 degrees compared to only 10.5 average value for the decreases. Three patients increased 45 degrees or more in their maximum combined acidity which must be considered abnormally high.

The tendency, then, with regard to combined acid is for it to increase following lobotomy. This trend seems to occur also in general but to a lesser extent with removal of areas of frontal cortex, except for that portion towards the frontal pole.

Changes of gastric acidity in the psychic phase of secretion as produced by insulin or epinephrine glycemic stimulation of parasympathetic or sympathetic centers fail to reveal any definite trend following extirpation of various areas of frontal cortex (tables 16, 17). The fact that only 7 out of 24 patients showed increases compared to 16 decreases of maximum free acid values in the insulin test is of only doubtful significance. Even less so is the fact that there were only 8 increases compared to 12 decreases of maximum free acid values in the epinephrine tests. Range of change and average values were comparable in both directions in each type of test. Analysis of data by area removed also showed no trend for specific frontal area extirpations with the exceptions of areas 10 and 11. The removal of area 11 tended to be followed by a decreased free acidity in both the insulin and epinephrine tests whereas there was a similar trend in the opposite direction for area 10.

Changes in the maximal combined acid values in the insulin test during the psychic phase indicate that only 2 out of 24 patients showed an increase compared to decreases in 22 patients below that of the average maximal combined acid value of 5 controls (table 16). In the epinephrine test only 4 patients showed increases compared to decreases in 17 patients below the average maximal combined acid value of 5 other controls (table 17). These changes in both tests were not characteristic of any specific areas. The range of increase and decrease and the average maximal values for these are comparable in each test.

It is perhaps of only incidental interest that the highest combined acid value obtained in both insulin and epinephrine tests occurred in patients who had area 47 removed, once alone and once in combination with other areas.

Thus, changes produced in the psychic phase of gastric acidity following topectomy as measured by insulin and epinephrine tests indicate a definite trend towards decrease of combined acid with a much less definite trend in the same direction for free acid. Whether or not this is a real effect due solely to the removal of cortex or whether it signifies the same effect as occurred in the gastric phase of the control patients, namely a weighted distribution (by reason of the much greater care and supervision provided during the testing and operative period) cannot be determined from the available data.

SUMMARY

Controlled studies of gastric acidity changes were made in 24 patients in the topectomy series and 8 patients undergoing prefrontal lobotomy. No alterations were found in excess of what is considered day-to-day fluctuation in the normal. However, based upon the changes occurring in the peak, free and combined acidities following operation and compared to controls who were handled in an identical manner, the following trends were noted:

Following topectomy or leucotomy a tendency usually develops for the free acid in the stomach to increase in the gastric phase of secretion. This trend towards increased acidity is also true of the combined acid but especially so following lobotomy.

A decrease of acidity, especially of combined acidity, seems to occur in the psychic phase of secretion as determined by insulin and epinephrine Rehfuss tests following topectomy, but this statement is made guardedly since these tests were not fully controlled.

In topectomy, specific tendencies for acidity to decrease are suggested when certain areas towards the frontal pole are removed—for area 9, the free acidity, and for area 9, 10, or 11, the combined acidity, in the gastric phase; and for area 11, the free acidity in the psychic phase.

### EPINEPHRINE TOLERANCE STUDIES

The response to epinephrine was determined before and after operation in the 24 operatees. A series of control patients who, instead of being operated upon were at the same time given a general anesthetic and used as blood donors for the operatees, were tested at similar intervals.

One blood sugar was taken, then 1 cc. of 1/1000 solution of adrenalin chloride was given intramuscularly and samples for blood sugar evaluation were taken at intervals of one-half hour, one hour, one and one-half hours, and two hours. This test was done preoperatively, or before anesthesia in the controls, and repeated five to seven days, ten to sixteen days, and three months after operation or anesthesia.

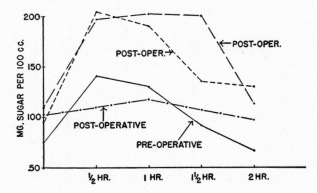

FIG. 74.  Blood sugar curves following administration of epinephrine to patient 36. Time
relationship to operation is indicated on the chart.

Preoperatively the peak of the sugar curves in the operatees ranged between 90 and 155 mg. per 100 cc. of blood. Peak values in the controls were of essentially the same range, 90 to 165 mg. per 100 cc.

In the operatees there was a trend toward an increase in the height of the curve in the seven-to-nine-day postoperative series and also, but to a slightly lesser degree, in the ten-to-sixteen-day postoperative series. In tests made three months after operation most of the peak values were below the preoperative level. Figure 74 in which the 4 curves of patient 36 are charted shows this trend. When the control cases are considered, however, these findings are much less significant because in these cases also there was considerable increase in peak value following anesthesia (fig.75).

When epinephrine tolerance was tested five to seven days after operation there was a considerable rise in the peak value in the operatee series. The greatest rise was 90 mg. per 100 cc. over the preoperative reading. In no instance was there a lower peak although one did not change. The range was therefore 0 to 90 mg. per 100 cc. over the preoperative peak. The average increase in peak value was 36 mg. per 100 cc. There was no correlation between area or amount of tissue removed and fluctuation in sugar response to the epinephrine.

As control in the first postoperative test 20 of the anesthetized patients who were not subjected to operation were used. Changes in peak value for this group ranged from −15 to +85 mg. per 100 cc., the average increase being 26.

For the second postoperative curve determined ten to sixteen days after operation all operatees were again tested. The change in peak value as compared to the pre-operative readings ranged from −10 to +85. The average change was +35. Six anesthetized patients were used as controls for this test. In this group changes from preanesthesia values ranged from 10 to 55 mg. per 100 cc., the average being +26.

Seven operatees were retested three months after operation. In 5 of the 7, peak value of the curve was less than it had been before operation. The range of the change was −35 to +20; the average change was −11. Four patients from the anesthetized group were used as controls. In only one subject was the peak lower than before anesthesia. The range of change was −10 to +40; the average change was +19 mg. per 100 cc.

### DISCUSSION

Our results show wide variations in response to the administration of epinephrine, as measured by blood sugar changes in both operatees and controls. Although the response on the first postoperative test was quite similar in the two groups, in the second test there was greater fluctuation and, on the aver-

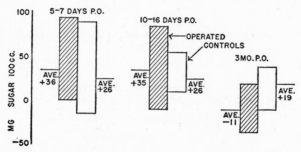

FIG. 75. Range of differences and average difference in peak values of sugar curve at various intervals following operation (or anesthesia in controls).

age, a greater increase in the operatees than in the controls. Results of the third test show a more striking contrast between the two groups. In the control group the average increase was only slightly less than it had been in the first two tests. In the operatee group average change from the first two postoperative tests was more marked. In contrast to 36 mg. per 100 cc. and 35 mg. per 100 cc. above the preoperative peak it was 11 mg. per 100 cc. below.

These results suggest that for a temporary period, following removal of frontal cortex, the sugar response following the administration of epinephrine is increased, but after a few months the response becomes less than it was before operation.

### BLOOD PRESSURE

Blood pressure readings were recorded for all operatees and ten controls before and after operation or anesthesia. One to four readings were charted preoperatively, or following anesthesia, on separate days for each of these patients. These readings were then averaged and treated as a single preoperative or preanesthesia value for each patient. Three determinations were made on each of the 10 controls on successive days during the third postanesthesia month (August 20, 21, and 22, 1947). Blood pressure was also recorded for the operatees on those same three days and, for both operatees and controls, these were averaged to give a single postoperative value for each in the third month after operation or anesthesia. In addition to these determinations, daily blood pressures were recorded for each operatee beginning the day of operation and continuing for approximately one month thereafter. For the first one or two weeks after operation, multiple readings were recorded (two to eleven daily) and these were averaged to give a single daily value. In the latter part of the first postoperative month only one blood pressure reading was recorded daily.

All pressures were determined on one arm by the usual sphygmomanometric method, a mercury manometer being used. All readings were taken early in the morning while the patient was in the reclining position and before he had gotten out of bed. In the case of the operatees whose pressure was measured several times daily immediately after operation, the pressures were always measured while the subject was in the reclining position although many of the patients were ambulatory between readings. Various observers, including ward nurses, determined the daily blood pressure reading for the operatees during the first postoperative month. The preoperative readings and those taken in the third postoperative month, however, were recorded by the same physicians and therefore are presumably subject to the same variations in technique for all patients at all times.

TABLE 18. AVERAGE CHANGES IN BLOOD PRESSURE READINGS MADE IN THIRD POSTOPERATIVE (OR POSTANESTHESIA) MONTH

| | Increase of 5 mm. or more | | Decrease of 5 mm. or more | | Number of patients showing less than 5-mm. change |
|---|---|---|---|---|---|
| | Number of patients | Average change in mm. | Number of patients | Average change in mm. | |
| Systolic pressure in | | | | | |
| Operatees.......... | 5 | 9 | 8 | 12 | 11 |
| Controls............ | 6 | 13 | 1 | 19 | 3 |
| Diastolic pressure in | | | | | |
| Operatees.......... | 12 | 9 | 4 | 10 | 8 |
| Controls............ | 8 | 13 | 1 | 17 | 1 |

In the subsequent discussion, diastolic values always refer to the point at which sound disappeared. The higher diastolic level (change in quality of the sound) was also determined before operation and in the third month after, but in evaluating pre- and postoperative changes the lower value has been used as one which is sharper and less liable to error through differences in individual technique.

In the group as a whole, no hypertensive patients were represented. In the control group the preanesthesia extremes of variation were 91/52 to 120/80; in the operatees the preoperative extremes were 93/56 to 126/75.

#### ANALYSIS OF DATA

In the third postoperative month the control patients showed an average increase of 5.8 mm. in the systolic pressure and a diastolic increase of 8.5 mm. The maximum variations of +24/+21 and −19/−17 were found in patients 15 and 34, respectively. Over the same period the average systolic pressure of the operatee group fell 1.9 mm. while the average diastolic value rose 3.1 mm. The maximum variations of +15/+15 and −15/−17 were found in patients 38 and 25 respectively. The number of patients participating in these changes as compared with those in the control group is presented in table 18 where the groups are arranged by increase or decreases of 5 mm.

or more, the remaining patients being placed in a "stable" group. It is apparent that the range of variation among the operatees is less than in the controls, whether the measurement is by relative numbers in any one deviating group or by average change (in mm. of mercury) recorded for that group. Thus we must conclude that three months after operation no general effect on blood pressure can be found.

In considering those blood pressure values obtained for the operatees during the month immediately after surgery we find that there was an average fall from the preoperative systolic level amounting to 6.5 mm. and a diastolic fall of 1.7 mm. The extremes in this group were +18/+20 and −21/−18, found in patients 19 and 42 respectively. It was felt that these average values might reflect the bed rest and general surgical trauma to which the patients had been exposed rather than a physiologic effect of area removal. Therefore the values of the first two weeks after operation were ignored and the average values of the succeeding weeks (June 16 to June 29, 1947) were compared with the preoperative averages. These differences are shown in table 19 along with the control values for the third postoperative month. If one assumes that two weeks are sufficient to allow for recovery from the general

TABLE 19.   AVERAGE CHANGES IN BLOOD PRESSURE READINGS IN THIRD AND FOURTH POSTOPERATIVE WEEKS IN OPERATEES

(As compared with their preoperative averages and control values for third postanesthesia month)

|  | Increase of 5 mm. or more | | Decrease of 5 mm. or more | | Number of patients showing less than 5-mm. change |
|---|---|---|---|---|---|
|  | Number of patients | Average change in mm. | Number of patients | Average change in mm. |  |
| Systolic pressure in |  |  |  |  |  |
| Operatees........... | 2 | 15 | 17 | 16 | 5 |
| Controls............ | 6 | 13 | 1 | 19 | 3 |
| Diastolic pressure in |  |  |  |  |  |
| Operatees........... | 3 | 11 | 14 | 10 | 7 |
| Controls............ | 8 | 13 | 1 | 17 | 1 |

effects of craniotomy then it is apparent that there is a trend toward lowering of the systolic and diastolic pressure among the patients operated upon in the first month after operation. This trend is apparent only in the number of patients involved and is not reflected in the average fall in mm. when that fall is compared with the control. (The control is of little value, consisting of only 1 patient.) More than half of the patients operated upon participated in a fall of more than 5 mm. of mercury as compared with one-tenth of the control patients, while the majority of control patients took part in a postoperative increase in pressure as compared to a very small number of operatees who showed a similar increase. Unfortunately, the control values are those of the third month and therefore not directly comparable, but this would not seem to invalidate the findings since the blood pressure changes in the two groups were strikingly different.

Not all operatees participated in the fall, however, and many variables were considered in an attempt to discover a factor or factors responsible for the lowered postoperative pressure. No differences could be attributed to the site of operation or amount of cortex removed, to the degree of clinical recovery, or the clinical diagnosis given the patient. Similarly, age and sex did not appear to be determining factors. A comparison of those patients who showed a systolic fall greater than 5 mm. with those who showed little change or an increase in pressure suggests that removal of the caudal and dorsal areas of frontal cortex (areas 6 and 8) does not usually produce a fall in blood pressure. The more rostral removals, on the other hand, were most often incriminated when pressure fell, but more patients must be studied before even this finding can be accepted.

### SUMMARY

The available data indicate that a small but apparently significant drop in both systolic and diastolic pressure occurred in more than half of the operatees. This fall in pressure was maintained throughout the first postoperative month, but by the third postoperative month no significant difference was present between the operatees and controls. These findings cannot be related to area removed or to any other single variable which was considered. Whether the temporary fall in pressure is dependent upon a combination of factors (such as the general region ablated plus weight of cortex removed) cannot be determined until more patients are studied.

## WEIGHT

### FLUCTUATIONS FOLLOWING ABLATION OF FRONTAL CORTEX

A record of each patient's weight was kept before and after operation or anesthesia. Each patient was weighed (clothed) from one to three times in the six weeks before operation or anesthesia and from three to nine times during

TABLE 20.  FLUCTUATIONS IN WEIGHT IN OPERATEES AND CONTROL PATIENTS THREE MONTHS AFTER OPERATION

|  | Number of patients | Average increase or decrease (lbs.) |
|---|---|---|
| Operatees showing more than 5 lbs. increase.............. | 12 | 15.5 |
| Operatees showing more than 5 lbs. decrease............. | 4 | 8.0 |
| Operatees showing less than 5 lbs. change................ | 8 |  |
| Control patients showing more than 5 lbs. increase........ | 8 | 12.4 |
| Control patients showing more than 5 lbs. decrease........ | 1 | 6.0 |
| Control patients showing less than 5 lbs. change........... | 15 |  |

the first four months after operation or anesthesia. Most patients had eight or nine weights recorded in the first four postoperative or postanesthesia months, the few exceptions being among the patients who were making home visits or whose behavior was too disturbed to make weighing practical. A single weight was obtained for each patient in the seventh postoperative or postanesthesia month. All weights were recorded in pounds.

A trend toward increase in weight was present preoperatively in the operatees; the control patients showed a similar trend during the preanesthesia period. The operatee group averaged 3.0 pounds gain in weight before operation with individual variations from −5 to +16 pounds. The control patients showed an average gain of 1.7 pounds with individual variations from −14 to +12 pounds. The preoperative and preanesthesia weight gains can presumably be explained on the basis of improved nutrition following transfer to the special ward, where nursing and attendant care were more plentiful than in other wards of the hospital.

TABLE 21. CORRELATION OF WEIGHT CHANGES THREE MONTHS AFTER OPERATION, WITH VARIOUS FACTORS IN PATIENTS' BACKGROUND

(The 8 patients with greatest changes and 8 with least change are used)

| Patient number | Average preoperative weight | Preoperative weight trend | Weight change lbs. ± | Weight change percent ± | Areas removed | Weight of brain removed (Gm.) | Clinical improvement | Diagnosis |
|---|---|---|---|---|---|---|---|---|
| 2♂ | 130 | Stable | +14 | +10.8 | 8 | 17.4 | 0 | Schizophrenia, hebephrenic |
| 8♂ | 161 | Stable | +12 | +7.5 | 8* 9* 10* 46* | 30.0 | 0 | Schizophrenia, paranoid |
| 19♂ | 133 | Rising | +17 | +12.8 | 45 | 11.8 | 0 | Schizophrenia with affective and Psychopathic features |
| 25♂ | 129 | Stable | +18 | +14.0 | 8 9 46 | 37.4 | 8 | Involutional psychosis, depression |
| 33♀ | 111 | Stable | +32 | +28.8 | 10* 44 45 46* | 29.6 | 8 | Schizophrenia, catatonic |
| 38♀ | 111 | Stable | +34 | +30.6 | 6 8 9 (vein ligation) 11 | None | 8 | Manic-depressive, manic |
| 42♀ | 134 | Unstable | +10 | +7.5 | 11 | 27.0 | 5 | Manic-depressive, manic |
| 49♀ | 122 | Unstable | +14 | +11.5 | 10 | 42.1 | 5 | Schizophrenia, paranoid |
| 3♂ | 156 | ? Rising | −1 | −0.7 | 9 | No Data | 2 | Involutional psychosis, mixed |
| 4♂ | 124 | Stable | +1 | +0.8 | 46 | 20.8 | 2 | Schizophrenia, paranoid |
| 21♂ | 152 | Stable | +4 | +2.6 | 10 | 25.4 | 6 | Manic-depressive, depressed |
| 22♂ | 141 | Stable | +1 | +0.7 | 9 10 46 | 49.4 | 5 | Schizophrenia, paranoid |
| 27♂ | 198 | Stable | +4 | +2.0 | 6* 8* 9* | 55.0 | 7 | Schizophrenia, hebephrenic |
| 31♀ | 100 | Stable | +3 | +3.0 | 9 | 33.1 | 1 | Involutional psychosis, paranoid |
| 32♀ | 120 | Unknown | −3 | −2.5 | 8 9 | 29.8 | 0 | Manic-depressive, manic |
| 40♀ | 101 | Stable | +2 | +2.0 | 24 32 | 14.2 | 0 | Schizophrenia, paranoid |

* Indicates partial removal.

**Analysis of Data.**  Differences were observed in the operatee and control groups in the postoperative period. Some of the patients upon whom operation was performed showed a decrease in weight of 1 to 10 pounds immediately after operation (patients 3, 13, 19, 21, 24, 27, 33, 36, 40, 42, 44, 47, 49). This appeared to be related to debilitation and temporary interference with nutrition consequent to surgery. Thereafter these patients returned to their preoperative weights or took part in further increases in weight along with the other operatees. The weight trend of the control patients did not change after anesthesia. The average increase (measured during the thirteenth to fifteenth postoperative weeks) was 6.8 pounds among the operatees and 4.2 pounds among the controls.

A tabulation of this material is presented in table 20 which indicates that a significant increase in weight was present in the operatees at the end of three months but that only half of the patients operated upon participated in it (patients 2, 7, 8, 18, 19, 24, 25, 33, 38, 42, 44, 49). On the other hand, 8 of the control patients showed similarly large gains but the weight of the majority (15) of control patients remained stable as compared with the average preanesthesia weights.

In the seventh postoperative month a single weighing indicated that 10 of the operatees had gained more than 5 pounds since the fourth postoperative month (patients 3, 8, 18, 19, 21, 27, 31, 33, 42, 49). Patients who were subjected to reoperation or lobotomy were excluded from this group. During this period the average gain for the group was 7.7 pounds and the extremes of variation were +40 pounds (patient 27) and −7 pounds (patient 13). During the same period the control group (excluding those who had had lobotomies) showed an average gain of 4.1 pounds. Only 5 of the 18 patients participated in a gain of 5 pounds or more. The limits of variation were +34 pounds (patient 37) and −15 pounds (patient 29).

In an attempt to evaluate the possible variables involved, table 21 was drawn up comparing various patients regarding their weight changes three months after operation. In it the 8 patients showing the greatest increase in weight at that time (10 pounds or more) are contrasted with the 8 patients showing the least change after operation. Data are included regarding sex, average preoperative weight, preoperative weight trend, number of pounds gained or lost, percentage of gain or loss measured on the basis of preoperative weight, areas of cortex and weight of cortex removed, degree of clinical improvement as measured by the weighted score and diagnosis. No one of these variables appears to be significant in itself. Which variables might be important in combination with one another cannot be determined from the limited number of patients studied.

**Summary.**  Both operatees and control patients showed a tendency as a group to gain small amounts of weight before operation or anesthesia. Seven months after operation the average weight gain among the operatees was 14.5 pounds; the average gain in the control group for the same period following anesthesia was only 8.3 pounds. Variations in weight were similar among individual patients of the two groups but an outstanding difference which emerged between the operatees and controls after operation or anesthesia was in the relative numbers of patients participating in a weight gain. A few operatees gained very large amounts of weight, but this was also true of some of the controls. Neither the type of operation nor the patient's response to it could be correlated with changes in weight.

FLUCTUATIONS FOLLOWING LOBOTOMY

Eight patients who were operated upon by the conventional lobotomy technique late in October, 1947, were also studied for changes in weight. Two of these patients (2 and 44) had had previous topectomies and the other 6 were selected from the original control group. All 8 patients were weighed ten times over a two and one-half-month period following lobotomy. During this period they showed an average gain of 4.25 pounds, an amount which is comparable to that seen in the topectomy group over a similar period. The individual extremes of variation among these lobotomized patients are also comparable, −8 to +16 pounds (44 and 11 respectively). A longer follow-up will be needed before direct comparisons can be made, but at this point it appears that the effects of lobotomy and topectomy on body weight are similar.

*Chapter 7*

# Laboratory Findings

## (*continued*)

CARL M. SAGERT, FRED A. METTLER, ELSIE EMMEL,
LAWRENCE ROTHFIELD, MALCOLM B. CARPENTER,
WILLIAM H. LONGLEY, Jr., JOHN J. WEBER,
AND H. HARVEY GASS

T HE present chapter is concerned with observations on the hemoglobin, formed elements of the blood (erythrocytes, reticulocytes, leucocytes), circulating minerals (calcium, potassium, and sodium), urea nitrogen, blood creatinine, and fasting reducing substances of the blood. (For a consideration of gastric acidity and sugar responses to special procedures see pp. 83-97.) Blood Wassermann reactions were negative on all patients (except in patient 46 who yielded a false positive reaction on one occasion). No tests were run on spinal fluid.

As is well known, a variety of autonomic effects have been reported upon stimulation of the frontal lobe or after removal of parts of it. While only distally affected by such autonomic changes, the substances investigated herewith might be expected to be susceptible to alteration as a result of drastic and prolonged autonomic imbalance, if such occurs after subtotal removal of frontal cortex. Moreover, there is a certain body of evidence to indicate that interference with the rostral portion of the brain does cause disturbances detectable in certain spheres of the present investigation. Mettler ('43) has reported alterations in the canine reticulocyte count after total, simultaneous, bilateral frontal decortication which were not found after occipital ablation. The phenomenon has been interpreted as a response to visceral vasostasis which precipitates a relative peripheral anemia. Whether such a phenomenon occurs after subtotal frontal decortication in the human being is unknown. Heath, working in the laboratories of the Department of Neurology, has encountered alterations in the blood sugar and profound disturbance in blood sodium levels after bilateral striatal ablation. Whether a cortical factor is of importance in such phenomena is unknown. Sweet, Kotzias, Seed, and Yakovlev ('48) have recently reported disordered metabolic phenomena following an ultimately fatal lobotomy. Whether such disorderly phenomena can be precipitated by cortical disconnection alone or, as seems more probable, were caused in this case by deep damage is not known. Finally, it might be supposed that the present investigation might throw some light on the not inconsiderable number of changes detectable by ordinary laboratory methods which have been reported to be related with psychic disturbances (as the well-known rise in blood sugar which is precipitated by emotional stress, the undisturbed differential leucocytosis found by Milhorat, Small, and Diethelm ('42) to also accompany psychic tension or the various alterations reported from Hoskins' laboratory at the Worcester State Hospital), although the probability of encountering alterations in these spheres by ablations so small and restricted as the present is, of course, remote.

<h2 style="text-align:center">PROCEDURE</h2>

Each of the patients in the operatee and control groups previously described (p. 21-23) received an average of three tests (given laboratory procedures were always performed by the same individual) during the sixty-day preoperative or preanesthesia period to determine the basic levels in each of the study categories reported herewith. After the visit to the surgery, whether the subject had been operated upon or not, follow-up studies were made to the extent demanded by the circumstances in each case. Thus, patient 15, who developed pneumonia, is excluded from the present studies from the time of the inception of his infectious disease. Also excluded from the control series (except in reticulocyte studies) are patients 41 and 48 on whom inadequate data are available. Further, in about half of the control patients the number of complete studies in the postanesthesia period was limited to one, if this fell well within the previous range of findings. However, about half of the control patients were followed just as fully as the operatees in order to detect any alterations which may have occurred as group phenomena had they appeared. In all patients (operatees as well as controls) in whom complete retests were done such tests were performed during the first two weeks after the visit to the surgery beginning with the fourth postoperative or postanesthesia day. In order to offset to some degree the factors resulting from mere blood loss and the effects of simple anesthesia in the operatees and also to obtain blood *pro re nata* for the patients actually operated upon the control patients were phlebotomized (to the extent of 500 cc.) while under narcosis induced by intravenous sodium pentothal. It should be pointed out at this place that it was not considered advisable to phlebotomize all the control patients nor invariably to employ more than minimal amounts of pentothal. Most of the operatees received some blood and plasma during the actual operation (see table 10) and a few also received intravenous saline or glucose or both on the day afterward. Patient 47 received intravenous saline and glucose on the third day after operation. It is unlikely that the laboratory findings were influenced by this but patient 33 received glucose and saline intravenously for four days after operation and also patient 24. The latter patient received additional intravenous fluid on the seventh day after operation. These two patients should be kept in mind in evaluating the results described in the succeeding pages.

<h2 style="text-align:center">RESULTS</h2>

<h3 style="text-align:center">HEMOGLOBIN</h3>

**Analysis of Combined Error.** All hemoglobin determinations were read on the Haden-Hausser hemoglobinometer and expressed to the nearest half gram as grams per 100 cc. of blood. In the preoperative period there was a total of 138 tests. Variations within an individual patient's determinations over 2 gm. occurred but three times; variations of between 1 to 2 gm. occurred nineteen times. We therefore conclude that any repeated variation of more than 1.5 gm. could be safely considered significant.

**Group as a Whole.** Preoperative hemoglobin levels ranged from 11 gm. per 100 cc. (4 cases, 1 operatee) to 15 gm. (2 cases, 1 operatee). Frequencies in intervening ranges were 11.5 (4, 1 operatee), 12.0 (7, all operatees), 12.5 (4, 2 operatees), 13.0 (9, 4 operatees), 13.5 (9, 4 operatees), 14.0 (6, 3 operatees), 14.5 (1, operatee).

**Controls.** Among the controls significant changes were encountered only in patients 5, 12, and 17 in whom the readings were as follows (readings obtained after visit to surgery marked with asterisk): for patient 5: 14, 13.5, 13.5, 12*, 12*, 11* gm.; for patient 12: 11, 11, 11, 9.5*, 9.5*, 10* gm.; and for patient 17: 12, 11, 11.5, 11*, 10*, 9.5* gm.

**Operatees.** All operatees showed postoperative drops of 1.5 gm. or more (only one patient, 40, showed such a minimal drop, 12.5, 12.5, 12, 10.5*, 9.5*, 10.5*). Drops of from 2.0 to 2.5 were exhibited by patients 4, 33, 38, 44, 47, 49; from 3.0 to 3.5 by patients 7, 13, 18, 21, 22, 25, 36, 42; from 4.0 to 4.5 by patients 2, 3, 19, 31; 5.0 to 5.5 by patient 6; and from 6.0 to 6.5 gm. by patients 8, 24, 27, 32.

### ERYTHROCYTES

**Analysis of Combined Error.** In the preoperative period 138 erythrocyte counts were made on the group considered here. Variation between any of three counts made on any given individual during this sixty-day period was less than 200,000 in 4 cases; from 300 to 400 thousand, 16 cases; 500 to 600 thousand, 14 cases. Variations of from 700 to 800 thousand occurred six times; between 900,000 and 1,000,000, five times; and between 1,100,000 and 1,200,000, once. Assuming that all these patients had an absolutely static cytology, presumably wholly erroneous counts, i.e. beyond a standard laboratory error of 500,000, may have therefore been anticipated in not over 8 percent of the readings. Since it is obvious that the cytology of the group was not constant we shall be perfectly safe if we require that data considered to be significant be outside this range.

**Group as a Whole.** Preoperative levels (in millions) ranged from 4.6 to 5.0 in 9 patients (3 operatees), from 4.1 to 4.5 in 22 patients (13 operatees), and from 3.6 to 4.0 in 14 patients (8 operatees); in one patient the level was 3.4.

**Controls.** Drops of over 500,000 were encountered in 4 cases: 700,000 in case 10 and 800,000 in cases 26, 34, and 46.

**Operatees.** Among the operatees the erythrocyte count dropped (in thousands) from 500 to 800 in patients 42, 44, 47, and 49; from 900 to 1,200, in patients 4, 7, 25, 33, 36, and 38; from 1,300 to 1,600 in patients 2, 3, 6, 8, 13, 18, 21, and 22; from 1,700 to 1,900 in patients 27 and 31; from 2,000 to 2,500 in patients 24 and 32. In patient 19, the drop was 2,800 thousand and in patient 40 it was 400 thousand.

**Interpretation of Results.** As might have been expected, the decreases in hemoglobin values and erythrocyte counts were quite comparable from case to case. It is evident that the observed phenomena could be due to either hemorrhage or visceral vasostasis. That it was due to hemorrhage is to some degree offset by the observation that with the exception of the cortical extirpations the operative procedures were relatively constant and one is forced to assume that particular ablations involved much greater losses of blood than others. While unquestionable variation existed in this respect there is no evidence that the largest drops occurred in the patients with the largest excisions and the smallest drops in those with the smallest excisions. An interesting comparison in this connection may be made between patients 38 and 40. Thus patient 38, in whom no excision was made, though the direction of drainage of the blood through the cortex was altered, showed a greater drop in erythrocytes (and hemoglobin) than did patient 40 in whom an ablation had been performed.

If one examines the location of the ablations which were followed by the most significant drops one is impressed by the fact that the smallest drops occurred in patients with lesions far forward or ventrally placed. Larger drops were not necessarily confined to patients having dorsocaudally situated ablations. It is interesting to observe that 8 of the 11 patients with minor drops were females. An interesting inverse correlation between the intensity of the psychotic manifestation and the amount of hemoglobin (and number of erythrocytes) was observed in several instances in patient 19.

### RETICULOCYTES

**Method.** Reticulocyte counts were performed by placing 1 drop of capillary blood on a clean, dry coverglass which was immediately inverted on a slide covered with a dried film of a saturated alcoholic solution of brilliant cresyl blue. After five minutes 1,000 red blood corpuscles were counted, and the number of reticulocytes observed in this sample was divided by 10 to arrive at the reticulocyte percentage.

**Procedure.** Before the visits to surgery three reticulocyte counts were made at intervals of at least two days on all but 1 operatee (33), on whom no preoperative records are available, and on all but 2 controls (15 and 29), on whom only 2 preanesthesia counts were made. Commencing on the fourth or fifth postoperative day, reticulocyte counts were repeated.

**Analysis of Laboratory Error.** No operatee or control showed a difference of more than 1.1 per hundred erythrocytes between any two preoperative or preanesthesia reticulocyte counts. The greatest range of normal day-to-day variation, plus experimental error, was therefore set at 1.1 per hundred erythrocytes.

**Group as a Whole.** In the entire group, 140 reticulocyte counts before the visit to surgery ranged from 0.1 to 1.6 percent. Individual patients showed average preoperative or preanesthesia reticulocyte counts ranging from 0.5 to 1.2 percent with frequencies as follows: 9 patients (3 operatees), from 0.5 to 0.69 percent; 20 patients (10 operatees), from 0.7 to 0.89 percent; 10 patients (3 operatees), from 0.9 to 1.09 percent; and 8 patients (7 operatees), from 1.1 to 1.2 percent. The average preoperative or preanesthesia reticulocyte count was 0.87 percent. Counts ranged from 0.2 to 1.4 percent in the control group and from 0.1 to 1.6 percent in the operatee group. Average preoperative or postanesthesia reticulocyte counts of individual cases ranged from 0.5 to 1.1 percent in the control group and from 0.6 to 1.2 percent in the operatee group. This indicates that the two groups were nearly identical prior to visit to surgery.

**Controls.** Following the visit to surgery reticulocyte counts in the control group ranged from 0.1 to 2.1 percent as compared with a previous range of 0.2 to 1.4 percent. Reticulocyte counts on the control group taken on the ninth day following the visit to surgery generally showed some slight rise but not exceeding the range of preanesthesia variation. No patients in the control group showed an increase in any one postanesthesia reticulocyte count of more than 1.1 per hundred erythrocytes over their preanesthesia average. Only 2 controls showed an increase in any one postanesthesia reticulocyte count of between 0.8 and 1.1 per hundred erythrocytes above the preanesthesia average. No controls showed a decrease in any one postanesthesia reticulocyte count of greater than 0.8 per hundred erythrocytes below their preanesthesia average. It can then apparently be concluded that the visit to surgery (loss of blood plus anesthesia) resulted in no determinable significant changes in the reticulocyte counts of any member of the control group. The greatest range of variation from pre- to postanesthesia period is 1.1 per hundred erythrocytes. Since this figure has also been accepted as the greatest range of experimental error and day-to-day variation, no changes of less than 1.1 per hundred erythrocytes in the operatee group, following operation, can be called significant.

**Operatees.** Postoperative reticulocyte counts on operatees range from 0.6 to 4.4 percent as compared to a preoperative range of 0.1 to 1.6 percent. Seven patients showed no increase (4, 25, 27, 42, 44) or a barely minimal increase (3, 22) of greater than 1.1 per hundred erythrocytes from their preoperative average on any one postoperative test. Fifteen patients showed a significant increase of greater than 1.1 percent over their preoperative average in any one postoperative test as follows: significant differences between preoperative average and highest postoperative count (peak response) of 1.1 to 2.0 per hundred erythrocytes in 5 patients (2, 32, 36, 40, 49); of 2.1 to 2.9 percent in 8 patients (6, 7, 13, 18, 19, 21, 24, 38); of 3.0 to 3.47 percent in 2 patients (8, 47). It is clear that there was a general rise in reticulocyte counts of the operatee group following operation· (fig. 76). Patient 31 is excluded from the above analysis because tests were not performed over the critical postoperative period.

Patient 33 has no preoperative record and can be judged solely by comparison with the general preoperative averages. Preoperative averages ranged from 0.5 to 1.2 percent. Since patient 33 showed a peak postoperative reticulocyte count of 3.0 percent (1.8 percent over the maximum preoperative average discovered), she is considered to have shown a significant, positive reticulocyte response.

**Interpretation of Results.** There was no apparent correlation between intravenous administration of whole blood or other fluids, during or after the operation, and reticulocyte response. Neither was a correlation apparent between volume of tissue excised and reticulocyte response. Although a general drop in erythrocyte count and hemoglobin values was noted in the operatee group it proved impossible to correlate specific reticulocyte responses with corresponding erythrocyte and hemoglobin changes

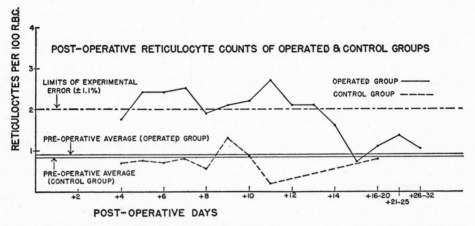

FIG. 76. In this figure it is obvious that the operatees, as a group, showed a definite post-operative reticulocytosis which fell to normal levels in about two weeks. The expression "limits of experimental error" should be interpreted in the light of a laboratory error of 1.1 reticulocytes per hundred erythrocytes, not 1.1 percent error of the normal level, which in this series was itself less than one reticulocyte percent.

owing to the limitations of the data secured (i.e. tests were not always made on identical days, and reticulocyte responses were, in general, followed for a longer period of time than were erythrocytes and hemoglobin). Further investigation into the inter-relationships of these responses, however, is most strongly indicated by the present study.

A correlation of reticulocyte responses and areal removals, on the other hand, produced the following interesting observations.

Area 46 was removed alone in 1 patient (4), and this patient showed no significant postoperative variation from his preoperative level. In 3 patients (4, 22, 25) from whom all of area 46 was completely removed (either alone or in combination with other areas) a barely minimal (22) or no significant increase over preoperative levels was observed. It would then be indicated that removal of area 46 does not exert in itself an influence tending to produce increases in the reticulocyte percentage of the blood. Although the reticulocyte response was notable in cases 13 and 36 in which area 46 was removed in connection with other areas it is apparent that these cases must owe their elevation to some factor other than removal of area 46.

In 3 cases (3, 22, and 25) in which area 9 was removed in combination with other areas, a barely minimal or no significant increase was noted. In 1 case (27) where the upper part of area 9 was ablated (together with the rest of the superior frontal gyrus) no significant increase was observed. It would thus seem that removal of area 9 exerts a very negligible effect, if any, on the reticulocyte percentage of the blood. As in the case of ablation of area 46 some other cases in which area 9 was removed, notably 13 and 32 (case 31 was excluded for the reason given above) the significant rises encountered in these cases must be due to some other factor.

Area 44 was removed alone in 1 patient (47), who showed the highest postoperative increase of the entire operatee group. The other patient (33) in whom area 44 was removed also showed a definite postoperative increase in reticulocyte percentage. Removal of area 44 can therefore be concluded to exert in itself an elevating influence on reticulocytes in the blood.

Area 45 was removed alone in 1 case (19), and a definite increase over the preoperative level was noted. In all cases where this area was completely removed definite increases were observed. Removal of area 45 thus apparently exerts an elevating influence on reticulocyte percentage in the blood.

Area 10 was removed alone in 1 case (21). In this patient a definite increase over preoperative reticulocyte levels was noted. When area 10 was notably encroached upon (7, 8, 21, 22, 33, 36, 49) 6 of these 7 patients showed significant postoperative increases over their preoperative reticulocyte levels. The remaining patient (22, in whom area 10 was completely removed in combination with areas 9 and 46) showed a minimal significant increase on the fourth postoperative day. Other postoperative reticulocyte tests on this patient were made on the seventh and ninth days following operation. This suggests the possibility that instead of the increase of just more than 1.1 percent over preoperative levels which was observed on the fourth postoperative day a more significant increase might have occurred on other postoperative days on which no reticulocyte counts were done. This possibility is borne out by the postoperative dates of most frequent postoperative peaks, to be given later in this section. Removal of area 10 then apparently has, in itself, an influence tending to produce increases in the reticulocyte percentage of the blood.

In those patients (6 and 24) from whom large amounts of area 6 were removed (except for the caudal part), significant increases were observed above the preoperative levels. In patient 27, in whom only the upper part of area 6 was removed as part of the superior frontal gyrus, no significant increase was noted during the period of postoperative reticulocyte counts. Postoperative reticulocyte counts were performed on this patient between the fourth and eighth postoperative days. If a significant increase (over 1.1 percent above preoperative levels) occurred in this patient before the fourth postoperative day or after the eighth postoperative day it would not have been observed by the procedure employed. The possibility exists that a significant increase might have taken place in this patient, in spite of our lack of evidence in that direction. These data, then, apparently indicate that removal of area 6 is sufficient in itself to produce a significant rise in reticulocyte percentage in the blood. The possibility is also indicated, but not definitely confirmed, that removal of the upper part of area 6 is not in itself a causative factor in increasing the reticulocyte percentage of the blood.

Area 24 was partly removed in one patient (40). A significant increase over the preoperative level was noted in this patient following operation.

Of 2 patients (18 and 42) in whom area 11 was removed without encroachment upon other areas, one (18) showed a significant increase in reticulocyte count, and the other (42) showed no significant rise. In one other patient (36) in whom area 11 was removed as part of a more extensive ablation, a significant rise occurred but this elevation can probably be attributed to other excised areas in this removal. No valid conclusions can be drawn about the effect of removal of this very small area until additional cases are accumulated.

Similarly, contradictory and inadequate data from supposed removals of area 8 require additional results before any attempt at correlating response with areal removal can be attempted.

No apparent correlation between areal removals and the day of first postoperative peak was noted. Postoperative peaks occurred as follows: fourth postoperative day, in patients 22 and 6; sixth postoperative day, in 8, 7, 3, and 49; seventh postoperative day, in 47, 18, 19, 24, 36, and 2; ninth postoperative day, in 13, 21, 38, and 40; tenth postoperative day, in 32. In all patients showing significant increases postoperative peaks in reticulocyte percentages in the blood were therefore reached by the tenth postoperative day, with the greatest incidence on the sixth, seventh, and ninth postoperative days.

All reticulocyte counts had returned to normal limits by the twenty-seventh postoperative day. In most patients the reticulocyte percentage returned to normal limits somewhere between the tenth and sixteenth postoperative day.

In evaluating the previously given correlations between reticulocyte responses and areal removals in each individual case, it must be borne in mind that the separate Brodmann areas removed in this series are not necessarily, and, indeed, are individually most unlikely to be the functional areas concerned with these responses. Thus, even though an area is excised which contains within itself a part of the tissue concerned with producing these variations, it may include so small a portion of the functional area that the limits of physiologic safety of the mechanism are not exceeded and no response is observed. It is apparent too, that although a single Brodmann area, when removed in its entirety, produces a positive response (as area 6), only a part of the excised tissue may be functionally concerned with the mechanism. The positive and negative effects ascribed to the removal of certain Brodmann areas do not in themselves delimit, therefore, the functional areas concerned with this mechanism, but merely serve roughly to indicate the outlines of any such areas.

### LEUCOCYTES

Since no postoperative infectious processes were detected one would expect that the degree of leucocytosis might be of value as indicative of any unusual degree of postoperative cortical malacia such as might have occurred as a result of inadvertent interference with blood supply of parts of the cortex which were not excised. Further one would expect in those cases which showed the most notable degrees of hemoglobin and erythrocyte decreases, that the inevitable postoperative leucocytosis would be to some extent offset. Finally, we have seen that Milhorat, Small, and Diethelm ('42) have encountered changes in the total leucocyte count, without shifting, in psychic disturbances.

**Analysis of Combined Error.** Of the 138 preoperative or preanesthesia leucocyte counts, individual variations, between three counts per patient, of from 0 to 3,000 occurred seven times; of from 4,000 to 6,000, twelve times; of from 7,000 to 9,000, twelve times; of from 10,000 to 12,000, nine times; and of 13,000 or over, six times. Such figures, in relation to an examination such as the leucocyte count, conducted over such a protracted period of time, especially where definite trends, either ascending or descending, are evident, are not of particular value in arriving at the factor of laboratory error but are nevertheless included for the sake of completeness.

**Group as a Whole.** Leucocyte levels ranged from 6,000 to 15,000 per cu. mm. (1 patient at the latter level was an operatee). The figures were as follows (in thousands): 6 to 8 (22 cases, 12 operatees), 9 to 11 (14 cases, 6 operatees), 12 to 14 (9 cases, 5 operatees).

**Controls.** Among the control patients, 4 of 19 exhibited a somewhat elevated leucocyte response after their visit to the surgery, 13 showed no change, and 2 displayed a decrease.

**Operatees.** In contrast to this lack of alteration, 15 (patients 2, 3, 6, 7, 19, 21, 25, 27, 32, 36, 38, 40, 42, 47, 49) of the 24 operatees exhibited an increased leucocyte count. Seven patients showed no change and 2 (4, 22) a decreased count. Of three counts on postoperative days two, four, and six the second was highest in 12 patients (of whom 10 were patients who established higher averages during this six-day period than they had previously exhibited).

**Interpretation of Results.** The extremely transitory nature of the response in these 12 cases argues against the existence of a continuing process of resorption of unviable tissue. Progressively increasing counts which established higher postoperative than preoperative averages occurred in patients 6 (the leucocyte count began to decline on the tenth postoperative day in this patient), 18, and 49 and it is possible that a certain amount of extension of the operative site continued in these patients.

There is nothing to indicate that variations in the "resting" leucocyte counts in these cases were directly influenced by neurophysiologic alterations. It is possible, of course, that fundamental changes were obscured by dilution of the formed elements of the blood, but this possibility cannot be profitably pursued here. Before discarding the leucocyte count as an indicator of cortically induced phenomena, however, future studies of this type should explore the possibilities of a more protracted period of counting. Further, blood counts should be correlated with the ingestion of glucose so that information bearing upon a possible alteration in the blood-sugar lymphocyte relationship reported by Freeman and Elmadjian ('47) can be obtained. So far as could be determined there was no relation whatsoever to area or amount of cortex removed. It is interesting to observe that there was no definite correlation between the behavior of the erythrocytes and leucocytes. Thus, of the 2 patients (22 and 40) who proved relatively stable with regard to red count, one (22) showed a decrease in the leucocyte level while the other exhibited an increase.

The differential count showed surprisingly little variation. The preoperative or preanesthesia ranges for the group as a whole were: nonsegmented neutrophils, from 1 to 10; segmented neutrophils, from 50 to 80; lymphocytes, from 20 to 50; monocytes, from 0 to 9; eosinophils, from 0 to 7 percent. Following operation or anesthesia there was very little alteration from the preoperative or preanesthesia level of variation characteristic of the case. It is true that patient 49 who showed a postoperatively higher leucocyte count exhibited a tendency toward a neutrophilic shift but the percentage changes still remained within the preoperative range for that patient.

REDUCING SUBSTANCES

**Determination of Combined Error.** Reducing substances in the blood were determined by the Folin-Wu method. While the clinical method is itself a thoroughly reliable one the vicissitudes of tests on blood-reducing substances are not inconsiderable. One is interested in knowing how well fasting conditions were maintained under the circumstances of the present investigation and how frequently deterioration of the sample may have occurred. Of 138 preoperative or preanesthesia determinations, discrepancies of 25 mg. or more per 100 cc. occurred in one of three tests on the same patient fifteen times (eight abnormal elevations, seven abnormal depressions). Of these eight elevations the increase was of the magnitude of 50 mg. or more in three instances, which presumably represent breaks in the fasting state. Therefore, one is probably safe in assuming that the determinations were within conventional limits of accuracy 90 percent of the time.

**Group as a Whole.** The preoperative fasting levels of the group as a whole were from 91 to 100 (mg. per 100 cc.), one third of the cases; from 81 to 90, one third of the cases; the remaining third (except 2 cases which lay between 61 and 70) lay between 71 and 80.

**Controls.** Only 2 control patients showed any deviation from their predetermined levels following their visit to the surgery. Both of these showed inconsequential rises.

**Operatees.** Eighteen of the operatees showed a very slightly elevated level of reducing substances in the blood as determined within the first six days after operation. Four showed no change, 2 exhibited a decrease.

**Interpretation of Results.** The magnitude of the rises seen was so small and indefinite that no specific correlations could be developed.

It is doubtful, in the absence of data on basal metabolism and a controlled intake of food, that one can absolutely deny that removal of frontal cortical areas exerts any effect upon blood-reducing substances but if such an effect exists in the first two weeks after operation it would appear to be upward and unspecific (that is, unrelated to the area removed).

From observations carried along for about six weeks after operation on 8 lobotomy patients it would appear that the postoperative glucose rise rapidly reaches a more or less steady plateau which begins to drop off shortly after about two weeks. Preoperative values may be reached soon after this or slightly elevated values may persist for over six weeks.

The lobotomy cases, considered as a group, showed about the same proportion of elevation as the topectomy series. That is, in 5 of the 8 patients there were definite elevations and in 3 little or no change (two slight elevations and one slight decrease).

These observations suggest that ablation of granular cortex may be followed by a modest rise in the blood sugar which rise generally is unsustained after two weeks. Inasmuch as some patients in the lobotomy as well as topectomy series failed to show a definite rise in blood sugar the effect is not necessarily due to the mere fact of operation. On the other hand, since 3 of the lobotomy patients failed to show such a rise, disconnection of granular cortex does not invariably cause it.

### UREA NITROGEN

**Determination of Combined Error.** Urea nitrogen was determined by the Summerson modification of the Karr method. There were marked variations in individual determinations in the urea nitrogen in the same patient in the preoperative or pre-anesthesia period. Although the patients received identical diets and extraneous food was prohibited we were unable to control the individual patient's consumption of what food was available. In the absence of such control (one patient, 10, is known to have been addicted to the consumption of his own urine) it must be recognized that the extent of the range of the combined errors is unknown.

**Group as a Whole.** In spite of variations in individual tests it was clear that the preoperative urea nitrogen levels in 43 patients were about as follows: 10 to 14 (mg. urea nitrogen per 100 cc. of blood), 27 cases; 15 to 19, 14 cases; 20 to 24, 2 cases.

**Controls.** Almost all controls showed a very slightly decreased urea nitrogen in the first two weeks after their visit to the surgery. The temporal pattern of high and low points determining this slightly decreased level was perfectly random.

**Operatees.** Six patients showed slightly decreased urea nitrogen levels in the first postoperative week. In 8 no trend could be detected. In 10 the urea nitrogen level rose somewhat.

**Interpretation.** With the commencement of operations more attention was paid to the diet of the operatees than controls and the latter apparently suffered some reduction in protein intake. The apparent random alteration in the operatees cannot be allowed to pass as such until analyzed for possible opposing cortical influences. None could be found. Neither could any correlation be found with the speed at which the patient began eating alone. There is no evidence to indicate that localized frontal cortical ablation influences urea nitrogen.

This conclusion is supported by urea nitrogen studies on 8 lobotomy subjects. No change was seen in 3 cases, a slight elevation in 2, and a slight decrease in 3—a random distribution. None of the elevations seen were of a notable magnitude.

### BLOOD CREATININE

**Determination of Combined Error.** Creatinine was determined by the alkaline picrate method on a Folin-Wu filtrate. Preoperative levels on the group as a whole varied from 0.95 to 1.45 mg. per 100 cc. of blood.

**Operatees.** In general the operatees showed an immediate drop in creatinine levels after operation. This drop was soon succeeded by a rise to greater than preoperative levels.

**Interpretation.** It is believed that the pattern seen in most of the operatees is nonspecific for the type of operation and merely a reflection of the general postoperative state.

· SERUM CALCIUM

**Analysis of Laboratory Error.** Ionic calcium in blood serum was determined by the method of Tisdall, as modified by Clark and Collip ('25). Variations of greater than 3 mg. per 100 mil. of serum between any two of the three preoperative tests in any one patient occurred ten times in 138 determinations, or less than 8 percent of the time. Any repeated variation of greater than 3 mg. per 100 mil. of serum from preoperative levels can therefore be considered significant.

**Group as a Whole.** Preoperative and preanesthesia levels ranged from 8 to 14 mg. per 100 mil. of serum with the following distribution: 8 to 10 mg. per 100 mil. in 20 cases; 10 to 12 mg. per 100 mil. in 23 cases; 12 to 14 mg. per 100 mil. in 3 cases.

**Controls.** One control (11) showed a significant decrease from his preanesthesia level. Another control (39) showed a barely significant increase over her preanesthesia level. No other control exhibited any change that even approached the limits of significant difference.

**Operatees.** One patient (24) showed a marked decrease in serum calcium following operation. However, it should be noted at this time that this patient's preoperative values fluctuated greatly, as follows: 13.9, 9.6, 16.75 mg. per 100 mil. His postoperative determinations were: 6.2, 6.5, 7.0 mg. per 100 mil. It should also be noted that he was in a catatonic stupor with attendant rigidity much of the time. It is obviously difficult, if not impossible, to set an accurate preoperative level with these data, and it is therefore difficult to call his decrease a significant one without further analysis or additional data. No other operatees showed significant or near significant changes from preoperative levels.

SERUM SODIUM

**Analysis of Laboratory Error.** Ionic sodium in blood serum was determined by the method of Kramer and Gittleman ('24-25). Variations of greater than 50 mg. per 100 mil. of serum between any two of the three preoperative tests in any one patient occurred eleven times in 144 determinations, or in less than 8 percent of the determinations. Any repeated variations in an individual case of greater than 50 mg. per 100 mil. from the preoperative levels can thus be termed significant.

**Group as a Whole.** Preoperative and preanesthesia levels ranged from 275 to 360 mg. per 100 mil. with the following distribution: 275 to 300 mg. per 100 mil. in 2 cases, 300 to 325 mg. per 100 mil. in 35 cases; 325 to 350 mg. per 100 mil. in 8 cases; 350 to 360 mg. per 100 mil. in 1 case.

**Controls.** One control (23) showed a nearly significant decrease from his preanesthesia level, while 3 others showed slight decreases following their visits to surgery. One control (37) showed a nearly significant increase, while one other control showed a slight increase from preanesthesia levels.

**Operatees.** One patient (27) showed an increase of nearly 50 mg. per 100 mil. from his preoperative average. Two others (6 and 31) showed slight increases from preoperative levels.

SERUM POTASSIUM

**Analysis of Laboratory Error.** Ionic potassium in blood serum was determined by the method of Kramer and Tisdall ('21). Variations of greater than 7.5 mg. per 100 mil. of serum between any two of the three preoperative or preanesthesia tests in any one patient occurred 8 times in 134 determinations, or in less than 6 percent of the determinations. Any repeated variation in an individual case of greater than 7.5 mg. per 100 mil. from preoperative or preanesthesia levels can therefore be called significant.

**Group as a Whole.**   Preoperative and preanesthesia levels ranged from 15 to 30 mg. per 100 mil. with the following distribution: 15 to 20 mg. per 100 mil. in 19 cases; 20 to 25 mg. in 22 cases; 25 to 30 mg. in 3 cases.

**Controls.**   No changes of greater than 5 mg. per 100 mil. from preanesthesia levels were noted in the controls, following their visit to surgery.

**Operatees.**   Only 2 operatees showed changes of more than 5 mg. per 100 mil. from preoperative levels. Patient 4 showed a significant increase (greater than 7.5 mg. per 100 mil.) over his preoperative level, and patient 7 showed a significant drop from his preoperative level.

## Conclusions

1. A survey has been made of the basic laboratory data of 46 patients in a mental institution. The general ranges were as follows: hemoglobin, 12 to 14 gm. per 100 cc. of blood; erythrocytes, 3.6 to 4.7 million per cu. mm. of blood; reticulocytes, 0.5 to 1.2 percent; leucocytes, 6 to 12 thousand per cu. mm. of blood; reducing substances, median fasting states 81 to 90 mg. per 100 cc., ranges in fasting state 71 to 100 mg. per 100 cc.; urea nitrogen, 10 to 19 mg. per 100 cc.; creatinine, 0.95 to 1.45 mg. per 100 cc.; calcium, 8 to 14 mg. per 100 cc.; sodium, 275 to 360 mg. per 100 cc.; potassium, 15 to 25 mg. per 100 cc.

2. Analysis of bilateral ablation of different portions of the frontal cortex, excluding area 4, failed to disclose any definite alterations in blood urea nitrogen, creatinine, sodium, potassium, or calcium.

3. Changes which were found in the leucocyte, erythrocyte, and reticulocyte counts and in values of hemoglobin and blood reducing substances are consistent with the belief that the cortex may exert an influence on these substances but before such a conclusion can be drawn the following conditions must be more rigidly met:

    a. Analyses must be conducted more frequently and over longer periods both pre- and postoperatively.

    b. Extraneous factors such as solid and fluid intake should be better controlled.

    c. Correlative tests (specifically, plasma volume, sedimentation rate, activity measures, and metabolic rate) should be introduced to help in evaluating the results.

# Chapter 8

# Audiometric Findings

PERRY J. GAMBILL

---

ALTHOUGH there is no reason to suppose that operations on the frontal lobe would exert any influence upon the acuity of hearing, audiometric examinations were instituted in the present study in order to detect the existence of any preoperative auditory difficulty which might, had it remained undetected until after operation, have obscured the results.

## PROCEDURE

All patients in both the control and operatee series were examined for patency of the auditory canal and the presence of otic abnormality. The nose and throat were, of course, also checked for the presence of acute infection. A routine audiogram was then made by the use of a standard commercial instrument but not in a sound-proof room.

A single determination was made roughly one week before, and two tests were made about three weeks and three months after, operation or anesthesia.

## RESULTS

The fact that it was necessary to remove foreign bodies, such as wads of paper, from the ears of 4 of the patients may be taken as indicative of the severity of the psychotic state in some individuals of the group. Impacted cerumen was removed from the ears of an additional 12 patients. One patient (4) had a large perforation of the tympanic membrane and a certain amount of discharge which yielded to therapy.

Prior to operation it was not possible to obtain satisfactory audiograms in 5 patients (24, 27, 33, 44, 47) of the group whose members were subsequently treated by topectomy. Of the control group, 10 patients (10, 11, 20, 30, 37, 39, 41, 45, 46, 48) could not be satisfactorily tested. There was thus a clear inequivalence between the two groups from the point of view of the ability of the members to report upon a test such as audiometry.

Following topectomy, patient 47 became testable before the first retest period and patients 27 and 33, untestable both preoperatively and at the first retest period, were testable at the second retest, three months after operation. The question naturally arises as to whether the improved cooperation of these 3 patients is related to topectomy or is merely a spontaneous phenomenon. Since only 1 (patient 39) of the 11 untestable control patients became testable in the same period it might be supposed that topectomy exerted some influence in rendering patients 27, 33, and 47 cooperative in spite of the apparent inequivalence of the two groups. One patient (6), testable before operation, was untestable at the first retest but testable at the second. Of the remaining 18 operatees, 7 (3, 4, 7, 21, 31, 42, and 49) showed no notable change between the preoperative and first retest audiograms, 2 (13 and 38) showed an eleva-

115

tion in the audiogram, and 9 (2, 8, 18, 19, 22, 25, 32, 36, and 40) exhibited very slight inconsistent average lowering of the audiogram line in the first retest followed by preoperative levels in the second.

Whether these changes in the level of the audiograms represent true increases and decreases of auditory acuity is doubtful for there was no consistent relation of them with air or bone conduction nor with middle nor end frequencies.

The rises in cases 13 and 38 are probably, like the alteration from untestable to testable condition, reflections of improved psychiatric condition.

One obtains the impression that the drops in the audiograms are similarly correlated with psychiatric rather than auditory changes and are probably a reflection of increased distractibility which many of these patients exhibited about the first retest period.

It is interesting to observe that while it was possible to obtain two-week postoperative audiograms in 18 of the 19 patients who were testable before operation it was only possible to obtain such retests in 3 of the 5 lobotomy subjects in whom preoperative testing had been possible.

No attempt has been made in the present study to correlate the findings presented herewith with areas or amount of tissue removed, or degree of psychiatric improvement as measured by the improvement scale of the psychiatrists, but since the pertinent case numbers have been cited it will be possible for the reader to develop such correlations should he care to do so.

It is perhaps worth mentioning in passing that dips in the region of 5792 cycles were rather common in all records (pre- and postoperative) obtained. Whether this represents a physical defect in the testing instrument employed, is a peculiarity of the psychiatric material tested, or can be correlated with vascular damage caused by antecedent shock therapy is not known. The point is raised since it may be encountered by subsequent investigators.

### Conclusions

Topectomy does not interfere with the ability of a patient to give a satisfactory audiogram so markedly as does lobotomy and may, in fact, render an uncooperative patient able to be tested.

There is no evidence that topectomy influences auditory function directly, but it does appear to exert an effect upon the manner in which a patient responds to audiometry. The response may be in the direction of a marked improvement which may appear within a matter of a couple of weeks or require as long as three months to appear. On the other hand, improvement may be unapparent or but slight. Impairment in the ability of an individual to give a satisfactory test occurred once in nineteen instances as a temporary phenomenon. Slight, temporary degradation in the audiograms occurred in nine of nineteen instances and appears to be related with distractibility rather than a true drop in auditory acuity.

The audiometer is a useful instrument for the purpose of making an objective measure of psychiatric condition or degree of psychiatric change.

## Chapter 9

# Vestibular Function

LEWIS A. SHEPPERD, NATHAN S. KLINE, AND JAMES Q. HOLSOPPLE

### INTRODUCTION

THE physiologic influence of the cerebral hemispheres on vestibular function has long been an unsettled problem. The higher centers are thought to exert an influence upon the manifestations of labyrinthine stimulations, according to current neurosurgical opinions; the Mettlers ('40) found evidence of labyrinthine disregard after removal of the caudate and a number of workers have been of the opinion that labyrinthine stimuli may activate certain parts of the thalamic nuclear group. The opportunity, therefore, to investigate the effects on the labyrinthine mechanism by the removal of specific frontal areas and known amounts of brain tissue is most timely since the course of the vestibular mechanism above the midbrain is poorly understood.

The effect of frontal topectomy and/or lobotomy on vestibular function in this series of patients was investigated by two different techniques, namely the *caloric* and *cinematic rotational* tests.

For purposes of clarity and comparison, the tests of vestibular function employed, their techniques, and respective findings will be described in two parts: (1) the caloric test and (2) the cinematic rotational test. The authors wish to point out that the caloric test for vestibular function was employed only on those patients upon whom topectomy was performed. The cinematic rotational test, on the other hand, was used on all the lobotomized patients pre- and postoperatively, one of the controls (17), and the topectomized patients postoperatively.

### CALORIC TEST

All patients, but one, in the operative series received a caloric test approximately five days preceding surgery. An attempt was made to eliminate the possible effects of immediate postoperative edema and anesthesia by performing most of the postoperative tests ten to fifteen days following surgery.

Four patients (6 [areas 8*, 6*, 6*], 27 [10*, 9*, 8*, 6*], 33 [10*, 46*, 45, 44*], and 44 [10*, lobotomy]) were uncooperative to the extent that reliable preoperative vestibular tests could not be performed. Owing to a change in the operating schedule, 1 (20) of the remaining 20 was taken to surgery before any preoperative tests were performed. Complete and fairly reliable records, however, were made on the remaining 19.

* Asterisks indicate areas which were not completely removed.

**Spontaneous Nystagmus.**    Each patient was tested preoperatively for spontaneous nystagmus. The Ballengers ('43) report that spontaneous nystagmus may be classified as: first degree, that which appears only on abduction of the eyes; second degree, that which appears when looking straight ahead; and third degree, that which appears in all positions. In this series of patients, reactions to preoperative tests for second- and third-degree nystagmus were negative when grossly observed.

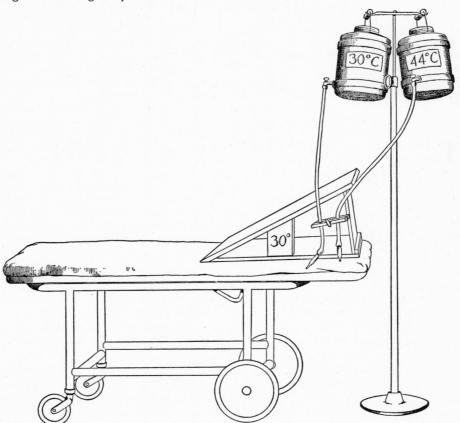

FIG. 77.    Caloric test apparatus. The illustration presents two 1-gallon jugs suspended 2 feet above the level of the midpoint on the back rest. This insures an approximate distance of 2 feet between the jug spigot and the patient's external auditory canals when the patient is placed on the table. The back rest is fixed at an angle of 30 degrees.

**Clinical Positional Nystagmus.**    After having ascertained the status of spontaneous nystagmus, attempts were made to elicit signs of gross clinical positional nystagmus. The positions used were those suggested by Nylén ('39) and also by Lindsay ('45), namely head-shaking, stooping and rising up, lying on the left side, lying prone, lying supine, and lying with the head hanging over the end of the table. Evidence of positional (first-degree) nystagmus was not found in any of the patients of this series by gross observation.

**Technique of Caloric Test.**    In deciding on a suitable caloric test, consideration was given to several factors. A test was required which would be informative and conclusive, yet one which possessed simplicity of technique and equipment. In addition, we required a minimal stimulus type rather than a maximal stimulus type, since it was shown by Kobrak as far back as 1922 that minimal caloric stimulation elicits more information about the state of the labyrinth than does maximum. Therefore, the method devised by Fitzgerald, Cawthorne, and Hallpike ('42) as modified by Glorig and Fowler ('47) was selected.

The apparatus was set up as follows: A 30-inch piece of uninsulated rubber tubing was attached to the on-and-off spigot of a gallon jug similar to the type commonly used at picnics (fig. 77). A nozzle having an inside diameter of approximately 2.5 mm. was attached to the other end of the tubing. The selected patient was placed in the supine position. By using a suitable backrest, the head was elevated, beginning at the waist, to an angle of 30 degrees. This resulted in the horizontal canal assuming a position in the vertical plane with the ampulla down. By the use of a suitable stand, the jug was suspended 2 feet above the level of the patient's ears.

It is important that illumination be correct. Light, natural or artificial, shining directly into the patient's eyes causes fatigue and reduces the degree of cooperation. It was found that a light of approximately 60 watts suspended above the line of sight and about 6 feet from the subject was most satisfactory. A small piece of black adhesive was placed on the ceiling as a point for eye fixation of the patient.

The technique required in performing the caloric vestibular test is quite simple. Each ear is tested with water at 30° C. and 44° C. The stimulation time is forty seconds. The measure of the response is taken as the time in seconds from the beginning of the application of the stimulus to the end of the visible nystagmus.

The stimulus time and the total time are kept by the operator with the aid of a stopwatch. Signals to stop irrigation are given the assistant at the end of forty seconds.

**Variable Factors Affecting Results of Test.**   In the performance of a caloric test as described, there were many variable factors in addition to those of age, sex, and barometric pressure. For example, variations of the body temperature occur in the same individual throughout the day. There may be a difference of 0.5° or even 1.0° F. in body temperature occurring between the maximum in the late afternoon or early evening, and the minimum at about four or five o'clock in the morning. At present, it is not known just how much these variables affect the results of vestibular tests.

Size, depth, and straightness of the canal are points which should also be considered. Thickness of the drum and the skin of the external auditory meatus is said to be a factor which may vary the latent period of the nystagmus. Even small pieces of wax might produce an "air-lock" just external to the drum. These would have the effect of insulating the tissues from the irrigating solution and thus produce a change in the duration of the nystagmus. There are numerous investigators who claim that the existence of previous otic disease and consequent scarring reduces the duration of nystagmus.

Of all the variable factors, probably the greatest rests in the determination of the end point of the nystagmus response. Investigators who have made observations of this type know only too well the problems involved. McNally ('47), and numerous other investigators claim that determination of the end point is difficult at best. In an effort to overcome this problem, Lewy ('47) has suggested the use of a head mirror for illumination and has the patient wear 16 to 20 diopter lenses. Others have found that the use of accessories such as Bartel's glasses result in making the end point even harder to evaluate. The experience accumulated in this series of patients was in accordance with this latter finding.

In an effort to improve the technique of determining the end point of nystagmus, Dr. Zigarelli made several unsuccessful attempts to obtain a nystagmogram by the use of his electroencephalograph. Although the beginning and early phase of the nystagmus were clearly outlined by the electric recorder, the final phase and end point were not clearly delineated because of artifacts originating from muscle movement, blinking, and various external sources which could not be filtered out by the electroencephalograph which was available.

The cinematic recording device, which will be described in the section dealing with the cinematic rotational test, may well prove to be the ideal instrument for recording this final phase and exact end point of nystagmus.

Granting that even under ideal conditions, the determination of the end point is uncertain, it may be assumed by the inexperienced that working with psychotic patients would make this determination even more unreliable. Only 4 patients, however, were uncooperative to the extent that caloric tests could not be performed. Consequently, it is believed that the determination made on the remaining patients in this series represent findings only slightly less reliable than those found by investigators working with normal and streptomycin-treated patients.

### DISCUSSION

In this series, thirty-eight tests were performed. In each test, of course, four stimulations are attempted. Our procedure was to repeat the irrigation in cases where the initial attempt for stimulation did not produce a discernible nystagmus. In cases where two irrigations with water at 30° C. did not produce a discernible nystagmus reflex, an attempt was made to elicit a response with ice water. In only one case (40) did stimulus with ice water elicit a response after attempts with water at 30° failed.

When more than one attempt was made to elicit either a cold or a warm response in one ear at one sitting, all such attempts for the cold were regarded as one "stimulation" and all such attempts for the warm were considered one "stimulation." Thus, an attempt to elicit a reflex which involved two irrigations with water at 30° C. and one irrigation with ice water represents one "stimulation." It will be seen then that there were 152 such "stimulations" in the group of thirty-eight tests.

In sixteen out of 152 attempts to elicit the nystagmus reflex, no discernible reflex could be detected. Since repeated attempts, with an interval allowed for return of the labyrinth to normal, were made on each of these patients, it is believed that nystagmus would have been observed even though of very small magnitude.

### RESULTS

The excitation of the semicircular canals in man is not uncommonly followed by nausea, vomiting, and pallor. In addition, there may be a fall of blood pressure of 10 mm. or more together with a slowing of the heart by eight or ten beats per minute. No attempt was made in this study to determine the effects on heart rate and blood pressure. Examinations, however, of the number of stimulations which resulted in dizziness or vertigo revealed no significant difference between preoperative and postoperative reactions.

An attempt was made to evaluate the amplitude of the nystagmus into a

TABLE 22.   DURATION OF NYSTAGMUS BEFORE AND AFTER OPERATION

| No. of pat. | Area excised bilaterally | Nystagmus time (seconds) Water at 30° C. Preop. | Postop. | Water at 44° C. Preop. | Postop. | Increase and decrease (seconds) Water at 30° C. | Water at 44° C. |
|---|---|---|---|---|---|---|---|
| **A. Patients in whom all stimulations elicited responses** |
| 2 | 8, 6ᵃ | L  102 | 117 | 97 | 127 | 15 | 30 |
|  |  | R  138 | 125 | 110 | 110 | −13 | 0 |
| 13 | 9ᵃ, 10ᵃ, 45, 46 | L  122 | 155 | 105 | 125 | 33 | 20 |
|  |  | R  122 | 125 | 140 | 145 | 3 | 5 |
| 18 | 11ᵃ | L  112 | 112 | 102 | 114 | 0 | 12 |
|  |  | R  92 | 117 | 94 | 100 | 25 | 6 |
| 19 | 45ᵃ | L  111 | 115 | 90 | 95 | 4 | 5 |
|  |  | R  95 | 112 | 102 | 100 | 17 | − 2 |
| 21 | 10 | L  151 | 153 | 118 | 158 | 2 | 40 |
|  |  | R  164 | 151 | 117 | 150 | −13 | 33 |
| 24 | 6ᵇ, 6ᵈ | L  100 | 135 | 105 | 133 | 35 | 28 |
|  |  | R  82 | 135 | 108 | 127 | 53 | 19 |
| 25 | 8, 9, 46 | L  120 | 150 | 113 | 151 | 30 | 38 |
|  | 10ᵃ | R  123 | 150 | 127 | 160 | 27 | 33 |
| 31 | 9 | L  90 | 116 | 93 | 120 | 26 | 27 |
|  |  | R  90 | 125 | 100 | 130 | 35 | 30 |
| 36 | 10, 11, 45 | L  105 | 130 | 89 | 120 | 25 | 31 |
|  | 46, 47 | R  97 | 145 | 100 | 95 | 48 | − 5 |
| 42 | 11 | L  108 | 102 | 105 | 102 | − 6 | − 3 |
|  |  | R  110 | 110 | 95 | 110 | 0 | 15 |
| 49 | 10, 11ᵃ, 46ᵃ | L  105 | 145 | 102 | 137 | 40 | 35 |
|  |  | R  125 | 150 | 113 | 95 | 25 | −18 |
| **B. Patients in whom one or more stimulations failed to elicit a response** |
| 3 | 9ᵃ, 6ᵃ | L  111 | 117 | 102 | 103 | 6 | 3 |
|  |  | R  140 | 145 | 117 | NR | 5 | — |
| 4 | 46 | L  105 | 110 | 115 | 117 | 5 | 2 |
|  |  | R  87 | 120 | NR | 135 | 33 | — |
| 7 | 8, 9ᵃ, 10ᵃ | L  132 | 105 | 70 | 92 | −27 | 22 |
|  |  | R  NR | NR | 90 | 100 | — | 10 |
| 8 | 10ᵃ, 46ᵃ | L  90 | 99 | 110 | NR | 9 | — |
|  | 9ᵃ, 8ᵃ | R  98 | 87 | 102 | 90 | −11 | −12 |
| 32 | 8ᵃ, 9, 10ᵃ | L  115 | 115 | 111 | NR | 0 | — |
|  |  | R  105 | 105 | 125 | 85 | 0 | −40 |
| 38 | 6, 8, 9, 10ᶜ | L  NR | 95 | NR | 98 | — | — |
|  |  | R  NR | 92 | NR | 105 | — | — |
| 40 | 24ᵃ | L  NR | 120 | 115 | NR | — | — |
|  |  | R  94 | NR | 110 | NR | — | — |
| 47 | 44 | L  94 | 105 | 80 | 90 | 11 | 10 |
|  |  | R  120 | 95 | NR | NR | −25 | — |

ᵃ Part only.
ᵇ Incomplete original removal (caudally).
ᶜ Venous ligation.
ᵈ Unilateral verification done.
N.R. No response.

classification of fine, medium, and coarse. All efforts, however, to make this differential by gross observation were unsuccessful. Generally, no variation was found between the magnitude of nystagmus preceding and following surgery.

It was found that preceding surgery 78 percent of the nystagmic responses of the patients fell within a range of ninety to one-hundred-thirty seconds' duration. Of the normal-subject studies by Fitzgerald and Hallpike, 80 percent were grouped in the same range. It will be seen, then, that the results in this series were distributed in essentially the same manner as in normal subjects.

Comparison of the length of nystagmic reflexes elicited before and after operation indicates that the performance of topectomies resulted, in general, in a slight increase in the duration of nystagmus.

TABLE 23.   AVERAGE INCREASE OF NYSTAGMUS*
VERSUS THE REMOVAL OF TISSUE†

| Sequence of maximum change | Patient number | Gms. removed |
|:---:|:---:|:---:|
| 1 | 24 | 31.2 |
| 2 | 25 | 38.4 |
| 3 | 31 | 33.1 |
| 4 | 36 | 73.5 |
| 5 | 49 | 42.1 |
| 6 | 21 | 25.4 |
| 7 | 13 | 31.6 |
| 8 | 2 | 17.4 |
| 9 | 18 | 29.0 |
| 10 | 19 | 11.8 |
| 11 | 42 | 27.0 |

* Measured in seconds.   † Measured in grams.

In Table 22, the first group of patients (group A) are those in whom all attempts to elicit a nystagmic reflex with water at 30° C. and 44° C. resulted in a satisfactory response. It will be seen that in 7 of the 11 patients in this group (13 [areas 9*, 10*, 45, 46], 21 [10], 24 [6*], 25 [8, 9, 46, 10*], 31 [9], 36 [10, 11, 45, 46, 47], 49 [10, 11*, 46*]) marked increased durations are to be observed when preoperative and postoperative examinations are compared.

In the second group (group B, table 22) those patients in whom one or more stimulations elicited no response evidenced the same trend toward increased duration though less well defined.

There is also a strong indication of a relationship between the increase in the duration of the nystagmus and the amount of tissue excised. In table 23, the patients of group A in table 22 have been listed in a column by their respective numbers in a descending order of the average increase in nystagmus between that shown in the preoperative and that in the postoperative caloric tests. By comparison with the known amount of tissue removed in grams for each patient, respectively, there is a product-moment coefficient of correlation of approximately 0.75 between increase in nystagmus and amount of tissue removed.

* Asterisks indicate areas which were not completely removed.

## CINEMATIC ROTATIONAL TEST

A new method of testing was introduced about three months after the original topectomies were performed but before any lobotomies had been done on the control subjects. The following presentation therefore includes data on (a) 95 nonpsychotic, nonpatient subjects (used to establish "base-lines" for comparison), (b) the topectomized patients three to four months postoperatively, (c) 1 psychotic control (17) at one-month intervals, and (d) the lobotomized patients, preoperatively; three weeks postoperatively; and three months postoperatively.

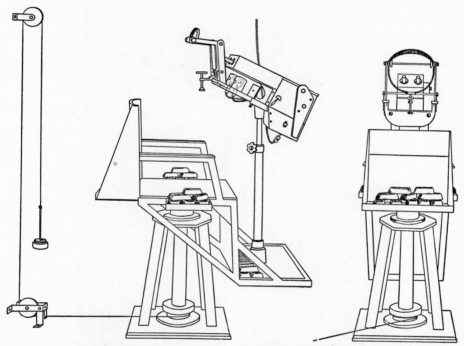

FIG. 78. Diagram of apparatus used in testing the vestibular function by the rotational cinematic method.

**Technique of Test.** The outstanding feature of the cinematic rotational technique is the use of a mechanical device that provides a permanent record of nystagmus and permits the detection of much smaller and finer movements than is ordinarily possible. An advantage of the rotational technique is that a constancy of stimulation is guaranteed.

Since the threshold for nystagmus in control subjects is rotation at roughly 2 degrees per second per second acceleration, it was felt that a rate of acceleration of 0.5 degree per second per second above threshold would be most diagnostic. This is in contradistinction to the usual Barany test where rate of acceleration is not held constant and which is usually about 20 degrees per second per second for a period (ten times threshold).

The apparatus consists of a specially constructed revolving chair (see fig. 78) on a permanent fixed base with ball-bearing swivel. The motivating force is a weight attached to a pulley so that the movements of the chair are controlled by gravity, thus assuring constancy. The rate of acceleration (and deceleration) can be varied by changing the number of weights. After a trial run of 100 subjects at rates of acceleration of 2.5 degrees per second per second, 5 degrees per second per second, and 7.5 degrees per second per second (unpublished data by Walter Leech), it was determined that 2.5 degrees per second per second acceleration appeared most suitable for our purpose. The machine was standardized for a 160-pound subject by placing a dozen 4-pound

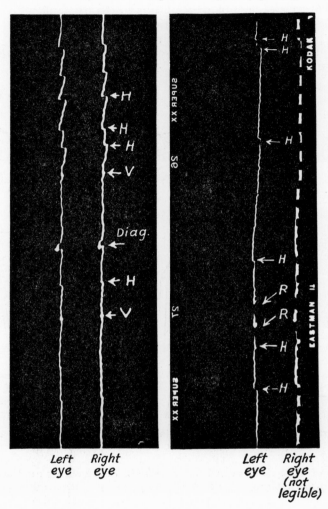

FIG. 79. Cinematic record of various types of nystagmoid movements. (*H*, horizontal; *V*, vertical; *Diag.*, diagonal; *R*, rotational.)

weights in special receptacles under each arm of the chair. By the removal of a number of these weights, or the addition of other weights, the rate of acceleration could be held absolutely constant.

Built into the machine was an American Optical Company Ophthalmograph using 35-mm. film. This revolved with the chair and provided a permanent record of eye movements before, *during*, and after rotation. The subject's head was placed on a chin rest. Additional stabilization was obtained by the use of braces over the frontal and temporal regions. This insured that the head would remain relatively immobile and at a 30-degree forward inclination so that the lateral canals were horizontal. The subject then fixed his eyes on a 2-mm. black spot on a card placed 25 cm. distant. A source of light on each side reflected onto the cornea, and the light from his corneal reflex was picked up and focused to a pinpoint by means of special lenses from which it was recorded upon the film (see fig. 79). A recording of both eyes could thus be taken simultaneously. The room was completely darkened except for the card at which the subject looked and the source of light on the cornea.

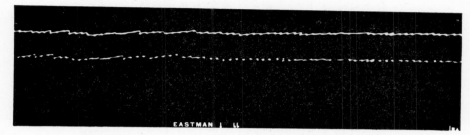

FIG. 80.  Cinematic record of extremely fine subclinical nystagmoid movements.

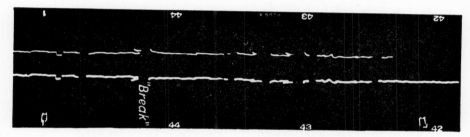

FIG. 81.  Cinematic record showing "break" due to convergence fatigue.

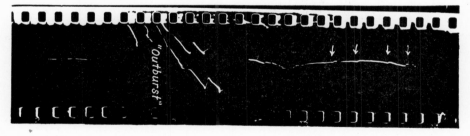

FIG. 82.  Cinematic record of "outburst" of nystagmoid movement.

After the subject was adjusted on the chair, a two- or three-minute period was allowed to elapse to eliminate any effects caused by head movements while getting into the chair. After focusing, the camera was turned on, and a thirty-second stationary run obtained with the subject at rest. Following this, the machine was released, and recordings were made during the periods of acceleration and deceleration. At the cessation of active deceleration, eye movements were recorded for an additional thirty-second postrotational period. Subjects were first rotated clockwise. Following this record, a two- to three-minute rest period was given, after which the subjects were rotated counterclockwise.

TABLE 24. ROTATIONAL AND POSTROTATIONAL NYSTAGMUS IN 95 NONPSYCHOTIC CONTROLS AND 7 PRELOBOTOMY PATIENTS

| | Areas excised bilaterally | Horizontal jerks | | Convergence difficulty | | Vertical jerks | | Reversals | | Tremor | | Average latent period in sec. | "Outbursts" | |
|---|---|---|---|---|---|---|---|---|---|---|---|---|---|---|
| | | Per min. | % of cases | Per min. | % of cases | Per min. | % of cases | Per min. | % of cases | Per min. | % of cases | | Per record | % of cases |
| Nonpsychotic controls (95) | | | | | | | | | | | | | | |
| Mean......... | None | 33.09 | 100 | .65 | 27.4 | .81 | 45.3 | 1.17 | 56.7 | .16 | 22.1 | 5.78 | .21 | 9.3 |
| S. D......... | | 16.55 | | 1.30 | | 1.49 | | 1.70 | | .44 | | 2.04 | 1.13 | |
| Prelobotomy patients | | | | | | | | | | | | | | |
| 5 ......... | Lobotomy | 55.80 | | 0 | | 0 | | 0 | | .32 | | 4.09 | 0 | 0 |
| 11......... | Lobotomy | 51.26 | | 0 | | .65 | | 3.57 | | 0 | | 4.58 | 0 | 0 |
| 20......... | Lobotomy | 29.85 | | 0.97 | | 0 | | 0 | | 0 | | 11.34 | 0 | 0 |
| 23......... | Lobotomy | 32.44 | | 0 | | .65 | | 0 | | 0 | | 5.99 | 0 | 0 |
| 28......... | Lobotomy | 70.40 | | 0 | | 0 | | 5.52 | | 0 | | 3.70 | 0 | 0 |
| 44......... | Lobotomy—uncoop. | | | | | | | | | | | | | |
| 46......... | Lobotomy—uncoop. | | | | | | | | | | | | | |
| Mean......... | | 47.95 | 100 | .19 | 20 | .26 | 40 | 1.82 | 40 | .06 | 20 | 5.94 | 0 | |

(NOTE: Patient 2 of the topectomy group was later leucotomized.)

The developed film could be read under magnification, so that even the finest degrees of subclinical nystagmus were observable (see fig. 80). On most of the records, independent readings were made by two observers with almost complete agreement. All types of nystagmus, horizontal, vertical, rotational, and dysjunctive could be noted (see figs. 81, 82). The amplitude of the corneal reflection could be accurately measured, and the end point determined explicitly. The data on amplitude proved to be of no significance except as noted. For practical purposes, to conserve film, the

TABLE 25. SPONTANEOUS NYSTAGMUS IN 95 NONPSYCHOTIC CONTROLS AND EIGHT POSTLOBOTOMY PATIENTS TESTED THREE WEEKS POSTOPERATIVELY

| | Horizontal jerks | | Convergence difficulty | | Vertical jerks | | Tremor | |
|---|---|---|---|---|---|---|---|---|
| | Per min. | % of cases | Per min. | % of cases | Per min. | % of cases | Per min. | % of cases |
| Nonpsychotic controls | | | | | | | | |
| Mean....... | 4.31 | 41.1 | .39 | 7.4 | .55 | 10.5 | .36 | 3.2 |
| S. D......... | 7.72 | | 3.24 | | 3.18 | | 3.25 | |
| Postlobotomy patients | | | | | | | | |
| 2........... | 48.66 | | 0 | | 6.49 | | 3.57 | |
| 5........... | 6.49 | | 0 | | 0 | | 0 | |
| 11........... | 22.71 | | 0 | | 0 | | 0 | |
| 20........... | 32.44 | | 3.24 | | 3.24 | | 0 | |
| 23........... | 29.20 | | 3.24 | | 0 | | 0 | |
| 28........... | 6.49 | | 0 | | 3.24 | | 1.62 | |
| 44*......... | | | | | | | | |
| 46*......... | | | | | | | | |
| Mean....... | 26.61 | 100 | .97 | 33.3 | 2.27 | 50 | 1.97 | 33.3 |

* Unreadable.

*frequency* during the thirty-second postrotational period was used instead of the determination of the absolute end point. The latent periods for acceleration and deceleration were also determined, and other qualitative aspects of the recordings reviewed.

## RESULTS

**Nonpsychotic Controls.** A group of 95 nonpsychotic control subjects were tested to establish baselines for comparison with the patient groups (see table 24). This nonpsychotic control group differed from the patient groups in that all the subjects were male veterans with a slightly different age distribution. Product-moment coefficients of correlation showed no significant positive relationship between either age or sex in test results, and for practical purposes, can therefore be safely disregarded. The influence of being veterans is undetermined but may have served to eliminate a "life history" that differed from that among the patient groups.

In these men, there was found to be spontaneous (probably congenital) subclinical nystagmoid jerks in 41.1 percent of the cases (see table 25). This provides a mean of 4.31 jerks per minute for the entire group and a mean of 8.17 jerks per minute for those in whom nystagmoid movements were found.

TABLE 26.   ROTATIONAL AND POSTROTATIONAL NYSTAGMUS IN 95 NONPSYCHOTIC CONTROLS AND 14 POSTTOPECTOMY PATIENTS

| | Areas excised bilaterally | Horizontal jerks | | Convergence difficulty | | Vertical jerks | | Reversals | | Tremor | | Average latent period in sec. | "Outbursts" | |
|---|---|---|---|---|---|---|---|---|---|---|---|---|---|---|
| | | Per min. | % of cases | Per min. | % of cases | Per min. | % of cases | Per min. | % of cases | Per min. | % of cases | | Per record | % of cases |
| Nonpsychotic controls (95) | | | | | | | | | | | | | | |
| Mean............ | None | 33.09 | 100 | .65 | 27.4 | .81 | 45.3 | 1.17 | 56.7 | .16 | 22.1 | 5.78 | .21 | 9.3 |
| S. D............ | | 16.55 | | 1.30 | | 1.49 | | 1.70 | | .44 | | 2.04 | 1.13 | |
| Topectomy patients* | | | | | | | | | | | | | | |
| 2............ | 8 | 78.83 | | 0 | | 0 | | 1.30 | | 0 | | 5.36 | 0 | 0 |
| 3............ | 9 | 31.47 | | 0 | | 3.89 | | 1.30 | | 3.24 | | 3.64 | 0 | 0 |
| 4............ | 46 | 35.74 | | 0 | | 1.95 | | 0 | | 0 | | 5.26 | 0 | 0 |
| 6A†............ | 8, 6 | 27.90 | | 0 | | 0 | | 4.22 | | 0 | | 8.49 | 2 | 0 |
| 6B............ | 8, 6 | 46.07 | | 0 | | 6.16 | | 0 | | 0 | | 6.83 | 0 | 0 |
| 13............ | 9, 45, 46 | 67.48 | | 0 | | 0 | | 0 | | .97 | | 6.63 | 0 | 0 |
| 21............ | 10 | 36.34 | | 0 | | 0 | | 0 | | 0 | | 7.00 | 0 | 0 |
| 24............ | 6 | 27.90 | | 0 | | 0 | | 0 | | 0 | | 7.40 | 0 | 0 |
| 25............ | 8, 9, 46 | 32.44 | | 1.30 | | 0 | | 1.30 | | 0 | | 7.10 | 0 | 0 |
| 27............ | 6, 8, 9 | 25.63 | | 0 | | 3.24 | | 0 | | 0 | | 9.46 | 0 | 0 |
| 33............ | 10, 44, 45, 46 | 50.61 | | 0 | | 0 | | 0 | | 0 | | 6.96 | 0 | 0 |
| 38............ | 6, 8, 9 | 49.64 | | .65 | | 0 | | 1.30 | | .32 | | 7.33 | 0 | 0 |
| 42............ | 11 | 61.32 | | 0 | | 11.68 | | .65 | | 0 | | 3.77 | 0 | 0 |
| 49............ | 10 | 31.14 | | 6.49 | | 3.24 | | 3.24 | | 0 | | 7.00 | 0 | 0 |
| Mean............ | | 44.99 | 100 | .65 | 23.1 | 2.31 | 46.7 | 1.03 | 53.8 | .36 | 23.1 | 6.44 | 0 | 0 |

* Tested three to four months postoperatively, except patient 6A—three weeks postoperatively.
† Not included in mean since different postoperative period. (See text.)

All subjects showed nystagmus after rotation with a mean occurrence of 33.09 jerks per minute with a standard deviation of 16.55.

Inability to maintain convergence on the fixation point (convergence difficulty) occurred spontaneously in 7.4 percent of the subjects (mean of 0.39 per minute for the group and 5.10 per minute for those in whom it occurred). During and following rotation convergence, difficulty was noted in 27.4 percent of the group with a mean occurrence of 0.65 per minute for the entire group and 3.8 per minute for those in whom it occurred.

TABLE 27.  SPONTANEOUS NYSTAGMUS IN 95 NONPSYCHOTIC CONTROLS AND 14 POSTTOPECTOMY PATIENTS

| | Areas excised bilaterally | Horizontal jerks | | Convergence difficulty | | Vertical jerks | | Tremor | |
|---|---|---|---|---|---|---|---|---|---|
| | | Per min. | % of cases | Per min. | % of cases | Per min. | % of cases | Per min. | % of cases |
| **Nonpsychotic controls** | | | | | | | | | |
| Mean...... | | 4.31 | 40 | .39 | 7.4 | .55 | 9.5 | .36 | 3.2 |
| S. D...... | | 7.72 | | 3.24 | | 3.18 | | 3.25 | |
| **Topectomy patients** | | | | | | | | | |
| 2......... | 8 | No record | | | | | | | |
| 3......... | 9 | Unreadable | | | | | | | |
| 4......... | 46 | 0 | | 0 | | 9.73 | | 0 | |
| 6A*...... | 8, 6 | 0 | | 0 | | 3.24 | | 0 | |
| 6B...... | 8, 6 | 0 | | 0 | | 0 | | 0 | |
| 13......... | 0 | 0 | | 0 | | 0 | | 0 | |
| 21........ | 10 | 6.49 | | 0 | | 0 | | 0 | |
| 24......... | 6 | No record | | | | | | | |
| 25......... | 8, 9, 46 | Unreadable | | | | | | | |
| 27......... | 9, 8, 6 | 0 | | 0 | | 0 | | 0 | |
| 33........ | 10, 46, 45, 44 | 3.24 | | 0 | | 0 | | 0 | |
| 38......... | 6, 8, 9 | 16.22 | | 0 | | 0 | | 0 | |
| 42....... | 11 | 0 | | 0 | | 0 | | 0 | |
| 49....... | 10 | 22.71 | | 6.49 | | 0 | | 0 | |
| 7........ | 8, 9, 10 | Unreadable | | 0 | | 0 | | 0 | |
| Mean..... | | 5.41 | 44.4 | .65 | 11.1 | 1.30 | 22.2 | 0 | 0 |

* Not included in mean since different postoperative.  (See text.)

Vertical jerks of a spontaneous nature appeared in 10.5 percent of the group with a mean of 0.55 per minute for the 95 subjects and a mean of 5.81 per minute in the 9 subjects in whom they appeared at all. During the following rotation, they increased to a mean of 0.81 per minute for the group and a mean of 2.14 per minute for the 45.3 percent in whom they occurred.

Note was also made of nystagmus that went against the prevailing direction induced by rotation, and such "reversals" were found to have a mean occurrence of 1.17 times per minute and occurred in 56.7 percent of the subjects with a mean of 2.29 per minute for those showing "reversals."

TABLE 28.  ROTATIONAL AND POSTROTATIONAL NYSTAGMUS IN 95 NONPSYCHOTIC CONTROLS AND 1 CONTROL PATIENT

| | Areas excised bilaterally | Horizontal jerks | | Convergence difficulty | | Vertical jerks | | Reversals | | Tremor | | Average latent period in sec. | "Outbursts" | |
|---|---|---|---|---|---|---|---|---|---|---|---|---|---|---|
| | | Per min. | % of cases | Per min. | % of cases | Per min. | % of cases | Per min. | % of cases | Per min. | % of cases | | Per record | % of cases |
| Nonpsychotic controls (95) | | | | | | | | | | | | | | |
| Mean......... | None | 33.09 | 100 | .65 | 27.4 | .81 | 45.3 | 1.17 | 56.7 | .16 | 22.1 | 5.78 | .21 | 9.3 |
| S. D......... | | 16.55 | | 1.30 | | 1.49 | | 1.70 | | .44 | | 2.04 | 1.13 | |
| Control patients Patient 17 | None | | | | | | | | | | | | | |
| Tested 10/10 | | 57.75 | | 0 | | 0 | | 1.30 | | 0 | | 7.10 | 0 | 0 |
| Tested 11/17 | | 62.94 | | 0 | | 0 | | 0 | | 0 | | 4.67 | 0 | 0 |

TABLE 29. ROTATIONAL AND POSTROTATIONAL NYSTAGMUS IN 95 NONPSYCHOTIC CONTROLS AND 8 POSTLOBOTOMY PATIENTS TESTED THREE WEEKS POSTOPERATIVELY

| | Areas excised bilaterally | Horizontal jerks | | Convergence difficulty | | Vertical jerks | | Reversals | | Tremor | | Average latent period in sec. | "Outbursts" | |
|---|---|---|---|---|---|---|---|---|---|---|---|---|---|---|
| | | Per min. | % of cases | Per min. | % of cases | Per min. | % of cases | Per min. | % of cases | Per min. | % of cases | | Per record | % of cases |
| **Nonpsychotic controls (95)** | | | | | | | | | | | | | | |
| Mean.......... | None | 33.09 | 100 | .65 | 27.4 | .81 | 45.3 | 1.17 | 56.7 | .16 | 22.1 | 5.78 | .21 | 9.3 |
| S. D........... | | 16.55 | | 1.30 | | 1.49 | | 1.70 | | .44 | | 2.04 | 1.13 | |
| **Postlobotomy patients** | | | | | | | | | | | | | | |
| 2............. | | 37.96 | | .65 | | 1.30 | | 9.73 | | .32 | | 5.44 | 1 | |
| 5............. | | 49.64 | | 0 | | 0 | | 0 | | .64 | | 7.08 | 0 | |
| 11............ | | 46.39 | | 0 | | .65 | | 4.87 | | 0 | | 3.94 | 6 | |
| 20............ | | 23.68 | | 0 | | 3.57 | | 9.41 | | 0 | | 2.56 | 10 | |
| 23............ | | 31.14 | | 1.30 | | 13.63 | | 3.89 | | .32 | | 3.20 | 2 | |
| 28............ | | 47.04 | | .65 | | 0 | | 0 | | 0 | | 7.30 | 7 | |
| 44*.......... | | | | | | | | | | | | | | |
| 46*.......... | | | | | | | | | | | | | | |
| Mean......... | | 39.25 | 100 | .42 | 50 | 3.18 | 66.7 | 4.64 | 66.7 | .23 | 50 | 5.25 | 4.33 | 83.3 |

* Unreadable.

Eye tremor, interestingly enough, dropped from a spontaneous mean for the group of 0.36 per minute (found in 3.2 percent) to 0.16 per minute during and following rotation (occurring in 22.1 percent of the group). This gives a mean of 1.14 per minute for spontaneous occurrence in those in whom it occurred and a mean of 0.72 per minute for those having eye tremor during and after rotation.

The average latent period before occurrence of nystagmus in the prevailing direction was measured following the initiation of acceleration and beginning of deceleration. The findings of these two types of latent period were averaged for both clockwise and counterclockwise rotation and the mean found to be 5.78 seconds with a standard deviation of 2.04 seconds.

TABLE 30.  SPONTANEOUS NYSTAGMUS IN 95 NONPSYCHOTIC CONTROLS AND 6 POSTLOBOTOMY PATIENTS TESTED THREE MONTHS POSTOPERATIVELY

| | Horizontal jerks | | Convergence difficulty | | Vertical jerks | | Tremor | |
|---|---|---|---|---|---|---|---|---|
| | Per min. | % of cases | Per min. | % of cases | Per min. | % of cases | Per min. | % of cases |
| Nonpsychotic controls | | | | | | | | |
| Mean............ | 4.31 | 41.1 | .39 | 7.4 | .55 | 10.5 | .36 | 3.2 |
| S. D............. | 7.72 | | 3.24 | | 3.18 | | 3.25 | |
| Postlobotomy patients | | | | | | | | |
| *2............... | 16.22 | | 0 | | 16.22 | | 0 | |
| 5†.............. | | | | | | | | |
| 11.............. | 0 | | 0 | | 32.40 | | 0 | |
| 20.............. | 0 | | 0 | | 8.10 | | 0 | |
| *23‡............. | | | | | | | | |
| *28.............. | 69.34 | | 0 | | 0 | | 0 | |
| Mean............ | 21.39 | 50.0 | 2.5 | 25 | 14.18 | 75.0 | 0 | 0 |

* Still hospitalized.
† Untested.
‡ Unreadable.

A phenomenon described as "outbursts" (short bursts of nystagmoid jerks of extremely marked amplitude) (see fig. 82) were found in 9.3 percent of these subjects. The mean occurrence of these outbursts was only 0.21 per record for the group as a whole, but 2.22 per record for those in whom they occurred.

**Topectomized Patients.**  The topectomized patients were not studied preoperatively by this technique. Patient 6 was tested three weeks postoperatively (see 6A in tables 26 and 27). This is a single case, but the patient is the only one of this group to show an "outburst." When retested after three to four months, no "outbursts" could be found.

In one respect, comparisons of the means of the topectomized patients with the control groups are meaningless, since the same operation was not performed upon each of the topectomized patients. In no individual patient did the data vary to a degree where they could be considered to be of statistical significance. It may be stated that as a group, topectomized patients tested by the cinematic rotational method three months after operation in no respect

TABLE 31.  ROTATIONAL AND POSTROTATIONAL NYSTAGMUS IN 95 NONPSYCHOTIC CONTROLS AND 8 POSTLOBOTOMY PATIENTS TESTED THREE MONTHS POSTOPERATIVELY

| | Horizontal jerks | | Convergence difficulty | | Vertical jerks | | Reversals | | Tremor | | Average latent period in seconds | Outbursts | |
|---|---|---|---|---|---|---|---|---|---|---|---|---|---|
| | Per min. | % of cases | Per min. | % of cases | Per min. | % of cases | Per min. | % of cases | Per min. | % of cases | | Per record | % of cases |
| **Nonpsychotic controls (95)** | | | | | | | | | | | | | |
| Mean | 33.09 | 100 | .65 | 27.4 | .81 | 45.3 | 1.17 | 56.7 | .16 | 22.1 | 5.78 | .21 | 9.3 |
| S. D. | 16.55 | | 1.30 | | 1.49 | | 1.70 | | .44 | | 2.04 | 1.13 | |
| **Postlobotomy patients** | | | | | | | | | | | | | |
| *2 | 42.82 | | 0 | | 17.79 | | 4.28 | | 0 | | .45 | 0 | |
| 5† | | | | | | | | | | | | | |
| 11 | 38.88 | | 0 | | 10.80 | | 0 | | 0 | | 2.62 | 2 | |
| 20 | 33.70 | | 0 | | 13.28 | | 0 | | 0 | | 3.80 | 1 | |
| *23 | 35.68 | | 0 | | 0 | | 0 | | 0 | | .85 | 0 | |
| *28 | 79.70 | | 2.59 | | 1.62 | | 11.87 | | .65 | | 1.50 | 5 | |
| *44† | | | | | | | | | | | | | |
| *46† | | | | | | | | | | | | | |
| Mean | 46.16 | 100 | .52 | 20.0 | 8.70 | 80.0 | 3.23 | 40.0 | .13 | 20.0 | 1.84 | 1.60 | 60.0 |

* Still hospitalized.
† Untested.

differed significantly in their vestibular responses from nonpsychotic control patients.

Spontaneous horizontal nystagmus at the three- to four-month test (40 percent in the nonpsychotic control group) occurred in 44.4 percent of the cases with a mean of 5.41 (nonpsychotic mean 4.31). Significant deviations were found in other respects. Vertical jerks occurred in 22.2 percent of the cases with a mean of 1.38 per minute for the group as opposed to 0.55 per minute for the controls. During rotation, the mean number of horizontal jerks per minute was 44.99 (less than 1 S.D. from the control mean). Vertical jerks showed an increase from 0.81 for the controls to 2.31 per minute. No "outbursts" were found.

**Psychotic Control.**   One psychotic patient (17) upon whom no operation was performed was tested at one-month intervals with constancy of findings well within statistical expectancy (see table 28).

TABLE 32. RELATION OF LATENT PERIOD AND HORIZONTAL JERKS PER MINUTE ON THE ROTATIONAL TEST TO SEQUENCE OF MAXIMUM CHANGE AS SHOWN BY THE CALORIC TEST

| Sequence of maximum change as found on table 23 | Latent period | Patient number | Horizontal jerks per minute |
|---|---|---|---|
| 1 | 7.40 | 24 | 27.90 |
| 2 | 7.10 | 25 | 32.44 |
| 5 | 7.00 | 49 | 31.14 |
| 6 | 7.00 | 21 | 36.34 |
| 7 | 6.63 | 13 | 67.48 |
| 8 | 5.36 | 2 | 78.83 |
| 11 | 3.77 | 42 | 61.32 |

**Lobotomized Patients.**   Prior to operation the lobotomized patients showed a mean rotational horizontal nystagmus of 47.95 jerks per minute, which is less than 1 S.D. from the nonpsychotic control mean (see tables 24 and 29). In this small sample other deviations from the nonpsychotic control group cannot be considered significant, so that no conclusions as to changes in vestibular function in mental disease as measured by this technique can be drawn. At present, a series of several hundred patients are being tested to determine if deviations of significance do occur.

After lobotomy the mean number of *rotational* horizontal jerks dropped from 47.95 to 39.25 per minute. Vertical jerks, reversals, and tremor increased considerably, but the small quantities involved made significance of deviation from the preoperative or nonpsychotic means of dubious importance. Latent period remained unchanged. All but one patient showed "outbursts" ranging from 1 to 10 per record. The interpretation of this is considered under "Discussion."

The small number of patients tested three months following lobotomy (see tables 30 and 31) make any findings of dubious value statistically. The latent period was within normal range in those lobotomy patients able to leave the hospital but not for those still hospitalized. On the other hand, those able to leave the hospital showed an absence of horizontal jerks and an increase of vertical jerks. A larger series is definitely indicated before even tentative conclusions can be drawn.

## DISCUSSION

Inadequate records were obtained of *spontaneous* nystagmus at the three-week postoperative test in the lobotomy group which is unfortunate since the postlobotomy records deviate extensively from the nonpsychotic control means. One hundred percent of the postlobotomy group, as opposed to 40 percent of the nonpsychotic controls, showed spontaneous horizontal nystagmus with a mean of 26.61 jerks per minute compared with the nonpsychotic control mean of 4.31 jerks per minute. Convergence difficulty, vertical jerks, and tremor showed no significant deviations when tested three months postoperatively.

In the topectomy patients, comparison of the correlation of the average increase in nystagmus compared to amount of tissue removed (table 23) at the immediate postoperative testing shows a most interesting change at the three- to four-month test. The second test was by a different method and shows quantity, not increase of nystagmus, but those patients noted in table 23 who were tested by the rotational technique showed a complete reversal from the earlier test with correspondingly reduced latent periods (table 32).

The records of the 9 men among the nonpsychotic controls who showed "outbursts" were compared to the controls without "outbursts." Although there was an increase in the number of horizontal jerks, both spontaneously and during rotation, the differences were not of statistical significance. Other differences showed a similar lack of statistical significance.

In all groups there was found to be a 0.43 positive product-moment coefficient of correlation between the length of the average latent period and the number of horizontal jerks per minute during and following rotation. The results are summarized in table 33.

## CONCLUSIONS

1. The caloric test has the advantage over the cinematic rotational test and other rotational tests in that with it each labyrinth can be studied separately; it is less complex, less expensive, and can be performed without the construction of special apparatus.

2. Both the caloric test and the cinematic rotational test are superior to the galvanic test in that they stimulate the end organ without exciting the retrolabyrinthine connections.

3. The cinematic rotational test has the distinct advantage in that (a) the end-point determination is much more accurate than in the caloric test, (b) the test itself is less disturbing to the patient than the caloric, (c) a constancy of stimulation is guaranteed, and, (d) a permanent record is obtained.

4. Neither the caloric nor the cinematic rotational test requires extensive skill or highly trained personnel for carrying out the respective procedures.

5. Testing of the labyrinthine mechanism in psychotic patients by the caloric test or the cinematic rotational test does not present any great difficulties.

6. Extensive control tests are indicated for these procedures in order to

TABLE 33. SUMMARY OF VESTIBULAR FINDINGS SHOWING MOST IMPORTANT VARIATIONS IN NONPSYCHOTIC CONTROLS AND IN PRE- AND POSTLOBOTOMY AND TOPECTOMY PATIENTS

| | Rotational and postrotational | | | | | Spontaneous | | | | | | |
| --- | --- | --- | --- | --- | --- | --- | --- | --- | --- | --- | --- | --- |
| | Horizontal jerks | | Average sec. of latent period | Outbursts | | Horizontal jerks | | Convergence difficulty | | Vertical jerks | | Time from operation to test |
| | Per min. | % of cases | | Per rec. | % of cases | Per min. | % of cases | Per min. | % of cases | Per min. | % of cases | |
| **95 Nonpsychotic** | | | | | | | | | | | | |
| Controls................. | 33.09 | 100 | 5.78 | .21 | 9.3 | 4.31 | 40 | .39 | 7.4 | .55 | 9.5 | No operation |
| S.D.................... | 16.55 | | 2.04 | 1.13 | | 7.72 | | 3.24 | | 3.18 | | |
| Prelobotomy patients........ | 47.95 | 100 | 5.94 | 0 | 0 | | | not tested | | | | No operation |
| Postlobotomy patients—3 weeks | 39.25 | 100 | 5.25 | 4.33 | 83.3 | 26.61 | 100 | .97 | 33.3 | 2.27 | 50.0 | 3–4 weeks |
| Postlobotomy patients— 3 months............ | 46.16 | 100 | 1.84 | 1.60 | 60.0 | 21.39 | 50 | 2.5 | 25.0 | 14.18 | 75 | 3–4 months |
| Postopectomy patients........ | 44.99 | 100 | 6.44 | 0 | 0 | 5.41 | 44.4 | .65 | 11.1 | 1.30 | 22.2 | 3–4 months |

determine the exact degree of influence that such variables, as age, sex, and barometric pressure, have on their respective results. If the standard of variation could then be determined, it would permit the measurement of the comparative variability of these procedures with the coefficient of variation in other tests of medical interest. Until this is accomplished, the value of the vestibular records must be classified as largely descriptive.

7. In general, topectomy resulted in a slight increase in the duration of nystagmus in this series of patients. For all intents and purposes, the finding of the product-moment coefficient of correlation of 0.75 strongly indicates that there is a positive relationship between the amount of tissue removed and the test of quantity or measurements at least, when measured three to four weeks postoperatively.

8. Consideration is being given to the possibility of incorporating a cinematic recording device with the caloric test. Comparisons will be made between the two tests with permanent records obtained for further diagnoses.

9. There appears to be an important relationship between the time at which tests are administered postoperatively and the results of the tests themselves. This fact may account for many of the apparently contradictory findings reported in the literature. This consideration leads directly into a discussion of the increased horizontal jerks, conjugate deviation, and vertical jerks as reported in table 30. The postlobotomy patients were tested three to four weeks postoperatively while the topectomy patients were tested three to four months postoperatively. The tremendous increase in spontaneous nystagmus in the postlobotomy group may be due to either the fact that testing was done shortly after operation or to the fact that a quantitatively greater amount of tissue was inactivated in the lobotomy patients than in the topectomy patients.

10. The nature of "outbursts" has led to considerable discussion. Owing to the recording method, it has not been possible to date to determine what occurs clinically. At one point, it was hypothesized that "outbursts" might be caused by nystagmus occurring during autokinetic movement. Against this hypothesis was the fact that they occurred in all but one of the lobotomized patients, none of whom at the time of the test showed any autokinetic movements (see chapter 9).

11. The vestibular findings in this series of patients, we feel, are not supported by a sufficiently clear preponderance of evidence. This chapter is, in the main, reportorial. It is felt that definite acceptance or rejection of any of our conclusions had best await further investigation and research. Pending such investigations, however, we believe that the foregoing résumé is worthy of consideration and should be thought of in the nature of a preliminary report.

*Chapter 10*

# Visual Apparatus:
# Visual Fields and Acuity,
# Color Vision, Autokinesis*

ROBERT G. HEATH, MALCOLM B. CARPENTER,
FRED A. METTLER, AND NATHAN S. KLINE†

---

R EPORTS are to be found in the literature of disturbances in vision in
primates following experimental removal of frontal cortex. For this reason
we carried out several tests before and following operation to detect if any
changes in the visual system occurred as a result of operation. (For changes
in casual movements of the bulbus see pp. 431 *et seq.*)

## VISUAL FIELDS AND ACUITY

**Topectomy Cases.** *Technique.* For testing visual acuity the standard Snellen
charts were used at 20 feet. For doing visual fields 1- and 5-mm. white test objects were
used with a standard black tangent screen. Patients were tested before operation and
again eighteen to twenty days following operation.
*Changes Resulting from Operation.* Preoperatively, 2 of the 23 patients showed
field defects from old corneal scarring. In one of these patients (19) there was an
upper, outer quadrantic field cut in the left eye. The other, patient 42, showed a
paracentral scotoma. These defects were not influenced by operation.
Of the 23 patients on whom topectomy was performed, 6 were so disturbed before
operation that neither fields nor acuity could be tested. In one additional patient it
was possible to evaluate acuity, but he was uncooperative for fields. After operation,
4 of these 7 patients were sufficiently improved that fields and acuity could be tested.
*Summary of Results.* No patient showed a field defect following operation that
was not present before. Visual acuity remained the same in most and improved in a
few. In no case was it impaired by operation.
In 12 of the patients, fields and acuity were the same following operation as before.
Three of the 7 patients who were too disturbed for preoperative testing remained
uncooperative after operation.
In 8 patients, performance was better following operation. In this group are included
the 4 who cooperated sufficiently to permit testing following operation but not before.
They are patients 22 (areas 9, 10, and 46), 25 (areas 8, 9, and 46), 27 (partial involve-
ment of areas 6, 8, 9, and 10), and 33 (areas 10, 44, 45, and 46). Four other patients

* For casual movements of the bulbus see p. 431 and for critical flicker fusion see chapter 19.
† Appreciation is expressed by Dr. Kline to Mrs. Jane Olmer and to Mr. A. Viggiano for
their technical assistance in his work.

showed improvement in visual acuity. Patients 2 (area 8), 7 (areas 8 and parts of 9 and 10), and 8 (middle frontal gyrus) showed an increase in acuity from 20/30 to 20/15. Patient 18 (area 11) showed a minimal increase from 20/20 to 20/15.

One patient, 40 (area 24), cooperated adequately for visual fields before operation but was too disturbed to be tested postoperatively. Her visual acuity remained the same.

**Lobotomy Cases.** There were 8 patients in this group. Three were disturbed and could not be tested before or after operation. Only one of the remaining 5 patients (11) was able to cooperate for the tests as well twelve to fourteen days following operation as before. The other 4 showed no field defects but they could not center their attention adequately for the examiner to locate the blind spot or accurately to outline the periphery of the field. Two patients in this group had previously had topectomy. One (44) also refused to cooperate before or following that procedure. The other patient (2) was more alert following removal of area 8 bilaterally than he had been before that operation. It was only after lobotomy that he became too distractible to be tested.

### DISCUSSION

Kennard ('39) reported visual field defects in primates following unilateral removal of area 8 (Vogt chart) that were indistinguishable from those seen following destruction of the occipital cortex. These were reported to last two to four months. Kennard also noted defects in the peripheral field of vision following bilateral removal of area 8 but not complete blindness.

Findings by other workers in the field were contrary to those of Kennard. Mettler ('44) and later Lashley and Clark ('46) denied that disturbances of true vision occurred after ablation of frontal cortex.

In this study there were no marked changes in the visual fields following topectomy. Peripheral vision was at least as good as before. Several of the patients had area 8 removed. Patients who were made more cooperative by operation frequently showed improvement in visual acuity and several who were too uncooperative to undergo visual-field examination before operation performed well after. Only 1 of the 5 lobotomized patients who before operation cooperated adequately was sufficiently cooperative following operation to permit the taking of fields.

### ISHIHARA COLOR VISION TESTS

In this test twenty-five numbers are concealed in a field of contrasting colors and there are seven designs that the subject is asked to trace through a field of various colors. Colors are so arranged that various types of color blindness can be detected from the responses. None of the patients was color blind. Mistakes were made but they were of a bizarre type which indicated an inability to concentrate rather than an organic difference in the visual system. As in the case of the visual-field and acuity tests, there was in several of the patients some difference in response before and after operation.

Thirteen of the 24 operatees gave essentially the same responses following operation as before. In 5 patients there were three to eight fewer errors after operation than before. Patient 25 (areas 8, 9, and 46) made 8 less errors. Others with lesser improvement were patients 32 (areas 8 and 9), 33 (areas 10, partial, 46, partial, 45, and 44), 49 (area 10), and 47 (area 44).

Five patients made more errors after operation than before. They were patients 38 (venous ligation), 7 (areas 8, 9, and 10), 4 (area 46), 3 (partial removal of areas 6, 8, and 9), and 19 (area 45). Three patients in this group improved clinically and 2 did not.

## DISCUSSION

Results of the Ishihara test fell within the realm of pure chance. The minimal differences between the pre- and postoperative testing indicated no disturbance in the visual system. Five patients performed slightly better and 5 slightly poorer.

### AUTOKINESIS

That a single point of light of not too great intensity will appear to move spontaneously when seen in dark surroundings has been known for some time. Systematic investigation of the nature of this phenomenon has been undertaken in relation to many fields and recently the claim has been advanced that there are significant statistical differences in different types of mental disease as far as the extent and nature of movement of this light is concerned. Since the extent and direction and pattern of movement is a spontaneous production of the subject, it was felt that the comparison of control subjects with both the topectomy and the lobotomy group would be of major interest.

**Apparatus.** The source of light is a hole of pinpoint size placed in an otherwise lightproof box containing a 15-watt standard bulb. The pinpoint is not directly in line but several inches above the center of the bulb itself. Fifteen feet from the source of light is a recording table. The table is built at an inclination comfortable for writing and fed over the top of it was a roll of ordinary wrapping paper which is held fast by a steel bar across the bottom with a cutting edge. This enables records to be easily removed, filed, and automatically prepares the board for the next record. The recording table itself is about 30 inches square. No other apparatus except a pencil, an automatic timer, and the lightproof room is required.

**Technique.** The subject is brought into the test room with the lights on. The source of light, however, is kept behind a curtain except when the lights are out. The subject is seated at the recording table and an "X" is placed by the experimenter in the center of the record sheet. The next step is to place the pencil in the subject's hand in an ordinary writing position resting on the "X." No explanation of what to expect is given at this time in order to influence the subject's reaction as little as possible. This procedure ordinarily occupies at least two or three minutes so that any ordinary stimulation of walking or turning is nullified. The lights are then turned off and simultaneously the autokinetic light is exposed. (Results allowing time for dark adaptation were not significantly different and therefore the adaptation period was abandoned.) The subject is then instructed to "describe what you see." Except in very rare instances, the usual object seen is "a small light." The color of the light may be described at this time spontaneously. The next instruction is "tell me anything at all that happens to the light." Instructions, of course, are worded this way in order to avoid suggesting movement. When movement, if it does occur, is indicated, the time elapsing between when the subject sees the light and when motion begins is noted (stop watch). When the subject mentions that the light is moving he is then told to "draw on the paper, the *distance* and *direction* in which the light moves; in other words, try to follow the light exactly as it is moving." The subject is also told to keep describing the movements or any other changes in the light. If the subject notes that the light stops (care is taken not to suggest that this will occur), he is told to place a circle at that point. He continues as before if the light should again move. If the subject comments that the pencil with which he is following the light has moved off the paper, and *only* if this occurs, he is asked to bring the pencil back to

TABLE 34. PATTERN ANALYSIS OF CONTROL, TOPECTOMY, AND LOBOTOMY SUBJECTS

**Control group (100 subjects):**

| Pattern | No movement | Simple | Unidirectional One reversal | Circular | Zigzag | Multiple | Nondescript |
|---|---|---|---|---|---|---|---|
| Frequency | 2 | 20 | 15 | 34 | 14 | 13 | 2 |

**Topectomy group:**

| Patient No. | 3 | 4 | 6 | 7 | 13 | 21 | 25 |
|---|---|---|---|---|---|---|---|
| Pattern | Unidirectional one reversal | Unidirectional one reversal | Circular | Nondescript | Nondescript | Zigzag | Unidirectional |

| Patient No. | 27 | 33 | 38 | 42 | 49 |
|---|---|---|---|---|---|
| Pattern | Unidirectional | Multiple | Unidirectional one reversal | Unidirectional | Unidirectional one reversal |

**Lobotomy group:**

| Patient No. | 2 | 5 | 11 | 20 | 23 | 28 | 44 | 46 |
|---|---|---|---|---|---|---|---|---|
| Pattern: | | | | | | | | |
| 3 wks. postop | No movement | No test* | Unidirectional one reversal | Zigzag* | Unidirectional | No movement | No movement | No movement |
| 3 mos. postop | No test | Unidirectional* | Circular | Unidirectional one reversal | Nondescript | Unidirectional | Nondescript | Unidirectional one reversal |

* Returned home before expiration of three-month postoperative period.

approximately the center of the paper and continue as before. Conversation that might influence or distract the subject is kept to a minimum. If no movement is noted after five minutes, the subject is told this time to note carefully whether or not the light moves and a second five-minute run is completed.

When the automatic timer, which has been set for exactly five minutes, rings, the curtain is pulled over the source of light with the room left totally dark. The subject is then asked to estimate the total distance which the light has moved since he first saw it "if the movement were stretched out in a straight line." The subject is next asked to estimate what part of the time the light was in motion and finally a check is made as to the color which the light appeared to be, if it had not been previously mentioned. If it had been previously mentioned, one makes certain it remained the same. The approximate speed of movement (slow, moderate, or fast) and the amount of forward and backward movement as it appeared is also obtained. Only after all this information has been gathered are the lights turned on.

**Results.** One hundred control subjects had already been tested for another experiment and the results obtained from these are given as a baseline. The control group differed from the test tabulation in that all of the controls were male, all veterans, and none had histories of known psychoneuroses or psychoses. Other data had already shown that there was no correlation between age and autokinesis so that this factor did not need to be accounted for.

On each of the subjects the following information was obtained: (1) Estimated distance. (2) Estimated part of the time in motion. (3) Color of the light. (4) Time before movement began after light was first seen. (5) Estimate of forward and backward movement. (6) Estimated speed of movement (slow, moderate, or fast). (7) Total distance in inches drawn on record. (8) Number of stops. (9) Greatest distance from the starting point (direct distance between starting point by direct measurement in a straight line to point farthest removed from starting point). (10) Greatest distance between any two points (maximum breadth). (11) Number of times pencil moved off paper. (12) Direction of movement. (13) Number of reversals. (14) Length of the test. (15) Age of the patient. (16) Whether done with monocular or binocular vision. (17) Whether the subject was wearing glasses (and if so, were they bifocals). (18) Occupation. (19) Handedness of the subject. (20) Eyedness (this was tested for by having the patient hold a card with a small hole in it and requesting him to look at a distant object). (21) Pattern as drawn on the recording sheet. (22) Other remarks that were felt might be contributory.

For the purpose of analysis, what appear at the present time to be the four most significant factors, are presented. These are: (1) pattern, (2) color, (3) total distance recorded by the pencil, (4) maximum breadth (greatest distance between any two points on the drawing pattern).

Table 34 presents the data on pattern for the control group, the topectomy group, and the lobotomy group (at both the three-week and three-month retests). The small number of cases in the two latter groups studied at the present time makes reliable statistical analysis very difficult. Table 35 presents the data on color. Table 36 presents the data on maximum breadth. Table 37 presents the data on total distance.

The most significant contrast between the control group and the test group is that 98 percent of the control group showed some movement whereas none of the lobotomy patients at the three-week testing showed any real autokinetic movement. A single movement on a single occasion (which is often caused by

TABLE 35. COLOR ANALYSIS OF CONTROL, TOPECTOMY, AND LOBOTOMY SUBJECTS

| | | | | | | | | | |
|---|---|---|---|---|---|---|---|---|---|
| **Control group (100 subjects):** | | | | | | | | | |
| Color.............. | White | Silver | Star | Yellow | Orange | Red | Blue | Green | Changeable |
| Frequency.......... | 35 | 2 | 1 | 37 | 7 | 9 | 4 | 1 | 4 |
| **Topectomy group:** | | | | | | | | | |
| Patient No......... | 3 | 4 | 6 | 7 | 13 | 25 | 27 | 33 | 38 |
| Color.............. | Gold | Bluish white | White | Changeable | White | White with blue | White with blue | White | Yellowish white |
| Patient No......... | 42 | 49 | | | | | | | |
| Color.............. | White | Yellow | | | | | | | |
| **Lobotomy group:** | | | | | | | | | |
| Patient No......... | 2 | | 5 | 11 | 20 | 23 | 28 | 44 | 46 |
| Color 3 wks. postop.... | White | | Amber | Red | Not recorded | Reddish yellow | "Cigarette" | Not recorded | Orchid |
| Color 3 mos. postop.... | Not recorded | | No test* | Red | White | Flame | White | No test | No test |

* Returned home before expiration of three-month postoperative period.

TABLE 36. MAXIMUM BREADTH DRAWN BY CONTROL TOPECTOMY AND LOBOTOMY SUBJECTS

| | 0–1.9 | 2–3.9 | 4–5.9 | 6–7.9 | 8–9.9 | 10–11.9 | 12–13.9 | 14–15.9 | 16–17.9 | 18–19.9 | 20–21.9 | 22–23.9 | 24–25.9 |
|---|---|---|---|---|---|---|---|---|---|---|---|---|---|
| **Control group (100 subjects):** | | | | | | | | | | | | | |
| Maximum breadth† | 0–1.9 | 2–3.9 | 4–5.9 | 6–7.9 | 8–9.9 | 10–11.9 | 12–13.9 | 14–15.9 | 16–17.9 | 18–19.9 | 20–21.9 | 22–23.9 | 24–25.9 |
| Frequency | 8 | 14 | 15 | 12 | 18 | 6 | 4 | 8 | 6 | 3 | 3 | 2 | 1 |
| **Topectomy group:** | | | | | | | | | | | | | |
| Patient No. | 3 | 4 | | 7 | 13 | 21 | 25 | 27 | 33 | 38 | 42 | | 49 |
| Maximum breadth† | 3.5 | 2.9 | | 10.0 | 5.8 | 6.0 | 1.6 | 28.0 | 14.3 | 3.1 | 18.1 | | 11.9 |
| **Lobotomy group:** | | | | | | | | | | | | | |
| Patient No. | 2 | 5 | | 11 | 20 | 23 | 28 | 44 | 46 | | | | |
| Maximum breadth:† | | | | | | | | | | | | | |
| 3 wks. postop. | 0 | 0 | | 0 | 0 | 0 | 0 | 0 | 0 | | | | |
| 3 mos. postop. | 0 | no test* | | 1.8 | 4.8 | .5 | 0 | no test | 0 | | | | |

\* Returned home before expiration of three-month postoperative period.
† Maximum breadth in inches.

TABLE 37.  TOTAL DISTANCE DRAWN BY CONTROL, TOPECTOMY, AND LOBOTOMY SUBJECTS

| | 0–9.9 | 10–19.9 | 20–29.9 | 30–39.9 | 40–49.9 | 50–59.9 | 60–69.9 | 70–79.9 | 80–89.9 | 90–99.9 | over 100 (141) |
|---|---|---|---|---|---|---|---|---|---|---|---|
| **Control group (100 subjects):** | | | | | | | | | | | |
| Total distance† | | | | | | | | | | | |
| Frequency | 24 | 26 | 18 | 12 | 8 | 4 | 0 | 1 | 5 | 1 | 1 |
| **Topectomy group:** | | | | | | | | | | | |
| Patient No. | 3 | 4 | 6 | 7 | 13 | 21 | 25 | 27 | 33 | 38 | 42 |
| Total distance† | 10.6 | 8.0 | 1.7 | 120.0 | 33.1 | 29.5 | 1.8 | 29.4 | 45.6 | 7.5 | 31.0 |
| Patient No. | | | | | | | | | | | 49 |
| Total distance† | | | | | | | | | | | 21.5 |
| **Lobotomy group:** | | | | | | | | | | | |
| Patient No. | 2 | 5 | 11 | 20 | 23 | 28 | 44 | 46 | | | |
| Total distance:† | | | | | | | | | | | |
| 3 weeks postop. | 0 | 0 | 0 | 0 | 0 | 0 | 0 | no test | | | |
| 3 months postop. | 0 | no test* | 2.2 | 9.5 | .5 | 0 | no test | no test | | | |

* Returned home before expiration of three-month postoperative period.
† Total distance in inches.

a gross head movement) is not considered to be autokinetic movement. Of the 5 lobotomy patients retested three months after operation, 3 did show autokinetic movement. Two of these 3 patients had been discharged from the hospital.

### DISCUSSION

The type and nature of the pattern is undoubtedly one of the most significant features in any record. The classification of patterns presents a difficult problem. After a general review, seven classifications were decided upon. Two of these are not true patterns since one is "no movement" and another "nondescript patterns." A third classification includes those subjects

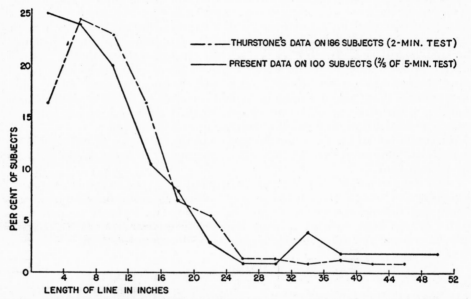

Fig. 83. Comparison of the total distance drawn in the autokinetic test by Thurstone's 186 subjects and by our 100 control subjects.

who utilize more than one pattern. This leaves only four true patterns: (1) unidirectional over-all movement, (2) unidirectional over-all movement with a single reversal, (3) circular, (4) zigzag.

There has been some conjecture that there may be an order of complexity of patterns which is roughly as enumerated in (1) to (4). This question is under investigation at the present time. On this hypothesis the patterns of the topectomized patients appear to be "simpler" than those of the controls. One difficulty involved is that the comparison is between previously psychotic patients and nonpsychotic controls. The patterns of several hundred psychotic patients are also being reviewed at the present time to provide a better baseline. Certainly if the opportunity is presented to repeat a study of this kind a record should be obtained pre- as well as postoperatively. This is true, of course, not only of patterns but for all factors investigated.

The meaning of the color distribution is not clear. The finding that subjects saw the light as other than white came as quite a surprise to the investigators. There had been some expectation that it might be seen as yellow but the fact that yellow predominated and that there was a veritable spectrum of other hues, is interesting.

The total distance is the simplest and most obvious measurement to make and in many respects appears to be the most differentiating. The actual total distance is certainly to some extent determined by the frame of reference in which the subject is asked to draw the apparent movement of the light. Comparing the present experiment with that of Thurstone ('43) it will be noted that Thurstone's subjects were tested for only two minutes while ours were tested for five minutes. Therefore, if two-fifths of our movement were plotted, it should give an approximate equivalent of the data obtained by Thurstone on his 186 subjects. This data is presented in figure 83 and the close agreement seems to indicate that a frame of reference may not be as important as we felt at one time, since our recording sheet is approximately two and a half times the size of that used by Thurstone. Further experimentation is under way to determine what role the frame of reference (as determined by the size of the drawing board) actually does play. The fact that 98 percent of the control subjects showed movement and none of the lobotomy patients showed movement three weeks postoperatively, has already been mentioned. Even after three months those who did show movement were all in the zero group which indicates a quantitative reduction of movement. Certainly a larger series of cases is needed before any definite conclusion can be drawn.

Maximum breadth is again partly dependent on the frame of reference and analysis of "minimum breadth" as well as maximum is being undertaken at the present time.

Other data as well as that presented are being subjected to rather thorough statistical analysis but it is felt that a more substantial series must be obtained before any significant conclusions can be drawn. The formula proposed by Voth ('47) has been rejected as being impractical for our purpose, in part at least, because of the difference in technique in obtaining the data.

## Conclusions

1. Bilateral, simultaneous ablation of various Brodmann frontal areas, and combinations of these, does not produce, in the human being, any impairment in the visual field nor in acuity of peripheral vision.

2. Color vision is not adversely influenced.

3. Improvements in the present patients' reports in these spheres is to be regarded as a reflection of improvement in psychiatric state rather than as visual improvement.

4. Lobotomized patients when tested three weeks postoperatively show a complete absence of autokinetic movement.

5. Three months postlobotomy there is recovery of autokinetic movement in some of the patients. This appears to be quantitatively reduced in the sense that the total distance observed is smaller than that for control subjects and qualitatively reduced in that the patterns drawn are "simpler."

6. There is no loss of autokinetic movement in patients tested three months posttopectomy but there is a suggestion that the patterns are "simpler" than in a group of nonpsychotic control subjects.

7. Both a more substantial series of cases and a more detailed statistical analysis are being undertaken at the present time to clarify the meaning of certain rather suggestive findings.

## Chapter 11

# Gastrointestinal Motility

### DANIEL G. MELVIN

PRE- and postoperative studies were made to determine any deviation in intestinal pattern, any increase or decrease in propulsive movement, or any other abnormality that might occur in psychotic patients subjected (a) to cortical ablation and (b) lobotomy.

**Method of Study.** The usual roentgenologic techniques were followed insofar as the patient's psychotic behavior permitted. Lack of cooperation introduced serious complications. When possible, the patients were observed fluoroscopically as they drank the barium mixture and the fluoroscope was utilized to great advantage in watching the progress of the meal through the gastrointestinal tract. Several of the patients refused to take any of the barium, others took two or three swallows, and several others took only approximately half of the mixture. This lack of cooperation on the part of some of the patients necessitated tube feeding. Others had to have the examination postponed for one or two days because of regurgitation of the barium or for other reasons. Serial films were made in the posteroanterior, anteroposterior, and right and left oblique projections of the stomach and duodenum. The small intestine was studied serially by films made in the anteroposterior and posteroanterior projection. As expected, numerous films were ruined because of movement of the patient and it was necessary to repeat many of the studies on this account. Spot films with compression were not attempted on these patients because the examiner had found on previous occasions that this procedure on the usual psychotic patient caused the subject to become so disturbed that it was impossible to obtain adequate results. Twenty-four- and forty-eight-hour films were not made.

**Preoperative Findings.** In table 38 the critical data for all of the patients are listed. For present purposes we are concerned with only the first line of figures (the data obtained just prior to the visit to the surgery) for each patient. Thus the emptying time of the stomach in most patients occurred between the third and fourth hours (from two to three hours in 10 patients, from three to four in 17, from four to five in 12, from five to six in 7, and from six to seven in 1; in 1 patient emptying was delayed until nine hours and forty-five minutes). The small intestine emptied in most patients between the eighth and ninth hour (from seven to eight, in 8, from eight to nine, in 12, from nine to ten, in 8, from ten to eleven, in 5, from eleven to twelve, in 3, from twelve to thirteen, in 5, from thirteen to fourteen, in 5, and from fourteen to fifteen, in 1; in 1 patient the intestines emptied in five and a half hours). Table 39 gives a general description of roentgenologic findings in all the cases studied.

TABLE 38. CRITICAL ROENTGENOLOGIC DATA PREOPERATIVELY (OR BEFORE VISIT TO SURGERY) AFTER TOPECTOMY AND AFTER LOBOTOMY

| Case No. | Age | Sex | Operation [a] | Emptying time of stomach | Emptying time of small intestines | Operative removal |
|---|---|---|---|---|---|---|
| 1 | 55 | M | | 4 hrs. 45 min. | 11 hrs. 45 min. | Control |
| 2 | 46 | M | P. (1) | 5 hrs. 15 min. | 11 hrs. 45 min. | 8, 6[b], (lobot.[c]) |
| | | | T. (2) | 8 hrs. 15 min. | 13 hrs. 30 min. | |
| | | | P.F.L. (3) | 3 hrs. 30 min. | 11 hrs. 45 min. | |
| 3 | 61 | M | P. (1) | 4 hrs. 45 min. | 10 hrs. | 9[b], 6[b] |
| | | | T. (2) | 3 hrs. 15 min. | 8 hrs. 30 min. | |
| 4 | 55 | M | P. (1) | 5 hrs. | 12 hrs. | 46 |
| | | | T. (2) | 5 hrs. | 8 hrs. 30 min. | |
| 5 | 35 | M | P. (1) | 6 hrs. | 12 hrs. | Control (lobot.[c]) |
| | | | P.F.L. (2) | 3 hrs. 15 min. | 8 hrs. 30 min. | |
| 6 | 32 | M | P. (1) | 3 hrs. 15 min. | 13 hrs. | 8[b], 6[d], 6[e] |
| | | | T. (2) | 4 hrs. 30 min. | 14 hrs. | |
| | | | T. (3) | 3 hrs. 30 min. | 10 hrs. 15 min. | |
| 7 | 40 | M | (1) | 3 hrs. | 9 hrs. 45 min. | 8, 9[b], 10[b] |
| | | | T. (2) | 4 hrs. 30 min. | 8 hrs. 45 min. | |
| 8 | 29 | M | P. (1) | 4 hrs. | 9 hrs. 45 min. | 10[b], 46[b], 9[b], 8[b] |
| | | | T. (2) | 2 hrs. 30 min. | 9 hrs. 30 min. | |
| 9 | 44 | M | | 3 hrs. | 12 hrs. 45 min. | Control |
| 10 | 44 | M | | 3 hrs. | 11 hrs. 30 min. | Control |
| 11 | 44 | M | P. (1) | 4 hrs. | 9 hrs. | Control (lobot.[c]) |
| | | | P.F.L. (2) | 2 hrs. 30 min. | 7 hrs. | |
| 12 | 57 | M | | 4 hrs. 45 min. | 9 hrs. 30 min. | Control |
| 13 | 43 | M | P. (1) | 3 hrs. 45 min. | 10 hrs. 15 min. | 9[b], 10[b], 45, 46 |
| | | | T. (2) | 3 hrs. 30 min. | 9 hrs. 15 min. | |
| 14 | 47 | M | | 4 hrs. 30 min. | 10 hrs. 15 min. | Control |
| 15 | 55 | M | | 4 hrs. 30 min. | 8 hrs. 45 min. | Control |
| 16 | 50 | M | | 3 hrs. 45 min. | 9 hrs. 15 min. | Control |
| 17 | 60 | M | | 9 hrs. 45 min. | 14 hrs. 15 min. | Control |
| 18 | 39 | M | P. (1) | 5 hrs. | 10 hrs. 30 min. | 11[b] |
| | | | T. (2) | 4 hrs. 30 min. | 6 hrs. 45 min. | |
| 19 | 50 | M | P. (1) | 3 hrs. 30 min. | 12 hrs. 45 min. | 45[b] |
| | | | T. (2) | 3 hrs. 15 min. | 11 hrs. 45 min. | |
| 20 | 28 | M | P. (1) | 5 hrs. | 12 hrs. 45 min. | Control (lobot.[c]) |
| | | | P.F.L. (2) | 2 hrs. 30 min. | 7 hrs. | |
| 21 | 42 | M | P. (1) | 3 hrs. 15 min. | 10 hrs. 30 min. | 10 |
| | | | T. (2) | 2 hrs. 45 min. | 7 hrs. | |
| 22 | 50 | M | P. (1) | 3 hrs. 30 min. | 13 hrs. 45 min. | 9, 10, 46 |
| | | | T. (2) | 3 hrs. 30 min. | 12 hrs. | |
| 23 | 29 | M | P. (1) | 4 hrs. | 13 hrs. | Control (lobot.[c]) |
| | | | P.F.L. (2) | 3 hrs. 30 min. | 10 hrs. 30 min. | |
| 24 | 41 | M | P. (1) | 2 hrs. 45 min. | 8 hrs. 45 min. | 6[d] (6[e]) |
| | | | T. (2) | 6 hrs. 45 min. | 12 hrs. 45 min. | |
| 25 | 58 | M | P. (1) | 3 hrs. 15 min. | 8 hrs. 15 min. | 8, 9, 46, 10[b] |
| | | | T. (2) | 3 hrs. 15 min. | 11 hrs. 15 min. | |
| 26 | 35 | M | | 3 hrs. 45 min. | 13 hrs. | Control |
| 27 | 34 | M | P. (1) | 5 hrs. | 13 hrs. | 10[b], 9[b], 8[b], 6[b] |
| | | | T. (2) | 2 hrs. 30 min. | 9 hrs. 15 min. | |
| 28 | 27 | M | P. (1) | 2 hrs. 15 min. | 7 hrs. 30 min. | Control (lobot.[e]) |
| | | | P.F.L. (2) | 3 hrs. 30 min. | 8 hrs. 30 min. | |
| 29 | 20 | M | | 2 hrs. 15 min. | 7 hrs. 30 min. | Control |

TABLE 38.   CRITICAL ROENTGENOLOGIC DATA PREOPERATIVELY (OR BEFORE VISIT TO SURGERY) AFTER TOPECTOMY AND AFTER LOBOTOMY—(*Continued*)

| Case No. | Age | Sex | Operation [a] | Emptying time of stomach | Emptying time of small intestines | Operative removal |
|---|---|---|---|---|---|---|
| 30 | 45 | M | | 2 hrs. 15 min. | 7 hrs. 30 min. | Control |
| 31 | 51 | F | P. (1) | 5 hrs. | 9 hrs. 45 min. | 9 |
| | | | T. (2) | 7 hrs. 45 min. | 14 hrs. 30 min. | |
| 32 | 41 | F | P. (1) | 3 hrs. | 8 hrs. 45 min. | 8[b], 9, 10[b] |
| | | | T. (2) | 3 hrs. 30 min. | 9 hrs. 15 min. | |
| 33 | 27 | F | P. (1) | 4 hrs. 30 min. | 8 hrs. 30 min. | 10[b], 46[b], 45, 44[b] |
| | | | T. (2) | 6 hrs. 15 min. | 13 hrs. 45 min. | |
| 34 | 33 | F | | 4 hrs. 45 min. | 7 hrs. 15 min. | Control |
| 35 | 59 | F | | 3 hrs. | 9 hrs. 30 min. | Control |
| 36 | 53 | F | P. (1) | 3 hrs. 45 min. | 8 hrs. 30 min. | 10, 11, 45, 46, 47 |
| | | | T. (2) | 9 hrs. 45 min. | 13 hrs. 30 min. | |
| 37 | 38 | F | | 2 hrs. | 8 hrs. | Control |
| 38 | 38 | F | P. (1) | 2 hrs. 15 min. | 7 hrs. 15 min. | 6, 8, 9, 10[f] |
| | | | T. (2) | 3 hrs. 30 min. | 6 hrs. 30 min. | |
| 39 | 44 | F | | 3 hrs. 15 min. | 7 hrs. 15 min. | Control |
| 40 | 29 | F | P. (1) | 3 hrs. 15 min. | 9 hrs. 15 min. | 24[b] |
| | | | T. (2) | 6 hrs. 30 min. | 9 hrs. 45 min. | |
| 41 | 46 | F | | 2 hrs. 15 min. | 7 hrs. 15 min. | Control |
| 42 | 40 | F | P. (1) | 2 hrs. 15 min. | 7 hrs. 15 min. | 11 |
| | | | T. (2) | 4 hrs. 15 min. | 10 hrs. 15 min. | |
| 44 | 38 | F | P. (1) | 5 hrs. 15 min. | 8 hrs. 30 min. | 10[b] (lobot.[c]) |
| | | | T. (2) | 6 hrs. 30 min. | 10 hrs. 15 min. | |
| | | | P.F.L. (3) | 3 hrs. 30 min. | 8 hrs. 45 min. | |
| 45 | 41 | F | | 5 hrs. 15 min. | 8 hrs. | Control |
| 46 | 29 | F | P. (1) | 3 hrs. 30 min. | 8 hrs. 30 min. | Control (lobot.[c]) |
| | | | P.F.L. (2) | 3 hrs. 15 min. | 9 hrs. | |
| 47 | 31 | F | P. (1) | 5 hrs. 15 min. | 8 hrs. 30 min. | 44 |
| | | | T. (2) | 5 hrs. | 14 hrs. 15 min. | |
| 48 | 26 | F | | 2 hrs. 45 min. | 5 hrs. 30 min. | Control |
| 49 | 39 | F | P. (1) | 2 hrs. 30 min. | 8 hrs. 30 min. | 10, 11[b], 46[b] |
| | | | T. (2) | 3 hrs. 30 min. | 9 hrs. 30 min. | |

[a] P.=preoperatively or preanesthesia; T.=after topectomy; P.F.L.=after lobotomy. Numbers in parentheses refer to number and sequence of the gastrointestinal studies so designated.
[b] Part only.
[c] Done five months after original operation or anesthesia.
[d] Incomplete original removal (caudally).
[e] Venous ligation.
[f] Unilateral verification done five months after original operation.

**Postoperative Findings in Topectomy Series.**   The control patients were not reexamined following their visit to surgery. The operatees were restudied approximately two weeks after operation, the shortest interval being ten days and the longest thirty. This is not the best procedure to follow. Mettler, Spindler, Mettler, and Combs ('36) have shown that the motility changes which occur after bilateral removal of canine frontal cortex vary with time. The emptying time of the stomach is at first delayed owing to pylorospasm. The pylorospasm may last from three to twenty-one days. When it disappears the fundamental activity of the remainder of the gastrointestinal tract becomes apparent in a reduction of emptying time wherever recorded. Such activity is apparently present from the onset but the pylorospasm prevents the test material from going through and the overactivity of the intestines is therefore not detected. In the present studies most examinations undoubtedly fell beyond the presumable period of greatest pylorospasm but it is recognized that one is dealing with a period of potential instability.

Directing our attention to the second line in table 38, that marked T, one may find the data obtained following topectomy. It may be observed that parts of and whole similar areas were removed in certain cases. Patient 8 had parts of areas 8, 9, 10, and 46 removed and patient 25 all of areas 8, 9, and 46 and part of area 10. Patient 18 had part of area 11 removed and patient 42 all of this area. Patient 7 had all of area 8 and part of areas 9 and 10 removed; patient 32 had parts of areas 8 and 10 and all

TABLE 39. GENERAL ROENTGENOLOGIC FINDINGS IN CASES STUDIED

Cases 1, 7, 8, 12, 13, 15, 18, 20–22, 25–27, 29, 30, 36, 38, 41, 45, 46—Gastrointestinal tract normal.

Cases 2, 3, 4, 6, 23, 24, 37, 39, 47—Gastrointestinal tract normal except for some spasticity of the colon.

Case 5—Cecum is in the pelvis. Some ptosis of the colon present.

Case 9—Gastrointestinal tract normal. Colon shows some ptosis.

Case 10—Gastrointestinal tract normal. The cecum is inverted.

Case 11—Gastrointestinal tract normal. There is some ptosis of the colon.

Case 14—Gastrointestinal tract normal. The cecum is low in the pelvis and the ascending colon is extremely long.

Case 16—Marked spasticity of the colon and some redundancy of the sigmoid.

Case 17—The stomach was normal in position and contour. There is no evidence of ulcer or other pathologic condition. The duodenal bulb shows marked deformity although no ulcer niche could be demonstrated. It took the stomach nine hours and forty-five minutes to be emptied. The intestinal pattern was normal and there is marked spasticity of the colon. Impression: Duodenal ulcer.

Case 19—Some ptosis and spasticity of the colon. The cecum is in the pelvis.

Case 28—Gastrointestinal tract normal except for some ptosis of transverse colon.

Case 31—The cecum is low in the pelvis. The transverse colon is markedly ptosed.

Case 32—The cecum is low in the pelvis. Some spasticity and ptosis of the colon, otherwise normal.

Case 33—Gastrointestinal tract normal except for ptosis and spasticity of the colon.

Case 34—The stomach is normal in position, size, and shape. The duodenal bulb is consistently deformed, though no definite niche can be demonstrated. Intestinal pattern is normal. Impression: Duodenal ulcer.

Case 35—Evidences of a posterior gastrojejunostomy performed for duodenal ulcer are noted. There is also some spasticity of the colon.

Case 40—Gastrointestinal tract normal. Colon is normal.

Case 42—Gastrointestinal tract normal. Some scoliosis of the spine to the right.

Case 44—Gastrointestinal tract normal except for some spasticity of the colon.

Case 48—Gastrointestinal tract normal. Marked ptosis and redundancy of the colon, some spasticity.

Case 49—The cecum is in the pelvis. Transverse colon shows marked ptosis.

of area 9 removed. Patient 27 had parts of areas 6, 8, 9, and 10 removed and patient 38 all of areas 6, 8, 9, and 10. Patient 21 had all of area 10 removed and patient 44 part of this area. Prior to operation, patient 8 showed an emptying time of the stomach of four hours and of the small intestines of nine hours; after operation the stomach emptied in two hours and thirty minutes and the small intestine in nine hours and thirty minutes. In patient 25, prior to operation the stomach emptied in three hours and fifteen minutes, the small intestine in eight hours and fifteen minutes; after operation the stomach emptied in three hours and fifteen minutes, the small intestine in eleven hours and fifteen minutes. In patient 18, prior to operation the stomach emptied in five hours, the small intestine in ten hours and thirty minutes; after operation the stomach emptied in four hours and thirty minutes, the small intestine in six hours and forty-five minutes. In patient 42, before operation the stomach emptied in two hours and fifteen minutes, the small intestine in seven hours and fifteen minutes; after operation the stomach emptied in four hours and fifteen minutes, the small intestine in ten hours and fifteen minutes. In patient 7, prior to operation the stomach emptied in three hours, the small intestine in nine hours and forty-five minutes; after operation the stomach emptied in four hours and thirty minutes, the small intestine in eight hours and forty-five minutes. In patient 32, before operation the stomach emptied in three hours, the small intestine in eight hours and forty-five minutes; after operation the stomach emptied in three hours and thirty minutes, the small intestine in nine hours and fifteen minutes. In patient 27, prior to operation the stomach emptied in five hours, the small intestine in thirteen hours; after operation the stomach emptied in two hours and thirty minutes, the small intestine in nine hours and fifteen minutes. In patient 38, before operation the stomach emptied in two hours and fifteen minutes, the small intestine in seven hours and fifteen minutes; after operation the stomach emptied in three hours and thirty minutes, the small intestine in six hours and thirty minutes. In patient 21, before operation the stomach emptied in three hours and fifteen minutes, the small intestine in ten hours and thirty minutes; after operation the stomach emptied in two hours and forty-five minutes, the small intestine in seven hours. In patient 44, prior to operation the stomach emptied in five hours and fifteen minutes, the small intestine in eight hours and thirty minutes; after operation the stomach emptied in six hours and thirty minutes, the small intestine in ten hours and fifteen minutes.

**Interpretation of Results of Topectomy.**    The three general regions within the frontal lobe which have been reported to exercise a particular effect upon the autonomic system are the orbital cortex (Bailey and Sweet, '40), the agranular precentral region (Sheehan, '34; Hesser, Langworthy, and Kolb, '41), and the cingular cortex (Smith, W. K., '45; Ward, '48).

With regard to the orbital cortex, it will be observed that the postoperative pattern was opposite in the 2 cases in which area 11 was removed by itself.

Patients in whom the front part of the agranular region (area 6) was removed without encroachment particularly upon cortex situated far forward, notably patients 6 and 24, showed an increased emptying time of the stomach with a reduced or unchanged emptying time of the intestines. Removal of the neighboring cortex (area 8) tended to produce the same effect. Other than these, no trends could be observed with regard to ablations which had areal factors in common.

The series contained only 1 patient (40) from whom medial cortex was removed. In this patient a notable lengthening of gastric emptying time occurred. More observations on this type of case are indicated.

In summary it may be stated that no definite pattern of disturbed gastro-intestinal motility was manifest in the operatees as a group, although 11 patients showed lengthening of both gastric and combined gastrointestinal times as against 6 who showed shortening of both, 13 showed lengthening of gastric emptying time alone as against 6 who showed shortening, and 13 exhibited increased combined gastrointestinal emptying time as against 11 who showed shortening. However, the difficulties attendant upon an investigation of this type on psychotic patients are such that unless large numbers are studied only very pronounced changes might be apparent. More cases should be studied and individual cases should be studied more frequently.

No evidence of trends in one direction or another could be correlated with removals of areas or parts of areas 6, 8, 9, 10, 11, and 36 or combinations of these. The observed data with regard to the single cases in which areas 24, 44, 45, and 46 were removed alone is recorded in table 38.

**Postoperative Findings in Lobotomy Series.** During the period from October 27 to November 1, 6 of the control patients (5, 11, 20, 23, 28, and 46) and 2 of the topectomy subjects (44 and 2), had prefrontal lobotomies performed. No additional studies were made before these operations to determine whether the initial data were still valid. Still the changes which were observed approximately two weeks after this operation were of such a marked degree that it seems important to report them. Moreover, a definite trend was apparent.

Following lobotomy, patients 5, 11, 20, 23, and 46 all showed a hastening of the emptying time of the stomach. These patients also showed a hastening of the emptying time of the small intestine with the exception of patient 46 who showed an increase of emptying time of thirty minutes. Patient 28 showed a delay of emptying time of the stomach of one hour and fifteen minutes, and of the small intestine of one hour. Patients 2 and 44 who had topectomies performed prior to the prefrontal lobotomies showed a marked decrease in emptying time of the stomach after the latter operation, although they had shown an increase in emptying time following the former procedure. In patient 2 the increase of emptying time after topectomy was three hours, in patient 44 one hour and fifteen minutes. After prefrontal lobotomy the emptying time of the stomach showed a decrease for patient 2 from eight hours and fifteen minutes to three hours and thirty minutes, for patient 44 from six hours and thirty minutes to three hours and thirty minutes. In neither of these patients was emptying time of the small intestine altered to any appreciable degree following lobotomy. As can be seen by table 38, in patient 5 the stomach emptied in six hours before lobotomy and in three hours and fifteen minutes after the operation. A decrease in emptying time of the small intestine of three hours and thirty minutes was also noted in this patient. In patient 11 the stomach emptied in four hours before operation and in two hours and thirty minutes after operation. A decrease in emptying time of the small intestine of two hours was also noted in this case. In patient 20 the stomach emptied in five hours before operation and in two hours and thirty minutes after operation; there was a decrease in emptying time of the small intestine of five hours and forty-five minutes. In patient 23 the stomach emptied in four hours before operation and in three hours and thirty minutes after operation; there was a decrease in emptying time of the small intestine of two hours and thirty minutes. Patient 46 showed a decrease in emptying time of fifteen minutes for the stomach and, as shown above, an increase of thirty minutes for the small intestine.

**Interpretation of Results of Lobotomy.** Data obtained from the lobotomy series confirms the initial discovery of Mettler, Spindler, Mettler, and Combs ('36) who first described increased gastrointestinal motility after bilateral removal of the canine cerebral cortex. The observations at hand do not, however, support the implication of Fulton's interpretation of Hesser, Langworthy, and Kolb's results, i.e. that morbid hunger is equivalent to increased gastrointestinal activity and that gastrointestinal activity is more marked after removal of area 6 than after ablation of areas 9, 10, 11, and 12 (Fulton, '43, p. 441). It is indeed interesting, as reference to table 38 will disclose, that removal of even considerable portions of the frontal cortex rostral to area 8 may not cause such a phenomenon though a mild hastening may put in its appearance under such circumstances. Mettler ('44) has previously pointed out that phenomena which may become just discernible when one of the subdivisions of the frontal granular area is bilaterally removed may be greatly enhanced by the inclusion of others of the same general type in the operation and a thorough lobotomy may safely be assumed to produce results closely approximating bilateral removal of most of the granular frontal cortex.

Attention is directed to the possibility, if it is true that ablation of area 6 slows gastrointestinal motility, that the frontal lobe possesses two systems exerting essentially opposing effects upon that function.

In conclusion, although exceptions apparently occur in a small proportion of cases, one should be prepared to expect hastening of both gastric and intestinal motility after lobotomy but there is no reason to suppose that bilateral removal of one or even two or three Brodmann areas will produce that effect.

*Chapter 12*

# Electroencephalography

JOSEPH F. ZIGARELLI

THE ablation of discrete cortical areas of the human frontal lobe afforded a singular opportunity to study the effectiveness of the electroencephalogram in localizing superficial cerebral lesions. Areas ablated left a discontinuity in the cortical cytoarchitecture with minimal involvement of the subjacent white neuronal connections. The aim of the study was to determine: (1) whether or not such discrete cortical lesions could be localized in routine electroencephalography, (2) what available standard methods of localization would be best suited for localization of these lesions, (3) what local and general variation of wave pattern and frequency would result, (4) the constancy and persistence of any abnormality, if present, and (5) what correlation could be determined as to the source of the existent wave patterns.

Previous studies on monkeys revealed no persistent change in electroencephalogram following cortical ablation (Kennard and Nims, '42). However, transient diffuse slowing and low amplitude were noted to be present until the fourth postoperative day. These changes were not unlike records of cerebral injury (Jasper, Kershman, and Elvidge, '44). Because of the small size of the monkey cranium no localization studies could be accomplished.

Electroencephalographic study of thirty human beings who had undergone prefrontal lobotomies revealed definite abnormalities postoperatively (Cohn, '45). The immediate response of the brain to a focal injury was maximum slow-wave activity in that region. There was a diminution of abnormal discharge within one to three months. The findings were likened to electroencephalographic changes seen in patients with acute head injuries (Jasper, Kershman, and Elvidge, '44).

## TECHNIC

The apparatus used was a four-channel Rahm electroencephalograph. The patient was comfortably seated. The head, in an erect position, rested on a headrest. Eyes were closed. All outside interference was controlled by proper insulation. The room was quiet, dimly lighted, and maintained at a comfortable room-temperature. The patient was informed of the painlessness of the procedure and reassured as the electrodes were placed.

The electrode placements (fig. 84) varied from the standard placements of Gibbs and Gibbs ('41), Penfield and Erickson ('41), and Davis ('41). The frontal electrode was placed 4 cm. above the orbital ridge, in line with the pupil of the eye as the patient looked directly forward. The motor lead was placed 4 cm. laterally from the midline of the vertex, in line with the external auditory meatus. The occipital lead was placed 4 cm. rostrally from the inion and 3 cm. laterally from the midline. The temporal lead was placed 6 cm. directly above and from the center of the zygomatic arch. The parietal lead was placed 8 cm. directly above and from the center of the mastoid process. The (indifferent) lead was placed on the ear lobe. These electrodes were applied in the following manner. The area was cleaned thoroughly with acetone. A small amount of bentonite paste was rubbed into the area. An adequate mound of bentonite paste* was then placed at the desired position. The electrode was then placed in the center of this mound and inserted through it to the scalp. The twelve

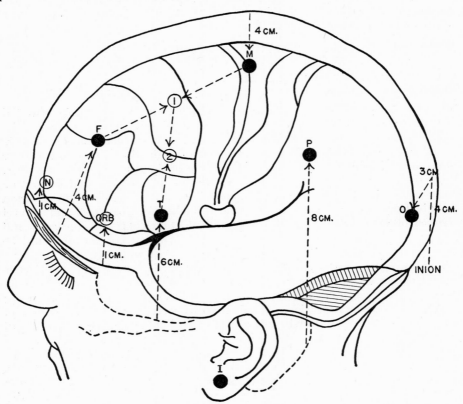

FIG. 84. Electrode placements used in this study. Solid black circles represent routine electrode placements. Plain circles represent additional electrodes used for more definitive localization. Basic drawing taken from Jasper.

electrodes (five bilaterally on the skull and two on the ear lobes) were then connected with the proper channels of the electroencephalograph. For the routine electroencephalogram the recordings shown in table 40 were taken. During the entire recording, the patient was under direct observation of the operator. All movements observed were tabulated on the record. If the patient proved uncooperative, various methods were used in an attempt to obtain the desired relaxed motionless state of the patient.

Further attempts at localization necessitated the placement of additional electrodes in the frontal areas. These electrodes were placed as follows: The (1) lead was placed equidistant and in line with the frontal and motor leads. The (2) lead was placed equidistant and in line with the (1) lead and the temporal lead. Another lead was

* Formula: bentonite powder and saturated solution of calcium chloride mixed to form paste of soft claylike consistency.

TABLE 40. ROUTINE PROCEDURE USED FOR ELECTROENCEPHALOGRAPHY

Apparatus: Four-channel Rahm electroencephalograph

1. Calibration

| | Time | Channel No. 1 | Channel No. 2 | Channel No. 3 | Channel No. 4 |
|---|---|---|---|---|---|
| 2. Amplitude: | ½ min. | L F O | L F O | L F O | L F O |
| | ½ min. | R F O | R F O | R F O | R F O |
| 3. Bipolar: | 1 min. | L F O | R F O | L M O | R M O |
| | 2 min. | L F M | L M O | R F M | R M O |
| | 1 min. | F F | M M | O O | T T |
| 4. Monopolar: | 1 min. | L F | R F | L M | R M |
| | 1 min. | L T | R T | L O | R O |
| | 1 min. | L P | R P | L M | R M |
| 5. Triangulation: | 2 min. | L F M | L M T | L T F | O O |
| | 2 min. | R F M | R M T | R T F | O O |
| | 1 min. | L M P | L P T | L T M | M M |
| | 1 min. | R M P | R P T | R T M | M M |
| | 1 min. | L M O | L O P | L P M | F F |
| | 1 min. | R M O | R O P | R P M | F F |
| 6. Hyperventilation: | 3 min. | L F M* | L M O* | R F M* | R M O* |

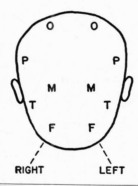

RIGHT    LEFT

* Unless other leads show a pathologic condition.

placed 1 cm. above the nasion and two additional leads were placed 1 cm. above the outermost edge of the orbital ridge bilaterally.

## RESULTS

### TOPECTOMY SUBJECTS

**Preoperative Findings.** Of the 48 patients in the topectomy series (24 operatees and 24 controls) 45 had routine electroencephalograms made three to four weeks prior to the first scheduled operation. At this time the operatees had not been selected. Three of the 48 patients were too uncooperative for electroencephalographic study to be made. Six patients required the presence of an assistant and one was given intravenous sodium amytal. Repeat electroencephalograms were required on 9 of the cooperative group. On 12 of the male patients a minute amount of India ink was tattooed at the selected electrode sites one week prior to the recording. The pain of this operation was not severe, yet the method was abandoned because of the noticeable apprehension of 3 of the patients at the time of the recording. Careful measurement on each electrode placement accomplished the desired accuracy.

The readable electroencephalograms obtained were placed into three groups: normal, abnormal, and normal with predominance of fast irregular activity. There were thirty-one normal records, four abnormal, and ten normal with predominance of fast irregular activity.

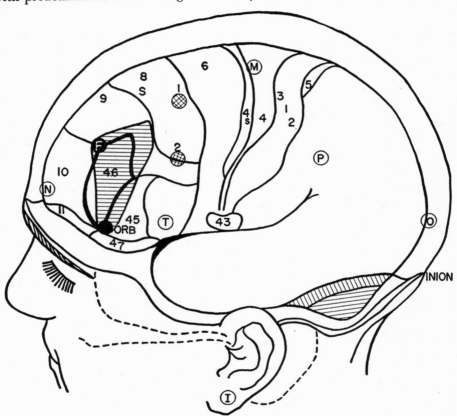

FIG. 85.  Patient 4. Area 46 had been removed. Solid black circles (frontal and orbital) represent electrodes revealing definite abnormality. Blocked electrodes *1* and *2* showed slight amount of abnormality.

Following the selection of 24 operatees, repeat electroencephalograms were performed one to five days preoperatively on all selected patients except the 3 uncooperative patients who were selected. These records were added to the original records to be used for comparative study with the postoperative recordings.

In all patients, at the time of and during the recording, a brief description of the subject's overt behavior was made. Following the electroencephalographic examination an attempt was made to obtain the patient's mental content during the recording. A definite correlation between the affective state

TABLE 41. DATA OBTAINED ON ELECTROENCEPHALOGRAPHIC STUDY OF OPERATEES*

| Pt. No. | Shock therapy | | | Year last | Preoper. EEG[a] | | Int. in days[c] | Postoper. EEG | | | 3 mos. postop. EEG | | | Areas removed |
|---|---|---|---|---|---|---|---|---|---|---|---|---|---|---|
| | Ins. | Met. | ECT | | Norm. | Norm. with fast irreg. act. | | Norm. | Abno. | Abno. with local. | Norm. | Abno. | Abno. with local. | |
| 2 | | | | 1940 | x | | 25 | | x | | | | | 8, 6[b] |
| 3 | 14 | -19 | | 1946 | x | | 22 | | | x | x | | | 9[b], 6[b] |
| 4 | | | 26 | 1946 | | x | 20 | | | x | | x | | 46 |
| 6 | 114 | 14 | 43 | 1944 | x | | 24 | x | | | x | | x | 8[b], 6[b] |
| 7 | 35 | | 33 | 1946 | | x | 25 | x | | | x | | | 8, 9[b], 10[b] |
| 8 | 39 | | 36 | 1946 | x | | 22 | | | x | | | | Mid. fro. gyr. |
| 13 | 56 | | 12 | 1944 | x | | 24 | | | x | | | x | 9[b], 45, 46, 10[b] |
| 18 | 35 | | | 1944 | x | | 29 | x | | x | x | | x | 11[b] |
| 19 | 17 | | | 1940 | x | | 26 | x | | | x | | | 45[b] |
| 21 | | | | | | x | 23 | x | | x | x | | x | 10 |
| 22 | 11 | | | 1944 | x | | 30 | x | | x | x | | | 9, 10, 46 |
| 24 | | 28 | | | | x | | | | | | x | | 6[b] |
| 25 | | | 21 | 1946 | x | | | | | | x | | | 8, 9 and 46, 10[b] |
| 27 | 53 | | 13 | 1946 | x | | | | | | x | | | Sup. fro. gyr. |
| 31 | 28 | | 15 | 1941 | | x | 23 | | | x | | | | 9 |
| 32 | | 22 | | 1937 | | x | 30 | x | | x | | x | x | 8[b], 9, 10[b] |
| 33 | 42 | | 34 | 1946 | x | | | | | | x | | | Inf. fro. gyr. |
| 36 | | | 22 | 1945 | x | | 17 | | | x | x | | | 10, 11, 45, 46, 47 |
| 38 | 9 | | 9 | 1943 | | x | 20 | | | x | | x | | 6[d], 8[d], 9[d], 10[d] |
| 40 | 41 | | 1 | 1945 | x | | 19 | | x | | x | | x | 24[d] |
| 42 | | | | | x | | 24 | x | | | x | | | 11 |
| 44 | 37 | 6 | 28 | 1943 | x | | | | | | x | | | 10[b], 47 |
| 47 | 41 | 12 | 20 | 1942 | | x | 25 | x | x | | x | | | 44 |
| 49 | | | | | x | | 21 | | x | | x | | | 10, 11[b], 46[b] |

[a] No preoperative electroencephalogram was abnormal.
[b] Partial removal of an area.
[c] Int. in days = interval in days between operation and first postoperative electroencephalogram.
[d] Venous ligation.
*In comparing this table with table 78 see page 78.

of the patient and the configuration of the electroencephalogram was noted. Ten tense, anxious patients showed a predominance of low-voltage fast activity. In 2 depressed, apathetic patients there was a predominance of alpha activity with a suggestible amount of slowing in one record. Active mentation and apparent hallucination in 2 patients produced low-voltage fast activity.

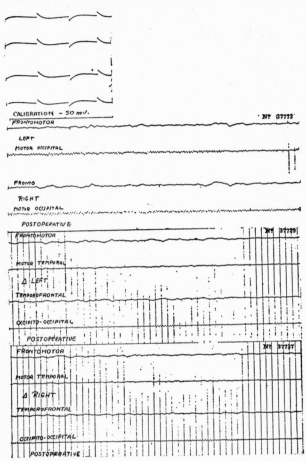

FIG. 86.   Patient 4 (area 46). (See fig. 85.) Solid black circles (frontal and orbital) represent electrodes revealing definite abnormality. Blocked electrodes *1* and *2* showed slight amount of abnormality. Bipolar recording and triangulation are abnormal.

Forty-three patients had some form of shock therapy from six months to seven years prior to electroencephalographic recording. Three of the four abnormal records obtained were from patients who had metrazol therapy.

**Immediate Postoperative Findings.**  Of the 24 postoperative patients, 19 were sufficiently cooperative for electroencephalographic recording. Of the 5 uncooperative patients, 3 had also been uncooperative preoperatively. Two of the cooperative patients required assistance during the examination. Six recordings had to be repeated. The electroencephalograms were taken seventeen to thirty days postoperatively. Of the nineteen readable recordings obtained, thirteen were abnormal (table 41). In ten of these there were definite localizing signs (figs. 85-92). The remaining six recordings were within normal limits (figs. 93-95).

At the time of the postoperative recording no information was had as to the operative procedure and what had been accomplished. Each recording followed the preoperative routine and, following this, special frontal and prefrontal leads were utilized for more definitive exploration (fig. 84).

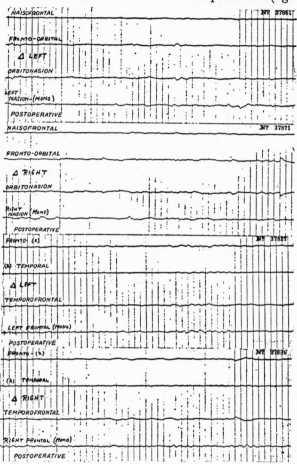

FIG. 87.   Patient 4 (area 46) (cont'd.). (See figs. 85, 86.) Above triangulation recordings are abnormal.

In the routine electroencephalogram, triangulation was most helpful in revealing some abnormality (figs. 85-92). In ten of the abnormal records some indication of abnormality was evident in triangulation. The frontal motor leads revealed abnormalities in nine of the thirteen records. The frontal monopolar leads revealed abnormality in seven records. The transverse frontofrontal leaders were abnormal in six of the abnormal electroencephalograms. The fronto-occipital leads were abnormal in four of the records. In the three remaining abnormal records the abnormality was discovered by triangulation by specially placed prefrontal and frontal electrodes.

Hyperventilation was attempted in all patients. However, this technique introduced so much movement artefact that it proved of no practical value in revealing abnormality or in localization in these patients. In most records hyperventilation increased the abnormal activity.

In all abnormal records the abnormality consisted of slowing with low to moderate voltage. The slowing ranged from marked base-line sway to six per second activity. The configuration of the wave pattern was irregular. Sharp

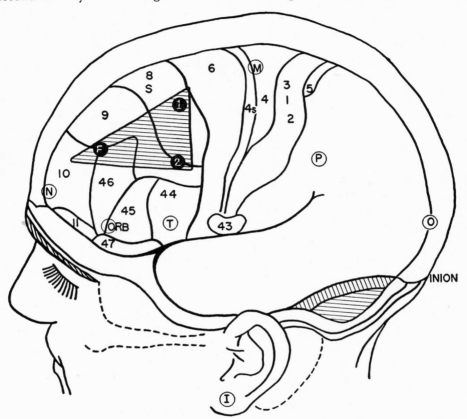

FIG. 88.    Patient 8. The middle frontal gyrus had been removed. Solid black circles (frontal, electrodes *1* and *2* represent electrodes revealing definite abnormality.

waves and spikes were notably absent from all records except one. Variation in the percentage of alpha activity was of no practical value, although there was comparative increase of alpha activity in four of the postoperative records.

**Findings Three Months after Operation.**    Three months postoperatively, electroencephalograms were made on 22 of the 24 operatees. Two patients continued to be uncooperative. Of the 13 patients having abnormal electroencephalograms, seventeen to thirty days postoperatively, 9 continued to show abnormalities. However, there was a definite decrease in the percentage amount of abnormalities in the records. Of the 10 patients who had abnormal records with localizing signs, all continued to show abnormality. Two records did not have any localizing signs, but continued to be abnormal. Two of the 3 abnormal records, in which abnormality without localization was shown previously, returned to normal. The remaining abnormal electroencephalogram which had not previously shown localizing signs continued to be the same. The 6 postoperative patients who had normal recordings seventeen to thirty days postoperatively showed no electroencephalographic abnormalities three months postoperatively.

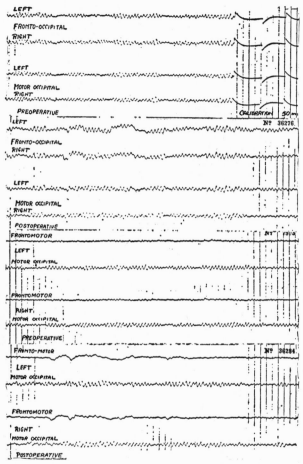

FIG. 89.   Patient 8 (middle frontal gyrus). (See figs. 88, 90-92.) Comparative preoperative and postoperative bipolar recordings. Postoperative recordings are abnormal.

The three electroencephalograms obtained from the previously uncooperative patients showed mild irregularities. Only one could be classified as abnormal without localizing signs.

Electroencephalograms were done on 8 selected patients of the control group, twenty-four days and three months postoperatively. No gross abnormalities were noted in comparing these records with the preanesthesia electroencephalograms.

In 4 cooperative postoperative patients, electroencephalograms (fronto-occipital and motor-occipital leads bilaterally) were taken with the subject's eyes open, with his eyes open and the patient imagining a scene, with eyes open and patient attempting to solve a mathematical problem, with eyes closed and patient imagining a scene, and with eyes closed and patient attempting to solve a mathematical problem. When the patient had his eyes open there was an eradication of alpha activity with a sporadic return of alpha activity within two minutes. When the patient imagined a scene or was solving

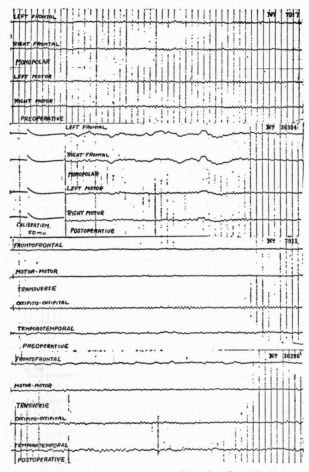

FIG. 90. Patient 8 (middle frontal gyrus) (cont'd.). (See figs. 88, 89, 91, 92.) Comparative preoperative and postoperative monopolar and transverse bipolar recordings. Postoperative recordings reveal abnormality from the frontal electrodes.

a mathematical problem, alpha activity failed to return. With the patient's eyes closed and the patient imagining a scene there was no interference with alpha activity. With the patient's eyes closed and the patient attempting to solve a mathematical problem there was no interference of alpha activity with the simpler problems but an eradication of alpha activity with the more difficult problems.

In 2 postoperative patients with normal electroencephalograms, recordings from monopolar leads placed in the center of cortically ablated areas produced alpha activity (figs. 93-95).

**Findings Six Months after Operation.** Six months postoperatively, electroencephalograms made on 22 of the 24 operatees revealed similar findings to those made three months postoperatively, except in patient 42. In this patient the three-month electroencephalogram revealed no abnormalities. The six-

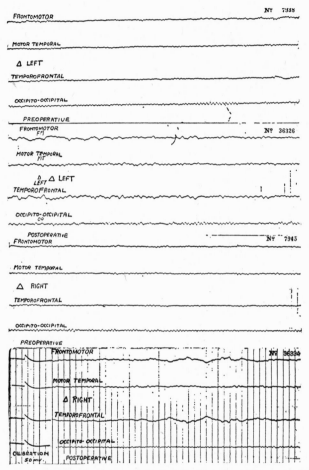

FIG. 91. Patient 8 (middle frontal gyrus) (cont'd.). (See figs. 88-90, 92.) Comparative preoperative and postoperative recordings. Postoperative triangulation recordings reveal abnormality bilaterally localized to frontal electrodes.

month postoperative record revealed abnormal wave configuration with localization to temporal and supraorbital regions bilaterally.

LOBOTOMY SUBJECTS

Electroencephalograms were made three to four weeks postoperatively on the 8 patients who underwent lobotomies. In all patients the records showed abnormality with localization to frontal areas bilaterally. The abnormality consisted of irregular, moderate to high voltage, slow activity from frontal, prefrontal, and temporal leads. Repeat electroencephalograms made four months postoperatively in all these patients revealed some diminution of electroencephalographic abnormality, but all records could be classified as abnormal with localization to frontal areas.

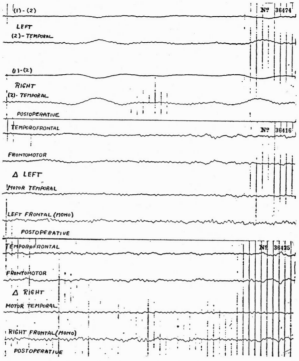

FIG. 92. Patient 8 (middle frontal gyrus) (cont'd.). See figs. 88-91.) Solid black circles (frontal 1 and 2 electrodes) reveal definite abnormality. Postoperative bipolar and triangulation recordings are abnormal.

### CONVULSIONS

Patients 8, 13, 40, and 42 experienced convulsive seizures following topectomy; patient 38 had a convulsive seizure following venous ligation. Patient 8 has had approximately one grand mal convulsion beginning six weeks postoperatively and occurring once every two weeks since that time. Patient 13 had two grand mal convulsions occurring on March 3, 1948, and April 20, 1948. Patient 38 had one grand mal seizure in the first few days after operation. Patient 40 has had three convulsive seizures on December 13, 1947, January 16, 1948, and February 10, 1948. Patient 42 had five convulsive seizures, one on January 23, 1948, and four consecutive grand mal seizures occurring on April 15, 1948.

In all these patients, the preconvulsive electroencephalograms showed abnormality. In patients 8, 13, and 38 the electroencephalograms showed abnormality with localization and in patient 40, abnormality without localization. In patient 42, electroencephalograms made twenty-four days and three months postoperatively failed to reveal any abnormality, but six months post-

operatively and following her convulsive seizures on April 15, 1948, the electroencephalogram showed abnormality with localization to the frontal areas.
Patient 22 was reported to have had one grand mal seizure which was not
witnessed by any medical personnel. There has been no recurrence of the
convulsive seizure in this patient. His electroencephalogram showed and has

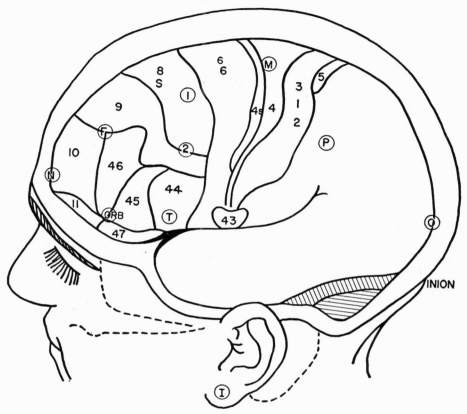

FIG. 93. Patient 22. Areas 9, 10, and 46 had been removed. No electrodes revealed any
abnormality.

continued to show no abnormality. Patient 20, who underwent a lobotomy,
experienced one grand mal convulsive seizure on April 15, 1948. Patient 5
also had seizures in the period immediately after lobotomy (on Nov. 2 he
had five grand mal seizures). Electroencephalogram on this patient showed
abnormality with localization to frontal lobes.

## DISCUSSION

Human cortical ablations can generally be localized by routine electroencephalography. However, in 6 patients with large cerebral lesions, the
electroencephalogram failed to reveal abnormality. Two of these patients had
area 11 removed; the position of area 11 on the inferior surface of the frontal
lobe may account for the failure to localize the lesions in these patients. The
remaining 4 patients had areas 8 and 6; 8, 9, and 10; 9, 10, and 46; and 10
removed respectively. These areas are covered by routine electrode placements.

In August, 1944, Kershman (Jasper, Kershman, and Elvidge, '44) reporting on 64 patients with cerebral trauma stated that the electroencephalogram would always reveal cerebral injury. Putnam and Schwab, in the discussion following this paper, stated that normal electroencephalograms could occur in the presence of known cerebral disorder. Cohn ('45) noted that in 3 of his 30 patients with lobotomies there were no electroencephalographic abnormalities one month postoperatively. Kennard and Nims ('42) found no abnormalities in monkeys with known cerebral lesions following the transient immediate postoperative changes.

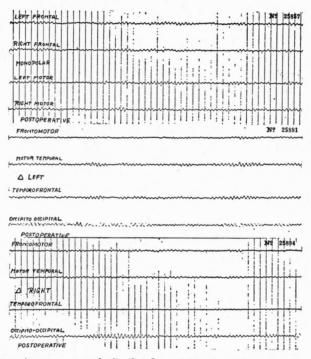

FIG. 94.   Patient 22 (areas 9, 10, and 46). (See fig. 93.) No electrodes revealed any abnormality. Monopolar recording and triangulation are normal. Calibration is the same as in fig. 95.

These observations cannot be discounted. The variability of response of the electroencephalogram may be due to the variability of the reparative index of the cerebrum of various individuals. This is supported by the observation that electroencephalographic abnormalities decrease with increase in postoperative time. Electroencephalographic findings in cerebral vascular accidents lend added support to this contention.

Much work has been done experimentally and clinically on the technique in localizing intracranial disease (Gibbs and Gibbs, '41; Penfield and Erickson, '41; Davis, '41; Williams and Gibbs, '39). Walter ('36; Walter and Dovey, '44) introduced the use of bipolar phase reversal technique and noted that superficial cerebral tumors spreading inwards exhibited one to three per second activity. Cobb ('44) emphasized the use of phase reversal in localizing cerebral lesions. Jasper and Hawke ('38) introduced the triangulation technique in 1938 which has had variable acceptance (Williams and Gibbs, '39). In the present investigation, triangulation was of most value in localizing cerebral disease. Bipolar recordings were next most helpful.

The electroencephalographic abnormality in this study consisted of slowing with low to moderate voltage and with the configuration of the wave patterns being irregular. These findings correspond to those found with damage to the cortical cytoarchitecture from injury or new growth (Jasper, Kershman, and Elvidge, '44; Yeager and Luse, '45; Scarff and Rahm, '41). The abnormalities

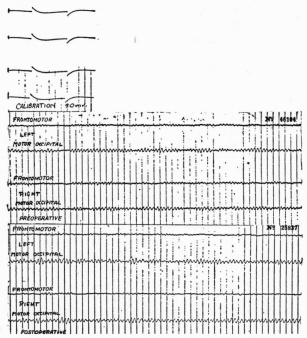

FIG. 95.   Patient 22 (areas 9, 10, and 46) (con'td.). (See figs. 93, 94.) No electrodes revealed any abnormality. Comparative preoperative and postoperative bipolar recordings are normal.

persisted in 10 of the 22 postoperative patients tested three months postoperatively. However, there was a definite decrease in the amount of abnormality shown in these records. These findings are in accordance with those of Cohn ('45) and Marmor and Savitsky ('40).

As to the correlation of the existent wave patterns with the probable source, two contentions became apparent. First, the postoperative abnormality was related to the damaged cortex surrounding the cortical ablation as evidenced by the variability of response. This damage was not static and in the majority of patients was reversible. Second, in 2 postoperative patients the presence of the cortex was not necessary for the production of alpha activity. This raises the question as to the origin of the normal alpha activity. It was noted by Kennard ('43) that rhythm not unlike that of human alpha activity could be elicited from decorticated monkeys. Morison and Bassett ('45) noted that the intralaminar area of the cat's thalamus can maintain eight to twelve per second bursts even after decortication, section of the optic tract, and transection of the midbrain. They noted the similarity of this rhythm to that of human alpha. Case and Bucy ('38), in one of their patients, noted that normal alpha activity was present over a porencephalic cyst in the posterofrontal region where the cortex was thin and gelatinous. They explained this on the basis of electrical activity from the neighboring cortex. Scarff and Rahm ('41), in their human corticographic studies, obtained alpha rhythm from an electrode placed on the optic nerve. This finding suggested fiber tract transmission to these workers.

Our findings of the presence of alpha activity in the center of a known area of cortical ablation adds further evidence to the question whether or not the human alpha activity originates in the cortex. Notwithstanding the work of Dusser de Barenne and McCulloch ('36), and that of Hoagland and Kaufman ('46), if one is to maintain the theory that the alpha activity originates in the cortex, one must offer the explanation of radiation of alpha activity from the surrounding cortex or conduction along fiber tracts (Scarff and Rahm, '41; Case and Bucy, '38). However, it is the opinion of the author that the finding of alpha activity over a large cortically ablated area indicates more accurately that the origin of the alpha activity is from the deeper centers with the cortex playing a secondary role. Further experimental work is indicated to ascertain this hypothesis; however, it is felt that the cortex may play the role of a filter. If there is no physiologic or anatomic abnormality in the cortex, the basic normal subcortical rhythm is recorded evenly. If there is some abnormality produced physiologically or organically in the cortical cytoarchitecture, some abnormality will be noted (Dusser de Barenne and McCulloch, '36; Hoagland and Kaufman, '46; Brazier and Finesinger, '45). If the abnormality is in the deeper subcortical structures, the basic rhythm is altered and is not materially influenced by the presence or absence of cortex, as Hursh ('45) found in his study of the origin of the spike and wave complex. He considered the thalamus or hypothalamus as tentative sites for the pacemaker of the spike and wave complex. The origin of the alpha activity in these structures is a very likely possibility, but this is only a conjecture in the present state of our knowledge.

In future studies of this nature it is recommended that use be made of stereoscopic skull x-rays in connection with the electroencephalographic work. X-rays taken preoperatively and postoperatively with the electrodes in place could be correlated with the outline of the cortical ablation when silver clips have been used in the operative procedure. Clean surgical excision, with minimal use of the cautery, is essential for comparative study.

## Conclusions

1. Discrete cortical ablations can be localized in routine electroencephalography.

2. In the presence of known cortical damage, the electroencephalogram may show no abnormality.

3. Triangulation technique proved most effective in localizing these superficial lesions.

4. The electroencephalographic abnormality consisted of slowing with low to moderate voltage and irregular wave configuration. These findings are similar to electroencephalographic changes following injury to the brain from other causes.

5. The abnormality persisted in 10 of the 22 patients studied, but all showed a diminution in amount of abnormality three and six months postoperatively.

6. The postoperative electroencephalographic abnormalities were related to the damaged cytoarchitecture surrounding the cortical ablation.

7. The human cortex is not essential for the production of alpha activity.

# SECTION III

# Psychologic Investigation

## Chapter 13

# Design of the Psychologic Investigation

### JOSEPH ZUBIN

TOPECTOMY offered the psychologist both an opportunity and a challenge to study some of the basic problems connected with frontal lobe function. The present chapter will list the particular questions to which the psychologic research team addressed themselves, describe the experimental design developed to answer certain questions, and explain the methods applied for evaluating the results. In the chapters which follow, the application of this design to various mental functions will be described and the results and conclusions presented. It is hoped that by presenting the basic design first, it will serve as a background against which the findings and conclusions may stand clear.

**The Problem.** The primary question for which we sought an answer was: Does excision of frontal lobe tissue influence behavior and mental life? This century-old problem has attracted many brilliant workers and the literature now abounds in reports of animal studies following cortical tissue ablation as well as of clinical studies of traumatic brain injuries, tumors, other brain diseases, and, more recently, lobectomies and lobotomies. Each type of brain damage is said to lead to a variety of changes in mental functioning or behavior in some but not all instances. There is, however, little or no agreement on the description of these changes and on their characterization. Some of the changes that have been reported in cases of verified brain tumors of the frontal lobes are personality changes, affective disturbance, euphoria, facetiousness, and memory or intellectual defects.

Reports on changes following more or less complete bilateral frontal lobectomy are for the most part based on single cases reported by isolated observers. Among the changes mentioned are difficulty in registering more than one impression at a time, diminished ability to perform mental synthesis, impaired memory, decrease in arithmetic ability, disorders in sense of humor, loss or decrease in ability to abstract or to generalize, impairment of the abstract attitude, reduction in biologic intelligence, constricted or restricted personality, lack of clarity in thought, decrease in ability to form new associations, greater emotional expressiveness, and diminished perceptual efficiency. In addition to these widely varying reports, both Hebb ('45) and Jefferson ('37) have independently reported that in cases studied by them there was an improved personality and intellectual ability following bilateral lobectomy.

Removal of frontal lobe tissue in animals has resulted in a variety of symptoms in the different species studied. For example, Bianchi ('22) reported that in dogs and monkeys there were motor disabilities, changes in inhibition and attention, and interference with "higher intellectual functions" following prefrontal lobe excision. Mettler ('44) has reported that the removal of frontal lobe tissue in monkeys leads to a change in "outgoingness" and to an increase in activity. Jacobsen ('35) reported that in the chimpanzee there were disturbances in delayed reaction, in sustained attention, and in frustration tolerance following frontal lobectomy.

Prefrontal lobotomy or leukotomy, that is, the severing of the tracts connecting the frontal lobe with the thalamus, has now been carried out on several thousand mental patients. The results vary from a mental condition which is worsened to a restoration of sanity or normality said to be better than that which existed before the onset of the mental illness. Various investigators have attempted to characterize the mental change going on with the return to normality. These changes have been described as decreased attention, emotional re-patterning, attitudinal changes towards life, decreased planning ability with recourse to trial and error, a diminution of superego tendencies, lack of deliberativeness and sustained attention, decreased sex urge, quantitative loss in intellectual function, constriction of the mental field, and bleaching of affect from self-consciousness or the diminution of the consciousness of self.

There have been a number of studies reported where standard or specially devised psychologic tests have been applied to patients in whom there was some structural change or alteration of the frontal lobes. Many of the findings are unclear and some of them are contradictory. They may be summarized as follows:

1. Most investigators report that there are changes in the performance on sorting tests, on the Rorschach Test, and on figures in which there is reversible perspective.

2. There is a general consensus that standardized intelligence tests do not show any significant alteration after operation. The Porteus Maze Test, however, has been reported to show a significant pattern of change following operation.

3. Changes in emotional responsiveness or affectivity have been reported with considerable variation from report to report.

In general the findings are not too definite, leaving the psychologist with very little to guide him in the selection of a battery of tests that might turn out to be crucial in determining changes following operation.

However, a review of the above literature does bring into relief the important questions that need to be answered. These may be listed as follows:

1. Are there any objectively demonstrable psychologic changes which invariably accompany bilateral removal of the frontal lobe tissue?

2. Does the amount of tissue excised relate to the magnitude of psychologic change?

3. Are the psychologic changes related to specific areas of the frontal lobe or are they concomitants of removal of any part of the frontal lobe?

Had the operation been performed on healthy normal persons in whom there was unquestioned normality of frontal lobe function, our problems in interpreting the results would have been considerably reduced. It is debatable whether the frontal lobes of psychotic patients are functioning normally. Any alteration in their postoperative behavior could arise from the operation itself or from a change in their psychosis. This interference with the psychotic process may be connected with the operation or may be only coincidental with it. Furthermore, the patients whom we studied had been in the back wards of the mental hospital and were essentially "hopeless" cases. Their sudden exposure to so-called "total push" of the experimental ward may of its own accord bring about either permanent or temporary changes in psychologic function. In designing the testing procedure and its evaluation both the primary as well as the secondary problems had to be borne in mind.

**The Testing Program.** The first step in setting up the testing program was to select the experiments and tests. It was felt necessary to use as wide a variety of psychologic procedures as could be applied. The physical circumstances surrounding the operatees caused certain tests to be inappropriate. Other than this we did sample as wide a variety of psychologic test performances as has ever been tried. All in all we considered approximately 100 tests or experiments for inclusion in the battery. Limitations of time, space, and personnel resulted in selection of thirty-five tests. The tests were grouped into seven major categories and an attempt was made to have each category represented as fully as possible. In this way a representative sampling of tests in the following areas were selected: (1) Intelligence, (2) Sorting and Abstraction Tests, (3) Learning and Retention, (4) Personality, (5) Visual Perception, (6) Attention, (7) Time Judgment.

Only five of the tests which were selected were of the standardized type: Wechsler-Bellevue Intelligence Test, Porteus Maze Test, Benton Visual Retention Test, Eisenson Aphasia Test, and the Harris Laterality Test. The remaining tests were either entirely new, being devised expressly for this project, or were in various stages of standardization or adaptation.

A set of directions for administering and scoring each procedure was devised before the administration of the test began and these directions were closely followed. Each of the examiners was given adequate practice in the use and scoring of these tests and frequent conferences were held to eliminate difficulties that arose in the course of the administration.

The selection of patients has been described in previous papers. It should be mentioned, however, that the availability of the results of certain of our tests permitted the establishment of matched pairs of individuals from which one could be selected for operation, and the other designated as a control.

The testing procedure was as follows: During the month before the first operation was undertaken, all the patients, both those that were subsequently operated upon as well as those who served as controls, were tested with the entire battery. This testing is designated as the O (original) testing. Most of these tests were repeated upon each individual three weeks after the operation. This repetition of the test is designated as the R1 testing (first repetition). A third period in which all tests were applied was undertaken approximately three months after the date of operation. This will be designated as the R2 testing (second retest). Because the operations were distributed over several weeks the scheduling of the test and retest had to be arranged so as to allow approximately equal intervals between the O, R1, and R2 testings for each patient.

Since the nature of this project required a test before operation and subsequent repetition of tests it was necessary to consider what changes might be expected from the effect of repetition itself. It might be expected that most patients would show an improvement arising from the practice effect when the same test is administered a second or a third time. In order to avoid the error of attributing changes resulting from practice to the influence of the operation a control group was utilized. This control group served as a check on practice effects as well as on the expected improvement arising from the "total push" exerted on all the patients.

The operation may enhance the gain from practice and total push, leave it unaffected, or interfere with it. It may also cause a basic deterioration or a facilitation of mental functioning independent of the practice effect. Each of these changes actually occurred in our results but each had to be interpreted in the light of the factors associated with it.

Since our experiments contrast two groups—operatees and controls—there are other measures than group averages that need to be considered. One of the significant characteristics of a distribution of scores obtained from a group of individuals is variation or variability. These individual differences within the group exist not only in the original score but also in the differences obtained when the same test is repeated; some individuals showing increased scores with repetition, others very little change, and some decreased scores. In general, continued repetition of a test might result either in greater variation or less variation in the group, and a consideration of the spread of the scores made by any group is important for an understanding of the outcome of the experiment. Whenever the operatee group becomes more variable, contrary tendencies within it due to some patients who gain and others who lose may account for the increase in variability. These contrary trends may neutralize each other so that the average gain for the whole operatee group may not differ from that of the controls but the scatter within the groups may be differential. On the other hand, the operatees may become less variable than the controls in which event the effects of the operation may have been to produce greater similarity among the patients upon whom operation was performed than was observed in the control group. The cause of this increase in similarity has to be determined from a study of the associated factors. Finally, patients vary not only from each other but also from their own level of performance from time to time. This last form of variation is called "intraindividual variability" or "scatter."

Another possible alteration which the operation may produce is a change in the relationship between the tests. Thus tests which had shown rather high correlation before operation may decline in their relation after operation. When this happens it may be concluded that the way in which the patients ranked or arranged themselves before has somehow been altered or disrupted. Tests which showed no preoperative correlation may show one after operation. This would mean that something had happened which tended to make the patients alike in the two things which are being measured.

**Analysis of Results.**   The techniques for analyzing the results depended mainly on standard statistical procedure as far as group comparisons were concerned but new techniques had to be introduced for dealing with analysis of individuals. In comparing the two contrasted groups, the method of analysis of variance was used for the comparison of averages. The scores of the operatees and controls were compared at O, $R_1$, and $R_2$ to determine whether any statistically significant difference occurred at any of these points. Then the differences between $R_1$ and O and $R_2$ and O were statistically treated to determine whether the group gains and losses could have occurred by chance or whether the change was beyond that which may be attributed to chance variation. In some tests, especially those on which the patients had been matched, no differences were apparent at the O testing, and hence whatever difference was found at the postoperative testing could be related to the influence of the operation. When, however, the two groups were not equal initially on a given test, no satisfactory conclusion could be drawn from the postoperative and postanesthesia differences until some correction was introduced for the initial inequality. The correction utilized in this study was the method of analysis of covariance which consists essentially of equating the two groups through an application of correlation methods.

When the psychologist is confronted with so many variables as this project affords, his natural tendency is to try to reduce the number of variables to a more comprehensible number. The technique for accomplishing such a reduction is known as factor analysis. In view of the limited number of patients, it was considered unwise to try a factor analysis over all the variables but partial factor analyses were performed in several psychologic areas such as learning tests, intelligence tests, and sorting and abstraction tests. It should be borne in mind, however, that factor analysis is not a method which leads to certain and unique results. The selection of tests and the mathematical processes involved provide opportunities, conscious and unconscious, for finding what the preconceptions of the factor analyst may dictate. Consequently we have used it sparingly in this study.

In determining whether an observed change would be associated with or attributed to the effects of operation or to the influence of the psychosis, the following approach was utilized. Whenever a change was observed in the entire operatee group regardless of degree of psychiatric improvement, and it did not occur in the control group, the change in question was regarded as associated with the effects of the operation rather than with changes in psychosis. Changes that occurred only in the improved cases, regardless of whether the subjects were operated upon or not, were attributed to the effect of changes in psychotic states. This latter change could be an indirect result of the operation or could have been merely coincidental with it. In deciding whether a given change was related to the removal of specific areas of the frontal lobe, a variety of methods were used which will be detailed as each specific instance arises.

Not all of the 48 patients were included in the final analysis because of such factors as inaccessibility, lack of cooperation, or incompleteness of record. We shall for the most part limit ourselves to the 32 cooperative patients who were included in the following analysis of the data. Of these 32, 19 were in the operatee group, and 13 in the control group.

The primary aim of the psychologic experiment was to answer the question of·how excision of frontal lobe tissue affects behavior and mental life. Certain safeguards have been introduced into the design so as to eliminate the influence of factors which might obscure the relationship or produce spurious ones. Some of the disturbing factors could not be successfully eliminated or controlled in this project but their detection and identification will serve to enable future workers from experiencing the same difficulties.

In expressing statistical significance we shall adhere to the convention of speaking of the .05 level of confidence and the .01 level of confidence. These refer to the accepted risks involved in claiming a given difference to be significant. Thus, a difference which could arise by chance only five times in 100 experiments is regarded as satisfying the .05 level of confidence and one that could arise by chance one time in 100 is regarded as satisfying the .01 level of confidence. It is customary to consider both of these levels as indication of statistically significant differences.

The term "variance" refers to a measure of variability or scatter which is equal mathematically to the square of the standard deviation. Analysis of variance and covariance refer to the techniques for ruling out incidental influences from affecting the primary differences attributable to the operation.

Once the experimental design was established and the methods for analysis determined upon, and the data collected, they were subjected to the most rigorous treatment at our disposal. Much of the data presented no special difficulties. But some baffling problems arose which had not been foreseen in our design. Even those data which lent themselves to treatment did not always present consistent findings. In these cases we had to depend on the scientific art of arriving at sufficient conclusions from insufficient data.

*Chapter 14*

# Intellectual Function[*]

HENRY EUGENE KING

———————

THERE is present in the medical and psychologic literature today a vast amount of material on the effects of injury to or removal of frontal lobe tissue in man. Despite the quantity of this material there is great confusion on fundamental points due largely to the fact that there have been few, if any, systematic approaches to the clinical material. Contradictory reports have served to obscure the picture of the symptomatic and psychologic effects resulting from the loss of frontal tissue.

One of the most basic questions which can be raised is that of the effects of the removal of frontal lobe tissue on the intellectual functions in man. A unique opportunity has been provided to attack this problem in a systematic and quantitative fashion in conjunction with the Columbia-Greystone Associates' pre- and postoperative studies of a group of psychotic patients from whom various portions of the frontal lobes were surgically removed.

The question raised in this study is that of the effects of the removal of frontal lobe tissue on intelligence, as measured by a battery of psychometric tests, when compared to a comparable group of patients not subjected to operation.

### HISTORY OF THE SPECIFIC PROBLEM

Our present-day concept of the role of the frontal lobes in man's behavior and activities has been derived principally from three sources: (1) Experimental work on the lower animals. (2) Isolated clinical observations on brain tumor cases and patients with traumatic injury of the brain. (3) The more recent fund of information from the effects of lobotomy undertaken for the "relief of psychic pain" as described by Freeman and Watts ('42).

The first of these sources, the animal experiments, stemmed largely from the work of Flourens (1842) and of Fritsch and Hitzig (1870). The results of the experiments of these early investigators began the controversy, which has persisted to the present day, as to whether the brain functions as a whole or whether its various portions have specific functions.

Flourens' experiments on the brains of animals led him to the belief that intelligent behavior in animals was an indivisible function depending upon the activity of the entire brain. He conceived of the nervous system as a single unified system. Essentially the same point of view was arrived at by Goltz (1881) who contended that intelligence could not be dissociated into subordinate functions which have separate localization in the brain.

[*] This chapter was submitted in partial fulfillment of the requirements for the degree of Doctor of Philosophy in the Faculty of Pure Science, Columbia University.

In contrast to this was the report of Fritsch and Hitzig (1870) who stimulated directly the exposed brains of dogs and found that electrical stimulation produced isolated muscle movements. Later evidence bore out the fact that damage to these stimulable areas produced paralysis in the same regions of the body. On the basis of this evidence it was believed that similar centers for the higher psychologic functions might be found to exist in the cortex. Munk's (1890) experiments led him to state his theory that there are a number of primary sensory spheres—visual, auditory, olfactory—in which were stored elaborated images and ideas associated with a particular modality of sensation. Intelligence or intellect was thought of as an aggregate of these spheres brought together by neural interconnections.

The primary method utilized in these localization studies was that of ablation or removal of cortical tissue and then observing the resulting alterations in behavior, postmortem studies of brain disease in cases with marked physical and mental symptomatology being a variation of the same technique. Ferrier's (1886) introduction of the method of direct electrical stimulation made possible many additional and corroborative studies of localization in the brain. The use of these two methods by a series of investigators working in many different laboratories has established the brain centers for vision and audition as well as delimiting those areas concerned with simple motor activity and somesthesia.

The localization of these primary areas, while important, sheds little light on the more complicated functions such as memory, learning, and intelligence. In an attempt to get at these factors the method of cerebral ablation has been used by recent investigators to study the effects on such higher functions as can be measured in animals. Notable are the pioneer experiments of Bianchi ('22) with bilateral extirpation of the frontal lobes in monkeys which resulted in what he described as alteration of character, involving both the emotions and intellect, in which there appeared to be a quantitative relation between the amount of tissue removed and the degree of alteration in behavior.

Franz ('07) was probably the first to utilize a quantitative method in a direct attempt to get at the effects of brain operation on the intelligence of animals. He trained cats and monkeys in specific tasks to a standard criterion of success prior to removal of various portions of the brain, and observed the degree of disruption in the previously well-established performance. He found that lesions in portions of the brain other than frontal did not affect performance, but that destruction of the frontal lobes resulted in the loss of recently formed habits. He also found that habits so lost could be relearned by the lobectomized animals at about the same rate that they were learned originally.

Lashley ('29) has studied the effects of brain operation on well-established learning patterns in rats, on the assumption that learning measures constitute our best measures of animal intelligence. His were especially careful experiments utilizing objective measures of performance, large groups of animals, and careful histologic study of the lesions involved. He used mazes of graded difficulty as a learning task. Lashley's conclusions from his experiments were that the retention of maze habits was decreased by the loss of cerebral tissue, the ability to learn maze habits following such destruction was also reduced, the loss was proportionate to the amount of tissue removed, and that reduction occurred regardless of the location of the lesion on the cortex. There was also some evidence that the lesions acted selectively, causing relatively greater reduction on difficult maze habits than on the simpler ones.

Jacobsen ('35, '36), Jacobsen and Nissen ('37), and Jacobsen, Wolfe, and Jackson ('35) also ran carefully controlled quantitative experiments using chimpanzees and came to the conclusion that there was no impairment of learning ability following frontal lobe damage. There was, however, measurable a marked deficit in recent memory, these deficits bearing a more or less quantitative relationship to the amount of tissue removed.

There is obvious lack of agreement apparent in the results reported by different investigators as to the effects of removal of cerebral tissue on the higher psychologic functions. The older studies made no use of quantitative measures of behavior and were more or less impressionistic. The lack of agreement among them is indicative of the absence of any gross and regular alteration which is universally present. The more recent quantitative studies, however, which are much more objective and sensitive to minor alterations, have been seen to be in strong disagreement; the evidence of Franz and of Jacobsen has been interpreted as supporting the notion of localized function and the conclusions of Lashley as giving weight to a theory of generalized cerebral function. The explanation has been offered that the discrepancy is due to the fact that different species were studied by the different investigators, and that since the brain of the monkey and that of the rat are differently organized they could hardly be expected to give similar results. It is all the more apparent, therefore, that the evidence concerning the cerebral localization of the higher psychologic functions which has been gained from animal experimentation is not directly applicable to man. Any extrapolations of the animal data are problematical since no uniformity of function has been demonstrated to exist in the cerebral organization of the higher psychologic functions in infrahuman species.

A more direct approach to the problem of cerebral representation of higher psychologic function is provided by the second line of evidence cited. If we wish to know the relation between the function of the frontal lobes and human intelligence we may study patients in whom there has been damage to the frontal lobes to see whether or not this is accompanied by an impairment in intelligence.

Since brain tumors are common there has been ample opportunity to observe the mental symptomatology which accompanies this type of pathologic damage to the frontal lobes. There are extensive accounts in the literature of the symptoms presented in cases of frontal lobe tumor. As pointed out by Freeman and Watts ('42) there are certain drawbacks present in the study of tumor material which render it of doubtful value in attempting to localize to the frontal lobe the basis for the symptoms expressed. The primary difficulty is the fact that a tumor is a progressive affair and the complications of increasing compression and infiltration over an undefined area of the brain may cause symptomatology not based on frontal lobe involvement alone. Also tumors are usually unilateral and to what extent compensation by the other lobe is taking place is an unknown variable. Generally speaking the effects noted are largely personality defects, such as lowered initiative, poor attention, moral obtuseness, and indifference, and the presence of these symptoms lower the validity of any measures of intelligence which may be made. Some observations have indicated definite intellectual impairment (Strauss and Keschner, '35), and some (Donath, '25) an inability to synthesize, the patient seeming to lack the ability to discern the essentials of an event and to combine the units of a situation into a composite picture.

Because of the likelihood of involvement of portions of the brain other than frontal lobe in all tumor cases, the evidence of the reports of tumor will not be discussed further here as a possible method of localizing the effects of brain disease upon intelligence. For the same reason the information available from cases of frontal lobe atrophy and bilateral softening of the frontal lobes cannot be utilized.

The evidence available from traumatic injury to the frontal lobes is somewhat more convincing. The criticisms applied in the case of tumors, atrophy, and brain softening are not applicable since the damage is more or less circumscribed and local. Accidents and war injuries have provided an adequate amount of material for study. Personality alterations, intellectual defects, and vegetative symptoms were noted in the early studies (Harlow, 1868) and the reports of the large number of head injuries in World War I has substantiated this to some extent. The latter consists of cerebral injuries to men who presumably possessed normally adapted personalities prior to injury. Although a good many differences exist in the various reports of symptomatology (Berger, '23; Feuchtwanger, '23) it is apparent that personality changes of one sort or another result from frontal damage, the nature of the symptoms expressed perhaps stemming from the pre-injury personality (Freeman and Watts, '42). Incontinence, gluttony, sleepiness, disorientation, inappropriate humor, coarseness and obscenity, childishness, indifference, stealing, lack of interest in anything are among the symptoms frequently reported. Intellectual defects as such have been rarely reported, although it was difficult to differentiate between some of the cases of extreme apathy and dementia.

Perhaps the most generally agreed upon aspect of the war injury studies was the fact that symptoms are much more marked in cases with bilateral damage to the frontal lobes than in cases of unilateral involvement.

There are several reasons why the studies of traumatic brain injury cases have not been too revealing psychologically. The primary criticism is the fact that no measures or objective estimates of the pretrauma intelligence and personality are available. Despite the presence of symptoms following injury, it is difficult to arrive at any well-grounded evaluation of the degree of change in the absence of adequate knowledge of the pretraumatic characteristics of the patient. There is, in addition, the uncertainty of amount of brain damage because of the "shattering" effect of the nature of the injuries.

The reports of studies of frontal lobectomy in man have afforded a far more encouraging mode of attack upon the functions of the frontal lobes than has any of the evidence reviewed thus far. Present-day surgical techniques allow the excision of large portions or a complete lobe for the removal of tumors located within or beneath the lobes. Thus the opportunity is provided to study cases in which there is relatively clear-cut surgical removal of tissue, and, in some instances, to obtain measures of intelligence prior to the excision of tissue.

Several studies have been made of cases with unilateral lobectomy which contain evidence bearing upon the intellectual functioning of patients with part or all of one lobe removed. Several patients operated upon by Penfield and examined psychologically by Hebb ('39) showed no marked inferiority of performance on intelligence tests administered several years postoperatively. Neither language nor non-language intelligence seemed markedly impaired. German and Fox ('32) reported one case of right frontal lobe resection in which there was definite impairment in intelligence, characterized chiefly by a paucity of motor response.

Usually cited as the most complete study in this field is that of Rylander ('39). Thirty-two patients were studied who had been operated on for some type of frontal lobe tumor over a period from two to seven years prior to his examination. Data was also obtained on an equal number of normals making up a control group composed of individuals of the same age, sex, occupation, and social status, usually relatives of the patients. An assortment of psychologic tests was used and statistical treatment of the data revealed certain significant differences between the two groups, the subjects upon whom operation had been performed doing less well on the intelligence tests and on tests requiring the use of the higher intellectual functions than did the controls. No evidence was obtained for the dominance of either lobe, but larger excisions were believed to result in greater deterioration than did the smaller ones. Rylander ('43) later made similar studies of patients with resections of parietal, temporal, and occipital lobes and failed to find any evidence that damage to these areas results in the intellectual impairment observed when the frontal lobes are operated upon.

Stookey, Scarff, and Teitelbaum ('41) reported a series of 23 cases of unilateral lobectomy in which intellectual functioning was examined after operation. No impairment of intellectual functions resulted when the lesion was completely removed. Lidz's ('39) thorough report of a single case studied preoperatively as well as post-operatively also failed to reveal any impairment on intelligence tests or tests of the higher intellectual functions resulting from loss of one frontal lobe.

Although these investigations have differed in clinical material and approach it can be seen that there is no common agreement as to the effects of unilateral excision of the frontal lobe upon intelligence. The absence of preoperative measures in the larger groups studied, the paucity of cases of those with pre-and postoperative measurement, and the general absence of adequate control cases make evaluation even more difficult.

The evidence for the effects of bilateral removal of the frontal lobes upon intelligence consists largely of extensive reports of single cases. What had been learned from cases of traumatic injury was the fact that bilateral damage was far more productive of change than unilateral lesions. Surgical removal of both frontal lobes is, however, rather rare. We are forced, therefore, to fall back upon reports of isolated cases rather than group data.

The most famous of these reports is that of Brickner ('36) who studied a case of extensive removal of the frontal lobes over a period of years. No preoperative measure of intelligence was made but numerous postoperative testings showed a rather low level of intelligence not altogether in keeping with the subject's education and business ability preoperatively. In the case reported by Ackerly ('35) of extensive frontal removal, on the other hand, average intelligence on psychometric measures was shown following operation.

A detailed study by Nichols and Hunt ('40) of a patient having bilateral lobectomy showed no defective performance on intelligence tests, but exhibited a rigidity of the categorical attitude and a restriction of integration and of the number of lines of endeavor the subject could successfully keep separated simultaneously. Mixter, Tillotson, and Wies ('41) reported a case of removal of both frontal poles in a young boy who yielded low intelligence test scores following operation. Hebb and Penfield ('40) reported a case in which bilateral lobectomy was more extensive than in Brickner's case. Preoperative intelligence measures were made and compared with postoperative test results, and showed a slight improvement in intellectual function.

Again we observe the lack of universal agreement among the different investigators. It is not difficult to see, however, that the faults inherent in the information obtained from the bilateral lobectomies render the interpretations dubious. The cases are isolated and handled by different investigators with little comparability in lesion or intellectual measurement. There has been no use of control data. Rarely have preoperative measures been possible and when they were they were made at a time when obvious and urgent brain disease necessitated the operation. There has frequently been a strong possibility of postoperative brain disease as well in cases of incomplete removal of the tumor. In view of these complicating factors there is little wonder that the opinions of different writers are in conflict.

The introduction of the technique of prefrontal lobotomy by Moniz ('36) has made possible a circumventing of some of the difficulties presented by pathologic change in the brain in tumor, wound, and lobectomy studies. This operation, clearly discussed by Freeman and Watts ('42), is undertaken for the relief of distressing mental symptoms in some of the psychoses. Patients who undergo this operation are free from any brain disease prior to the operation and are subject only to such damage as results from the procedure. The complicating factor is, in this case, the fact that the patients are psychotic. This is not an insurmountable barrier, however, since it is quite possible to obtain psychometric records from such patients.

The use of this operation as a therapeutic procedure has been widespread, and has provided adequate material for studies of its effects upon intelligence. Essentially what is done is the bilateral sectioning of the thalamocortical tracts: a severing of the white matter of the frontal lobes. The gross destruction of these connecting pathways affects frontal cortical areas in a nonlocalized fashion, but is confined to the frontal lobes. Since a major portion of the frontal lobes is presumably rendered inactive its absence may give us some idea as to its normal contribution to intelligence.

Reports have been published by several investigators utilizing various techniques for the estimation of the effects of this type of frontal damage on intelligence. Many of these are not based on psychometric measures but upon general impressions and are not too useful for our purposes. In the recent work of Frank ('46), Kisker ('44), Robinson ('46), Hunt (in Freeman and Watts, '42), and Ström-Olsen, Last, Brody,

and Knight ('43) objective measures have been employed in arriving at their conclusion that the impairment of intelligence measured by the Binet type test resulting
from this operation is either negligible or none at all. Porteus ('33), on the other
hand, has always held that intelligence is not well measured by the usual Binet type
of psychometric examination, and has devised his own maze test for getting at what
he termed social intelligence. He reports (Porteus and Kepner, '44) that lobotomy
patients give definite evidence of impaired intelligence on his test and that this is
related to their planning ability. The results of Robinson ('46) with this test, though
few in number, tend to confirm this statement. The patients studied by Ström-Olsen,
Last, Brody, and Knight ('43) showed no such impairment on the Porteus Mazes.

This brief consideration of the fund of evidence with regard to frontal lobe
function which has come from the study of lobotomy cases indicates a marked advance
over that gained from the animal work, tumor and trauma study, and the lobectomy
evidence. The fact that lobotomy allows the study of the effects of cortical damage
on brains with no demonstrable disease helps answer some of the bewildering questions
raised by the earlier studies. There are, however, certain questions which remain
unanswered from this evidence as well. There is the fact that the damage incurred
in lobotomy is nonlocalized within the frontal lobes, and the uncertainty as to the
use of interconnecting pathways other than those interrupted. There is also the
uncertainty as to the amount of cerebral damage done, and as a correlate of this
we still lack information as to the relative effects of small and great cerebral damage
upon intelligence.

The present study has been designed to fill in some of these gaps in the
information available in order to arrive at a satisfactory point of view as to
the relation between the frontal lobes and intelligence. Much has been learned
from the preceding studies as to what requirements must be fulfilled before
the results obtained may be used with confidence. Every effort has been made
to profit from lessons learned from the history with regard to the use of objective measurement, the nature of the measures employed, the inclusion of
adequate control groups, selection of groups with no previous brain disease,
and the study of the effects of lesions of differing size and location on the cortex
as well as many lesser considerations.

*The problem with which this study is concerned is the demonstration of
the effect or lack of effect of bilateral surgical removal of portions of the
frontal lobes upon intellectual function.* The results should indicate to what
extent intelligence is dependent upon the function of the frontal lobes, either
as a whole or in parts. The relation of the amount of tissue excised to performance should be made clear. Since tests of intelligence based upon differing theoretical grounds were applied, the effects of topectomy upon tests utilizing different theoretical approaches may be observed.

An attempt was made to apply each test in the battery to each patient on
three occasions: (1) Preoperative testing—performed one month before operation. This will be referred to as the O (original) test period hereafter. (2) First
postoperative testing—performed three weeks after operation. This will be
referred to as the R1 (retest one) test period. (3) Second postoperative testing
—performed four months after operation. This will be referred to as the R2
(retest two) test period.

All tests were administered in the same way for each test period. The results
reported here constitute only a fraction of the results obtained with the entire
battery. Only one aspect of the entire psychologic evaluation of such brain
injury can be included here.

As is to be expected in a study dealing with psychotic patients the usable number of test results is diminished since the condition of some patients is not amenable to valid psychologic examination. Since it was desired to work with data which were clouded as little as possible by the mental status of the patients, high standards were set for acceptance. The test results retained for analysis in this study met the criteria of completeness of survey (all three testing periods), were considered by the examiner to be representative efforts of a cooperative patient, and were uncomplicated by distracting symptoms such as delusional intrusion, silliness, and mutism. These considerations have reduced the group to 32 patients. The composition of the operatee and control groups finally selected is described in table 42.

TABLE 42. BACKGROUND VARIABLES IN THE OPERATEE AND CONTROL GROUPS UTILIZED IN THE PRESENT STUDY

| Variables | Operatees | Controls |
|---|---|---|
| Number of cases | 19 | 13 |
| Male | 11 | 10 |
| Female | 8 | 3 |
| Age, average | 41.8 | 42.4 |
| Age, range | 27–60 | 18–58 |
| Education, average years | 9.42 | 9.23 |
| Education, range | 6–19 | 4–19 |
| Wechsler-Bellevue IQ, average | 101.7 | 105.2 |
| I.Q., range | 74–131 | 83–121 |

The groups thus set up with the experimental variable of topectomy lends itself admirably to the investigation of the effects of this type of cerebral damage upon psychologic characteristics.

### EXPERIMENTAL PROCEDURES

**Wechsler-Bellevue Test of Adult Intelligence.** As a primary measure we wished to include a test which samples a wide variety of human performance which has been found to be valid when correlated with the available criteria of intelligence, such as educational success. Such a test attempts to assess an individual's intelligence in terms of the evaluation of his mental productions, by their number and excellence and the speed with which they are effected over a variety of types of tasks.

The Wechsler-Bellevue is a well-known instrument of just this sort. Since it has been standardized upon adult groups it was chosen in preference to other tests as being particularly suited to our group. It samples a large number of abilities and provides measures of both verbal and nonverbal intelligence. One of the advantages of this type of measurement is the fact that the many subtests of which it is made up may be independently analyzed to yield information on the specific function they are designed to measure. In this way it acts as a substantial battery of tests yielding information on quite a variety of types of performance. Such a subtest analysis was desired in the examination of the relative performance of our groups. Another advantage of this test is the fact that use of its weighted scores makes possible study of the variability of individuals in its execution.

The test was administered in standard fashion according to Wechsler ('44) and scored by the standard criteria provided. Our only innovation was the addition of an extra score,* which in no way disturbs the remainder of the test.

**Porteus Mazes.** As indicated in the survey of the literature, Porteus ('33) has always held that intelligence is not well measured by the usual Binet-type psychometric examination and has devised a maze test for the measurement of intelligence. It is Porteus' contention (Porteus and Peters, '47) that one can never arrive at a measure of "social intelligence" or such aspects of intelligence as "foresight" and "planning" and "social sufficiency," by validating tests against educational standards. His test, which is composed of a series of paper-and-pencil mazes of graded difficulty, was validated against such social criteria as measured by rating scales (Porteus, '33). This is a well-known test, widely used by clinical psychologists.

In a recent publication, Porteus and Peters ('47) have expressed the opinion that study of lobotomy cases has given corroborative evidence for the validity of their scale. Since specific claims have been made that this test measures planning, initiative, and common sense judgment in practical situations, it would be expected to reflect alterations of these traits of intelligence in postlobotomy cases if, indeed, these traits are as modified as the accounts of clinical observations would lead us to believe.

We have included the Porteus Maze Test in our battery because of its fundamental difference in approach to the assessment of human intelligence. The test was administered in standard fashion as directed by Porteus ('33, '42) and scored by the standard criteria.

**Continuous-Problem Task.** Frequent mention is made in the literature of the lack of intellectual initiative, diminished powers of attention and concentration, and the poor quality of sustained effort on tasks requiring intelligent behavior which is exhibited in cases of frontal lobe damage (Conkey, '38-9; Robinson, '46; Rylander, '39). Some measure of these factors is, of course, afforded by the tests previously described (e.g. Wechsler-Bellevue Digit Symbol), but it was believed that a task designed to bring out some of these important aspects should be included in our battery. The task selected for this role, the Continuous-Problem Task, was adapted to suit our needs. Since it is a new test it must be described here in some detail.

A machine was designed† for the use of the Army Air Forces in World War II, which would afford a measure of complicated choice reaction, a factor used in the selection of pilots. This particular type of instrument was never used, since the war ended before its construction was completed. With some modifications it was found well suited to our needs.

The apparatus consists of an upright panel board of signal lights arranged as shown in figure 96a. There are four distinct groups of five white lamps each arranged in a similar pattern for each group. In the center of each group is a red and green bullet lamp.

Attached to the base of this and at right angles is a panel board of switches arranged as shown in figure 96b. There are four distinct groups of five switches each arranged in a similar pattern for each group. As can be readily seen, the arrangement of each

* On the test of Digit Symbol Substitution the score consists of the number of such substitutions made correctly in one and one-half minutes. This measure was obtained, and, in addition, the subject was allowed to finish the sixty-seven substitutions and a time score was obtained for this unit of performance.

† Complex Reaction Time Test. Model A, designed and built by the Vector Manufacturing Company, Houston, Texas.

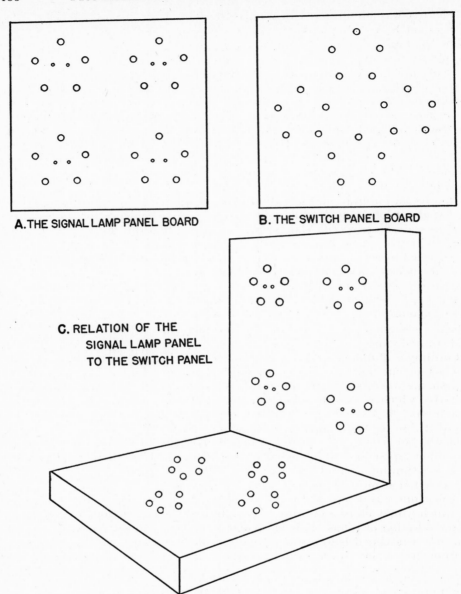

FIG. 96. The Continuous-Problem Task.

group is similar to that of the lamps on the signal board but the placement of the four groups on the board is different.

The relation of the signal panel to the switch panel is diagrammed in figure 96c.

By means of a solenoid stepping switch and an elaborate wiring system various patterns of signal lamps may be illuminated in series circuit with *one* of the switches. Breaking by this particular switch will extinguish the lamp pattern and automatically light up another pattern.

Forty such light patterns are presented consecutively by the machine, each new pattern being automatically set·up as the old one is extinguished. A counter is built into the machine which records the number of patterns which have been presented. Each pattern consists of the illumination of one red bullet, one green bullet, and one white lamp, and involves one switch in circuit with these. The operation of the machine is explained in the paragraphs describing instructions given to the subject.

The task was *not* presented to the patient as a problem. Each step in the task was fully explained and he was allowed to practice with it and gain confidence in its operation to a given degree of competency.

In order to teach the patient the task he was instructed as described below. Variations in the instruction to meet the patient's level and repetitions in any required amount were allowed since our concern was the subject's ability to perform the task, not his ability to learn it. The patient was seated before the apparatus and the first pattern inserted.

"Here's a board with lights (indicate), and here's a board with switches (indicate). These switches control these lights and if you turn the *correct one* the lights will go out but if you turn the wrong one nothing will happen. Now the lights themselves will tell you how to find the correct switch—but before we go into how they do that take a look at these switches. You see they are in four groups (indicate by holding hand over all switches in a group). These are named for the way you are sitting; right—on your right, left—on your left, up from you and down toward you.

"Now look at these lights. You see that there is one red one lit, one green, and one white. First look at the red and green lights. These will tell you what group the correct switch is in. *The way you go from green to red is the name of the correct group.* (Demonstrate—to get from green to red you must go up on signal board, then correct switch is in group named 'up'.) The direction will always be up, down, right or left, there won't be any diagonals.

"To find out which one in this group is the correct switch is easy. The white light tells you which one. You see that each of these groups (indicate light groups) is shaped like each of these (indicate switch groups). To turn off the lights just pick the switch in the correct group which is in the same position as the white light that is lit. This is the correct switch, and when you twist it all the lights will go out."

These instructions were modified or repeated until the patient had a grasp of the principles involved. He was allowed to practice until he reached the criterion of ten consecutive correct problem (pattern) solutions with no aid from the examiner. Satisfying this criterion, it was assumed that he had reached the required level of proficiency in the operation of the machine.

Once the patient had demonstrated mastery of the principles involved the test proper was begun. He was directed to operate the machine as rapidly as he could (continuous problem solving) until told to stop. His performance, as measured by the number of correct solutions and errors committed, was measured for a period of four minutes. A one-minute rest period was allowed and then another measure was taken, and so on until four test periods of four minutes each were obtained. The problems are randomly presented and are of approximately equal difficulty, and the measure thus obtained is a good reflection of performance in unit time. Supplementary qualitative measures were made of the presence of blocking and the length of such pauses, the nature of the errors made, and the like.

What we desired to observe by this task was the patient's ability to bear in mind principles once learned in the face of a minor stress situation—a confusing spacial relationship and timed performance—for a prolonged period of time. The fact that performance on this task is strongly influenced by intelligence was determined by exploratory testing with normals and was confirmed by its correlation with the preoperative Wechsler-Bellevue I.Q. of this patient population (+.51).

**Summary of Procedures.** The assessment of the intelligence of the operatee and control groups before and after frontal topectomy has been made utilizing these three measures: the Wechsler-Bellevue Test which yielded information on a variety of abilities and which could be added to give an estimate of intelligence, the Porteus Maze Test which had made its strongest claims as a measure of the type of intelligence required for social adjustment, and the Continuous-Problem Task which would serve as an index of the degree to which effort was sustained on a task requiring intelligent behavior. The application of these measures based upon differing concepts of intelligent behavior was designed to obtain as complete a coverage as possible of the intellectual functioning of these groups.

## RESULTS

In treating the group data obtained on the three testing intervals the method of analysis of variance has been applied throughout. Since intelligence was one of the bases upon which these groups were matched the means of the operatee and control groups were very similar on the preoperative data for the over-all measures. Breakdown of the total scores into their constituent subtests could hardly be expected to fall into well-equated groups and the method of covariance has been applied throughout to correct for these discrepancies in preoperative means.

### WECHSLER-BELLEVUE TEST

**General Measures.** The first question to be answered is that of the effect of operation upon the total estimate of intelligence yielded by this test. Several measures have been computed in order to obtain a full answer. These have been called general measures, since they are additive scores made up of performance on the many subtests. The results of this analysis may be seen in table 43.

The primary measure was that of full I.Q. which represents an estimate of intelligence derived from weighed scores obtained on both the verbal and performance portions of the test.

A gain in mean score was shown by both groups on each testing interval. The increase of the control group was slightly larger than that of the operatees at $R_1$, otherwise there was approximately equivalent gain, presumably the effects of practice with repetition of the test. The means and the variances of the groups did not differ significantly at $R_1$ or $R_2$, or on $R_1$-O or $R_2$-O.* Analysis of the total weighted score, which would eliminate the Wechsler correction for age, showed no differences existing between the groups.

It was of interest to know whether or not operation had any differential effect upon the verbal and performance items of this scale. Examination of the mean scores revealed the fact that in both instances there was a greater gain by the control group on $R_1$, so that each was contributing to this effect seen in total score. In general, the gains made by the two groups on verbal score were equivalent but on performance items the control group exceeded the

---

* These are difference scores. The original score has been subtracted from the retest score since the latter was usually larger and this facilitated computation. These scores were utilized primarily as a searching tool to detect alteration in groups not equated originally, and as an indispensable aid in the analysis of individual performance.

TABLE 43. MEANS AND F RATIOS OF OPERATEE AND CONTROL GROUPS ON THE GENERAL MEASURES AND SCATTER SCORES OF THE WECHSLER-BELLEVUE TEST

| Subtest | Group | Means | | | Analysis of variance F ratios | | | | Analysis of covariance F ratios | |
|---|---|---|---|---|---|---|---|---|---|---|
| | | 0 | R1 | R2 | | 0 | R1 | R2 | R1 | R2 |
| Full I.Q. | OP | 101.7 | 105.6 | 108.6 | Betw. var.'s | 1.3 | 1.0 | 2.3 | | 0.5 |
| | C | 105.2 | 112.8 | 115.3 | Betw. means | 0.5 | 1.8 | 1.1 | | 2.1 |
| Total wtd | OP | 97.6 | 103.9 | 108.4 | Betw. var.'s | 1.5 | 1.1 | 1.7 | | 2.3 |
| | C | 103.5 | 116.6 | 120.2 | Betw. means | 0.5 | 1.8 | 1.6 | | 2.8 |
| Verbal wtd | OP | 55.7 | 57.6 | 59.7 | Betw. var.'s | 1.5 | 1.3 | 1.5 | | 1.7 |
| | C | 63.2 | 67.9 | 68.9 | Betw. means | 2.0 | 3.2 | 2.4 | | 0.3 |
| Perf. wtd | OP | 42.0 | 46.3 | 48.7 | Betw. var.'s | 1.3 | 0.7 | 1.5 | | 1.6 |
| | C | 40.4 | 48.8 | 51.4 | Betw. means | 0.2 | 0.3 | 0.5 | | 3.2 |
| Total raw | OP | 160.3 | 169.9 | 178.1 | Betw. var.'s | 1.6 | 1.0 | 1.7 | | 2.6 |
| | C | 168.1 | 186.8 | 196.4 | Betw. means | 0.3 | 1.3 | 1.5 | | 2.8 |
| Verbal raw | OP | 76.5 | 78.8 | 81.5 | Betw. var.'s | 1.3 | 1.4 | 1.4 | | 1.0 |
| | C | 86.4 | 91.9 | 94.0 | Betw. means | 2.1 | 3.0 | 2.5 | | 0.4 |
| Perf. raw | OP | 83.8 | 91.1 | 96.6 | Betw. var.'s | 1.6 | 0.7 | 1.6 | | 1.7 |
| | C | 81.7 | 94.9 | 101.4 | Betw. means | 0.1 | 0.2 | 0.4 | | 2.2 |
| Total scatter | OP | 5.5 | 6.1 | 5.6 | Betw. var.'s | 0.3 | 0.6 | 0.9 | | 1.0 |
| | C | 7.7 | 7.6 | 7.0 | Betw. means | 3.4 | 1.3 | 1.4 | | 0.1 |
| Verbal scatter | OP | 4.8 | 6.1 | 5.6 | Betw. var.'s | 0.6 | 2.5 | 0.8 | | 0.6 |
| | C | 6.2 | 5.2 | 6.4 | Betw. means | 1.3 | 0.001 | 0.3 | | 0.1 |
| Perf. scatter | OP | 5.3 | 5.9 | 5.7 | Betw. var.'s | 0.6 | 1.5 | 0.6 | 1.6 | 0.7 |
| | C | 5.4 | 6.3 | 6.2 | Betw. means | 0.003 | 0.1 | 0.1 | 1.0 | 0.1 |

NOTE: There were 19 patients in the operatee group and 13 in the control group.
In this and succeeding tables the following data applies:
The terms "between means" and "between variance" which appear in the tables of F ratios are defined as follows:

$$\text{between variances} = \frac{Vop}{Vc}$$

$$\text{between means} = \frac{Vb}{Vw}$$

*For the analysis of variance:* (where: operated group N = 19) control group N = 13)

F ratios between means $\left(\frac{Vb}{Vw}\right)$ must exceed 4.17 to be significant at the .05 level of confidence.

F ratios between variances $\left(\frac{Vop}{Vc}\right)$ must exceed 2.63 to be significant at the .05 level of confidence.

*For the analyses of covariance:* (where: operated group N = 19) control group N = 13)

F ratios between means $\left(\frac{Vb}{Vw}\right)$ must exceed 4.18 to be significant at the .05 level of confidence.

F ratios between variances $\left(\frac{Vop}{Vc}\right)$ must exceed 2.69 to be significant at the .05 level of confidence.

All values which were found to be significant by the above criteria are marked with an asterisk.
*For the critical ratios:* The values which the critical ratio must exceed in order to be significant at the .05 level of confidence varies somewhat with the size of the groups compared. The values obtained have been tested against Fisher's t tables (Fisher, R. A., and Yates, F., 1943, Statistical tables for biological, agricultural and medical research. London, Oliver & Boyd, Ltd.), and those C.R.'s which were found to be significant are marked with an asterisk.

operatees. Again the differences of the means and the variances at R1, R2, R1-O, and R2-O were not statistically reliable.

It was felt that the weighting of the scores imposed by the Wechsler scoring system to achieve equivalence between tests might conceal minor differences existing in the data. The raw scores were therefore computed for the total test, and for the verbal and performance items separately. Analysis showed that exactly the same situation existed as was found with the weighted scores.

The I.Q.'s determined preoperatively for the topectomy group showed a rank order correlation of +.90 with the R1 measure, and +.92 with the R2 testing. Correlations of similar order were obtained between testing intervals for the control group and when all participants were considered together.

The conclusion is apparent that there were no group differences in the general measures achieved on the Wechsler-Bellevue Test attributable to frontal topectomy, either in total measure or when verbal and performance items were considered separately.

Scatter. Any individual taking a test of this type, which is constructed of many subtests, will earn a series of scores on the subtests that will differ from each other to a larger or smaller extent. This is expressible as his "scatter"— which is measured by taking deviations around the average of all the subtest scores. Psychotics have been found to be variable in some intelligence test performances, and their "scatter" on intelligence tests of this sort has been used by some workers as a diagnostic aid in assessing their mental status.

In order to see whether or not frontal topectomy had a measurable effect upon such individual variability an analysis was made of the performance of each individual at each of the three testing intervals. Considering an individual's spread of subtest scores around his average as an indication of his tendency to vary on the different tests, the variance (or square of the standard deviation) of each individual's performance was computed. The variances thus obtained were treated as scatter scores, representing an index of individual spread, and pre- and postoperative comparisons were made.

The means for all the scatter scores showed that the operatee and control groups were not exactly equated preoperatively, but that neither group was altered appreciably in the postoperative testing. Application of covariance to allow for the initial discrepancy made it clear that there were no significant differences in the means or variances of the groups at R1 and R2 which could be attributed to the operation. The same result was obtained when similar treatment was applied to the verbal and performance scatter scores separately. Some fluctuations of the means and spread of the groups occurred but these differences were not statistically reliable. In summary we may say that the tendency of an individual's subtest scores to scatter around his mean did not seem to be altered in any way by frontal topectomy.

Subtest Analysis. In addition to the over-all measures it affords, the Wechsler-Bellevue Test yields information on a variety of specific abilities. The subtests of which it is composed are devised to sample a wide variety of types of human performance. Half of the measures are tests of what is called verbal ability (words, use of words and numbers to express ideas, etc.) and half are tests of what is called performance ability (spatial arrangements, use of objects, expression of ideas through motor performance). It contains tests of General Information, General Comprehension, Digit Span, Arithmetic, Similarities, Vocabulary, Picture Arrangement, Picture Completion, Block Design, Object Assembly, and Digit Symbol Substitution.

TABLE 44.   MEANS AND F RATIOS OF OPERATEE AND CONTROL GROUPS ON THE SUBTESTS OF THE WECHSLER-BELLEVUE

| Subtest | Group | Means | | | | Analysis of variance F ratios | | | Analysis of covariance F ratios | |
|---|---|---|---|---|---|---|---|---|---|---|
| | | 0 | R1 | R2 | | 0 | R1 | R2 | R1 | R2 |
| Info. | OP | 14.4 | 14.4 | 15.4 | Betw. var.'s | 1.9 | 2.8* | 1.6 | | 2.7 |
| | C | 17.1 | 17.2 | 17.9 | Betw. means | 3.7 | 3.4 | 2.7 | | 0.1 |
| Compr. | OP | 10.3 | 10.7 | 10.7 | Betw. var.'s | 1.3 | 0.9 | 0.7 | | 0.6 |
| | C | 11.5 | 12.2 | 13.3 | Betw. means | 0.8 | 1.0 | 3.8 | | 4.1 |
| Digits | OP | 10.4 | 11.2 | 11.2 | Betw. var.'s | 1.0 | 0.9 | 1.4 | | 0.6 |
| | C | 11.5 | 12.1 | 11.4 | Betw. means | 0.02 | 1.0 | 0.03 | | 2.1 |
| Arith. | OP | 6.8 | 7.1 | 7.3 | Betw. var.'s | 1.4 | 1.6 | 1.4 | | 1.4 |
| | C | 8.4 | 9.3 | 8.5 | Betw. means | 2.9 | 4.3* | 1.6 | | 1.3 |
| Simil. | OP | 11.5 | 11.1 | 13.0 | Betw. var.'s | 0.8 | 0.9 | 1.0 | | 0.6 |
| | C | 11.6 | 12.8 | 15.0 | Betw. means | 0.01 | 1.6 | 1.6 | | 2.7 |
| Vocab. | OP | 23.1 | 23.9 | 24.0 | Betw. var.'s | 1.1 | 0.9 | 1.4 | | 2.0 |
| | C | 26.4 | 27.1 | 28.6 | Betw. means | 1.9 | 1.1 | 3.2 | | 1.6 |
| P. Arr. | OP | 8.5 | 9.9 | 10.6 | Betw. var.'s | 3.3* | 0.9 | 1.2 | | 0.5 |
| | C | 8.6 | 11.1 | 11.5 | Betw. means | 0.01 | 0.4 | 0.3 | | 0.4 |
| P. Comp. | OP | 9.9 | 11.0 | 11.1 | Betw. var.'s | 0.7 | 0.9 | 0.9 | | 1.4 |
| | C | 9.6 | 11.4 | 11.2 | Betw. means | 0.1 | 0.2 | 0.003 | | 0.2 |
| Block Des. | OP | 18.9 | 19.3 | 21.5 | Betw. var.'s | 1.0 | 0.6 | 1.0 | | 1.1 |
| | C | 21.3 | 22.1 | 23.4 | Betw. means | 1.1 | 1.3 | 0.5 | | 0.1 |
| Object. Assem. | OP | 17.0 | 18.0 | 18.7 | Betw. var.'s | 0.6 | 0.3 | 0.8 | 0.6 | 1.4 |
| | C | 14.9 | 18.2 | 19.9 | Betw. means | 2.7 | 0.03 | 1.9 | 0.8 | 6.4* |
| Dig. Symb. | OP | 29.6 | 32.1 | 34.9 | Betw. var.'s | 2.6 | 0.9 | 2.0 | 0.5 | 2.9* |
| | C | 27.2 | 32.0 | 35.5 | Betw. means | 0.4 | 0.0 | 0.02 | 0.2 | 0.9 |
| Suppl. Dig. Symb. | OP | 217.5 | 196.6 | 204.3 | Betw. var.'s | 0.9 | 0.4 | 3.2* | 0.4 | 4.7* |
| | C | 232.1 | 218.6 | 185.8 | Betw. means | 0.2 | 0.4 | 0.2 | 0.2 | 1.6 |

NOTE: There were 19 patients in the operatee group and 13 in the control.
* Significant at .05 level.

An analysis has been made of the performance of the operatee and control groups on each of these measures. Since each test was considered separately the analysis has been carried out with raw scores in order to obtain maximal sensitivity. These results are given in table 44.

When the twelve subtests were treated by an analysis of variance the following differences were found between the operatee and control groups which were significant at the .05 level of confidence. Reliable differences between means existed for the tests of Arithmetic (at R1), and Object Assembly (on R2-O). Comparison of the variance or spread of the groups showed reliable differences existing for the tests of Picture Arrangement (at O), Digit Symbol

Substitution (on R2-O), and Supplementary Digit Symbol Substitution (at R2 and on R2-O).

Since the operatee and control groups were not well equated preoperatively on the many subtests an analysis of covariance was applied to correct for the initial discrepancy and the number of statistically significant differences was reduced to three: (1) A difference between means of the operatee and control groups which was significant at the .05 level of confidence for Object Assembly (at R2) in favor of the control group. (2) A difference between the variances of the operatee and control groups which was significant at the .05 level of confidence for Digit Symbol Substitution (at R2), indicating that the operatee group was more variable. (3) A difference between the variances of the operatee and control groups which was significant at the .01 level of confidence for Supplementary Digit Symbol Substitution (at R2), indicating that the operatee group was more variable.

It is apparent, therefore, that the operatee and control groups showed significantly different performance on tests of two specific abilities. Further inquiry was made into these tests in order to determine the direction of change, and, if possible, the nature of the change.

The test of Object Assembly requires the subject to assemble into a meaningful whole parts of well-known configurations (a manikin, a face, and a hand). The mean score of both operatee and control groups showed a gain with repetition of the test with the control group increasing more than the operatees at R1. Since this test is scored for both time and accuracy of performance, it was possible to analyze each of these components separately to ascertain its contribution to the total effect observed. It was observed that the control group showed "better" scores (less time, more accuracy) throughout than did the operatee group. This was especially marked at R1, and apparently the group difference seen at R1 in total score was attributable to a general effect. There was no indication that either the time or the accuracy score was solely responsible for the difference seen in the total; they seemed to act together in producing the difference.

It will be noted that the difference between the groups was produced by greater gains of the control group as compared to the operatees, rather than by an actual drop below preoperative level of performance by the operatee group.

Digit Symbol Substitution (and its Supplementary score) is a test of the speed and accuracy of transcription of digits and symbols which are associated in a key visible to the subject at all times. It would appear to be a task requiring persistent effort which is influenced to some extent by learning effects in the case of handling the symbols. It does not, however, lend itself to breakdown into these possible components.

As may be seen from the means for this test listed in table 44, the control group showed a greater gain in performance in unit time, and the supplementary score corroborated this by showing greater reduction in the time required to complete the unit task by the control as compared with the operatee group. The significant difference reported was not between means, however, but in the variance of the groups. The variance of the operatee group at R2 was 81.17 and for the control group 27.82. This large discrepancy, which was verified by covariance, indicated a much greater variation of performance between members of the operatee group than between members of the control group. The same effect was obtained when the supplementary score was analyzed. This conclusion is somewhat weakened by the fact that a contrary situation was found to exist for both measures at R1. The control group showed greater variance than the operatees although the difference did not reach the point of significance.

It can be stated that in general this test showed "better" performance (more substitutions in less time) by the control group postoperatively than by the operatee group but that the spread of the groups was an uncertain element making comparisons between the groups on this basis problematical.

TABLE 45.  RELATION OF SCORES ON THE THREE BASIC TESTS TO BACK-
GROUND AND EXPERIMENTAL VARIABLES
(Relationship expressed as a critical ratio)

|  | Wechsler-Bellevue full I.Q. | | Porteus M.A. | | Continuous-problem task (correct minus error) | |
|---|---|---|---|---|---|---|
|  | R1–0 | R2–0 | R1–0 | R2–0 | R1–0 | R2–0 |
| AGE (Upper third–lower third)........ N=6        N=6 | 0.56 | 1.31 | 1.07 | 1.32 | 0.73 | 0.83 |
| SEX (Male–female)................... N=11  N=8 | 1.05 | 1.77 | 1.70 | 1.34 | 0.15 | 1.19 |
| BRAIN WT. EXCISED (Upper third–lower third)........ N=6        N=6 | 0.28 | 0.10 | 1.07 | 0.72 | 0.07 | 0.83 |
| SOCIAL IMPROVEMENT (Third most imp.–third least imp.). N=6        N=6 | 0.51 | 0.51 | 0.37 | 0.44 | 0.04 | 0.71 |

* Significant at the .05 level.

The results of the analysis of the various subtests clearly substantiated the findings with the over-all measures. There was no marked change in the structure of the specific abilities which in total score give an estimate of intelligence. The survey of a variety of specific abilities afforded by a subtest analysis has revealed only two which are altered postoperatively to a statistically reliable degree.

**Comparisons within the Operatee Group.**  In addition to contrasting the operatee and control groups certain comparisons have been made within the operatee group with respect to the special considerations of age, sex, brain weight and area excised, and social improvement. The method of critical ratio has been applied in comparing the means of these smaller subgroups. In each case a comparison was made of the means of the difference scores (R1-O, R2-O) of the subgroups. The results may be read in table 45.

*Age.*  It is possible that an operation of this type might have differential effects on individuals of different ages. A comparison of the mean I.Q. obtained by the oldest one-third of this group with the mean I.Q. of the youngest one-third revealed no reliable difference between the groups.

*Sex.*  To examine the possibility of a differential effect of operation on the sexes the mean I.Q. obtained by the males was contrasted with the mean I.Q. of the females. No reliable difference was found to exist.

*Area Excised.* A question of the greatest importance is the examination of the possibility of differential effects resulting from the excision of different cortical areas. For this comparison the mean of the difference scores obtained by the individuals with the area in question removed has been compared with the mean of the difference scores for the control group. The results, together with the number of the area involved and the N of the group receiving the operation, are given in table 46.

This table may be summarized by the statement that the removal of different cortical areas did not show differential effects upon the general measures or the scatter measures obtained on the Wechsler-Bellevue Test.

TABLE 46. MEANS AND CRITICAL RATIOS FOR THE AREA SUBGROUPS ON THE WECHSLER-BELLEVUE FULL I.Q. AND THE SCATTER SCORES

| | | Full I.Q. | | | | Scatter scores | |
|---|---|---|---|---|---|---|---|
| Area No. | N | Mean R1–0 | CR | Mean R2–0 | CR | Mean R2–0 | CR |
| 8................ | 5 | 2.00 | 1.58 | 4.80 | 1.88 | 1.59 | 1.37 |
| 9................ | 6 | 1.33 | 1.28 | 7.20 | 1.10 | 0.25 | 0.61 |
| 10................ | 4 | 7.50 | 0.01 | 11.50 | 0.46 | −0.19 | 0.28 |
| 46................ | 4 | 4.25 | 0.86 | 9.00 | 0.36 | 2.41 | 1.72 |
| 11................ | 3 | 7.67 | 0.03 | 7.70 | 0.70 | 0.16 | 0.42 |
| Controls.......... | 13 | 7.54 | | 10.08 | | −0.70 | |

* Significant at .05 level.

*Brain Weight Excised.* As indicated earlier in this study, the relation of the amount of tissue removed to performance is an important consideration. A comparison of the mean I.Q. obtained by the one third of the patients with the greatest tissue removal with the mean I.Q. of the third with the least amount of tissue removed revealed no indication of a difference between the groups. This was confirmed by the correlation of −.14 between brain weight excised and the change (gain) in I.Q.

*Social Improvement.* It is of interest to know whether social improvement on the part of the patients was accompanied by an increase in I.Q. or reduced scatter on this test of intelligence. An index of social improvement following operation was available in the form of a rather objective rating scale prepared by the psychiatrists of the Columbia-Greystone project. A comparison of the mean I.Q. of the one third of the patients rated "most improved" and the mean I.Q. of the third rated "least improved" revealed no differences between the groups. The same groups compared on the basis of scatter scores also showed no differences.

**Notes on Special Areas.** Two of the operatee patients in whom there was bilateral removal of area 44, which is the so-called speech area of Broca, were of special interest. A brief profile of these patients should indicate the effect of this removal on what is called "verbal intelligence."

Patient 47. An extremely verbal patient who maintained a stream of speech at all times had area 44 removed bilaterally. She began to speak immediately after recovery from operative anesthesia. Once the postoperative sluggishness had passed off there was no slowdown in speech apparent to observers as compared to her pre-operative condition. Some eccentricities in spelling occurred immediately following operation which disappeared within a few days. She was subsequently examined carefully and completely for aphasia but no traces of aphasic disturbance could be detected. Her scores on the Wechsler-Bellevue Test showed a slight gain and analysis revealed that the patient had superior scores on the verbal tests as compared to the performance items both before and after operation.

Patient 33. This patient had been mute for several months prior to having Broca's area removed bilaterally. She began to speak about one month after operation and, spoke clearly and distinctly. Her performance on the Wechsler-Bellevue Test showed equal ability on the verbal and performance items of the scale. The measure was made four months after operation. Test results for this patient are not included in the body of this study since her mutism prior to operation prevented adequate measurement.

### SUMMARY OF FINDINGS WITH THE WECHSLER-BELLEVUE TEST

1. No significant differences between the operatee and control groups were found to exist on the over-all measures of verbal subtests, performance subtests, or when the two were considered together in the form of an I.Q.

2. The tendency of an individual's scores on the subtests to "scatter" around his mean (intraindividual scatter) was not affected by the operation.

3. When the subtests were considered separately as a survey of specific abilities the operatee and control groups showed a statistically significant difference in performance on the test of Object Assembly and Digit Symbol Substitution.

4. No relation could be established between the scores obtained postoperatively and the factors of age, sex, area or brain weight excised, or social improvement.

5. Scores obtained on the verbal and performance items of the test were not affected by the excision of areas usually associated with speech production and sequential motor activity.

### THE PORTEUS MAZES

The measures obtained by this test are indices of total performance. The test consists of a series of paper-and-pencil mazes of graded difficulty. The subject begins at a simple level (five-year level) regardless of his age and works through the series. He is credited with additional mental age (beyond the five-year level at which he began) for each maze successfully completed. The amount of credit received depends upon the number of trials required to succeed on each maze. His score on the test as a whole is the sum of the credits received at each year level, and this is his mental age (M.A.). The maximal M.A. measured by the test is eighteen years.

Two other scores are available on the Porteus Mazes. The first of these is the test quotient (T.Q.), a score derived by dividing the M.A. by C.A. with certain additional allowances made for the age of the subject. Since all of our patients were above the maximal age for the transformation table this score is to all intents and purposes merely another way of writing the mental age. A qualitative score is also available, although not an intelligence measure *per se*. The nature of faulty performance (crossed lines, cut corners, lifted pencil, etc.) is scored by the allotment of a numerical weighting to each of these minor errors not scored in the M.A. These are totalled to give an estimate of the degree of error not scored in the M.A. and this is called the Q score.

The latter two scores are not treated in the body of this study. Since the T.Q. is a direct transformation of the M.A. its inclusion was not required. The Q score is not a measure of intelligence but more of a personality indicator. In the hope that it would shed light on general performance on the maze test it was carefully taken and fully analyzed. At no time did the results obtained differentiate between the operatee and control groups or add to the understanding of maze performance in general. It has, therefore, been omitted as a consideration from the treatment herein.

Our primary interest, then, was to observe the effects of topectomy on M.A. which is the intelligence measure afforded by the test.

TABLE 47.   MEANS AND F RATIOS OF THE OPERATEE AND CONTROL GROUPS ON THE PORTEUS MAZE TEST

| Score | Group | Means | | | | | Analysis of variance F ratios | | | | Analysis of covariance F ratios | | |
|---|---|---|---|---|---|---|---|---|---|---|---|---|---|
| | | 0 | R1 | R2 | R3 | | 0 | R1 | R2 | R3 | R1 | R2 | R3 |
| M.A. | OP | 13.2 | 12.0 | 13.3 | 13.6 | Betw. var's | 0.8 | 3.1* | 1.7 | 0.9 | 2.3 | 1.2 | 1.3 |
| | C | 13.2 | 14.2 | 15.0 | 14.4 | Betw. means | 0.0 | 4.8* | 3.0 | 0.5 | 6.2* | 3.8 | 0.2 |

* Significant at .05 level.

Examination of the mean (see table 47) scores made by the operatee and control groups revealed a rather striking trend. Figure 97 presents this graphically.

The means of the two groups were almost identical at O, since M.A. was one of the bases upon which the patients were matched. At the R1 testing the controls showed a slight gain in performance while the operatee group showed a distinct loss which reduced the mean score to a level 1.21 years of M.A. below the preoperative level. At the R2 testing the controls continued to show a slight gain with repetition of the test and the operatees also showed a gain which brought their mean score back up to its preoperative level. Because of the interest of this finding the test was given again eight months postoperatively and this has been called R3.* Mean score at this testing showed that the control group maintained its previous level while the operatee group continued to gain although it was still somewhat below the level of the control group.

Treatment of the data by the analysis of variance showed that the difference in performance of the operatee and control groups at the R1 testing was statistically significant at the .05 level of confidence for differences between means and between variances. An analysis of covariance was applied to correct for original discrepancies between the variances of the groups and this accentuated the difference between means at R1 but reduced the difference between variances to a point below significance. The high covariance F ratio

* Data were obtained on all of the operatees and 10 of the 13 controls. The minor fluctuation of the mean of the control group at R3 is perhaps attributable to the reduced number of cases.

seen in table 47 for the R2 testing reflects the fact that the groups still differed markedly at this testing although not significantly. The low covariance F ratio at R3 reflects the fact that the means were in close approximation by this testing interval.

**Within-Test Analysis.** An attempt was made to look into the test performance to determine the nature of the impaired performance of the operatee group although the test does not lend itself readily to fractionation. One aspect that could be investigated was the number of maze trials that were required to achieve the M.A. assigned. Tabulation of the number of trials

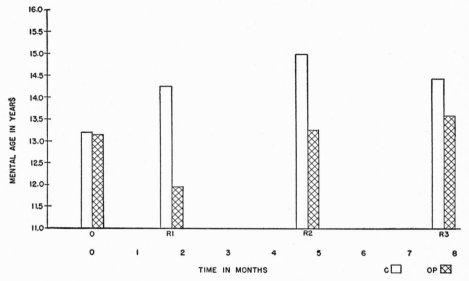

FIG. 97.   Plot of the mean scores obtained on the Porteus Maze Test by the operatee and control groups over the four testing intervals.

required by the operatee and control groups up to the point of failure failed to show differences between the groups. A tabulation was made of the number of trials required for each year level by each individual at each testing. From this tabulation it was apparent that "spottiness" of performance, such as missed years at low levels with success at higher levels or excessive number of trials required throughout the test, was not responsible for the lower mental ages achieved. The effect was apparently an earlier cutting off or lower ceiling on M.A. achieved by the operatee group. Stated in other words this means earlier failure at the upper age levels of the test by the operatee group. Introduction of additional scoring systems for performance on the upper age levels of the test failed to clarify the location or reasons for this earlier cutting off.

**Comparisons within the Operatee Group.** Comparison within the operatee group has been carried out as well as the contrasting of the group as a whole with the controls. As in the case of the Wechsler-Bellevue Test, these special considerations were age, sex, brain weight and area excised, and social improvement. The method of critical ratio has been applied in comparing the means of the difference scores (R1-O, R2-O) of these smaller subgroups. The results may be read in table 45.

*Age.* The mean scores obtained by the oldest third of the operative group did not differ significantly from those of the youngest third.

*Sex.* No statistically reliable difference in mean score was found for the male and female groups contrasted.

*Area Excised.* The area comparisons are of especial interest since the group as a whole exhibited impaired performance. The mean difference scores obtained by the different individuals with the area in question removed have been compared with the mean difference scores of the control group. The results, together with the number of the area involved and the N of the group receiving the operation, are given in table 48.

TABLE 48.  MEANS AND CRITICAL RATIOS FOR THE AREA SUBGROUPS ON THE PORTEUS MAZES

| Area No. | N | Mean R1–0 | CR | Mean R2–0 | CR | Mean R3–0 | CR |
|---|---|---|---|---|---|---|---|
| 8................. | 5 | −3.00 | 2.69* | −1.10 | 1.32 | −0.10 | 0.41 |
| 9................. | 6 | −1.33 | 1.65 | −0.08 | 0.62 | 1.33 | 0.52 |
| 10................ | 4 | −0.87 | 1.14 | −1.00 | 1.18 | 2.13 | 0.91 |
| 46................ | 4 | −0.62 | 0.99 | 1.62 | 0.40 | 1.13 | 0.33 |
| 11................ | 3 | −1.67 | 0.40 | 2.00 | 0.56 | 1.33 | 0.40 |
| Controls.......... | 13 | 0.96 | | 1.81 | | 0.55 | |

* Significant at .05 level.

The greatest effects observed were on the R1-O scores. The means of areas 8, 9, 10, and 46 showed the deficit in varying amounts while the means of area 11 reflected a gain. The excision of area 8 seemed to be more productive of deficit than the other areas and the difference in score between individuals having this area removed and the control group is statistically reliable.

At R2-O the mean of areas 8 and 10 continued to show deficits while areas 9, 46, and 11 showed a gain.

At R3-O the mean of area 8 still showed a slight deficit while the means of all other areas showed appreciable positive direction.

This finding may be summarized by the statement that removal of areas 8, 9, 10, and 46 resulted in impaired performance on this test when measured at a period three weeks after operation, but damage to area 11 had no apparent effect. Those patients having area 8 removed showed the greatest degree of impairment both in original amount and duration of impaired performance.

*Brain Weight Excised.* The mean obtained by the one third of the group with greatest tissue removal was compared with that of the one third sustaining the least amount of tissue removed. The groups did not differ reliably. This corroborated the nonsignificant correlation of +.23 which existed between brain weight excised and change (gain) in M.A. on R1-O; on R2-O the correlation was −.06.

*Social Improvement.* Comparisons were made of the mean score of the "most improved" and "least improved" group which did not show the groups to be reliably different. Inspection of the data, however, showed that the pattern of scores made by the individuals was more instructive than a comparison of means. Inquiry into the pattern of performance over the four testing periods showed a marked relation between performance on this test and social improvement.

**Considerations of the "Drop and Rise" Pattern.**   The results of the group data clearly indicated an impairment in maze test performance following frontal topectomy. A plot of the mean scores obtained by the operatee and control groups at each testing interval showed the pattern presented in figure 97.

The most striking aspect of the relative performance of the two groups was the drop in mean score of the operatee group at the $R_1$ testing with subsequent gain at the later testing intervals. Examination of the score pattern for each individual showed this to be a general effect, not attributable to the marked deviation of a few individuals.

Since the operatee group as a whole had shown social improvement as measured by the improvement index discussed above an effort was made to relate this finding to the alteration of performance on this test. This meant a relation of the impairment phenomenon observed in each individual's performance to his social improvement. The answer was not long in forthcoming. Those individuals whose pattern of performance most resembled the pattern of group performance were found to be the ones who had shown the greatest degree of social recovery.

In order to make this statement quantitative the following criterion of selection was applied in selecting those individuals in the operatee group whose pattern of performance most resembled that of the group as a whole.

> Any individual whose scores showed a loss in mental age of one year or more at the $R_1$ testing which was regained such that a score at least as high as his preoperative score was obtained at $R_2$ and who maintained this gain by an $R_3$ score which was at or above his preoperative level was said to exhibit the required similarity.

When this criterion was applied to the patients in the operatee group 6 patients were selected. Five of these 6 patients are in the group of 6 patients rated by the psychiatrists as showing the greatest social improvement. All of them are at home and working. When this criterion was applied to the control group no patients were found to satisfy it.

When evaluated on an eight-point scale of social improvement, on which a higher number indicates greater improvement, these 6 patients obtained a mean of 5.83 as compared to a mean of 1.0 for all other operatees and a mean of 0.67 for all controls.

Comparisons of the mean score of these 6 patients with the mean score of all other operatees showed that they were not reliably different in age, amount of brain tissue excised, preoperative social rating, preoperative I.Q. or M.A., or change in I.Q. ($R_1$-O and $R_2$-O on Wechsler-Bellevue Test).

A comparison of the areas removed from these 6 patients showed that no one area was regularly represented. Areas 8, 9, 10, and 46 were all involved but area 11 was conspicuous by its absence. The lack of impairment in patients with area 11 removed has been commented upon previously.

In summary it may be stated that a performance pattern of a particular type has been found which was strongly associated with social improvement. This association held for the operatee group as a whole as well as for individual performance. It was characterized by a distinct impairment of the preoperative level of maze test performance when measured at $R_1$ followed by gains in performance at R2 and R3 which reached and exceeded the level of preoperative performance.

1. The operatee and control groups showed a different pattern of performance over the four testing periods. Although the groups were equated at O the operatee group exhibited a distinct impairment in performance at R1 while the control group showed a gain. This difference was found to be statistically reliable. At R2 the controls continued to gain and the operatee group recovered its preoperative level; at R3 the controls showed a slight loss while the operatee group continued to gain although its mean score still did not reach that of the control. The difference between the groups at R2 and R3 was not statistically reliable.

2. The nature of the impaired performance by the operatee group appeared to be simply earlier failure at the upper age levels of the test.

3. No relation could be established between the scores obtained postoperatively and the factors of age, sex, or brain weight removed.

4. Bilateral damage to cortical areas 8, 9, 10, and 46 resulted in impaired performance on this test when measured three weeks following operation, but damage to area 11 had no apparent effect. Those patients with area 8 removed showed the greatest degree of impairment both in original amount and duration of impaired performance.

5. The particular pattern of performance on the test made by the operatee group was found to be associated strongly with psychiatric ratings of social improvement. This association held for both the operatee group as a whole and in the case of individual performance.

### CONTINUOUS-PROBLEM TASK

This is not a test of intelligence in the same sense as the procedures previously described. As explained in the section on experimental procedures, the principal reason for its inclusion was to obtain a "work sample" of the patient's ability to perform on a task requiring close attention and sustained effort over a period of time. Perhaps its greatest advantage is the fact that it requires continued effort and attention over a prolonged period (sixteen minutes). A more complete explanation of the reasons for its inclusion has been given above.

Three scores were obtained on the proficiency of performance: (1) the number of problems solved within the time allotted, (2) the number of errors made in solving the problems, (3) the number of correct problem solutions minus the numbers of errors made. This should take into account both of the aspects of performance described in numbers (1) and (2) above. The results of the O testing showed that the correct and error scores were unrelated ($r = -.03$), therefore each has been included as a separate index and the two were also combined into a single measure.

The first of these scores was an important one since we were concerned with the application of the subject to his task and this is reflected principally in the amount of performance rather than its accuracy (as for example, in Digit Symbol Substitution). In order not to neglect the accuracy of performance, however, it has been separately scored and also introduced as a corrective factor in the correct minus error score. Since the errors made were rather numerous, amounting to roughly one third of the number of correct solutions, the scores have been directly combined. Their relative size prevents the overshadowing of the influence of the smaller score.

The first question to be answered was the effect of operation on performance of this type as measured by the number of correct problem solutions. The results of this comparison may be read in table 49.

The mean scores of the operatee and control groups were fairly equal originally. Both groups showed an increase at R1, but the gain of the controls was greater than that of the operatees. At R2 both groups again showed an increase in mean score and once again the increases of the control group exceeded those of the operatee group. These differences were treated by analysis of variance and covariance, to allow for the original discrepancies noted, and were not found to be statistically reliable.

TABLE 49.   MEANS AND F RATIOS OF OPERATEE AND CONTROL GROUPS ON THE CONTINUOUS-PROBLEM TASK

| Score | Group | Means | | | Analysis of variance F ratios | | | | Analysis of covariance F ratios | |
| --- | --- | --- | --- | --- | --- | --- | --- | --- | --- | --- |
| | | 0 | R1 | R2 | | 0 | R1 | R2 | R1 | R2 |
| Correct.......... | OP | 154.2 | 172.7 | 217.5 | Betw. var.'s | 1.0 | 2.5 | 1.9 | 1.8 | 1.3 |
| | C | 167.3 | 211.8 | 252.5 | Betw. means | 0.2 | 1.5 | 0.9 | 1.3 | 0.7 |
| Error............ | OP | 53.1 | 70.2 | 57.7 | Betw. var.'s | 1.0 | 1.4 | 0.6 | 0.6 | 0.6 |
| | C | 45.9 | 41.5 | 38.1 | Betw. means | 0.2 | 1.6 | 1.5 | 1.9 | 1.3 |
| Correct minus error | OP | 102.6 | 103.1 | 160.0 | Betw. var.'s | 1.4 | 3.9* | 2.1 | 1.0 | 0.8 |
| | C | 121.3 | 165.8 | 214.4 | Betw. means | 0.3 | 3.3 | 1.0 | 3.6 | 0.8 |

NOTE: There were 19 patients in the operatee group and 13 in the control.
* Significant at .05 level.

When the groups were contrasted with respect to the number of errors scored the following trends were seen (table 45). The mean scores of the groups were approximately equal originally but at R1 the control group showed a decrease in errors while the operatee group showed an increase. At the R2 testing the controls again showed a decrease and the operatees also showed a decrease in mean score, but this was not sufficient to reach the preoperative level. Treatment of the data by an analysis of variance and covariance showed that these differences were not statistically reliable. It should be noted, however, that this score is the second instance in which the operatee group dropped below its preoperative level of performance with subsequent regain (see impairment on Porteus Maze performance).

When the two scores were combined into one (C minus E) the trends noted above were accentuated since they were in opposite directions. When considered on the basis of this combined score the groups were not too well equated at O (see table 49). The operatee group made no gain at R1 while the control group showed a marked increase. Both groups increased in mean score at R2 about the same amount but the operatee group still scored appreciably below the level of the controls. When these scores were treated by an analysis of variance and covariance the groups were not found to be reliably different but the trend of the groups to differ is strong. It can be seen that adjustment of the error score to numerical parity with the larger score of correct solutions in this combination would certainly differentiate the two groups reliably. To do this, however, is to place more emphasis on the accuracy of performance than it deserves.

It was apparent that the topectomy group suffered no marked impairment in its ability to perform a task of this type. Certain trends, however, were clearly evident and these generally showed "better" performance (more problems solved, fewer errors made) on the part of the control group than by the operatees.

TABLE 50.  MEANS AND CRITICAL RATIOS FOR THE AREA SUBGROUPS ON THE CONTINUOUS-PROBLEM TASK

(Correct minus error score)

| Area No. | N | Mean R1–0 | CR | Mean R2–0 | CR |
|---|---|---|---|---|---|
| 8 | 5 | −35.60 | 2.00 | 3.40 | 1.49 |
| 9 | 6 | −13.50 | 1.55 | 46.50 | 1.56 |
| 10 | 4 | 12.75 | 0.72 | 25.25 | 0.97 |
| 46 | 4 | −18.75 | 1.43 | 12.25 | 1.20 |
| 11 | 3 | 59.00 | 0.54 | 71.00 | 0.74 |
| Controls | 13 | 48.90 | | 93.00 | |

\* Significant at .05 level.

**Within-Test Analysis.**  In addition to the scores described above observations were recorded as to the nature of the errors, that is whether the wrong group of switches was selected or the wrong switch within the group, and the tendency to block, defined as a pause in performance of ten seconds or more. These tabulations showed that the preponderant source of error for both operatee and control groups was the selection of the wrong group rather than the wrong switch within the group, and the fact that blocking was minimal in both groups.

**Comparisons within the Operatee Group.**  As in the case of the tests previously treated, comparisons within the operatee group have been carried out as well as contrasting the group as a whole with the controls. The C-E score has been utilized throughout since it was considered to be the best measure for the reason stated above. A similar analysis was carried out for the other scores and no contradictions appeared. Subgroups within the operatee group have been contrasted with reference to the considerations of age, sex, brain weight and area excised, and social improvement. The result of this treatment of difference scores may be read from the table of critical ratios, table 45.

*Age.*  The mean scores obtained by the oldest third of the operatee group did not differ significantly from those of the youngest third.

*Sex.*  No statistically reliable differences were found when the mean scores of the male and female groups were contrasted.

*Area Excised.*  Table 50 presents the results, together with the number of the area involved and the N of the groups receiving this operation. As in the case of area comparisons on our other tests, the mean scores of an area subgroup has been compared with the mean of the controls.

It can be seen from the subgroup means listed in table 50 that the patients with areas 8, 9, and 46 removed exhibited the greatest degree of impairment on R1-O while those with areas 10 and 11 excised showed no decreases. These differences were not statistically reliable. On R2-O the means reflect a gain on the part of all subgroups and, here again, the patients with area 8 removed showed the greatest degree of retardation. This finding is in keeping with results obtained with the Porteus Mazes and the tendencies shown in the Wechsler-Bellevue, namely that those patients having area 8 removed showed the greatest degree of impairment both in original amount and duration of impaired performance.

*Brain Weight Excised.* The means obtained by the one third of the group with the greatest tissue removal was compared with that of the one third sustaining the least amount of tissue removed. The groups did not differ reliably nor markedly in trend. This agreed with the correlation of −.24 which exists between brain weight excised and change (gain) in C-E scores on R1-O and −.16 on R2-O.

*Social Improvement.* Comparisons were made of the mean scores of the "most improved" and "least improved" groups which did not demonstrate the groups to be reliably different. Comparisons of the patterns of individual performance over the three testing intervals, such as those made with the Porteus Mazes, were unproductive principally because of the wide variations in individual performance.

### SUMMARY OF FINDINGS WITH THE CONTINUOUS-PROBLEM TASK

1. No significant differences were found in the performance of the operatee and control groups on this task as measured by the number of problems correctly solved in unit time, the number of errors made, or these two measures combined.

2. Contrary trends were observed in the operatee and control groups which generally showed "better" performance (more problems solved, fewer errors made) on the part of the control group as compared to the operatees.

3. No relation could be established between the scores obtained postoperatively and the factors of age, sex, brain weight removed, or social improvement.

4. Bilateral excision of cortical areas 8, 9, and 46 resulted in impaired performance on the test but damage to areas 10 and 11 had no apparent effects. As was observed with the Porteus Mazes and to some extent in the Wechsler-Bellevue, those patients having area 8 removed tended to show the greatest degree of impairment both in original amount and duration of impairment.

### DISCUSSION AND CONCLUSIONS

It has been the purpose of this study to frame properly an experiment which would reveal the effects of partial removal of the frontal lobes upon intellectual function. The unique opportunity afforded to study cases in which there was to be bilateral removal of relatively specific areas of the frontal cortex has made it possible to circumvent many of the difficulties which have beset previous investigations of the relation of the frontal lobe to intelligence. The results of this study have clarified the effect of the experimental variable by making use of a series of cases, by the inclusion of adequate controls, by utilizing subjects with no organic brain disease, and by the use of objective measurement for pre- and postoperative assessment of ability. The fact that given areas were removed and that the weights of these removals were known has also made it possible to present evidence as to the relative importance of particular portions of the frontal lobes and the quantity of cortical tissue removed. In order to make the assessment of intelligence as broad as possible tests were included which are predicated upon differing theoretical grounds in an effort to obtain a more complete appraisal of intellectual ability. The answers to the questions raised are, for the most part, clear.

The fundamental question to be answered is that of the permanent effects of topectomy upon intellectual function as measured by the tests utilized. The general findings of this survey with regard to a total picture of intellectual function indicated no alteration which can be regarded as permanent. The performance of the operatee group compared to that of the control on the over-all measures of intellectual ability afforded by the Wechsler-Bellevue Test, the Porteus Mazes, and the Continuous-Problem Task indicated no permanent interference with the functions measured by these tests which could be attributed to the effects of frontal lobe operations.

With regard to the possibility of differential function by the various portions of the frontal lobe, the results obtained indicated that the excision of no one cortical area, of the areas sampled in this series of operations, influenced intellectual function *permanently* any more than any other. The removal of area 8 produced the most pronounced of the transient effects noted, but even these could not be regarded as permanent on the basis of the data obtained. Since the groups formed with a given area removed are small this finding must be regarded as an indication rather than a proof that the various cortical areas do not exert a differential influence upon intelligence.

No evidence has been found in the performance of intellectual tasks by this group of operatee patients which would indicate that the amount of frontal tissue removed exerted a differential effect on the performance of these intellectual measures.

It would appear, from the results obtained in this investigation, that the frontal lobes do not play a very active role in measurable intelligence, and that interference with their function, whether by specific locus or proportion of their total size, has no *permanent* repercussion in tasks requiring intellectual ability.

Although the general measures of intelligence utilized have indicated no permanent alteration of intellectual function, certain trends and significant changes have become apparent in the course of this study which are not without interest. In addition to exhibiting recognizable trends the data have shown that the groups may be reliably differentiated on tests of certain specific abilities, and have demonstrated transient alterations in the performance of the tests which merit discussion.

There was a consistent tendency for the control group to show a greater gain in score on retesting than was exhibited by the operatee group. This discrepancy between the groups was generally greater at $R_1$, but clearly present on both $R_1$ and $R_2$. Reference to the mean scores listed in tables 43, 44, 47, and 49 will show that this is true of the principal measures on all three of our tests and is apparent in the great majority of the subtests on the Wechsler-Bellevue. Since practice effects are to be expected on repetition of a test, it would seem that the operatee group was not able to profit from its previous experience with the tests to as great an extent as were the controls. Another possible explanation could be that an actual loss in ability has occurred but there has been no interference with practice effect, and that this serves to mask the actual loss. Although it is not possible to answer this question on the basis of the data available it would appear unlikely that such a "loss" on each test would be so neatly covered by the practice effect.

Another point which deserves further comment is the fact that some, but not all, of the performance tasks showed reliable differences to exist between the operatee and control groups. The Wechsler-Bellevue subtest of Object Assembly, for example, showed differences between the groups while the tests of Block Design, Picture Arrangement, and Picture Completion did not. This might be thought to be a result of the time factor involved, in terms of some sort of motor disturbance, but analysis of the Object Assembly Test showed that both the time and accuracy scores were contributing to the total effect. Further, the Block Design Test is also scored in terms of the time as well as accuracy in the manipulation of objects into a pattern, and this test showed the groups to be well equated. The Porteus Mazes, which clearly differentiated the groups, was another instance. This test does not involve a time factor at all, but is scored in terms of accuracy only. It would appear that some factor other than speed of performance alone was interfered with in the performance of these tasks.

It is interesting to note that certain consistent relations seem to hold between such alterations as were found on our tests and some of the cortical areas of the frontal lobe. In considering these relationships it must be borne in mind that the groups formed with a given area removed are small and that conclusions drawn from the data can only be tentative at best.

It has been pointed out repeatedly in the presentation of results that removal of cortical area 8 seemed to exert a depressing influence upon performance. Those patients with area 8 excised showed a greater degree of impairment both in original amount and in the duration of impairment (see tables 48 and 50). The performance of patients having this area removed differed reliably from that of the controls for the Object Assembly subtest and the Porteus Maze Test, and remained retarded at $R_2$-O, although the differences noted at this test interval were not reliable. The tendency for depressed performance by those patients having this area removed was observable on the Continuous-Problem Task and it is also noteworthy that the patients with this area removed showed the smallest amount of gain on the Wechsler-Bellevue Full Scale I.Q. The removal of area 9 also tended to show decreased performance (see tables 48 and 50) but these were not reliable differences. The influence of the excision of areas 10 and 46 was found to be variable, while the removal of area 11 seemed to have the least effect of all. Once again, caution must be urged in the interpretation of these findings because of the smallness of the groups and the surgical impossibility of precise removal of areas which can only be positively differentiated by histologic examination.

The transient effects which have been noted in the performance of the operatee group on the Porteus Maze Test are interesting. The operatee group has been demonstrated to exhibit a definite impairment immediately following operation from which it gradually recovered, and this loss with subsequent regain has been seen to bear a rather close relationship to the social recovery of the patients upon whom operation was performed. This agreement held for both the operatee group as a whole and in the case of individual performance.

Porteus has recently reported (Porteus and Peters, '47) the effects of frontal lobotomy upon Maze Test performance in which he observed much the same phenomena as have been reported here. It is the belief of the author of the test that the Maze Test is very significantly sensitive to changes in the social adaptation aspects of intelligence following lobotomy. It is Porteus' belief that subsequent to lobotomy there is a marked diminution in foresight and planfulness which is gradually regained and that his test, which he has always claimed would measure these very traits, reflects this loss and regain. Why this process should be related to social improvement is not altogether clear. Various explanations could be offered, such as the operation breaking up old habits of social adaptation and planning, and the subsequent formation of new habits which may be more socially acceptable, but this would be speculation beyond the available data. Of this much, however, we may be relatively certain, and that is that operation on the frontal lobes resulted in impaired ability to exercise the type of intelligence measured by the Porteus Mazes. This initial loss was gradually regained and those patients most typically exhibiting this pattern of loss with subsequent regain are among those most benefited from the operation from a therapeutic point of view.

The evidence obtained from the results of this study on the role of the frontal lobes in intellectual function has tended to bear out some of the opinions discussed in the survey of the literature and to be in opposition to others. The general finding of an absence of measurable effect resulting from the loss of frontal tissue is in agreement with the reports of studies of lobectomy cases by Hebb, Lidz, and Ackerley and with the results obtained in the study of lobotomy cases by Frank, Kisker, Robinson, Hunt, and Ström-Olsen *et al.* The results did not reflect the permanent impairment of intelligence as it has been reported in the studies of lobectomy cases made by Rylander, Brickner, German and Fox, and others.

In addition, the general absence of demonstrable loss in intelligence resulting from damage to the frontal brain would make it appear that this region is not as intimately involved in human intelligence as it has been reported to be in animal intelligence by Lashley, Franz, and Jacobsen.

On the whole, it would appear that the frontal lobes do not play as important a role in intellectual functioning as has sometimes been assumed. It would be unfounded, of course, to state definitely that the frontal lobes play no part in the intelligence of an individual, but it can be stated that in the presence of known frontal lobe damage no permanent alterations were manifested on the varied measures of intelligence utilized in this study.

## SUMMARY

1. Observations have been made on the effects of bilateral surgical removal of portions of the human frontal lobes upon intellectual functions. Pre- and postoperative assessment of intelligence was made by means of the Wechsler-Bellevue Test of Adult Intelligence, the Porteus Maze Test, and the Continuous-Problem Task, which were administered to a series of patients subjected to topectomy and an equivalent control group one month prior to the time of operation, three weeks after operation, and four months after operation.

2. The removal of cortical tissue from Brodmann's areas 8, 9, 10, 11, and 46 did not result in any alteration of intellectual function, as measured by these tests, which could be regarded as permanent.

3. The results obtained indicated that the excision of no one cortical area,

of the areas sampled in this series of operations, influenced intellectual function permanently any more than any other. The removal of area 8 was found to produce the most pronounced of the transient effects noted.

4. No evidence was found in this series which would indicate that the amount of frontal tissue removed exerted a differential effect on the performance of the intellectual measures utilized.

5. In the performance of the Porteus Maze Test the operatee group has been demonstrated to exhibit a definite impairment immediately following operation from which it gradually recovered, and this loss with subsequent regain was seen to bear a close relationship to the social recovery of the patients undergoing operation. This association held for both the operatee group as a whole and in the case of individual performance.

*Chapter 15*

# Learning and Retention*

ANNE KENNARD STAUFFER

IT WAS the purpose of this portion of the study to investigate the effects of bilaterally symmetrical excision of portions of the human frontal cortex upon the learning and retention of verbal material. These functions have been among the most frequently mentioned of the higher mental processes commonly attributed to the frontal lobes.

The operatee patients included in this portion of the study were patients 2, 3, 4, 6, 7, 8, 13, 18, 19, 21, 25, 31, 32, 36, 38, 40, 42, 47, 49, a total of 19; the control patients were 1, 5, 9, 11, 12, 14, 17, 23, 26, 29, 34, 35, 39, a total of 13. For details concerning these individuals see chapter 20. This particular group is the same as that reported by Henry Eugene King in chapter 14, table 42.

## EXPERIMENTAL DESIGN

**Test Material.** The test material sampled a wide variety of types of learning, ranging from material relatively free of previous associations to material high in associative value, and from isolated words to continuous passages.

As examples of material of limited associative value of the discrete type, lists of Semi-Meaningful Paired Associates were selected, in which the name of a common household commodity was paired with a nonsense pseudo-brand name, e.g. "bell-delit." At the opposite extreme were passages of Verbal Directions, in which simple directions were given for carrying out specific, uncomplicated activities, such as going to the grocery store. Between these two extremes were the Meaningful Paired Associates, in which common words bearing no apparent associative relationship to each other were paired, e.g. "building-rather." Each of the Paired Associates lists consisted of six items, and each set of Verbal Directions included twenty items.

The schedule of testing was as follows: Three lists of Semi-Meaningful Paired Associates, three lists of Meaningful Paired Associates, and one set of Verbal Directions were learned before operation. Retention of this material was tested at $R_1$, using the methods of recall, recognition, and relearning. One new list of each type of Paired Associates and a new set of Verbal Directions were learned at $R_1$. Tests for retention of this material were given at $R_2$. In addition, a third set of Verbal Directions was newly learned at $R_2$.

* This chapter was submitted in partial fulfillment of the requirements for the degree of Doctor of Philosophy in the Faculty of Pure Science, Columbia University.

**Procedures and Scoring.** The following procedures were used for both types of Paired Associates tests: the Semi-Meaningful and the Meaningful.

During each of the two learning periods (O and R1), one list was learned each day. At O, half of the patients proceeded through three Meaningful lists before beginning the Semi-Meaningful, while the other half began with Semi-Meaningful and followed with Meaningful. The three lists of each type were always learned in a constant order. At R1 half of the patients learned the Semi-Meaningful list first, the other half the Meaningful.

The procedure used in the learning of the Paired Associates was as follows: A practice list was first presented, with appropriate instructions, to familiarize the patient with the procedure and type of material. The first list to be learned was then presented. The first member of the pair was exposed for approximately ten seconds, followed by exposure of the second member. Both words were read aloud by the patient. After a brief pause the remaining pairs were presented in the same manner. After each trial the cards were shuffled and the list repeated. As each pair was learned to the criterion of one successful anticipation of response word, the card containing the pair was removed. In this manner the factor of overlearning was eliminated, since each pair on the list was learned to the same criterion of success. This procedure has been called the "Method of Adjusted Learning" by Woodworth ('38) and Gillette ('36). Learning difficulty was measured by the total number of individual item exposures required before each of the six items was correctly anticipated. Each patient's learning score at O was the average for three lists, and at R1 the score was based on only one list.

The tests of retention were given in the following order: recall, recognition, and relearning.

In testing for *recall*, the cards were presented in random order, the examiner concealing the response word with his hand, and the patient was asked to recall the paired associate for each stimulus word. The score was the number of correct recalls. For testing *recognition* of the response word, each original stimulus word was typed on a card, followed by four choices, one of which was the original response word. The score was the number of correct choices. In the case of *relearning*, the material and procedure described above for learning were again utilized. The score was the number of item repetitions required for relearning, adjusted for any correct recalls and recognitions which had preceded the relearning. The difference between the relearning score and the previous learning score was the measure of saving.

The methods and scores for the Verbal Directions were essentially similar to those described above, modifications being introduced only where required by the difference in type of material.

In the *learning* task, the passage was read aloud by the examiner, the patient then being asked to repeat as much as he could remember. This procedure was repeated until either (a) the entire passage was correctly reproduced, or (b) a prearranged number of trials (at least eight) had been given. The number of items correctly reproduced on each trial was recorded. Learning ability was measured by the rate at which the learning took place, in terms of items learned per trial. The most desirable learning score, for purposes of comparison with results on the paired associates, would have been a measure of trials required for the correct reproduction of the entire passage. In a considerable number of cases, however, perfect reproduction was not achieved within the limits of the testing period. A rate score was, therefore, selected as a more suitable measure for this test.

In the *recall* test, the subject was asked to recall as much as possible of the set of directions previously learned, the score being the number of items correctly recalled. For measuring *recognition*, a special form of the test was prepared in which a key word in each memory item was omitted and replaced by three choices, one of which was the correct word. The score was the number of correct choices made. For measuring rate of *relearning*, the procedure described above for learning was repeated.

The variation exhibited by each patient in learning the three lists of Semi-Meaningful Paired Associates preoperatively was determined by computing the variance of each patient's three learning scores about his mean learning score. A similar measure was obtained for the three Meaningful lists. After operation, the same procedure was applied to the relearning scores.

The operatee and control groups were compared in their performance in each of the aspects of the learning and retention tasks noted above. The statistical methods of analysis of variance and covariance were employed throughout to test the significance of apparent group differences in performance. In addition, the possible relation of performance to other variables was examined, including sex, age, intelligence, area excised, amount of brain tissue rendered nonfunctional, and social improvement.

## RESULTS

**Correlational Inspection of Preoperative Scores.** All preoperative scores obtained in the entire battery of psychologic tests were intercorrelated. The three scores included in the measures of learning were (1) Semi-Meaningful

TABLE 51.   CORRELATIONS OF MEANINGFUL, SEMI-MEANINGFUL, AND VERBAL DIRECTIONS WITH CERTAIN OTHER SCORES IN THE BATTERY OF PSYCHO-LOGIC TESTS

|  | Meaningful | Semi-meaningful | Verbal directions |
|---|---|---|---|
| Word Association | | | |
| Reproduction reaction time....... | .56 | .43 | −.36 |
| Word Association | | | |
| Association reaction time......... | .46 | .40 | −.25 |
| Wechsler-Bellevue | | | |
| Information.................... | −.32 | −.42 | .54 |
| Block design................... | −.41 | −.41 | .54 |
| Arithmetic..................... | −.41 | −.49 | .36 |
| Similarities.................... | −.52 | −.48 | .47 |
| Vocabulary.................... | −.39 | −.33 | .58 |
| Full scale I.Q................. | −.35 | −.37 | .54 |
| Analogies test.................... | −.47 | −.38 | .40 |
| Capps shift test................... | −.52 | −.46 | .50 |
| Addition time................... | .49 | .46 | −.16 |

NOTE: Only those scores are listed which correlated significantly at the .01 level of confidence, with at least one of the learning scores.

Paired Associates, (2) Meaningful Paired Associates, and (3) Verbal Directions. The intercorrelations were: (1) and (2) +0.72; (2) and (3) −0.48; (1) and (3) −0.26. It should be remembered that the Paired Associates learning scores represented difficulty of learning, as opposed to the Verbal Directions score which indicated positive ability in terms of rate. The signs of correlation coefficients must be interpreted accordingly. Therefore, this represents a progressive relationship from most similarity (Paired Associates) to least similarity (Semi-Meaningful—Verbal Directions). The correlations of the Meaningful, Semi-Meaningful, and Verbal Directions with certain other scores in the battery are given in table 51.

As is evident, the learning scores are highly correlated with certain intelligence test scores and with the abstraction tests (Analogies, Capps) as well as with speed on the Addition Test.

In general, learning ability, as measured in this study, is associated to some degree with other mental processes involved in intelligence (intellect), ability to abstract, and speed of performance. The learning shown in the acquisition of Meaningful and Semi-Meaningful Paired Associates and Verbal Direction material involved similar abilities.

**Reliability of Measures.** The reliability index for the lists of Semi-Meaningful Paired Associates was obtained by correlating the scores for the total group of patients at the O testing on List 1 with the scores on Lists 2 and 3 combined. In a similar manner the reliability of the Meaningful lists was computed. This yielded reliability coefficients of $+.76 \pm .05$ and $+.73 \pm .06$ for the Semi-Meaningful and the Meaningful lists respectively. It may be concluded that these tests were sufficiently reliable to warrant group comparisons.

No measure of reliability of the Verbal Directions Test is available.

**Learning Ability.** The first question to be answered was: Did the topectomy alter ability to learn verbal material? If the operation interfered with or otherwise altered learning ability, it would be expected that the learning of new material after operation would differ from the learning of similar material before operation. This was not found to be the case, i.e. the operatee group showed no significant mean gain or loss when compared with the controls on any of our three tests. When the preoperative levels of the two groups were equated statistically, the status remained unchanged.

In the case of Verbal Directions, the difficulty of the learning tasks seemed to increase in both the operatee and control groups, but the difference in the rate of decline was not differential between  he two groups. For this reason the increase in difficulty is to be regarded as a function of the material used rather than as a result of the operation.

Certain differences in the spread of scores within the operatee and control groups did appear after operation. At $R_1$, the operatee group was significantly more variable than was the control on the Semi-Meaningful Paired Associates and the Verbal Directions, but less variable on the Meaningful Paired Associates. It should be noted, however, that in the only new learning task given at $R_2$ (Verbal Directions), the difference between the groups in spread of scores was no longer apparent, indicating that the differences found at $R_1$ were temporary in nature.

It seemed possible that the individual gains and losses in learning ability might have been related to some of the background factors on which data were available. Therefore, comparisons were made of the postoperative difference scores ($R_1$-O, $R_2$-O) within the operatee group with respect to sex, age, and preoperative Wechsler-Bellevue Full Scale I.Q. A critical ratio was obtained for each comparison of means. No one of these indicated a reliable difference in learning scores.

The effects of the operation could have been shown by (1) specific involvement of localized cortical areas in the learning process, or (2) relation of the mass of tissue destroyed to changes in learning scores. The present study permitted analysis of postoperative changes in terms of both of these considerations.

In order to find whether learning or retention was altered by excision of specific cortical areas, mean difference scores were obtained for patients subjected to removal of Brodmann's areas 8, 9, 10, 46, and 11 respectively. Each mean was compared with the theoretically possible range of the control group mean, for the .05 level of confidence. It could thus be determined whether the mean of any single area subgroup differed significantly from the mean of the control group. Though certain regularities did emerge, the findings were not striking. Three weeks postoperatively (R1) in patients from whom areas 8 and/or 9 had been removed, there was evidence of significant losses in learning of the Semi-Meaningful Paired Associates, but gains in the Meaningful Paired Associates and the Verbal Directions scores. However, in the Semi-Meaningful learning the average losses were clearly due to the disproportionate decrease by one or two, but not all, of the persons comprising the small subgroups employed in these comparisons. The individual scores were somewhat more consistent in the case of the Meaningful Paired Associates and Verbal Directions. In the R2 data for Verbal Directions, however, these trends though still apparent were not statistically reliable, again suggesting the instability of the relations noted at R1.

On the basis of cytologic studies an estimate was made of the amount of brain tissue presumably rendered nonfunctional in each case, including not only the actual mass excised but also that probably rendered nonfunctional by other means in the course of operation. Since these were but approximate estimates of functional interference, we have divided the patients into those with greater and those with lesser amounts of tissue destroyed. The difference scores for these two groups were then compared by the method of critical ratios. These ratios showed a significant difference in favor of those having the greater amount of tissue rendered nonfunctional for the Verbal Directions Test at R2, and a general tendency in this group toward superiority in all three learning tests at R1. Apparently destruction of a sufficient amount of tissue tended to facilitate learning, especially learning of logically coherent material.

The final possibility to be considered was that individual improvements in learning ability might have been due to improvement in the patient's mental condition, and dependent on the operation only insofar as the operation resulted in recovery from psychosis. Psychiatric studies indicated that approximately half of the operatee group showed social improvement, on the basis of their making satisfactory adjustments outside the hospital. The evidence indicated that the majority of these improvements could be attributed to the operation. The learning and retention scores were therefore analyzed with respect to social improvement. On the basis of the psychiatric data, the operatees were divided into two groups, improved and unimproved, and the mean scores for these groups were compared by critical ratios. The individual changes in learning of Semi-Meaningful and Meaningful Paired Associates showed no regular relations to recovery from psychosis. On the Verbal Directions, although the improved and unimproved groups did not differ significantly, the improved patients tended to do better than the unimproved and than the controls.

**Retention of Preoperatively Learned Material.** The retention of the material learned before operation was tested at R1, using the methods of recall, recognition, and relearning. The recall on the Meaningful as well as the Semi-Meaningful Paired Associates was so slight that no statistical treatment of the data was advisable. In the recall of preoperatively learned Verbal Directions the operatee and control groups were very nearly equal. The recognition method likewise yielded no differences between the groups.

In retention as measured by relearning, both the operatee and control groups showed positive saving for the Semi-Meaningful and Meaningful Paired Associates, but there was no significant difference between them in this respect.

On the Verbal Directions Test, however, both operatee and control groups sustained a loss rather than positive saving. As in the case of the rate of learning, this general result may be a reflection of discrepancies between the two forms of the test since both groups were affected in the same direction. However, the operatees did not show as great a loss as did the controls. This difference remained significant, at the .05 level of confidence, when differences in initial rates of learning were held constant. In explanation it might be suggested that the specific type of material to be remembered may be the factor which determined the differences; specifically the retention of pairs of discrete elements was not significantly altered, while the retention of logically connected passages appeared to have been facilitated in the operatee group.

TABLE 52.   MEAN SCORES AT R2 FOR RECALL AND RECOGNITION OF POST-OPERATIVELY LEARNED MATERIAL

| Group | N | A. Recall | | B. Recognition | |
|---|---|---|---|---|---|
| | | Verbal directions (form B) | Semi-mean. paired ass. (List 4) | Meaningful paired ass. (List 4) | Verbal directions (form B) |
| Operatees............. | 19 | 7.42 | 3.47 | 2.26 | 9.11 |
| Controls............... | 13 | 3.54 | 3.07 | 1.54 | 7.15 |
| F Ratio............... | | 6.82 * | .49 | 2.14 | 5.97 * |

* Significant at the .05 level of confidence.

Was the retention of material learned before operation related to any of the background or associated experimental variables? Neither sex, age, nor I.Q. was found to be differential in its effect on the retention of preoperatively learned material. No significant relation or consistent trend could be shown as far as excisions of specific areas were concerned. Likewise no regular relationship with amount of tissue rendered nonfunctional could be established. The patients who showed social improvement were significantly better than were the unimproved in their mean score for recognition of the Verbal Directions, although their savings score was significantly poorer. Recognition and relearning of the Paired Associates material were not related to improvement or lack of improvement.

**Retention of Postoperatively Learned Material.** Although, as has been shown, there was little or no evidence that learning ability or retention of preoperatively learned material was altered by topectomy, there remained the possibility that the operation might alter the ability to retain material learned after operation. New material learned at R1 was tested for retention at R2 and the scores of the operatees and control groups were compared.

The recall and recognition scores on the Verbal Directions Test were significantly better for the operatee group. The recognition scores for Meaningful and Semi-Meaningful Paired Associates were also better for the operatees than for the control patients although the differences were not statistically significant. These data are shown in table 52.

These scores were found to be unrelated to sex, age, or I.Q.

When the individual scores were examined, it was found in the Verbal Directions and Meaningful Paired Associates that retention was rather markedly and consistently better in patients from whom areas 9 and/or 10 (and possibly 11) had been excised. Social improvement (which was usually associated with removal of areas 9 and 10) was accompanied by significantly better recall for Verbal Directions and a tendency toward better recognition for both Verbal Directions and Meaningful Paired Associates. These associations were not shown by the scores based on the saving method of measuring retention; they were not shown by the various scores obtained from the Semi-Meaningful Paired Associates. In general it seemed that the increased efficiency in retention which did show at certain points was associated with social recovery from psychosis. The recovery seemed to be associated with the loss of psychotic anxiety (chapter 20) which in turn followed excision of areas 9 and 10.

**Intra-Individual Variability.** Even though the operation produced no alteration in ability to learn or relearn this material, as judged by group mean scores, it seemed possible that some change in the individual's consistency of performance on a given occasion might have occurred as part of the recovery from psychosis. An approach to this question was made possible in the case of the Paired Associates by the learning of three comparable lists of each type (Semi-Meaningful and Meaningful) at O and relearning of the same lists at $R_1$ and $R_2$. Comparison of the individual variance scores of the operatees and control patients, however, revealed no change in intra-individual variability. No relation to any of the background or associated experimental variables could be established.

DISCUSSION

Despite the many puzzling aspects of our results, the general answers to the major questions raised seem clear.

*Was learning ability altered by the operation?* Within the conditions of this experiment, no significant alteration was apparent. No impairment was found which could be attributed to the operation *per se*, or to any of the associated variables we have considered.

The individual gains in learning of logically connected material did tend to be associated with both social improvement and the amount of tissue rendered nonfunctional. Which of these two factors is primary and which secondary cannot be determined definitely on the basis of the available data, but the weight of the evidence indicates that the gains in learning are probably due to the operation only insofar as it facilitated social improvement.

Certain phenomena found in $R_1$, including changes in group variability and relations of gains and losses in learning to removals of specific areas, were transient in that they were no longer evident at $R_2$. Although at that time data for learning ability were obtained on the Verbal Directions Test only, it is not unreasonable to assume, in the light of the general findings, that $R_2$ results for the Paired Associates would have supported or at least not proved inconsistent with those for the Verbal Directions.

*Was retention altered by the operation?* In the retention for preoperatively learned material there was clearly no significant impairment, and for the most part no relation to any of the associated variables. Those positive results which did appear, namely better relearning in the operatee group and certain relations to social improvement, were found only in the Verbal Directions, which in general seems to have been our most sensitive test.

Here we were again dealing with results obtained at R1, only three weeks after operation. It might have been expected that the results of this testing period would show inconsistencies, since some of the patients had not yet attained their final degree of stability. This was indeed found to be the case, and such findings as did emerge were not generally borne out later at the R2 testing. For this reason the differences found at R1 probably should be discounted. The only tenable conclusion is that retention at R1 was not interfered with by the operation, and whether it was facilitated remains in doubt.

We may now turn to the measures at R2 for retention of the material learned after operation. These probably indicate the more lasting effects of the operation, so far as they may be discerned in this experiment. Here we found no significant difference in retention as measured by the saving method, but clear-cut superiority of the operatee group in recall and recognition of the Verbal Directions. The better scores here, as well as in recognition of the Meaningful Paired Associates, tended to accompany social improvement, and to be related to removals of Brodmann's areas 9 and 10. Garrison has demonstrated that removals of areas 9 and 10 were highly associated with loss of psychotic anxiety and with social improvement (chapter 19). Thus we may interpret the superiority in retention as part of the recovery from psychosis and only secondarily dependent on the removal of brain tissue.

The finding of superiority in the operatee group at R2 in recall and recognition, without a corresponding advantage in saving, appears somewhat inconsistent with the usual findings for these methods on normal persons. Somewhat similar discrepancies between these measures of retention have been noted by Coffin ('46) and Hansen ('46) in patients receiving electro-convulsive therapy, in whom retention as measured by recognition was relatively unimpaired during treatment while the saving method indicated very little retention.

Two possible explanations of the present result may be offered. First, an essential difference between the recognition and saving methods seems to be the factor of interference from previous associations with the test material, which is probably relatively unimportant in recognition but more important in relearning. In giving the relearning tests it was sometimes noticeable that the operatees tended to exhibit qualitatively more interference effects than did the controls. In the present study the operatees may have been generally more capable of better retention, but heightened sensitivity to interference effects may have depressed the overt retention as measured by relearning to the level of the controls.

A second possibility is that the psychotic process may have interfered pre-operatively with recall and recognition while having no very definite effect on retention as measured by relearning. With the amelioration of the psychotic process after operation, recall and recognition show an improvement in the operatee group but the relearning method can show no improvement since it was not defective preoperatively. Both of these explanations are speculative at this time.

At a number of points our findings suggest the possibility that the sensitivity of learning and retention to the effects of topectomy may be a function of the type of material used. There was a tendency for the more meaningful and connected materials to show changes where the less meaningful and disconnected did not. It was noted that certain effects appeared either more frequently or markedly in the Verbal Directions alone, or in the Verbal Directions and the Meaningful Paired Associates without being noted in the Semi-Meaningful.

The results on tests of immediate memory as shown in the Word Association Test reported in chapter 17 indicated that the topectomy operation did not interfere, but instead enhanced immediate memory as measured by reproduction. These findings are in line with the present results. Thus neither immediate memory nor retention for previously implanted associations suffered impairment as a result of operation.

## SUMMARY

1. Ability to learn verbal material, as measured in this study, was not altered by topectomy.

2. Ability to retain material learned before operation suffered no demonstrable impairment.

3. Ability to retain logically connected material learned after operation, as measured by recall and recognition, was facilitated. These gains appeared to accompany social improvement, and are therefore regarded as only secondarily dependent on the removal of brain tissue.

4. Retention as measured by the saving method failed to show improvement. Two possible explanations for this have been considered: (1) the operatee group may have been rendered more susceptible to interference effects, a factor more prominent in relearning than in the other methods; (2) the psychotic process, alleviated by the operation, may previously have impaired recall and recognition but not relearning.

5. The more meaningful and connected materials tended to be generally more sensitive to the effect of topectomy.

6. Intra-individual variability of learning within a given testing period was not altered by topectomy.

APPENDIX

A sample of each of the three types of material employed in the learning tasks is given below.

### Semi-Meaningful Paired Associates

LIST 1

| bell | — | delit |
|---|---|---|
| clock | — | lumag |
| fork | — | zapom |
| gown | — | ridaz |
| mop | — | bakad |
| towels | — | lactil |

### Meaningful Paired Associates

LIST 1

| allow | — | village |
|---|---|---|
| building | — | rather |
| twenty | — | nature |
| neighbor | — | although |
| table | — | season |
| present | — | almost |

### Verbal Directions

#### FORM A—OVERSEAS PACKAGE*

/You can buy some cards/ at the bookstore/. He can use them to play solitaire/ or, if there are enough people,/ to play bridge/. Buy some candy and some gum/. You might include a few small books/. Cigarettes are hard to get in Japan/ so send some of those too/. Be careful not to get too many things because/ it all has to go in a box/ about ten inches/ by eight inches/ by three inches/. Wrap it in heavy paper/. When you address/ the box be sure to include his serial number/ or it might get lost/.

* Each portion between /'s constitutes one item.

## Chapter 16

# Ability to Abstract[*]

WILBUR RICHARD KING

---

THE idea that the damage to the frontal lobes impairs the "abstract behavior"[†] of an individual grew out of the work of Gelb and Goldstein ('25) during and after World War I. Goldstein ('36b) said that his view of the psychic function of the frontal lobe was first set forth in a paper published in 1923 (Goldstein, '23), and that subsequent investigation has confirmed his earlier findings. This review of Goldstein's work up to the present time will follow, in the main, the chronologic order of his publications.

Gelb and Goldstein ('25) published their first experimental investigations of the brain-damaged victims of World War I. In this paper they introduced the sorting-test methods and concluded that all the mental changes of brain-injured patients could be traced to a unitary, basic abnormality, namely an impairment in "abstract behavior." Their first test was the sorting of the colored Holmgren wools. However, in the appendix of this report they list the object-sorting test which they used analogously to the color experiments. It is pertinent to note here that Goldstein has changed his sorting tests and evaluations of his results very little in the past twenty years. He has merely added more elaborate descriptions to his original findings.

In 1936 Goldstein published his first papers in this country. In one paper (Goldstein, '36) he enlarged the scope of his "categorical behavior" theory to explain the verbal behavior of aphasic patients. He denies the conditioned response interpretation of the name-object relationship, as he states: "we find the seemingly so simple function of naming objects does not present a simple superficial connection between a thing and a word." He would add a certain something called the abstract attitude toward the word, and it is this abstract aspect that is impaired in aphasic behavior and not a lack of words or lack of ability to call up word images, as it is generally assumed. Again the results of the color-sorting test (Holmgren wools) were cited as the experimental basis for his conclusions.

The second paper (Goldstein, 36a) was a preliminary discussion of his holistic philosophy which eventuated in his book, "The Organism" (Goldstein, '39).

However, his third 1936 paper (Goldstein, '36b) is an often-cited reference as therein he definitely allocated impairment of abstract behavior to the frontal lobes and not to any other part of the brain. In summarizing the symptoms found in cases of frontal lobe lesion, he stated: "(1) There are disturbances in different fields of psychic performance, in each field perhaps, but the disturbance of no one field can be regarded as the basic cause of other disturbances. (2) No field is disturbed throughout its extent.

[*] This chapter was submitted in partial fulfillment of the requirements for the degree of Doctor of Philosophy in the Faculty of Pure Science, Columbia University.

[†] The term "abstract behavior" is used in the sense in which Goldstein has defined it.

There are always some performances which the patient is able to execute. (3) The basic change is not a change of any one field or any one performance, but a change of total behavior, with a lack of a particular behavior, which lack finds expression in certain performances in all fields and leaves intact certain performances in all fields."

In point 3 above, he referred directly to the lack of abstract attitude. The fact that the abstract attitude is localized in the frontal lobes was clearly brought out by his following statement: "We find identical symptoms in lesions of the frontal lobe and in diffuse cortical affections which implicate always, as well, the frontal lobe. The symptoms observed in cases of frontal lobe lesions are therefore not manifestations of an assumed general cortical affection; on the contrary, the characteristic symptoms in diffuse cortical affections are manifestations of the damage to the frontal lobe."

Bolles and Goldstein ('38) reported that the impairment of the abstract attitude was a characteristic of certain, but not all, schizophrenic patients. Goldstein ('39a) elaborated upon the impairment of the schizophrenic patient by speculating that somatic therapy may remove the abstract impairment and thus make the patient more amenable to psychotherapy.

Finally, Goldstein and Scheerer ('41) published a description of their tests and formulated the criteria for abstract and concrete behavior in their most objective form. The five tests used to assess abstract and concrete behavior included: (1) the Cube Test (a modification of Kohs Blocks Test), (2) Color Sorting Test (modification of the Holmgren Wool Test), (3) Object-Sorting Test (essentially similar to P.I. Sorting Test used in this study), (4) Weigl Color-Form Sorting Test, and (5) the Stick Test. All were tests that Goldstein had been using clinically for some years.

In his most recent publication Goldstein ('44a) offered answers to some of the criticisms which have been published with respect to his theory of the abstract attitude. In the present article reference will be made primarily to the two last publications of Goldstein (Goldstein and Scheerer, '41; Goldstein, '44a).

## THE ABSTRACT BEHAVIOR OF ATTITUDE*

Goldstein ('44) defines the abstract attitude as basic for the ability:

1. To assume a mental set voluntarily (not phenomenologically evident).
2. To shift voluntarily from one aspect of the situation to another (the shift factor in this study).
3. To keep in mind simultaneously various aspects.
4. To grasp the essential of a given whole; to break up a given whole into parts and to isolate them voluntarily. (Approximated by the isolation factor in this study.)
5. To generalize; to abstract common properties; to plan ahead ideationally; to assume an attitude toward the "more possible," and to think or perform symbolically. (Common to most of the factors in this study.)

Again according to Goldstein some of the characteristics of the abstract attitude are the following:

1. The normal person is capable of assuming both attitudes, whereas the abnormal individual is confined to but one type of behavior—the concrete (Goldstein and Scheerer, '41).
2. Some tasks can be performed only by virtue of the abstract attitude; for others, the concrete attitude is sufficient.
3. Concreteness is manifest in verbal behavior and characterized by the following (Goldstein, '40):
   a. Whole language changed from an active, spontaneous productive means for expressing ideas, feelings, etc., to a passive, more or less compulsive, stereotyped, and unproductive reaction.

* These definitions and statements in this section are selected quotations or paraphrasings from Goldstein's articles.

b. Amount of speech reduced, especially spontaneous speech.

c. Patients have greatest difficulty in beginning to speak.

d. Speaking has to be elicited through outside stimuli.

e. When stimulated to speak, patients have difficulty in stopping and use many stereotyped utterances, etc.

By use of sorting tests, Goldstein arrived at an analysis of behavior that led to this distinction between "two modes of behavior"—the abstract and the concrete. "The abstract and concrete behaviors are dependent upon two corresponding attitudes which are psychologically so basic that one may speak of them as levels" (Goldstein and Scheerer, '41). The abstract and concrete attitudes are capacity levels of the total personality. "Each attitude constitutes one definite behavioral range which involves a number of performances and responses. These latter, when taken individually at their surface value, may appear to be discrete entities of quite a diversified nature, e.g., attention, recall, recognition, synthesizing, symbolization, etc."

Goldstein's claims have met wide acceptance in neurology and in abnormal and clinical psychology. Many regularly employed clinical tests used to appraise organic brain damage are modifications of Goldstein's original tests. The differentiation between organic brain involvement and purely functional psychopathology is often of real importance in determining therapy.

In different studies Goldstein has pointed out that abstract behavior involves several mental processes. These processes are usually grouping, isolation, and shift. By *grouping* is meant the ability to bring together as belonging together, miscellaneous objects or words in which there is one common element, which can be abstracted e.g., all red or all metal. By *isolation* is meant the picking out of one or more objects or words from a miscellaneous assortment because the objects or words isolated do not have a common attribute possessed by all other members of the group. By *shift* is meant the ability to regroup objects or words which have been grouped on the basis of one kind of pertinence into a different grouping on the basis of a second kind of pertinence upon request.

In this study we proposed to view not only abstract behavior in general but abstract behavior as shown by performance grouping, isolation, and shift and by verbal grouping, isolation, and shift.

## EXPERIMENTAL PROCEDURES

**Subjects.**   As is the case with most studies dealing with mental patients, the usable number of cases is reduced because the condition of some patients is not amenable to valid psychologic examination. Since this study was particularly concerned with results uncomplicated by the mental condition of the patients, the standards for acceptable test results were set fairly high. The test results retained in this study were only those meeting the following criteria: (1) complete test protocols for all three testing periods, (2) test results considered by the examiner to be representative of a cooperative subject, and (3) test results uncomplicated by extremely disconcerting symptoms, such as silly responses and delusional intrusion. These considerations took their expected toll and the final number of subjects used in the main body of this study was 30, 13 controls and 17 operatees. Table 53 gives the relevant background data on this group of 30 patients.

**PI Sorting Test.***   The procedure used with the object sorting test in this study differed somewhat from previous usage and to indicate that uniqueness as here used we will designate it as the PI Sorting Test.

* The sorting test method originated by Gelb and Goldstein ('25) has been modified in a variety of ways in this investigation.

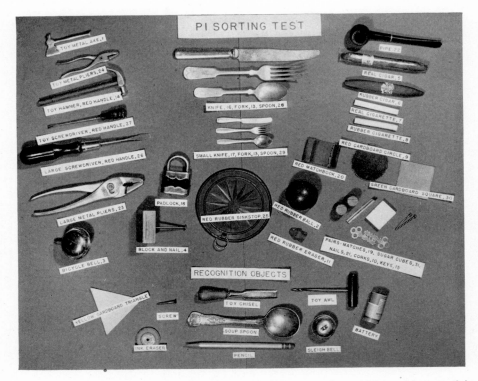

Fig. 98. The objects which made up the PI Sorting Test, together with the objects used in the Recognition Test.

As previously mentioned, Gelb and Goldstein ('25) introduced the sorting-test method in their study of impairment of abstract behavior. Weigl ('41) gave the first extensive report on the use of an object-sorting test. Rothmann ('34) reported on the use of an object-sorting test for an analysis of a case of circumscribed head injury. Goldstein ('44a) stated that "This test originated in common work in my laboratory." Five years later, Rylander ('39) used an object-sorting test derived from Rothmann's study in his study of the function of the frontal lobes. Rylander referred to his test as Rothmann's test although he modified the procedure to "make the test more comprehensive and sensitive."

TABLE 53.  STATUS OF PATIENTS IN THE OPERATEE AND CONTROL GROUPS WHOSE TEST RESULTS HAVE BEEN UTILIZED IN THE MAIN BODY OF THE PRESENT STUDY

| Variables | Operatees | Controls |
|---|---|---|
| Number | 17 | 13 |
| Male | 11 | 10 |
| Female | 6 | 3 |
| Age, average | 44.7 | 45.8 |
| Age range | 29–61 | 20–60 |
| Education, average years | 9.12 | 8.23 |
| Education, range | 6–16 | 2–12 |
| Wechsler-Bellevue I.Q. | 103.9 | 104.5 |
| I.Q. range | 89–131 | 81–125 |

Prior to Rylander's ('39) study, Bolles ('37) reported on the first use of the object-sorting test in this country. She stated that "the particular objects used were patterned after those used by Weigl." Subsequently the object-sorting test has been used by many different investigators in America and England and is considered a standard procedure in the clinical study of organic brain cases.

The PI Sorting Test was composed of the following thirty-one articles illustrated in figure 98: 1, small metal toy axe; 2, red rubber ball (medium size); 3, metal bicycle bell; 4, block with a nail partially hammered into it; 5, real cigar; 6, rubber cigar; 7, real cigarette; 8, rubber cigarette; 9, red cardboard circle; 10, two corks; 11, pencil-eraser top; 12, large table fork; 13, small toy fork; 14, small hammer with red handle; 15, two keys for a padlock (item #18); 16, large table knife; 17, small toy knife; 18, padlock; 19, two large burnt matches; 20, red match book without matches; 21, two nails; 22, a dark-brown-colored pipe; 23, large pliers; 24, small toy pliers; 25, red circular sink-stop; 26, large red-handled screwdriver; 27, small red-handled screwdriver; 28, regular table spoon; 29, small toy spoon; 30, green cardboard square; 31, two cubes of sugar.

Four separate tasks or procedures were carried through with this test.

*PI—Part 1 (PI Sorting Test—Grouping).* All thirty-one objects were placed on a table top in front of the subject. There was no order in the way in which the objects were presented.

First, the subject was asked, "Do you know what all these objects are? If you don't know what to call any one of them, ask." This was done to make sure that the subject was familiar with and knew the name and use of each article. Next the subject was told to "pick out any one of the items you wish." This item selected by the subject was placed apart from the rest and then he was told to "pick out all the objects which belong with this one." After the subject selected all the items that "belong together," he was asked to "tell me why they belong together." A record was kept of both the verbalized reason and the objects selected by the subject. (This part of the test does not enter into the scoring.)

Following the first sorting wherein the reference object was picked out by the subject, the subject was asked to "pick out the things that belong with" six reference objects selected by the examiner. The subject's verbalizations and objects selected for each of these six sortings were recorded. The six reference objects used in every case were, in order, item numbers 12, 22, 3, 9, 24, and 2. This part was scored in terms of the total number of objects put together on these six groupings.

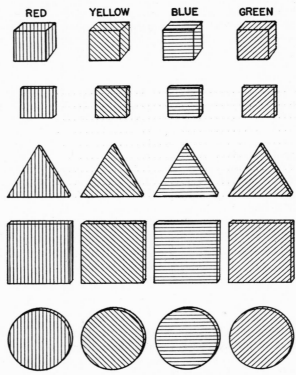

RED     YELLOW     BLUE     GREEN

FIG. 99.   Plastic objects used in Weigl Test.

*PI—Part 2 (PI Sorting Test—Shift).*   The examiner stated: "I am going to put some things together which all belong together for some reason. You are to tell me what the reason is that they all belong together. All right, this is the first group. Why do these things belong together? In what respect are they all alike?" The verbalized reason for each of the eleven following sortings was recorded.

    1. Articles predominantly red: items 14, 26, 27, 9, 2, 20, 25.
    2. Articles predominantly round (these articles were also all red, and if the subject gave this reason he was told, "That is correct. Now can you give me another reason why these belong together?"): items 2, 9, 25.
    3. Articles which were paper: items 20, 9, 30.
    4. Smoking materials: items 5, 6, 22, 19, 20.
    5. Articles which were white: items 31, 7, 8.
    6. Articles which were square: items 4, 30, 20, 31.

7. Articles which were rubber: items 6, 8, 2, 25, 11.

8. Toys: items 29, 17, 13, 24, 26, 14, 1, 3, 2.

9. Articles which were made of metal: items 16, 17, 12, 13, 28, 29, 23, 24, 26, 27, 15, 1, 3, 18.

10. Tools: items 26, 27, 23, 24, 14, 1.

11. Silverware: items 28, 29, 16, 17, 12, 13.

Note that the bases of grouping were respectively: color, shape, material, use, color, shape, material, use, material, use, use. The score on this part of the test was the total number of correct names given the eleven groups.

*PI—Part 3 (PI Sorting Test—Isolation).* The examiner stated: "Now I am going to put some things together out of which all belong together for some reason, except one object. There will be one object in the group which will be different from the others for some reason. If you take away that one thing that is different, all the rest will be alike for some reason. All right, this is the first group." (First group assembled.) "Pick out the one thing that is different from all the others." (Later.) "Why is it different?"

The following five groups of objects were assembled in the order indicated. Parenthetic expression indicates the grouping basis after removal of the object not belonging which is the number in parenthesis. The score was the number of items correctly isolated in the five presentations.

1. (Wood): 4, 22, (11), 14, 26, 27.

2. (Tools): (28), 14, 26, 23, 27, 24, 1.

3. (Long-thin): 23, 24, 12, 16, 26, 28, 22, 14, (25), 27, 7, 8.

4. (Brown): 4, (20), 22, 10, 7, 8.

5. (Pairs): 31, 15, 7, 8, (30), 19.

*PI—Part 4 (PI Sorting Test—Recall).* This was a recall test. The examiner collected all the objects in a box and put it out of the sight of the subject. Then he stated: "Now tell me the names of all the ones you remember." (If the subject paused, "And what else do you remember?") The score was the total number of the thirty-one objects correctly recalled.

Four different measures of abstract behavior were obtained from the PI Sorting Test. They were:

1. Grouping score (Part 1) was total number of objects the subject included with all reference objects. This was a performance measure of the grouping factor.

2. Shift score (Part 2) was the number of correctly identified common properties of the eleven groupings. The total possible score was 11. This was a verbal measure of the shift factor. It was assumed that in order to obtain a "good" score on this part of the PI Sorting Test it was necessary for the subject to change his "abstraction" reference with each consecutive grouping.

3. Isolation score (Part 3) was the number of correct "nonbelonging" objects isolated from five different groupings. The total possible score was 5. This was a performance measure of the isolation factor.

4. Grouping score (Part 4) was the number of objects the subject recalled by verbal statement. The total possible score was 31. This recall test may, according to Goldstein ('44), be called a verbal grouping score.

**Weigl Test.** The materials for this test consisted of twelve flat plastic figures of three different forms: squares, triangles, and circles (see fig. 99). Each of these forms had one side colored either red, yellow, blue, or green while the other side was white. In addition, twelve ¾-inch square wooden cubes of four colors (also red, yellow, blue, and green) were used. The directions were as follows:

First sorting: The pieces were placed with the colored side up in random order in front of the subject and he was told: "Put all those together that belong together for some reason." If the subject asks, "Do you mean by color or form?" he is told to do whichever he prefers. If he does not seem to understand he was told: "Put all those together that are alike for some reason." After the subject had sorted the figures, he was asked: "Why do they belong together that way?"

Second sorting: If the subject sorted the colored figures in any fashion as a response to the initial instructions, the colored figures were again placed randomly in front of him and he was told: "Now, put all those together that belong together for a different reason." If he complied with these instructions, and his two types of sorting were color and form, the test was considered completed. Otherwise, the following additional procedure was continued.

If the subject sorted for color but not form, the geometric figures were presented white-side up so that the stimulus field was uncomplicated by color. Again, the subject was told: "Now, put together those that belong together."

If the subject sorted for form but not color in his initial two sortings, he was then presented with the colored wooden cubes and the same instructions: "Now, put those together that belong together." In this presentation, the objects were sorted in terms of color uncomplicated by form.

If the subject succeeded on any of the above single bases of sorting, he was then presented again with the original colored figures and given the same instructions in order to see if he could profit by his simple sorting.

Finally, if the subject still failed to sort for one or none of the categories of form or color, the examiner demonstrated the failed sorting without giving any verbalized reason. After the demonstration, the subject was asked to sort as the examiner did and give the reason for the sorting.

The above modification of the Weigl Test was used in the hopes of quantifying gradations of shifting ability. The subjects' performances were scored on the following scale:

A. Sorted correctly according to both categories immediately.
   1. Simultaneously sorted for both color and form in a two-way arrangement, or alternately without the examiner requesting the second sorting. (Score=10.)
   2. Sorted for one category and then upon request for the other. (Score=9.)
B. Sorted according to only one category initially.
   1. Was able to sort for second category on original figures after practice on the isolated variables (turning figures on white side if unable to shift from color to form, or introducing cubes if unable to shift from form to color). (Score=8.)
   2. Was able to sort for second category after demonstration. (Score=7.)
   3. Was unable to sort for second category even after demonstration. (Score=6.)
C. Was unable to sort for either category initially.
   1. Was able to sort for both categories after practice on isolated variables. (Score=5.)
   2. Was able to sort for only one category after practice on isolated variables but succeeded on second sorting after demonstration. (Score=4.)
   3. Was able to sort for both categories only after demonstration. (Score=3.)
   4. Was able to sort for only one category even after demonstration. (Score=2.)
   5. Was unable to sort for either category even after demonstration. (Score=0.)

This test was used as an evaluation of the performance shift factor as recommended by Goldstein and Scheerer ('41).

According to the above scoring system, the presence of the ability to shift as Goldstein has formulated the concept would be indicated by a score of 9 or 10, inability to shift by a score of 8 or lower.

**Essential Differences Test.**  The Essential Differences Test was taken from Wegrocki's ('40) study on the "Generalizing Ability in Schizophrenia." The test consisted of thirty-four groups of four words. The subject was told: "In this test you are to underline that word in each line which you think is most different from the remaining three; but the three words left must all be in some way related and similar. For example, of these four words—apple, peach, carrot, and pear—which one would you underline?"

If the subject's answer indicated that he understood that carrot was a vegetable while the remaining items were fruit, the examiner proceeded with the second example, using the words: bitter, sour, sweet, white—following the same procedure as above. When the subject showed satisfactory understanding of the instructions, he proceeded with the rest of the test until he had answered every item. The test was used as a power test with no time limit. The score used was the number of correctly answered items. The criterion of a correct

TABLE 54. CORRELATION MATRIX OF THE INTERCORRELATION OF AGE, YEARS OF SCHOOLING, I.Q., AND THE SEVEN TESTS ON THE PREOPERATIVE TEST SCORES OF THE COMBINED CONTROL AND OPERATEE GROUP (N = 30)

| Variables | 1 | 2 | 3 | 4 | 5 | 6 | 7 | 8 | 9 | 10 |
|---|---|---|---|---|---|---|---|---|---|---|
| 1. PI–1.............. | — | .09 | .23 | .27 | .40 | .32 | .07 | .16 | .43 | .52 |
| 2. PI–2.............. | .09 | — | .52 | .27 | .06 | .28 | .09 | .27 | .10 | .12 |
| 3. PI–3.............. | .23 | .52 | — | .34 | .11 | .33 | .15 | .00 | .35 | .23 |
| 4. PI–4.............. | .27 | .27 | .34 | — | .39 | .32 | .31 | −.16 | .55 | .35 |
| 5. Analogies......... | .40 | .06 | .11 | .39 | — | .36 | .17 | .36 | .53 | .63 |
| 6. Ess. diff........... | .32 | .28 | .33 | .32 | .36 | — | .17 | .12 | .51 | .40 |
| 7. Weigl............. | .07 | .09 | .15 | .31 | .17 | .17 | — | .00 | .11 | .20 |
| 8. Age.............. | .16 | .27 | .00 | −.16 | .36 | .12 | .00 | — | −.09 | .47 |
| 9. I.Q.............. | .43 | .10 | .35 | .55 | .53 | .51 | .11 | −.09 | — | .51 |
| 10. Schooling........ | .52 | .12 | .23 | .35 | .63 | .40 | .20 | .47 | .51 | — |

item was that established by Wegrocki. In the present study this test was used as a measure of the isolation factor in verbal behavior. The subject had to "isolate" out the word that did not belong with the group. It was considered analogous to PI—Part 3 where the subject had to "isolate" the object that did not belong with a group in performance behavior.

**Analogies Test.** The Analogies Test was taken from Wegrocki's ('40) study. The test consisted of twenty-seven graded analogies in the form such as: "Horn is to blow as bell is to . . ." The subject was told: "This is an Analogies Test. Here is an example: Color is to red as taste is to (sweet). The idea is to write in such a word that expresses a relationship to taste that will be the same as that of red to color." The examiner continued his explanation until he was fairly certain the subject understood the instructions. He drew upon a special list of examples as often as necessary. The test was used as a power test as no time limit was imposed. The subject answered every item. The score was the number of correctly completed analogies. A total score of 27 was possible.

In this study, the Analogies Test was assumed to measure the verbal isolation factor, as it seemed to demand that the subject shift from one abstract relationship to another and then isolate the correct word that completed the relationship.

### RESULTS

**Correlational and Factorial Analysis of Test Battery.** An attempt was made to give to all 48 patients before operation all seven of these tests of the abstract attitude. Because of lack of cooperation on the part of some of the patients, valid results were obtained on only 30 patients. Our analysis is based on these 30 sets of scores.

In order to determine statistically the common score of these tests the original (O) scores were intercorrelated. A factor analysis was made of these intercorrelations together with their correlation with the background variables of age, years of schooling, and I.Q. as determined by the Wechsler-Bellevue full scale score. Thurstone's ('47) group centroid method was used.

Inspection of the correlation matrix (table 54) shows that nearly all the intercorrelations are positive. The age variable which generally was correlated negatively with the other tests was reflected so as to produce positive correlations for ease in computing the factors.

TABLE 55. FACTOR MATRICES BEFORE AND AFTER THE "PARTIALLING OUT" OF AGE, YEARS OF SCHOOLING, AND I.Q. RESPECTIVELY (N=30)

| Variables | Factor I | | | | Factor II | | | |
|---|---|---|---|---|---|---|---|---|
| | $r_{iI}$ | $r_{iI.8}$ | $r_{iI.8(10)}$ | $r_{iI.8(10)9}$ | $r_{iII}$ | $r_{iII.8}$ | $r_{iII.8(10)}$ | $r_{iII.8(10)9}$ |
| 1. PI–1............. | .608 | .595 | .362 | .308 | .015 | −.119 | −.038 | .035 |
| 2. PI–2............. | .276 | .210 | .363 | .321 | −.180 | −.264 | −.270 | −.225 |
| 3. PI–3............. | .369 | .388 | .311 | .215 | −.392 | −.516 | −.496 | −.450 |
| 4. PI–4............. | .527 | .614 | .424 | .296 | −.487 | −.511 | −.498 | −.428 |
| 5. Analogies........ | .766 | .738 | .583 | .535 | .154 | −.113 | −.022 | .084 |
| 6. Ess. Diff.......... | .590 | .586 | .496 | .366 | −.177 | −.338 | −.299 | −.188 |
| 7. Weigl............ | .239 | .251 | .115 | .171 | −.126 | −.166 | −.132 | −.160 |
| 8. Age............. | .309 | — | — | — | .647 | — | — | — |
| 9. I.Q............. | .694 | .762 | .554 | — | −.343 | −.376 | −.351 | — |
| 10. Schooling........ | .815 | .798 | — | — | .189 | −.174 | — | — |
| Minimum r required for P of .05............ | .36 | .37 | .37 | .38 | .36 | .37 | .37 | .38 |

Subscript symbols: i = variable; I = factor I; II = factor II.
Arabic numbers = variable numbers.
On left side of period (.) are listed the variables (by number) "partialled out" of factor loadings.

The two factors extracted are shown in table 55. The second factor residuals were too small to merit the extraction of a third factor. (At this point it is important to note that correlations and factor loadings of less than +.36 do not attain the .05 level of confidence.)

When the background variables of age and years of schooling are excluded from consideration it becomes apparent that factor I is primarily dependent upon I.Q. (.69) and the Analogies Test (.77). Both of these tests indicate that factor I probably is the general intelligence factor postulated by Spearman ('27), Garrett ('46), and Thurstone ('38). Factor II does not lend itself to such ready description. The two tests having the greatest factor loadings (−.39 and −.49) are PI-3 and PI-4 respectively, which have correlations of approximately the same magnitude with both factors.

In order to "purify" the abstraction tests, the variables of age and years of schooling which may be regarded as of incidental importance were "partialled out" of both the factor matrix and the correlation matrix. (The method of selecting the patients in this study was so dependent on such fortuitous circumstances as availability, accessibility, and consent for operation, as to preclude the possibility of obtaining a random sample of any well-defined population.) The resulting factor matrix is shown in table 55.

The removal of the age variable resulted in relatively little change in the correlations among the tests and the factors. However, the removal of the educational variable reduced the correlations between factor I and the Analogies Test and between factor I and the PI-1 (Grouping) Test, indicating that both tests are to some degree a function of years of schooling. The correlations among the other tests and the two factors changed relatively slightly.

In order to determine whether factor I is primarily a general intellectual factor, the I.Q. variable was "partialled out" of the factor matrix (see table

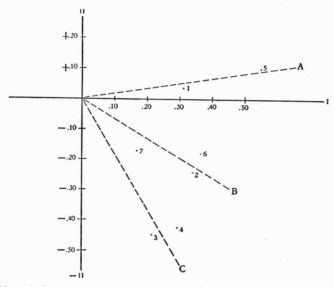

FIG. 100.  Plot of the factor loadings of the seven tests of abstraction with age, years of schooling, and I.Q. "partialled out" with reference to the centroid axes I and II. The numbered points refer to the projections of the seven-test vectors.

55). Removal of the I.Q. resulted in all the tests except the Analogies Test and the Essential Differences Test dropping to an insignificant level (below .36). Therefore it may be concluded that factor I was highly saturated with the factor of general intelligence. Factor II remained significantly correlated with PI-3 (Isolation) and PI-4 (Recall).

Figure 100 shows the plot of the seven factor loadings for the two factors remaining after age, years of schooling, and I.Q. were eliminated. Three fairly distinct clusters of tests are evident. These clusters are indicated by three major reference vectors (dotted lines on figure 100). Vector A is composed of the Analogies Test and PI-1 (Grouping) and may be tentatively designated as a grouping component. Vector B is composed of Essential Differences Test, PI-2 (Shift) and Weigl Test (Shift) and may be tentatively identified as a shift component. Vector C is composed of PI-3 (Isolation) and PI-4 (Recall) and may be tentatively called the isolation component. Disregarding the tentative titles of these test clusters, we feel that there is some (though not complete) evidence for the three-fold breakdown of Goldstein's abstract attitude. Although the reference vectors fail to correspond completely with the *a priori* logical analysis the results of factor analysis are suggestive of three underlying factors.

In conclusion, the results of the factor analysis indicate that the intercorrelations of the seven tests of abstraction, after age, years of schooling, and I.Q. have been "partialled out," may be tentatively resolved into three under-

TABLE 56.  MEANS AND F RATIOS OF THE NUMBER OF ITEMS SELECTED TO GO WITH THE DIFFERENT REFERENCE OBJECTS ON PI–1 (GROUPING) FOR THE OPERATEE AND CONTROL GROUPS ON THE THREE TESTING PERIODS

| Reference objects | Groups | N | Means | | | F ratios | | |
|---|---|---|---|---|---|---|---|---|
| | | | 0 | R1 | R2 | 0 | R1 | R2 |
| Large fork (2)......... | OP | 16 | 5.94 | 5.69 | 4.94 | .47 | .96 | .37 |
| | C | 13 | 4.92 | 7.15 | 4.31 | | | |
| Pipe (3)............. | OP | 16 | 4.69 | 4.87 | 3.94 | .63 | .92 | 1.07 |
| | C | 13 | 5.23 | 6.31 | 4.69 | | | |
| Bicycle bell (4)......... | OP | 16 | 3.75 | 5.62 | 4.75 | .00 | .02 | 1.46 |
| | C | 13 | 3.69 | 5.38 | 6.92 | | | |
| Red circle (5).......... | OP | 16 | 2.44 | 4.56 | 3.00 | 2.26 | .95 | .03 |
| | C | 13 | 3.31 | 3.62 | 3.07 | | | |
| Toy pliers (6).......... | OP | 16 | 4.94 | 6.31 | 7.06 | 1.07 | .65 | .10 |
| | C | 13 | 6.00 | 5.23 | 7.85 | | | |
| Rubber ball (7)........ | OP | 16 | 4.13 | 4.19 | 3.31 | 2.23 | .01 | 3.49 |
| | C | 13 | 3.54 | 4.08 | 4.77 | | | |
| Total................ | OP | 16 | 25.88 | 30.31 | 25.69 | .01 | .28 | .19 |
| | C | 13 | 26.85 | 33.38 | 31.62 | | | |

NOTE: F ratios must exceed 4.20 to be significant at .05 level.

lying components which are identified with the logically derived components of the abstract attitude as defined by Goldstein. These components show considerable intercorrelation. Hence this statistical analysis is in accord with the hypothesis that the abstract attitude is made up of intelligence, grouping, isolation, and shift. A more definite and precise establishment of the hypothesis, which would be desirable, will have to be done with data more critically collected than those which were used in this study.

**Grouping as Shown by Performance.**   The ability to abstract may be evidenced both by performance which does not necessarily involve speech and by verbal explanations given for grouping behavior. This is a useful separation even though the correlations presented in the preceding section show performance and verbal grouping to be correlated.

Grouping in performance was demonstrated by the number of objects which a subject would put together from an assortment of miscellaneous items when told: "Put together all the objects that go together with this one." Goldstein said that this mental operation suffers a loss after injury to the frontal lobes of the brain (Goldstein, '44a). Such brain-injured patients put only a very limited number of objects together while the person without brain injury puts together many objects.

After the PI-1 Sorting Test (Grouping) was presented to these patients the means and F ratios, given in table 56, for the two groups for the three testing periods—preoperative (O), first postoperative (R1), second postoperative (R2) —were obtained. The differences between the means of the operatee and control groups were not significant for any of the test periods. None of the F ratios

TABLE 57.   MEANS AND F RATIOS OF CONTROL AND OPERATEE GROUP ON THE VARIOUS TESTS FOR THE THREE TEST PERIODS
(F Ratios Must Exceed 4.19 to be Significant at the .05 Level for This Data)

| Group | N | Means | | | F ratios | | |
|---|---|---|---|---|---|---|---|
| | | 0 | R1 | R2 | 0 | R1 | R2 |
| Isolation (PI–3) | | | | | | | |
| OP........................ | 17 | 2.88 | 2.76 | 3.00 | | | |
| C........................... | 13 | 2.54 | 3.23 | 3.23 | .78 | 2.10 | .36 |
| Weigl | | | | | | | |
| OP........................ | 17 | 7.76 | 8.71 | 8.47 | | | |
| C........................... | 13 | 8.00 | 8.46 | 8.69 | .06 | .25 | .20 |
| Recall (PI–4) | | | | | | | |
| OP........................ | 17 | 24.41 | 24.35 | 24.94 | | | |
| C........................... | 13 | 25.08 | 24.77 | 25.85 | .11 | .05 | .39 |
| Essential differences | | | | | | | |
| OP........................ | 17 | 24.29 | 25.23 | 26.18 | | | |
| C........................... | 13 | 22.69 | 25.38 | 24.15 | .38 | .00 | .74 |
| Analogies | | | | | | | |
| OP........................ | 17 | 19.12 | 20.00 | 20.94 | | | |
| C........................... | 13 | 19.00 | 18.69 | 19.69 | .004 | .48 | .43 |
| Verbal shift (PI–2) | | | | | | | |
| OP........................ | 17 | 6.71 | 7.41 | 7.12 | | | |
| C........................... | 13 | 6.08 | 7.23 | 7.23 | .23 | .05 | .02 |

reported in table 56 are significant at the .05 level. Many of the F ratios are less than unity, indicating that the variance within the group is greater than the variance between groups. Since the PI-1 (Grouping) score was the only one of the seven test scores that did not directly reflect the presence of the abstract attitude by virtue of the magnitude of the score itself, a comparison of the means of the grouping scores (PI-1) between all the patients (N = 30) and 26 normals (hospital nurses and attendants) was made for the number of objects grouped with each of the six reference objects and the total grouping score. None of the F ratios approached significance, in fact all but one of the F ratios were less than one. We may conclude from this that the patients (preoperatively) and a comparable group of normals select the same number of objects in PI-1 (Grouping) and hence the patients are no more impaired in their abstract attitude in mean score than are the normals.

This grouping relationship might conceivably depend on the particular kind of objects selected for grouping. To investigate this quantitatively the data were analyzed as follows. Since selection was partially manifested in performance by the type of objects selected as well as the number of objects, the two groups were compared for significance of percentage differences in the number of times each of the thirty objects (thirty-one minus the reference object) was selected to go with a given reference object. For example, taking the fork (2) as the reference object, the number of subjects in the operatee group selecting the axe to go with the fork was compared with the number of subjects in the control group selecting the axe to go with the fork. Critical ratios were computed for both groups for all of the objects in relation to each reference object. Of these 540 critical ratios only three attained a significance of 2 or greater (significant at the .05 level). Hence, it may be assumed that the two groups were selecting approximately the same type of items to go with a given reference object consistently for all three testing periods. Therefore the variation within each group does not depend on the selection of special items at the expense of others.

The brain ablations conducted on this series of patients do not produce a sufficient restriction in the selection of the number of objects to be statistically significant as a group phenomenon. Neither did they result in a tendency to group certain items rather than others.

**Isolation as Shown by Performance.**   The next mental manipulation entering into abstraction to be considered is isolation. Isolation means, as previously explained, the picking out of an aggregation of objects an item which lacks a common quality possessed by all the others. This was demonstrated by the PI-3 (Isolation) Test. On this part of the test the subject selected from an aggregation of objects grouped by the examiner, the one object that did not "belong for some reason." His score was the number of correct isolations.

Table 57 shows that the means of the two groups are not statistically different for any of the test periods. Two of the F ratios show that the variance within the groups is greater than that between the groups for both preoperative and second postoperative periods.

In order to ascertain whether the variation could be attributed to the selection of a particular item, all of the item selections were analyzed separately for comparing percentages of the two groups selecting the right item for the three test periods. The difference between no pair of percentages compared was statistically significant. Hence the internal variation was not due to the preference in selecting one item rather than another.

Thus the isolation factor in the generalization process was not impaired by the brain operation when judged by group statistics.

**Shift as Shown by Performance.**   Shift in the process of abstraction refers to the ability to change from one method of grouping to a new and different method. It corresponds, in part, to a reversal of figure and ground in Gestalt studies of perception. The Weigl Test was used to investigate the ability to shift. In this test, as previously explained, the subject first sorted geometric, colored figures in one way, and then on request sorted the same figures in a second way. The usual scoring of the Weigl Test was modified to permit the degree of "shifting ability" to be estimated on a scale from 0 to 10. The means of the control and operatee patients were compared for the three test periods. Table 57 indicates that the means remained approximately the same for all testing periods.

**Grouping as Shown by Verbal Behavior.**   Goldstein ('44a) commenting on the work of Halstead ('40) said: "In the recall test, they recalled on the average considerably fewer objects . . . The patients are changed in their behavior. . . . They are restricted in the selection of the number of objects and number of grouping." In the PI-4 (Recall) Test the patients were asked, after all objects had been removed, to recall and name as many of them as possible. This recall is, according to Goldstein, evidence of grouping abstraction behavior shown verbally. The score was the number of objects correctly recalled.

Table 57 shows that means for both groups remain relatively constant for the three test periods. There is no evidence of loss or restriction in verbal recall as shown by group statistical treatment. Furthermore, no particular object (of total of thirty-one) was recalled significantly more often by one group than by the other.

**Isolation as Shown by Verbal Behavior.** Isolation as evidenced by verbal behavior in the abstraction process was studied in terms of the Essential Differences Test and the Analogies Test. In both tests the score was the number of correct answers. Since no time limit was imposed on either test the results should indicate the capability of the subject at the time the test was given.

The evidence for group differences on the Essential Differences Test is presented in table 57. The equivalence of the group means and insignificance of the F ratios are obvious. An item analysis of the individual items of the Essential Differences Test showed that no one item was dealt with in a differential fashion by the operatee group as compared to the control group.

The group results obtained from the Analogies Test are given in table 57 which shows the comparison of the means and F ratios before and after the operation. The means remained relatively constant with no significant F ratios. An item analysis of the twenty-seven items of the test yielded no intra-test pattern that differentiated the two groups.

**Shift as Shown by Verbal Behavior.** The PI-2 (Verbal Shift) Test required the subject to verbalize the common element in each successive grouping of objects placed before him. He must successively recognize the grouping principles of color, form, material, use, color, form, material, use, material, use, and use. To receive a high score in this test, the subject was forced to shift his grouping reference (presumably, his "abstract attitude") constantly. Four of the eleven groupings were "use" which is the easiest similarity to comprehend. This was done with the idea of reducing the possibility of chronic failure disturbing the subject's motivation.

Table 57 shows that the means of the two groups are very closely equivalent for the three testing periods. No evidence of loss in verbal shifting could be found in the group data. The same pattern of grouping principle preference occurred in both groups and was constant for all test periods. Use was the easiest principle to perceive, next material, then form, and finally color which seemed to be difficult for these patients to handle.

**Qualitative Estimates of the Abstract Attitude.** Goldstein and Scheerer ('41) stated: "The usual scoring method based on a scale of difficulty which has been standardized on a statistical basis offers no adequate instrument for determining the nature or the degree of impairment in a [brain injured] patient. Unless one takes into account the entire procedure, the specific reasons for the difficulty the patient encounters, one cannot simply read off from a score which task represents a greater difficulty and which is a lesser. Any statistical evaluation has to be based upon a qualitative analysis of test results; qualitative has to precede statistical analysis."

In light of this it was decided to apply qualitative estimates to the data. First,

Goldstein's and Scheerer's ('41) monograph, especially the section on the object-sorting test, was carefully abstracted for usable qualitative criteria of abstract behavior. These are listed below; each is followed by quotations from Goldstein to justify its use:

Any sorting or verbalization of a ready-sorted group of objects could be considered indicative of abstract behavior, if it fulfilled the following stipulations:

1. *"Use" is not the verbalized basis of sorting, but rather "color," "form," "material," or "pairs."*
   a. Concrete type of sorting described as: "Fitting the objects together according to factual usability in the present situation, e.g., eating utensils or smoking utensils." (p. 84.)
   b. ". . . . the most realistic type of concreteness almost never overcomes the aspect of use." (p. 92.)

TABLE 58.  MEAN FREQUENCY OF OCCURRENCE OF ABSTRACT ATTITUDE QUALITATIVELY ESTIMATED ON PI SORTING TEST

| PI Sorting test | Testing period | Operatee means (N = 17) | Control means (N = 13) |
|---|---|---|---|
| PI–1 (Grouping) . . . . . . . | 0 | .06 | .46 |
| | R1 | .65 | .85 |
| | R2 | 1.06 | 1.38 |
| PI–3 (Isolation) . . . . . . . | 0 | 3.18 | 2.77 |
| | R1 | 2.35 | 3.46 |
| | R2 | 3.47 | 3.54 |
| PI–2 (Shift) . . . . . . . . . . | 0 | .35 | .61 |
| | R1 | .23 | .31 |
| | R2 | .47 | .46 |
| PI (Total) . . . . . . . . . . . . | 0 | 3.59 | 3.84 |
| | R1 | 3.23 | 4.61 |
| | R2 | 5.00 | 5.38 |

NOTE: None of the mean differences are significant at the .05 level.

2. *No specific object named in the verbalization.*
   a. Concrete behavior described as: "Fitting the objects according to the way one subjectively experiences their appurtenance to a situation; e.g., a subject sorts the piece of wood and the nail together with the hammer, because, 'you put the nail in the wood with the hammer,' he then adds the white candle 'because you make a light when you hammer.' " (p. 84.)
3. *No situational reference mentioned in the verbalization.*
   a. Concrete behavior described as: "Fitting the objects according to one's past experience with them, e.g., having seen all toy objects in a toy store or all metal objects in a hardware store." (p. 84.)
4. *The verbalized basis of sorting not the same as the previous one, e.g., not sorted by material consecutively, but color and form as well.*
   a. Ability to shift essential to the abstraction process. (pp. 86-87.)
5. *Reference object not sorted alone nor with just one other object.*
   a. Criterion of concreteness was uniqueness, "a subject who responds very concretely will usually either refuse to group other articles with a given one or

will sort only a few articles with a given one or will sort only a few articles to go with it." (p. 87.)

    b. Criterion for concreteness was a preference for pairs (p. 88).

Using the above criteria, each sorting or verbalization of a ready-made sorting on parts of the PI Sorting Test was rated as concrete or abstract.

Table 58 shows the average frequency of the occurrence of abstract behavior qualitatively estimated as outlined above. It is evident that no one of the tests nor the total test combination gave evidence of impairment of the abstract attitude after operation. As a matter of fact, the averages indicate that for both groups there was an increase following operation, rather than a decrease.

**Does Impairment of the Abstract Attitude Depend on Interference of Functional Integrity of Specific Areas of the Frontal Lobes?** We have shown that certain tests of the abstract attitude are intercorrelated and probably (on a statistical basis) represent separate mental factors, namely, grouping, isolation, and possibly shift. We have further shown that no one of these tests shows a regular decrease in score (evidence of impaired ability to abstract) in the operatee group when compared to the control group. A qualitative scoring of the PI Sorting Test likewise failed to show impairment in the operatee group when compared to the control group.

Certain individual operatee patients did show decreased scores on the R1 or R2 testing when those scores were related to their O scores. Patients in the control group also showed decreases. That is, there is some variability shown in performance on repetition of the same tests on three occasions. This raised the question of, "How much decrease is indicative of an impairment of the abstract attitude?" It seemed logical to consider any decrease in score (O minus R1 and O minus R2) which equaled or exceeded the greatest decrease made by any member of the control group as a *marked deviation* and probably evidence of impairment.

In table 59 are given the areas excised in each patient. The entries in table 59 dealing with the Weigl test are (+), (−), or (?). A score of 10 or 9 was entered as (+) (could shift without or with prompting); a score of 8 or less was entered as (−) (could not shift without assistance). Where no score was obtained owing to lack of cooperation the entry is (?). If one groups the data given in table 59 with respect to areas removed the following conclusions may be drawn:

1. There was no regularity in specific decreases which were evoked through ablations of any specific area.

2. Five of 8 patients in whom some part of area 46 was removed were unable to shift their sorting on the Weigl Test at either postoperative test period. The other 3 patients (13, 33, and 49) did shift (score of 9) at the second postoperative test when requested, but did not do it spontaneously.*

3. Three of 9 patients (7, 31, 32) who had area 9 excised showed marked decreases in PI-1 (Grouping) score; patients' 3, 13, and 25 scores remained the same while the scores of patient 8 increased; no comparison could be made on patients 22 and 27 because they failed to cooperate in the O testing. Patients 7 and 32 had areas 8, 9, and 10 removed; patient 31 had out area 9. Patient 8

---

* Although this relationship to area 46 is interesting, it must be noted that 3 control patients (17, 29, and 30) had the ability to shift (score 9 or 10 on Weigl, O testing) and lost that ability (score 8 or less) on R1 and R2 testing. In other words, five area-46-removal patients lost the ability and 3 control patients did the same thing.

TABLE 59. MARKED DECREASES AND INCREASES IN SCORES (PROBABLE IMPAIRED ABSTRACT ATTITUDE) IN OPERATEES TOGETHER WITH BRAIN AREAS EXCISED, AND PSYCHIATRIC IMPROVEMENT SCORE*

| Pt. No. | Improvement Score | Areas excised | Weigl 0 | Weigl R1 | Weigl R2 | PI-1 R1 | PI-1 R2 | PI-2 R1 | PI-2 R2 | PI-3 R1 | PI-3 R2 | PI-4 R1 | PI-4 R2 | Anal. R1 | Anal. R2 | Ess. diff. R1 | Ess. diff. R2 |
|---|---|---|---|---|---|---|---|---|---|---|---|---|---|---|---|---|---|
| 2 | 0 | $6^a$, 8 | + | + | + | 0 | 0 | 0 | 0 | 0 | 0 | − | − | + | + | 0 | 0 |
| 3 | 2 | $6^a$, $9^b$ | + | + | + | − | − | + | − | 0 | 0 | − | 0 | 0 | + | 0 | 0 |
| 4 | 2 | 46 | + | − | − | 0 | 0 | 0 | 0 | 0 | 0 | 0 | 0 | 0 | 0 | 0 | 0 |
| 6 | 1 | $6^a$, $8^a$ | + | + | + | 0 | 0 | + | + | 0 | − | 0 | 0 | 0 | 0 | 0 | 0 |
| 7 | 5 | 8, $9^a$, $10^a$ | + | + | + | − | − | 0 | 0 | 0 | 0 | 0 | 0 | 0 | 0 | 0 | 0 |
| 8 | 0 | 8, $9^a$, $10^a$, $46^a$ | − | − | − | 0 | + | 0 | 0 | 0 | 0 | + | + | + | + | + | + |
| 13 | 6 | $9^a$, $10^a$, 45, 46 | − | − | + | 0 | 0 | 0 | 0 | 0 | 0 | 0 | 0 | 0 | 0 | 0 | 0 |
| 18 | −1 | $11^a$ | + | + | + | 0 | 0 | 0 | + | 0 | 0 | 0 | 0 | 0 | 0 | 0 | 0 |
| 19 | 0 | $45^a$ | − | + | + | 0 | 0 | − | 0 | − | 0 | 0 | 0 | 0 | 0 | 0 | 0 |
| 21 | 6 | 10 | + | + | + | − | − | − | − | 0 | 0 | 0 | − | 0 | 0 | − | 0 |
| 22 | 5 | 9, 10, 46 | ? | ? | ? | ? | ? | ? | ? | ? | ? | ? | ? | ? | ? | ? | ? |
| 24 | 1 | $6^a$ | + | − | − | − | − | − | 0 | 0 | − | − | − | 0 | 0 | ? | ? |
| 25 | 8 | 8, 9, 46, $10^a$ | + | ? | + | 0 | 0 | 0 | 0 | − | − | 0 | 0 | ? | 0 | 0 | − |
| 27 | 7 | $6^a$, $8^a$, $9^a$, $10^a$ | ? | ? | + | ? | ? | 0 | 0 | ? | 0 | ? | ? | ? | ? | ? | ? |
| 31 | 1 | 9 | − | + | + | 0 | 0 | ? | ? | 0 | ? | ? | ? | ? | ? | ? | ? |
| 32 | 0 | $8^a$, 9, $10^a$ | + | + | + | − | − | 0 | 0 | 0 | 0 | 0 | 0 | 0 | 0 | 0 | 0 |
| 33 | 8 | $10^a$, $44^a$, 45, $46^a$ | ? | ? | ? | ? | ? | ? | 0 | ? | 0 | 0 | 0 | ? | | ? | ? |
| 36 | 0 | 10, 11, 47, 45, 46 | + | − | + | 0 | 0 | 0 | + | − | 0 | 0 | 0 | + | 0 | 0 | 0 |
| 38 | 8 | $8^b$, $9^b$, $10^b$ | − | − | + | 0 | 0 | 0 | ? | 0 | 0 | 0 | 0 | + | ? | 0 | 0 |
| 40 | 0 | $24^a$ | − | + | + | 0 | 0 | 0 | 0 | 0 | ? | 0 | 0 | + | 0 | 0 | 0 |
| 42 | 5 | 11 | + | − | − | 0 | − | ? | ? | − | ? | 0 | ? | ? | | ? | ? |
| 44 | 0 | $10^a$, 47 | ? | ? | ? | ? | ? | ? | ? | 0 | ? | ? | 0 | ? | ? | ? | ? |
| 47 | 0 | 44 | − | − | + | ? | ? | ? | ? | ? | 0 | 0 | 0 | 0 | 0 | ? | ? |
| 49 | 5 | 10, $11^a$, $46^a$ | − | + | + | 0 | − | + | + | 0 | 0 | 0 | 0 | 0 | 0 | − | 0 |

Improvement score: −1 means slightly worse, 0 means no change, 1 through 8 ranges from improved to very much improved.
Weigl: + means could shift, − means could not shift, ? refused to cooperate.
Other tests: + means increase greater than all but one control, − means decrease greater than all but one control, ? means no control, ? means no test score.
$^a$ Part of area.
$^b$ Venous ligation over area.

*In comparing this table with table 78, see page 78.

had out areas 8, 9, 10, 46; patient 25, areas 8, 9, 10, 46; and patient 13, areas 9, 10, 45, 46. For this limited sample if grouping ability is impaired as a result of area 9 ablation it is spared if area 46 is removed at the same time.

4. One may abstract table 59 as follows: Consider only the four parts of the PI Test. Group the patients by areas removed so that all patients who have an area removal in common are assembled. Consider only the data where records were available, i.e., disregard (?). Count the number of (−) entries and (+) entries and determine the percentage of decreases and of increases. From this procedure table 60 was drawn up. These increases or decreases are deviations beyond those shown by control patients. Table 60 then shows that marked decreases indicated by the PI Test appear most frequently when area 6 is removed and appear with regularly diminishing frequency as one goes rostrally along the surface of the frontal lobe over 6, 8, 9, 10, 45, 46, to area 11.

TABLE 60. RELATION OF MARKED DECREASES AND IN-CREASES ON PI SORTING TEST SCORES TO AREAS OF THE BRAIN REMOVED

| Brain area | No. of patients | Opportunities for marked increases or decreases | Percent decreases | Percent increases |
|---|---|---|---|---|
| 6 | 3 | 24 | 29.1 | 16.6 |
| 8 | 6 | 48 | 27.1 | 4.2 |
| 9 | 7 | 56 | 25.0 | 10.7 |
| 10 | 8 | 64 | 20.3 | 9.4 |
| 45 | 3 | 24 | 16.6 | 12.5 |
| 46 | 6 | 40 | 12.5 | 15.0 |
| 11 | 4 | 32 | 3.1 | 6.2 |

5. In table 59 are entered the "psychiatric-social" ratings of improvement in status of the patients six months after the operation. It will be noted that they vary from −1 to +8, where −1 is slightly worse, O no change and on to +8 which represents "returned home, working and well adjusted." We have found no relation between general improvement and these results on the seven tests of abstract attitude.

6. To summarize the individual finding we have evidence of the following: (1) Weigl loss, i.e., inability to shift performance tends to be associated with area 46 ablation; (2) PI-1 loss, i.e. restriction in number of objects grouped together tends to be associated with area 9 ablation but does not occur if both 9 and 46 are removed; (3) marked decreases in grouping of objects, successful isolation of objects inappropriate in a group, naming of groups, and recall of objects, i.e. PI-1, 2, 3, 4, occur most frequently when area 6 or 8 is removed and less frequently as one goes rostrally over the frontal cortex.

Due scientific caution must be observed in generalizing from these findings of the relationship of brain areas to behavior functions. The number of cases is small. The anatomic overlap of areas is better than anything hitherto accomplished but still open to possible error. The findings have not been confirmed by repetition with other samples. These and other reasons urge caution. With such caution in mind we may put forth the following speculations:

1. Goldstein's idea that the abstract attitude depends on the intact frontal lobes rested on the correct clinical observation that some patients with frontal

lobe damage of one or another variety were unable to shift, as demonstrated by the Weigl Test and that other patients (sometimes the same persons) had difficulty in grouping items together which belonged together. As we have shown this is true of some "frontal lobe" patients but not of all. It is relatively true of area 46 cases with respect to the Weigl Test and is true of 3 of 6 of area 9 cases with respect to grouping performance on the PI Sorting Test.

2. Just how the restriction in ability to group shown by patients with area 9 removed is related to learning, memory, I.Q., and the like, as indicated both by our factor analysis and by other data of the Columbia-Greystone Project, is not clear.

3. It is not apparent why the Analogies and Essential Differences Tests failed to show decreased or increased scores which could be related to an area or areas.

DISCUSSION

Gelb and Goldstein isolated in certain brain-injured patients a defective mental process which they called a loss or impairment in "abstract behavior." Goldstein further elaborated and somewhat clarified this concept by subsequent clinical studies and by laboratory investigations. His finding met general acceptance in both clinical psychology and clinical neurology. Many psychologic tests which are at present in general use depend on this idea that defects in abstract behavior are valid indicators of organic brain damage probably limited to the frontal lobes. Most clinical workers have noted the occurrence of this phenomenon in certain patients in whom organic involvement of the frontal lobes was subsequently verified. However, repeatedly cases have been found where verified frontal damage was not evidenced by sorting-test defects. These were usually explained as owing to incorrect test application, mental "compensation" in which other methods were used to solve the tasks, or they were ignored. Some clinicians have felt that Goldstein was not too explicit and that his vagueness led them to miss seeing the phenomenon he was describing. Although Goldstein held that he was dealing with a unique mental process there were those who held that the process probably depended on such factors as I.Q., age, verbal fluency, memory, and experience, and it was a particular combination of processes that was defective in some respect rather than a unique element.

Goldstein's concept was rooted in the figure-ground reversibility of perception emphasized in Gestalt psychology. He generalized from this perceptual phenomenon to a much more general type or types of mental function. He has reported that this loss of abstract behavior is found in brain-injured patients, in patients with tumors of the frontal lobes, in patients with organic neural deterioration of the frontal lobes, in lobotomy patients, and in some schizophrenic patients who recover the ability when they recover from their psychosis.

He has never reported, nor has anyone else, on the application of the sorting tests and Weigl Test to a large number of normal persons differing in age, I.Q., verbal ability, and the like. Thompson ('41) did show that in children the scores on these tests increase with chronologic age and mental age. We have shown that they are in part dependent on these factors in psychotic and normal adults.

Still a more serious criticism of the Goldstein hypothesis is the fact that neither he nor anyone else, so far as we can determine, ever had the opportunity to apply these tests to patients on whom frontal ablation or lobotomy was to be done before the operation was performed and then to retest to find what changes if any were brought about by the operation.

Where do our findings fit into this background and what do they signify?

No one of the seven tests which we employed showed a significant decrease (or increase) in mean score when applied to this group of patients before and after topectomy. The general operation of topectomy, irrespective of areas removed, has no regular specific effect on the test results. Otherwise stated, the generality of abstract behavior does not depend on the generality of the frontal lobes.

One specific performance test, namely the ability to shift voluntarily from one way of sorting objects to another way of sorting the same objects (Weigl Test), does in 5 of 7 patients depend upon the integrity of area 46.

The ability to group objects with specific reference to some other object (PI-1—Grouping) shows a restriction in the number of objects so grouped after ablation which involves area 9, or 9 in combination with 8 and/or 10. When both area 9 and area 46 were removed the restriction did not occur.

Marked decreases in the four scores of the PI Sorting Test (Grouping, Isolation, Shift, and Recall) appeared in 29.1 percent of the R1 and R2 scores of area 6 patients and in a regularly diminishing order of magnitude as one moves rostrally down the frontal cortex over area 8 (27.1 percent), 9 (25 percent), 10 (20 percent), 45 (17 percent), 46 (13 percent) to 11 (3 percent).

We doubt that there is a general factor of abstract behavior in the rather inclusive way in which Goldstein described it. We seem to have found three relatively specific components or factors which persist even after the general intelligence factor is removed.

Our findings of loss of ability to shift (Weigl Test) associated with ablation of area 46 and grouping restriction associated with ablation of area 9 indicate that the clinical observation which Goldstein made does occur with a certain limited regularity. Goldstein generalized too far from isolated observations.

Further studies of patients subjected to brain operation should include not only tests of grouping performance and of ability to shift but other related tests which may clarify some of the questions which we have raised. Such tests will have to be given to the patient before operation in order to be sure that apparent decreases in scores are real.

## SUMMARY

1. The findings of Kurt Goldstein that the "abstract attitude" was impaired by damage to the frontal lobes were reviewed historically and restated in terms of this study.

2. Seven different tests were used to measure impairment to "abstract attitude" in mental patients undergoing a topectomy operation (ablation of specific frontal lobe areas according to Brodmann's architectonic scheme). Thirteen control and 17 operatee patients were tested preoperatively and at two different time intervals postoperatively.

3. A factor analysis of the preoperative scores with I.Q., age, and years of schooling included was made. When these background variables are "partialled out" of the two factors, the residual factor loadings show three possible underlying components which were made evident by three test clusters lying along three reference vectors in the plot of these factors. These three components

were tentatively identified with the logical constructs of shift, isolation, and grouping.

4. The preoperative as well as the postoperative results showed no significant statistical differences in the means of any of the seven tests between the control and operatee groups.

5. Qualitative estimates made in accordance with Goldstein's statements failed to show mean differences between the operatee and control groups.

6. Examination of individual losses (marked decreases in test scores from preoperative testing to postoperative testing, which decreases equaled or exceeded the change occurring in any control patient) disclosed three findings related to specific brain areas. They are: (a) a tendency for a loss in ability to shift in sorting behavior (Weigl Test) when area 46 was removed, (b) a tendency to restrict the number of objects grouped together (PI-1) when area 9 is removed which ability is spared if both areas 9 and 46 are removed, and (c) a tendency for the number of markedly decreased scores on the entire PI Sorting Test to diminish in frequency as one moves rostrally over the frontal cortex ablations from area 6 through 8, 9, 10, 45, 46 to area 11.

*Chapter 17*

# Word Association*

SHIRLEY REIDER RASHKIS

---

THE word association technique has an experimental history beginning in 1879 when Galton (1880) first published his observations on various aspects of his own association process. He exposed a list of stimulus words one at a time and allowed himself to make only two or three associations to each word which he then recorded, together with his reaction time. From the data obtained on four separate presentations of the list he observed the general stability of his associations and attempted to trace their origin.

The subsequent history of the word association technique was reviewed by Kohs ('14). He pointed out that Kraepelin, beginning in 1896, outlined a program of study of word association experiments in the field of psychopathology. Kraepelin investigated the effects of practice and of drugs on association, and his students continued the study of the manifold factors influencing the association process.

Jung ('18) applied the word association technique in a study of the psychoanalytic concept of the unconscious. He described and distinguished certain reactions to the stimulus word which he and his students thought were indicative of the fact that the stimulus word had touched upon an emotional complex. These reactions or characteristics of the associations he termed "complex indicators." The complex indicators were subject to verification by the facts which emerged from interviews with the subject. Among the indicators noted by Jung in his work with normal subjects and mental patients were: delayed reactions, unusual reactions, superficial reactions, repetition of the stimulus word, perseveration of the preceding response, failure to respond, emotional reactions, and failure to repeat the same response on repetition of the stimulus list, i.e. reproduction.

Kent and Rosanoff ('10) conducted a study to determine the differences between the reactions of psychotics and normal individuals on the Word Association Test. They compiled a stimulus list of 100 familiar English words. They then gave the list to 1,000 normal subjects of both sexes, recording in each case the first word that was given in response to the stimulus word. From the responses of these subjects they prepared a series of frequency tables, each table listing the stimulus word and the frequency of each word given in the responses of the 1,000 subjects. Kent and Rosanoff then administered the test to 247 psychiatric patients and compared their responses with those of the normal subjects. They found that the psychotics gave more individual reactions than did the normal individuals. However, there was no sharp distinction between the associations of the two groups, rather there was a gradual transition of disturbances in association from the normal to the abnormal state.

* This chapter was submitted in partial fulfillment of the requirements for the degree of Doctor of Philosophy in the Faculty of Pure Science, Columbia University.

Hull and Lugoff ('21) reported a study in which they attempted to determine which of the complex indicators designated by Jung were truly associated with emotional complexes and which gave evidence of diagnostic reliability. They indirectly tested the validity of an indicator on the basis of its association with each of several other indicators in the individual responses of 100 normal subjects to the Jung association list. The degree of association between any single indicator and all other indicators combined was considered a measure of the relation of the indicator to emotional complexes, i.e. of its diagnostic reliability. They concluded that, of the indicators examined, stimulus repetition, apparent misunderstanding of the stimulus word, long reaction time, and defective reproduction of the reaction word were probably real complex indicators and that stimulus repetition was the most reliable diagnostic indicator.

Huebner ('38) investigated the effect of repetition of the Kent-Rosanoff Word Association Test. In a study of two successive examinations of 60 schizophrenic patients and 60 control subjects, she observed that on repetition of the test the control subjects showed greater communality in their responses while the schizophrenic patients showed no tendency toward greater or less communality. Comparison of the original responses with those given on retest showed that a greater number of controls than schizophrenics tended to repeat the same common responses to the stimulus words. Huebner found on the basis of five successive examinations of the schizophrenic patients that the number of most common, individual, and unusual responses remained fairly stable and that there was a tendency for patients showing an increase in the communality of their responses from first to fifth examination to show a corresponding improvement in clinical condition.

Rapaport ('46) observed in a study with the Orbison list of stimulus words that psychotics, as compared with neurotic patients and normal subjects, gave fewer popular reactions and showed the highest incidence of long reaction times as well as the highest average frequency of association and reproduction disturbances.

Summarizing the studies of word association with psychotics, it may be stated that certain investigators have indicated that there is a tendency for various characteristics of responses, particularly communality, to differentiate the associations of the psychotic from those of the normal; and that the communality of associations for psychotic patients has been found to be fairly stable on retest.

The Word Association Test has recently been employed in the investigation of the psychologic effects of electric convulsive therapy. Zeaman ('47) compared the performance of a small group of patients on a word association test before and after certain members of the group received electric shock therapy. She found that clinical improvement for both the treated and untreated patients was reflected in a decrease in the number of complex indicators in the associations and an increase in the stability of associations as measured by reproduction. Janis ('49) reported in a similar study of the Word Association Test with electric shock and control patients that, following shock, the treated patients, as compared with the controls, showed a slight statistically significant increase in remote or idiosyncratic associations, stimulus repetitions, and multiword responses, as well as a statistically significant increase in defective reproductions of associations.

In studying the changes in word association following prefrontal lobotomy, Hunt ('42) found longer total test times, fewer extremely delayed responses, fewer failures in response, fewer peculiar and self-reference type responses, and less perseveration. Also working with prefrontal lobotomy cases, Kisker ('43) reported that the word association technique failed to show changes in performance which could be considered as characteristic of the postlobotomy patient.

## PROBLEM

The present-day concept of the frontal lobes as "association areas" is derived largely from the work of Franz ('07) on animals. Knowledge of frontal lobe function in human beings is based primarily on generally isolated clinical observations and on theories developed from animal experiments. On the assumption that word association is a function of the frontal lobes of man, it might be expected that removal of tissue from the frontal lobes would produce an observable interference with the word association process which would be evidenced by changes in the stability or reproducibility of associations.

Prefrontal lobotomy, which does not involve the actual excision of brain tissue, has been described by Freeman and Watts ('42) as resulting in an improved emotional and social adjustment in certain mentally ill patients. Assuming that bilaterally symmetrical removal of certain portions of the frontal lobes, i.e. topectomy, might bring about similar clinical evidence of improvement, it seemed worth while to ascertain if such changes in emotional and social adjustment would be reflected by changes in the emotional aspects and in the communality of responses to the Word Association Test. It might be assumed that certain characteristics of the responses to the Word Association Test, termed complex indicators by Jung ('18), would give evidence of changes in emotionality.

TABLE 61. THE SUBJECTS

| Group | N | Age Mean | Age Range | School years completed Mean | School years completed Range | I.Q. Mean | I.Q. Range |
|---|---|---|---|---|---|---|---|
| Operatees | 15 | 42.0 | 28–58 | 9.5 | 6–16 | 102 | 89–131 |
| Controls | 11 | 47.6 | 34–60 | 8.1 | 4–11 | 105 | 81–125 |

The following hypotheses were set forth on the basis of the considerations noted above:

1. Removal of brain tissue from the frontal lobes of man will produce changes in the associative process which will be reflected in changes in performance on the Word Association Test.

2. Improvement in emotional and social adjustment will be reflected in these changes by a decrease in the number of complex indicators and by an increase in the communality of responses.

3. Interference with the associative process by the removal of brain tissue will decrease the stability of associations. This will be evidenced by a decrease in the tendency of responses given prior to operation to persist following operation and by a change in the communality of responses.

4. The decrease in the stability of associations following operation will be further evidenced by a decrease in the accuracy of immediate reproduction of responses.

It was intended that the entire group of patients be used in the present study. Because of their mental condition complete data could not be obtained on all 48 patients, hence the findings were limited to 26 patients on whom complete preoperative or preanesthesia and postoperative or postanesthesia data were available.

The latter group consisted of 15 operatees and 11 control patients. There were 9 males and 6 females in the operatee group, and 8 males and 3 females in the control group. The range and mean age, education, and I.Q. of each group are presented in table 61.

METHOD

Three lists of stimulus words, lists A, B, and C, were used in the present study.

Word association lists A and B were derived from the Kent and Rosanoff ('20) Word Association Test. The two lists, A and B, were regarded as equivalent. They were selected in the following manner. The 100 words in the Kent-Rosanoff Word Association Test were ranked in the order of the frequency of the most common association to each word obtained by Kent and Rosanoff with 1,000 normal subjects. For example: *lamp*, most frequent response: light, frequency: 650, rank: 1; *eagle*, most frequent response: bird, frequency: 568, rank: 2. From this ranking the even-numbered words were made into list A and the odd-numbered words into list B.

Word association list A consisted of the following fifty words: *eagle, dream, justice, boy, bible, memory, cottage, swift, hungry, ocean, head, long, religion, whiskey, child, bitter, city, butter, loud, joy, heavy, tobacco, scissors, street, afraid, stem, table, music, man, soft, mountain, house, comfort, hand, fruit, butterfly, command, sweet, woman, white, rough, citizen, foot, needle, red, anger, high, sour, earth, soldier.*

Word association list B consisted of the following fifty words: *dark, sickness, deep, eating, black, mutton, short, smooth, chair, whistle, cold, slow, wish, river, beautiful, window, spider sleep, carpet, girl, trouble, cabbage, hard, stomach, lamp, yellow, bread, light, health, sheet, bath, blue, priest, stove, hammer, thirsty, square, doctor, thief, lion, bed, baby, moon, quiet, green, salt, king, cheese, blossom, working.*

Word association list C consisted of forty words which were obtained from the stimulus-word list of Orbison ('46). The words used were as follows: *world, love, father, hat, breast, curtains, trunk, drink, party, bowel movement, book, rug, boy friend, depressed, spring, bowl, suicide, paper, radiator, girl friend, screen, masturbate, frame, movies, cut, laugh, bite, dance, hospital, daughter, taxi, beef, mother, nipple, race, water, suck, horse, fire, intercourse.*

**Procedure.** The following procedure was employed in the administration of each of the word association lists:

The patient was seated at a right angle to the examiner to avoid distraction during the test performance, and was given the instructions: "I am going to call out a list of words, one at a time. After I say each word I want you to answer with the first word that comes to your mind, just as quickly as you can. You are to answer with just one word, no more. Also, do not repeat the words that I say. Remember, answer as fast as you can with the first single word that comes to your mind."

The patient was asked to respond to a preliminary list of sample words to accustom him to the procedure. The word association list was then administered. The examiner read each word distinctly and recorded the patient's complete response and reaction time. The stop watch was started at the same time the stimulus word was read, and stopped as soon as the patient began his response. The time limit was thirty seconds. Reaction times were recorded to the nearest second. The first time the patient responded with more than one word to a stimulus word he was reminded to respond with a single word. No further cautions were given. No stimulus words were repeated. The responses and reaction times to the first administration of each list of stimulus words will be referred to as *associations* and *association reaction times* respectively in the treatment of results.

On completion of the word association list the patient was instructed: "Now I am going to read the same list of words which I gave you before and I want you to answer each word with the same word you gave the first time."

The examiner then reread the word association list. The responses and reaction times were recorded as described above. The responses and reaction times to this second administration of each list of stimulus words will be referred to as *reproductions* and *reproduction reaction times* respectively in the treatment of results.

Word association lists A and C were administered during separate sessions about one month before operation, list A preceding list C. Lists B and C were given during separate sessions about four months following operation, list B preceding list C. List A was given preoperatively (O) and list B postoperatively (R2) in order to obtain comparable data without the interference of a learning effect. List C, in contrast to lists A and B, contained certain words which might be considered "emotionally toned." Since the equivalence of presumably "emotionally toned" stimuli could not be accurately judged, list C was administered in identical form preoperatively and postoperatively. This procedure made possible the study of the persistence of associations to list C, as will be described below.

In all subsequent discussion word association lists A and B will be referred to as Word Association Test A, and word association list C as Word Association Test C.

## RESULTS

### METHOD OF SCORING

**Complex Indicators.** The complex indicators studied in this investigation were: Multiverbality, Stimulus Repetition, Clangs, Rare Responses, Failure to Respond, and Delayed Association Reaction Time. These indicators were delimited and scored for each patient on Word Association Tests A and C preoperatively and postoperatively as follows:

(a) *Multiverbality:* Total number of associations of more than one word, excluding two-word responses containing a repetition of the stimulus word (ex. *bible*—"pertaining to God").

(b) *Stimulus Repetition:* Total number of associations containing complete or partial repetitions of the stimulus word (ex. *boy*—"boy, childhood"; *comfort*—"discomfort").

(c) *Clangs:* Total number of paralogical associations either rhyming with the stimulus word (ex. *light*—"tight"); having the same first consonant sound as the stimulus word (ex. *child*—"chili sauce"); or containing a main accented vowel assonant with the main accented vowel of the stimulus word (ex. *soft*—"lost").

(d) *Rare Responses:* Total number of associations on Test A which occurred in terms of frequency value (communality) in the lowest interval of a normalized distribution of the Kent-Rosanoff frequency tables; total number of associations on Test C not occurring in Rapaport's ('46) table of popular reactions.

(e) *Failure to Respond:* Total number of stimulus words to which the patient failed to give an association within the time limit (thirty seconds).

(f) *Delayed Association Reaction Time:* Total number of association reaction times of nine seconds or longer. (Nine seconds was 2 sigma above the mean reaction time of the combined operatee and control groups on both Tests A and C preoperatively.)

The total number of complex indicators for each patient on Tests A and C was also determined.

(g) *Total Number of Complex Indicators:* The sum of the scores on (a) to (f) inclusive.

TABLE 62.   COMPARISON BY ANALYSIS OF VARIANCE OF THE PREOPERATIVE AND POSTOPERATIVE MEANS AND THEIR DIFFERENCES FOR THE OPERATEE AND CONTROL GROUPS ON WORD ASSOCIATION TESTS A AND C

| Measures | Test | Preoperative (0) means | | F | Postoperative (R2) means | | F | Differences between the means (R2–0) | | F |
|---|---|---|---|---|---|---|---|---|---|---|
| | | $M_{OP}$ | $M_C$ | | $M_{OP}$ | $M_C$ | | $M_{OP}$ | $M_C$ | |
| Multiverbality......... | A | 1.53 | 4.00 | 8.15ᵃ | 4.80 | 3.18 | .30 | +3.27 | − 0.82 | 2.53 |
| Multiverbality......... | C | 2.40 | 2.27 | 1.02 | 5.00 | 3.18 | .76 | +2.60 | + 0.91 | .92 |
| Stimulus repetition..... | A | 5.13 | 1.91 | .15 | 1.93 | 0.64 | 3.80 | −3.20 | − 1.27 | .24 |
| Stimulus repetition..... | C | 4.27 | 2.27 | .38 | 2.73 | 1.45 | 1.62 | −1.54 | − 0.82 | .09 |
| Clangs............... | A | 0.53 | 0.82 | .49 | 0.73 | 0.73 | .01 | +0.20 | − 0.09 | .39 |
| Clangs............... | C | 0.33 | 0.27 | .04 | 0.73 | 0.18 | 4.39ᵃ | +0.40 | − 0.09 | 1.63 |
| Rare responses........ | A | 11.07 | 10.18 | .11 | 10.80 | 8.27 | .72 | −0.27 | − 1.91 | .50 |
| Rare responses........ | C | 26.33 | 23.45 | 1.96 | 25.60 | 23.73 | .81 | −0.73 | + 0.28 | .24 |
| Failure to respond..... | A | 0.27 | 0.82 | .13 | 0.13 | 0.00 | .94 | −0.14 | − 0.82 | 1.65 |
| Failure to respond..... | C | 0.20 | 0.73 | 2.05 | 0.27 | 0.46 | .29 | +0.07 | − 0.27 | .70 |
| Delayed assoc. RT..... | A | 4.73 | 7.27 | .87 | 3.93 | 7.45 | 1.35 | −0.80 | + 0.18 | .21 |
| Delayed assoc. RT..... | C | 5.27 | 5.09 | .01 | 5.07 | 7.27 | .70 | −0.20 | + 2.18 | 1.42 |
| Total No. compl. indic.. | A | 23.27 | 25.00 | .07 | 22.33 | 20.27 | .10 | −0.94 | − 4.73 | .41 |
| Total No. compl. indic.. | C | 38.80 | 34.09 | 1.04 | 39.40 | 36.27 | .45 | +0.60 | + 2.18 | .12 |
| Persistenceᵇ.......... | C | | | | 14.13 | 14.82 | .08 | | | |
| Communality......... | A | 308.60 | 311.91 | .03 | 309.87 | 324.27 | .50 | +1.27 | +12.36 | .45 |
| Communality......... | C | 131.67 | 139.45 | .75 | 135.53 | 144.82 | .92 | +3.86 | + 5.37 | .02 |
| Inaccurate reprod...... | A | 10.47 | 13.36 | .58 | 12.00 | 8.55 | 1.01 | +1.53 | − 4.81 | 4.83ᵃ |
| Inaccurate reprod...... | C | 7.73 | 7.18 | .02 | 7.73 | 5.82 | .43 | 0.00 | − 1.36 | .41 |
| Delayed reprod. RT.... | A | 4.73 | 3.64 | .31 | 5.07 | 7.82 | 1.21 | +0.34 | + 4.18 | 2.68 |
| Delayed reprod. RT.... | C | 4.80 | 3.18 | .88 | 3.60 | 6.00 | .99 | −1.20 | + 2.82 | 4.67ᵃ |

ᵃ Significant at .05 level of confidence.
ᵇ Persistence was only a postoperative measure; scored as described above.
NOTE: There were 15 patients in the operatee group and 11 in the control.

**Other Measures.**   The following measures were used in the study of the mnemonic aspects of association: Persistence, Communality, Inaccurate Reproduction, and Delayed Reproduction Reaction Time. These measures were delimited and scored for each patient on Tests A and C preoperatively and postoperatively as follows:

(a) *Persistence:* Number of stimulus words on Test C to which the same association was given preoperatively and postoperatively.*

(b) *Communality:* The association to each stimulus word on Test A was assigned a rating on the basis of its frequency of occurrence in the Kent-

* Test A was not scored for Persistence since identical stimulus words were not used preoperatively and postoperatively.

Rosanoff frequency tables, when these tables were converted to a normal distribution. Ratings were from 1 to 9, with 9 indicating the highest frequency or communality. The total communality score for each patient on Test A was the sum of the ratings for all of his associations to the Test. The association to each stimulus word on Test C was assigned a rating on the basis of its frequency of occurrence in Rapaport's ('46) table of popular reactions, when the frequencies in the table were converted to a normal distribution. Ratings were from 1 to 7, 7 indicating the highest frequency or communality. The total communality score for each patient on Test C was the sum of the ratings for all of his associations to the Test.

(c) *Inaccurate Reproduction:* Total number of reproductions of associations which were completely different from the original associations.

(d) *Delayed Reproduction Reaction Time:* Total number of reproduction reaction times on Test A of nine seconds or longer (nine seconds was 2 sigma above the mean reproduction reaction time of the combined operatee and control groups on Test A preoperatively); total number of reproduction reaction times on Test C which were eight seconds or longer (eight seconds was 2 sigma above the mean reproduction reaction times of the combined operatee and control group on Test C preoperatively).

### GROUP COMPARISONS

The preoperative (O) and postoperative (R2), means and the differences between the preoperative and postoperative means (R2-O) of the operatee and control groups for each of the measures on Tests A and C were compared by analysis of variance. The means and corresponding F ratios are presented in table 62. The data contained in table 62 justify the following statements:

The preoperative mean of the control group on Multiverbality, Test A, exceeded that of the operatee group at the .01 level of confidence. With the exception of this finding the operatee and control groups exhibited no significant differences preoperatively on Test A or Test C.

The postoperative mean of the operatee group on Clangs, Test C, exceeded that of the control group at the .05 level of confidence. There were no other significant differences between the groups postoperatively.

Comparison of the differences between the preoperative and postoperative means of the two groups indicates that the operatee group showed an increase in score on Inaccurate Reproduction, Test A, and a decrease in score on Delayed Reproduction Reaction Time, Test C, both of which were significant at the .05 level of confidence. On all other measures the differences between the preoperative and postoperative means of the two groups were not significantly different.

### COMPARISON OF INDIVIDUAL CHANGES

Table 63 gives the difference scores (R2-O) of the operatees and control patients for all of the measures on which Word Association Tests A and C were scored, in addition to the sex, age, I.Q., psychiatric improvement rating, and areas excised for each patient. The psychiatric-social ratings of improvement represent the status of the patients six months after operation. These ratings ranged from -1 to +8, -1 signifying slightly worse, 0 no change, and progressive positive ratings increasing improvement. A rating of +8 indicated the patient had returned home, was working and well adjusted.

TABLE 63. INCREASES AND DECREASES IN SCORE FROM PREOPERATIVE TO
TESTS A

| 1 | 2 | 3 | 4 | 5 | 6 | 7 | 8 | 9 | 10 | 11 | 12 | 13 | 14 |
|---|---|---|---|---|---|---|---|---|----|----|----|----|----|
| | | | | | | | | | | | | | *Test* |
| Pt. No. | Sex | Age | I.Q. | Improvement ratings | Areas excised | Multiverbality | | Stimulus repetition | | Clangs | | Rare responses | |
| | | | | | | A | C | A | C | A | C | A | C |
| **Operatee group:** | | | | | | | | | | | | | |
| 2 | M | 46 | 107 | 0 | 8 | + 5 | + 2 | 0 | 0 | 0 | 0 | − 1 | − 4 |
| 6 | M | 33 | 92 | 1 | 6, 8 | 0 | − 2 | − 1 | − 1 | +2 | −3 | +12 | − 9 |
| 7 | M | 40 | 93 | 5 | 8, 9, 10 | +19 | + 8 | − 1 | + 3 | −1 | 0 | + 3 | 0 |
| 8 | M | 29 | 90 | 0 | MFG[a] | − 1 | + 2 | 0 | 0 | +1 | +1 | + 8 | + 8 |
| 13 | M | 43 | 96 | 6 | 9, 10, 45, 46 | +25 | +13 | − 1 | + 6 | 0 | +1 | − 2 | + 1 |
| 18 | M | 39 | 127 | −1 | 11 | 0 | − 1 | − 1 | 0 | 0 | +1 | − 2 | + 5 |
| 19 | M | 50 | 102 | 0 | 45, 46 | + 1 | 0 | + 2 | +29 | 0 | 0 | − 4 | + 3 |
| 21 | M | 42 | 104 | 6 | 10 | + 3 | + 3 | + 3 | + 4 | +1 | 0 | + 2 | + 2 |
| 25 | M | 58 | 89 | 8 | 8, 9, 46 | − 2 | + 2 | −49 | + 1 | +2 | +1 | 0 | 0 |
| 31 | F | 51 | 96 | 1 | 9 | − 1 | 0 | − 5 | − 9 | 0 | +1 | − 3 | 0 |
| 32 | F | 41 | 131 | 0 | 8, 9, 10 | 0 | 0 | + 3 | 0 | 0 | +2 | − 3 | − 3 |
| 36 | F | 53 | 93 | 0 | IFG[b] | − 1 | + 6 | − 1 | + 1 | 0 | 0 | − 1 | − 7 |
| 38 | F | 38 | 106 | 8 | VT[c] | − 2 | 0 | − 1 | + 1 | −3 | +1 | −17 | − 6 |
| 40 | F | 28 | 91 | 0 | 24, 32 | + 4 | +12 | + 2 | + 2 | +1 | 0 | − 1 | − 2 |
| 49 | F | 39 | 111 | 5 | 10 | − 1 | − 6 | + 2 | − 2 | 0 | +1 | + 5 | + 1 |
| **Control group:** | | | | | | | | | | | | | |
| 1 | M | 55 | 119 | 0 | —— | − 1 | 0 | 0 | + 3 | 0 | +1 | + 1 | + 2 |
| 5 | M | 35 | 81 | 0 | —— | − 2 | − 1 | − 1 | − 1 | +1 | 0 | + 4 | − 2 |
| 9 | M | 45 | 113 | 4 | —— | + 2 | + 3 | + 1 | 0 | −1 | 0 | −13 | − 7 |
| 11 | M | 44 | 91 | 0 | —— | − 9 | + 1 | − 9 | −11 | 0 | 0 | + 3 | − 3 |
| 12 | M | 57 | 109 | 0 | —— | + 2 | + 4 | − 3 | − 3 | +2 | −1 | + 1 | +13 |
| 16 | M | 50 | 83 | 0 | —— | 0 | − 1 | − 1 | + 2 | −2 | −1 | − 1 | + 8 |
| 17 | M | 60 | 103 | 0 | —— | + 3 | + 4 | + 3 | 0 | −1 | 0 | − 3 | + 1 |
| 23 | M | 39 | 117 | 0 | —— | + 1 | 0 | 0 | 0 | 0 | −1 | + 2 | − 4 |
| 34 | F | 34 | 125 | 0 | —— | − 3 | − 1 | − 1 | + 1 | −1 | 0 | − 6 | − 4 |
| 35 | F | 59 | 111 | 0 | —— | − 1 | + 6 | − 2 | − 1 | +1 | 0 | − 3 | + 3 |
| 39 | F | 45 | 101 | 5 | —— | − 1 | − 5 | − 1 | + 1 | 0 | +1 | − 6 | − 4 |

[a] Middle frontal gyrus.
[b] Inferior frontal gyrus (areas 10, 11, 47, 45, 46).
[c] No excision, venous ligation over areas 8, 9, and 10.

In comparing individual changes in test performance following operation the question arose as to the amount of change in any patient's score which should be considered significant. Since both groups under scrutiny were small (operatees, N = 15; controls, N = 11), composed of mental patients, and patients subject to a variety of frontal lobe excisions, we set our standard high, namely no change in score shown by any operatee was considered significant unless it exceeded the changes made by all of the control patients. In table 63 the

POSTOPERATIVE TESTING OF INDIVIDUAL PATIENTS ON WORD ASSOCIATION AND C

| 15 | 16 | 17 | 18 | 19 | 20 | 21 | 22 | 23 | 24 | 25 | 26 | 27 |
|----|----|----|----|----|----|----|----|----|----|----|----|----|
| *Measures* | | | | | | | | | | | | |
| Failure to respond | | Delayed assoc. RT | | Total No. compl. indic. | | Persistence | Communality | | Inaccurate reproduction | | Delayed reprod. RT | |
| A | C | A | C | A | C | C | A | C | A | C | A | C |
| 0 | 0 | − 2 | + 8 | + 2 | + 6 | 17 | + 32 | +27 | + 2 | + 3 | + 4 | 0 |
| 0 | 0 | 0 | − 2 | +13 | −17 | 1 | − 59 | +37 | +14 | − 5 | + 3 | − 5 |
| −1 | 0 | − 4 | − 1 | +15 | +10 | 19 | − 9 | − 4 | + 6 | − 1 | − 3 | + 2 |
| −1 | 0 | − 3 | + 1 | + 4 | +12 | 12 | − 23 | −45 | +14 | − 6 | − 2 | 0 |
| −2 | −1 | −11 | − 3 | + 9 | +17 | 19 | + 1 | − 4 | −18 | −11 | −11 | − 2 |
| 0 | 0 | − 4 | − 1 | − 7 | + 4 | 20 | + 19 | −24 | − 1 | − 1 | + 2 | 0 |
| 0 | 0 | + 1 | + 1 | 0 | −25 | 14 | − 8 | −10 | − 1 | − 4 | + 3 | − 3 |
| 0 | 0 | − 2 | 0 | + 7 | + 9 | 14 | − 15 | + 1 | + 5 | + 4 | + 5 | − 3 |
| 0 | 0 | + 2 | − 1 | −47 | + 3 | 6 | − 4 | + 2 | + 3 | + 8 | − 4 | − 2 |
| 0 | 0 | + 3 | + 4 | − 6 | − 4 | 18 | + 16 | + 1 | − 1 | + 6 | + 2 | − 2 |
| 0 | 0 | − 1 | − 3 | − 1 | − 4 | 11 | − 7 | +12 | + 3 | 0 | + 2 | + 1 |
| 0 | +1 | − 1 | 0 | − 4 | + 1 | 17 | + 18 | +23 | − 3 | − 6 | − 4 | − 2 |
| 0 | 0 | − 4 | −10 | −27 | −14 | 20 | +113 | +19 | − 5 | − 3 | − 2 | −10 |
| +2 | +1 | +12 | + 5 | +20 | +18 | 15 | − 10 | + 8 | − 3 | +11 | + 7 | + 6 |
| 0 | 0 | + 2 | − 1 | + 8 | − 7 | 9 | − 45 | +15 | + 8 | + 5 | + 3 | + 2 |
| 0 | 0 | + 3 | + 6 | + 3 | +12 | 13 | − 2 | + 1 | − 2 | 0 | + 3 | 0 |
| −6 | −3 | − 4 | +13 | − 8 | + 6 | 22 | + 6 | +31 | −10 | − 3 | − 5 | +19 |
| −2 | 0 | − 6 | − 7 | −19 | −11 | 13 | +124 | +34 | − 6 | − 3 | 0 | + 3 |
| 0 | 0 | − 7 | + 1 | −22 | −12 | 17 | − 30 | +15 | − 1 | − 2 | + 1 | − 1 |
| 0 | 0 | +11 | + 1 | +13 | +14 | 5 | − 19 | −53 | − 5 | −10 | +20 | + 1 |
| 0 | +3 | + 7 | + 7 | + 3 | +18 | 18 | − 33 | −38 | − 8 | + 6 | +10 | + 5 |
| 0 | 0 | − 1 | + 1 | + 1 | + 6 | 9 | + 9 | − 2 | − 2 | 0 | + 2 | − 2 |
| 0 | −1 | + 5 | + 8 | + 8 | + 2 | 4 | − 13 | +24 | −20 | − 5 | +14 | + 5 |
| 0 | 0 | − 5 | + 1 | −16 | − 3 | 17 | + 43 | +23 | + 3 | 0 | − 1 | + 2 |
| 0 | −2 | − 1 | − 7 | − 6 | − 1 | 24 | + 6 | + 6 | + 1 | + 3 | + 1 | − 1 |
| −1 | 0 | 0 | 0 | − 9 | − 7 | 21 | + 45 | +18 | − 3 | − 1 | + 1 | 0 |

Bold face indicates increase in score greater than that shown by any control.
*Italics* indicates decrease in score greater than that shown by any control (excl. Persistence).

bold face figures indicate **marked increases** in score greater than those shown by any controls, the italicized figures indicate *marked decreases* in score greater than those shown by any controls. *Marked deviations* are increases or decreases in score greater than the comparable increases or decreases in score made by any control patient.

**Complex Indicators.** Frontal lobe operations bring about a clinically observable alleviation of mental symptoms and a social recovery in some mental patients. When such recovery does take place, the change has been described as "bleaching of affect" or a general decrease in emotionality. Previous studies with the Word Association Test have indicated that word association tends to be affected by emotional disturbances, and that evidences of these disturbances may be seen in the presence of complex indicators. Hence, it might be expected that those operatees in this study who showed improvement would give evidence of decreased emotional disturbance by decreased scores on the complex indicators.

Columns 7 to 18 inclusive of table 63 give the increases and decreases in score from preoperative to postoperative testing on the complex indicators for Tests A and C. Examination of the marked deviations on each of the indicators for Tests A and C separately in relation to the associated variables shows there was no regular relationship between marked increases or decreases in score on any single indicator for Test A or Test C and areas excised, social improvement rating, sex, age, or I.Q. Examination of the marked deviations shows further that there was no systematic relationship between the occurrence of marked deviations for the individual operatees on any single indicator and the occurrence of marked deviations for the same patients on any other indicator on either Test A or Test C.

Analysis of the total number of marked increases and decreases in score shown by the individual operatees on all of the complex indicators combined reveals that neither the total number of marked increases or decreases in score on Test A or Test C was consistently related to any of the associated variables.

Columns 19 and 20 of table 63 give the changes (R2-O) in the total number of complex indicators for Tests A and C respectively. Patients 7 and 40 showed a marked increase and patients 25 and 38 a marked decrease on Total Number of Complex Indicators, Test A. Patients 6, 19, and 38 showed a marked decrease on the same measure on Test C. Examination of the operatees who showed these marked changes reveals the following:

Patient 6 (male; age, 33; I.Q. 92; very slight social improvement; areas 6 and 8 excised) showed a marked increase in score on Rare Responses, Test A, and a marked decrease on Rare Responses, Test C, together with a marked decrease on Clangs, Test C. The two decreases on Test C accounted for the marked decrease on Total Number of Complex Indicators, Test C. The marked change for this patient on Test C, while in the direction expected by hypothesis, was not an accurate reflection of social improvement rating.

Patient 19 (male; age, 50; I.Q. 102; no social improvement; area 45 excised) showed a marked decrease of Stimulus Repetition, Test C, of such magnitude that it placed him in the group who showed an over-all decrease on Total Number of Complex Indicators, Test C. This change was inconsistent with the patient's failure to show a social improvement.

Patient 25 (male; age, 58; I.Q. 95; very marked 8-point social improvement; areas 8, 9, and 46 excised) employed a large number of stimulus repetitions on Test A preoperatively and only a single stimulus repetition postoperatively. The marked decrease in score on Stimulus Repetition, Test A, accounted for the marked decrease on Total Number of Complex Indicators, Test A, and was consistent with the patient's social improvement rating. It is to be noted that none of the indicators, with the exception of Stimulus Repetition, reflected the marked social improvement made by this patient.

Patient 38 (female; age, 38; I.Q. 106; very marked 8-point social improvement; no excision, venous ligation over areas 8, 9, and 10) showed a marked decrease in score on both Clangs and Rare Responses, Test A, and a marked decrease in Delayed

Association Reaction Time, Test C. These decreases accounted for the fact that on both Tests A and C patient 38 showed a marked decrease on Total Number of Complex Indicators, and were in accordance with the marked social improvement noted for this patient.

Patient 7 (male; age, 40; I.Q. 93; marked 5-point social improvement; areas 8, 9, and 10 excised) showed marked increases in score on Multiverbality, Tests A and C, the former of which resulted in a marked increase on Total Number of Complex Indicators, Test A. The change on Test A was not in accordance with the clinically observed improvement of this patient.

Patient 40 (female; age, 29; I.Q. 91; no improvement; areas 24 and 32 excised) showed a marked increase in score on Multiverbality, Failure to Respond, and Delayed Association Reaction Time, Test A, and a marked increase in score on Multiverbality, Test C. The marked increases on Test A accounted for the marked increase on Total Number of Complex Indicators, Test A. These changes were not consistent with the patient's improvement score of 0, insofar as the latter indicated that there was no clinical evidence of poorer emotional adjustment following operation.

From the above analysis it may be concluded that for only 2 of the 6 patients (25 and 38) who showed marked changes in the total number of complex indicators were the changes in good correspondence with social improvement ratings.

**Persistence and Communality.** It was previously noted in our discussion of table 63 that removal of portions of the frontal lobes resulted in improved mental status and social recovery in some psychotic patients. The hypothesis may be offered that this brain operation disrupts existing "association pathways" producing the opportunity for the formation of new associative connections. In the word association experiment we would then expect that associations given by the operatees preoperatively would show less stability, i.e., less tendency to persist after operation than would the associations given by the control patients. Furthermore, in keeping with their observed social recovery, the operatees would be expected to show greater increases in the communality of their associations postoperatively than the control patients.

Since Test C was administered in identical form preoperatively and postoperatively, it was possible to determine the persistence score for each patient on this test by computing the number of stimulus words to which he gave the same association preoperatively and postoperatively. The scores on Persistence, given in column 21 of table 63, indicate the number of persistent associations. The range of the number of persistent associations in the operatees was 2 to 20, out of a possible 40; in the control group the range was 4 to 24. One operatee, patient 6, was outside the control range. The very low score on Persistence of this patient was not confirmed by the score of patient 2, who had an operation similar to that of patient 6, nor by the scores of any other members of the operatee group.

Individual changes in score (R2-O) on Communality for Tests A and C are given in columns 22 and 23 respectively of table 63. Changes marked (+) indicate an increase, changes marked (−) indicate a decrease in the communality of associations. As noted in table 63, patients 6 and 49 showed a marked decrease in score on Communality, Test A, and patient 6 showed a marked increase on Communality, Test C.

The case of patient 6 was discussed above and it was pointed out that this patient made a slight social improvement (1-point) and made increased use of rare responses on Test A and less use of rare responses on Test C following operation. Rare Responses being inversely related to Communality, patient

6 appears in this latter analysis. The explanation of the marked contradiction between this patient's marked decrease in score on Communality, Test A, and marked increase in score on Communality, Test C, is not apparent. Patient 49 likewise showed a marked decrease in score on Communality, Test A, but not on Test C. The 5-point social improvement noted for patient 49 was inconsistent with her decrease in communality of associations.

Of the very few marked deviations on Persistence and Communality, neither the single marked deviation on Persistence nor those on Communality (Test A or Test C) were regularly related to any of the associated variables.

**Reproduction.** The Persistence measure described above gave evidence of the stability of associations from preoperative to postoperative testing. The stability of associations was also studied over a much shorter interval by the method of immediate reproduction. Columns 24 to 27 inclusive of table 63 give the increases and decreases in score from preoperative to postoperative testing on Inaccurate Reproduction and Delayed Reproduction Reaction Time for Tests A and C. Examination of the marked deviations of the operatees on these measures reveals the following facts:

Five patients, 6, 7, 8, 21, and 49, showed a marked increase in score on Inaccurate Reproduction, Test A. Included in this group were 3 patients, 7, 21, and 49, who had area 10 removed. The relationship between defective reproduction and removal of area 10, while noteworthy, was not statistically significant. The marked increases on Inaccurate Reproduction, Test A, were not regularly related to social improvement rating, sex, age, or I.Q. There were no marked decreases in score on Inaccurate Reproduction, Test A.

Patients 25 and 40 showed a marked increase and patient 13 a marked decrease in score on Inaccurate Reproduction, Test C. The marked deviations of these patients were not significantly related to any of the associated variables.

One patient, 13, showed a marked decrease in score on Delayed Reproduction Reaction Time, Test A, and 4 patients, 6, 19, 21, and 38, showed a marked decrease in score on Delayed Reproduction Reaction Time, Test C. Neither the marked decreases on Test A nor on Test C were systematically related to any of the associated variables. There were no marked increases in score on Delayed Reproduction Reaction Time on either Test A or Test C.

**Total Marked Changes.** When the total number of marked changes (the sum of the marked increases and decreases in score on Tests A and C combined*) shown by the individual operatees was related to social improvement rating, age, and I.Q., the following rank-difference coefficients of correlation were obtained:

Total marked changes—Improvement ratings: $r = .56 \pm .13$
Total marked changes—Age (youth): $r = .51 \pm .13$
Total marked changes—I.Q.: $r = -.26 \pm .17$

These correlations indicate a significant positive relationship (at the .05 level of confidence) between total marked changes and both improvement rating and age (youth); and a nonsignificant negative relationship between total marked changes and I.Q. Since these correlations are based on a small sample and are not very large, they must be noted with due caution.

When the total number of marked changes shown by those patients who had a common area removed was determined (disregarding whether the area

---

* Communality and Persistence were omitted from this total, the former because it was inversely related to Rare Responses, which was included among the complex indicators, and the latter because it did not provide a difference score.

was removed singly or in combination with other areas), the average total number of marked changes which was associated with the removal of that area was readily calculable. The separate areas removed, the number of patients having each area removed, and the average total marked changes for the individual areas are shown in table 64. This tabulation indicates that when the average total marked changes were listed in order of magnitude,

TABLE 64.  AVERAGE TOTAL MARKED CHANGES

| Areas excised[a] | No. of patients | Average total marked changes |
|---|---|---|
| 6 | 1 | 5.0 |
| 8 | 5 | 2.4 |
| 9 | 5 | 2.4 |
| 10 | 4 | 2.3 |
| 46 | 3 | 1.3 |
| 45 | 2 | 1.0 |
| 11 | 2 | 0.0 |

[a] Patient 8 (middle frontal gyrus removed), patient 38 (venous ligation over areas 8, 9, and 10), and patient 40 (areas 24 and 32 removed) were omitted from this tabulation because the operations performed on these patients could not be compared to the operations performed on any of the other operatees.

the areas whose removal was associated with these changes lay in a plane extending rostrally across the cortex. A similar gradient was obtained for the total number of marked changes on the complex indicators.

### COMPARISON OF TESTS A AND C

A comparison was made of Tests A and C with respect to the number and direction of the marked changes each had shown on the individual complex indicators and mnemonic measures. It was found that, in general, while Tests A and C were not equivalent tests, they were not in disagreement and showed approximately the same capacity to distinguish operatees from controls under the conditions of this study.

### SUMMARY OF RESULTS

1. The only statistically significant changes in the operatee group which might be attributed to removal of brain tissue from the frontal lobes were an increase in Inaccuracy of Reproduction on Test A and a decrease in the number of Delayed Reproduction Reaction Times on Test C.

2. Neither the marked increases or decreases in the occurrence of complex indicators in the associations of the operatees (on Tests A or C) were regularly related to areas excised, social improvement rating, sex, age, or I.Q.

3. There was no systematic relationship between marked changes in the communality of associations or the stability of associations (as measured by Persistence or by Inaccuracy of Reproduction) and areas excised, social improvement rating, sex, age, or I.Q.

4. There was a significant positive correlation for the operatee group between total number of marked changes in score (marked increases and de-

creases on Tests A and C combined) and social improvement rating (r = .56), as well as between total number of marked changes and youth (r = .51).

5. The average total number of marked changes which was associated with the removal of each of the various areas was found to be greatest for area 6 and decreased consistently in the nature of a gradient extending rostrally across the cortex.

DISCUSSION

Did removal of brain tissue from the frontal lobes produce changes in the association process which were reflected by changes in performance on the Word Association Tests? The only statistically significant differences between preoperative and postoperative performance on the Word Association Tests were an increase in Inaccuracy of Reproduction on Test A and a decrease in the number of Delayed Reproduction Reaction Times on Test C. In each instance the comparable change on the other test, though not statistically significant, was in the same direction. Since no other findings on the mnemonic measures, i.e. stability, were statistically significant and since the memory and learning scores obtained by Stauffer (chapter 15) with Paired Associates on these same patients failed to show regular changes following operation, we are not inclined to attribute our significant findings to changes in memory efficiency nor to attach any particular meaning to them.

As previously noted, the operatees, as compared with the controls, did not show a decrease in the stability of their associations as measured by Persistence. In interpreting this finding the manner in which persistence was measured should be recalled. When the same association was given to a stimulus word both before and after operation, that association was said to "persist." When the test was administered postoperatively, the patient was not instructed to give the same association he had given preoperatively. Memory was involved in persistence, then, to the extent that all verbal associations are dependent on previous learning or an habitual mode of response. Removal of portions of frontal lobe tissue did not affect this measure and presumably did not result in the disruption of old, well-established associations. The same point was borne out by the failure to obtain differential changes in the communality of associations.

Were there any changes in performance on the Word Association Tests which reflected the clinically observed social improvement of the operatees? When the total number of marked changes (on the several measures of Tests A and C combined) of the individual operatees were related to social improvement ratings, a significant positive correlation was obtained. However, neither the marked increases nor marked decreases in score on the test measures, either singly or in combination, were systematically related to social improvement ratings. It may be accordingly concluded that the operatees who improved tended to show more marked changes in performance on Word Association Tests than did the unimproved operatees, but their improvement was not regularly reflected in the direction of the changes they showed.

Were the changes in performance on the Word Association Tests in any way related to the specific areas of the frontal lobes removed? Neither the marked increases nor marked decreases in scores of the operatees on the test measures, either singly or in combination, were regularly related to areas excised. When the average total number of marked changes (on Tests A and C combined) which were associated with the removal of each of the areas were arranged in order of magnitude, a gradient was obtained. This gradient indicated that there were progressively more marked changes with the removal of the more caudal areas of the frontal lobes than with the removal of the more rostral areas.

The hypotheses which were set forth early in this chapter have been verified only in part. Removal of brain tissue from the frontal lobes of man *did* produce changes in performance on the Word Association Tests. These changes did reflect improvement in emotional and social adjustment, but not in the simple and direct manner we had anticipated. There was no decrease in the number of complex indicators, nor was there an increase in the communality of associations which could be significantly correlated with clinical estimate of social improvement. The manner in which social improvement was reflected in performance has already been discussed.

There was no clear-cut evidence of "interference with the associative process." There was no decrease in the stability of associations, as measured by their persistence or as reflected by changes in the communality of associations.

## SUMMARY

1. Word association experiments were conducted one month before and four months following operation with 15 mental patients from whom bilaterally symmetrical portions of the frontal lobes (approximating Brodmann's areas) were removed, and with 11 mental patients not subjected to operation, in order to determine whether there were changes in the emotional and mnemonic aspects of association which regularly followed operation.

2. The preoperative and postoperative responses to two word association tests were analyzed for changes in the occurrence of complex indicators, for changes in the communality of associations, and for the stability of associations as measured by persistence and by changes in immediate reproduction.

3. Comparison of the operatee and control groups revealed that the only statistically significant changes from preoperative to postoperative testing which could be attributed to the effects of operation were an increase in the inaccuracy of reproduction of associations on one of the two word association tests employed and a decrease in the number of delayed reproduction reaction times on the other word association test. Since no other changes in mnemonic function were obtained, no particular interpretation of these findings was suggested.

4. Changes in score of the operatees from preoperative to postoperative testing which exceeded the changes shown by any of the control patients (marked increases or marked decreases) were related to the variables of this investigation, which included: brain areas excised, clinical estimate of social improvement, sex, age, and I.Q. Neither the marked increases nor marked decreases in scores of the operatees on any of the test measures, either singly or in combination, were found to be significantly related to any of these variables.

5. There was a tendency for the operatees who improved to show more marked changes in score (increases and decreases combined) than did the unimproved operatees.

6. The average total number of marked changes in score, disregarding the direction of change, which was associated with the removal of each of the various areas, was found to be greatest for area 6 and decreased consistently in the nature of a gradient extending rostrally across the cortex.

*Chapter 18*

# Time Judgment

JOHS CLAUSEN

---

WITH the disorganization of personality brought about by psychosis one of the first changes is a disturbance in time sense or in the correct evaluation of the passage of time. Unlike space perception which is easily anchored in external reality, time perception has few anchorages save in subjective memory. A defect in time judgment may develop so subtly that neither patient nor physician is aware of it. A time judgment experiment was incorporated in the psychologic test program because of the frequency with which such defects occur in mental patients. Furthermore, Freeman and Watts ('42) have pointed out that factors such as foresight and planfulness, in which the time sense may be involved, are usually altered by prefrontal lobotomy.

## PROCEDURE

Previous studies with normal individuals and with schizophrenic patients have indicated that both groups tend to underestimate intervals shorter than thirty seconds and overestimate longer intervals. In this experiment, in order to keep the time judgment task within the patients' attention span and in order to avoid dealing with both long and short intervals, only five-, ten-, and 15-second intervals were utilized.

The apparatus used in this experiment consisted of an electrically driven stop clock which could be read to a hundredth of a second, attached in series with an electric lamp, buzzer, and key. When the key was depressed, the circuit was made, starting the clock and the lamp, also the buzzer if it was switched into the circuit. When the key was released the circuit was opened, the clock stopped and the light and the sound ceased.

Three types of time judgment tasks were used: reproduction, verbal estimation, and operative estimation. In the reproduction experiment the experimenter would hold down the key for a given interval (either five, ten, or fifteen seconds) and would ask the subject to duplicate this demonstrated time interval by holding down the key for an equal length of time. The second task, that of verbal estimation, consisted of having the patient guess and name the actual duration of a time interval, of five, ten, or fifteen seconds, set by the experimenter. The third task, that of operative estimation of time intervals, consisted of telling the patient to hold down the key for five, ten, or fifteen seconds to demonstrate how long he thought these intervals lasted. Each of the patient's performances was clocked and recorded to the nearest hundredth of a second.

In each of these three experiments, twelve readings were taken distributed in random order among the three time intervals. Half of these readings were taken

254

during quiet or unfilled time conditions and the other half with the buzzer sounding —filled time conditions. We found that no one of the three types of judging time was affected by the intervals being filled or unfilled.

## RESULTS

An examination of the intercorrelation between the scores obtained in these time judgment experiments and the other psychologic test results showed that operative estimation of fifteen seconds correlates above the .01 level of confidence with Number of Rorschach responses, Wechsler-Bellevue Similarities, Wechsler-Bellevue Picture Completion, Sorting Test Grouping (PI-1), and Years of Schooling. An intellectual factor seemed to be common to these tests. After operation all these correlations decreased except that with Years of Schooling. For example, Wechsler-Bellevue Similarities correlated +.46 with Time Judgment originally and +.07 after operation. Years in school correlated +.55 at O and +.44 at R2. It is difficult to explain why these significant correlations with an intellectual factor should disappear. It is interesting to contrast this result to Halstead's ('47) finding that his time judgment test correlated +.43 with his psychometric intelligence factor (C).

The intercorrelations between the three tasks indicated that the task of reproducing time intervals was basically different from that of either verbal or operative estimation. The last two, verbal and operative estimation, correlated —.60. Within each time judgment task the several subtests generally correlated significantly with each other but these correlations were not as large in the reproduction task.

In the reproduction of time intervals the patients tended to overestimate the duration of the five-second interval, holding the key down for an average of 5.59 seconds. For the ten- and fifteen-second intervals they tended to underestimate the duration, the average figures being 9.86 and 13.72 respectively. The operation failed to produce any constant alteration in the behavior of the operatee group when compared with the control. The control group, however, decreased in variability of time judgment while the operatee group failed to make such a decrease. This held true of both the filled and the unfilled intervals but did not hold true of all of the longer intervals. It may be concluded that reproduction of short time intervals was not affected by the operation.

In verbally estimating the length of time intervals, the patients tended to overestimate the absolute duration from two to three times its actual duration. On the average they named five seconds as 14.68; ten seconds as 27.59 and fifteen seconds as 34.41. On the postoperative retest the two groups did not differ significantly in their means but they did differ significantly in their variability. The operation produced several contrary trends within the operatee group, causing its members to vary from each other considerably in their postoperative change in time judgment. The individual patients in whom these contrary trends were produced did not have in common any such external criteria as area excised or degree of cortical damage. It may be concluded that the topectomy operation did not interfere with the ability to estimate time intervals verbally.

In the task of operative estimation of a five-, ten-, or fifteen-second interval both the control and the operatee group tended to underestimate the three intervals, releasing the key sooner than the absolute time interval required.

The average estimation of five seconds was 4.42, of ten seconds was 8.40, and of fifteen seconds was 11.47. After operation the ten- and fifteen-second intervals were still underestimated but the five-second interval was overestimated in both groups. The operation failed to produce a change in the mean difference between the operatee and the control groups, but the variability of the control group became somewhat greater on the retest. In general it may be concluded that the operation did not interfere with this type of time judgment.

For the reproduction and operative estimation the variability in the operatee group failed to decrease to the same extent as was the case in the control group. For verbal estimation the variability in the operatee group remained at the same level whereas there was an expansion in variability in the control group, largely caused by 2 patients.

## DISCUSSION

In general the operation did not produce any significant alteration in these aspects of the time judgment task. Certain discrepancies appeared between the three parts of the experiment. This was not surprising since, as we have shown, the time tasks do not involve the same underlying function. The reproduction of time intervals appears independent of the particular method of evaluating the passage of time which characterizes the subject. His own personal time units may be long or short but as long as these remain constant he will be able to reproduce accurately a given interval set by the examiner. In the other two tasks a direct link exists between the subject's personal time and clock time. If his personal time moves rapidly, he will take a shorter period for estimating the five-second interval and he will name an absolute five seconds more than its true clock value. This, then, is the reason that the correlation between reproduction of time intervals and the verbal and operative estimation of time intervals was low and the correlation between verbal and operative estimation of time intervals would be negative, which is what we found. Despite this basic difference in task, the operation failed to change any of these different time judgment functions.

## Chapter 19

# Critical Flicker Frequency*

### KATHLEEN MARY YOUNG

---

STIMULATION of the eye by regular intermittent flashes of light at frequencies ranging between 5 and 40 per second produces the sensory phenomenon of flicker. The frequency which just produces the impression of steady illumination, or the sensory effect called fusion, is known as the critical flicker frequency, or CFF.

The experiments reported in the literature on this phenomenon, dealing with the stimulus variables affecting the CFF, have been concerned for the most part with the theoretical implications of the findings for visual physiology. A brief survey of this literature will serve to indicate certain of the factors which affect the CFF.

Perhaps the most widely studied relationship has been that between flicker frequency and illumination intensity. Talbot's Law (Bartley, 41, pp. 117-119), which is concerned with the magnitude of the sensory impression, has been experimentally verified by different investigators. When the sensory effect is one of fusion, the level of illumination is equivalent to the original illumination multiplied by the fraction which the actual duration of illumination is of the total duration of a complete cycle of illumination and darkness. From this stated relationship, it is clear that a reduction in the duration of illumination results in a reduction of the perceived intensity. Another direct measurable relationship states that the critical frequency is proportional to the logarithm of the illumination intensity. In plotting this relationship, the CFF tends to rise with an increase in intensity, forming a plateau in the middle of the curve, then rises again with the intensity up to a certain point, from which it declines with further increases in intensity. The lower portion of the curve apparently represents the function of the rods, and the upper portion the function of the cones. Hecht and Smith ('36) report that the relation of critical frequency to intensity is a single function for foveal areas between 2 degrees, where the retina contains only cones, and a dual function for the larger regions, which contains rods as well.

The relative duration of the light and dark periods also affects the CFF. For a given intensity, the CFF is maximal when the light-dark ratio is equal. When the light time is longer, the CFF is lowered. In terms of intensity, then, the longer the light time, the higher the intensity required for a given CFF.

* This chapter was submitted in partial fulfillment of the requirements for the degree of Doctor of Philosophy in the Faculty of Pure Science, Columbia University.

Another factor influencing the CFF is that of the size of the test field. The larger the area, the higher the maximum CFF. This relationship has been explained in terms of the neural structure of the retina.

The above findings have been interpreted by Hecht ('34) in terms of a photochemical theory of visual processes. He states, "the general form of most of the existing relationships in the effects of intermittent illuminations are already apparent in the characteristics of the behavior of the initial photochemical event." Other investigators have utilized the material to demonstrate features of retinal processes.

The effects of age and sex and the influence of practice and set upon the CFF have also been reported (Knox, '45; Misiak, '47). There is a considerable decrease in the average CFF in old age, which has been said to be associated with degeneration of the optic nerve or cerebrum. No sex differences were found. The CFF, while fairly stable, can be modified within certain limits by practice and set.

There are few studies dealing directly with the effect of removal of cortical areas on the CFF. In animal experimentation, a study of flicker discrimination before and after removal of the visual cortex in the cat has been reported. (Morgan, '43). Flicker discrimination was found to be considerably impaired by the operation, particularly at high illuminations. With prolonged training, however, the animals subjected to operation regain their normal sensitivity at all levels of illumination, "so it cannot be held that the cortex is absolutely necessary for cone functions in flicker vision." For this reason, it has been suggested that what occurs with striate removal is an interference with the animal's ability to give its "attention" to visual stimuli, rather than with cone functions as such.

Poppelreuter ('17) has reported that patients sustaining injuries to the striate area of the occipital lobe show defects in visual efficiency on numerous tests of visual functions. By this, he meant that such a patient is somewhat visually inefficient and handicapped in performance. He can do the required tasks, but not with the speed or effectiveness commonly shown by a person with an intact cortex. It was his finding which suggested that the impaired CFF shown in the animal study might be dependent, at least in part, on factors other than the optic mechanism itself.

To date, there has been little reported dealing specifically with the effect on CFF of removal of cortical tissue in human beings. Recently, Teuber and Bender ('48) determined the CFF of a group of 28 naval casualties who had sustained injuries to the occipital lobes, and found that their CFF was significantly lower than the CFF of 20 normal subjects. They conclude that "neural rather than photochemical factors limit perception in brain-injured patients, and that the limiting factor is an abnormal slowness of the cerebral function subserving vision." Halstead's ('47) research, from which he reported that frontal lobe injury has a definite effect upon the CFF, served as the starting point for the present investigation. He formulated his findings in terms of a concept of "biological intelligence," as this concept is related to brain function. The concept of biological intelligence is perhaps best understood in terms of the operational definition which Halstead offers. An original test battery of twenty-seven tests was set up which satisfied the following criteria: (1) differentiation between brain-injured and normal individuals, (2) tests of personality functions, (3) tests of psychometric intelligence and, (4) tests of sensory capacities. From results on 237 subjects, thirteen tests were selected which seemed likely to reflect varied aspects of biological intelligence. A statistical factor analysis of these data yielded four factors. The flicker test was included in this battery, and its correlation with the memory component of the tactual discrimination test, and the central form and color components of the Halstead dynamic visual field tests comprised what Halstead has called P or the "power factor." Halstead wrote, "The P factor is a dynamic factor which, in terms of a single estimation, probably reflects the overall status of the brain . . . Its specific physiology is unknown, but it would not be surprising should it be found to parallel those vital processes which sustain the brain and cortex at a high level of efficiency." The basis for this statement lies in the fact that "the writer and his associates have been able to demonstrate a direct relationship between brain wave activity and certain essential features of the flicker fusion test." In applying the flicker test to a group of subjects including frontal and nonfrontal lobectomy subjects, normal and miscellaneous controls, he found that the frontal lobectomy subjects gave a significantly lower CFF than the rest of the subjects, and that they were less variable, that is more accurate, in locating the fusion point. These findings he interpreted as indicating that injury to the frontal lobes results in a less efficient functioning of the brain.

While the Halstead hypothesis concerning the use of flicker as a means of estimating the efficiency of brain functioning is an interesting construct, four aspects of his experimental procedure suggested that replication of the experiment would be worth while: (1) Halstead had no preoperative data on his subjects. (2) The extent and influence of the already existing damage to the brain, which necessitated the operation, was a circumstance whose influence on the performance is difficult to estimate. (3) In reporting the data on the flicker test, the CFF, and the average deviation measures of the miscellaneous controls are strikingly similar to that of the frontal lobectomy subjects, although Halstead gives no explanation for this. (4) His group contained data on psychiatric patients including scores on the same individuals before and after lobotomy as two separate and not directly compared entries.

In summary, the literature on the CFF has been concerned mainly with the study of retinal processes, and with an investigation of the factors affecting the CFF. There is evidence that the CFF is influenced by cerebral events, particularly since Halstead has assigned a definite effect on the CFF caused by frontal lobe injury.

In the light of previous research, the present investigation was designed to answer the following questions: (1) Is there a significant alteration in CFF following topectomy? and if so, (2) What anatomic, physiologic, or psychologic variables are associated with this alteration? and (3) Is there a decrease in the variability of the individual determinations of the CFF, i.e. is flicker discrimination more, or less, accurate following operation?

## DETERMINATION OF CRITICAL FLICKER FREQUENCY

**Subjects.** Not all of the 48 patients who were studied in the entire project were sufficiently cooperative to provide satisfactory reports from which to obtain CFF thresholds. We have limited the present report to results obtained with 17 operatees and 13 control patients. As table 65 shows, the two groups were fairly well equated as to background factors.

**Apparatus.** A stroboscopic tachometer (Strobotac, General Radio Co., Type 631 B) was used. This is essentially a gas-filled lamp which will give a flash of light having a duration of five to ten microseconds when a condenser is discharged through it. A variable condenser permits flashing at rates varying from 600 to 14,400 per minute. The speed of the flashing may be read directly from a scale graduated in flashes per minute. A knob permits the experimenter to control the rate of flashing.

A cardboard box measuring 15 by 15 by 9 inches, with a gray piece of cardboard, measuring 18 by 13 inches, covering the front, contained the Strobotac. The subject saw only the gray cardboard, which had a circular aperture, measuring 2 inches in diameter, cut out at its center and covered with milk glass. Within the box, the Strobotac was placed at a distance of 9 inches from the aperture. The subject sat so that there was a distance of approximately 2 feet from his eyes to the milk glass.

**Procedure.** The subjects were tested two or three weeks preoperatively, three weeks postoperatively, and four months postoperatively. Hereafter these three testing periods will be referred to as O (original testing), R1 (retest 1), and R2 (retest 2).

TABLE 65.  COMPOSITION OF THE GROUP, MEAN AND RANGE ON
BACKGROUND VARIABLES

|  | N | Age Mean | Age Range | I.Q. Mean | I.Q. Range | Years of schooling Mean | Years of schooling Range | Sex M | Sex F | Known visual anomalies |
|---|---|---|---|---|---|---|---|---|---|---|
| Operatees....... | 17 | 43.5 | 18–61 | 100.1 | 84–131 | 9 | 6–12.5 | 11 | 6 | None |
| Controls........ | 13 | 45.2 | 19–59 | 104.5 | 81–121 | 8.5 | 0–19 | 10 | 3 | None |

Each subject sat facing the circular glass window. His attention was directed to the flickering screen, and he was cautioned to look directly at the window. The directions were as follows: "You can see there a window of light which is flickering. Tell me when it stops flickering, and becomes a steady light." The frequency was then increased until the subject reported a steady light. After a notation of the frequency at the time of the report, the frequency was further increased, and the subject was told: "Now the window shows a steady light; tell me when it begins to flicker." The frequency was then decreased until the subject reported a flickering light, and the frequency at which this report occurred was noted.

The above procedure was repeated until five ascending readings (a report of fusion) and five descending readings (a report of flicker), a total of ten determinations, were made. The ascending and descending readings were made alternately.

The averages for the ascending and descending readings were obtained separately. These two averages were then averaged to obtain the *critical flicker frequency*.

## RESULTS

Four scores may be considered in the treatment of group results. Three of these are threshold determinations: (1) average threshold of the descending series, (2) average threshold of the ascending series, (3) the critical flicker frequency, which is the average of the combined ascending and descending series. The fourth score deals with each individual's variation around his own CFF, called intra-individual variability.

The data on the threshold scores, which have been treated statistically by analysis of variance, reveal:

1. The ascending and descending series do not differ from each other nor from the combined threshold in any significant manner on the measures obtained on the two groups. These results indicate that we are justified in considering the combined threshold (the CFF) hereafter.

2. There is no statistically significant difference in the mean CFF of operatee and control groups at any of the three testing periods.

3. At the R2 testing there is a statistically significant difference at the .01 level between the groups in variability within each group. From O to the R2 testing, the operatee group exhibits a trend towards decrease in variability, their CFFs clustering closer around the mean of the group at R2. The control group exhibits a contrary trend, so that at R2 their CFFs spread more widely around the mean of the group. Analysis by covariance indicates that this difference in variability is not due to the original levels of the measures.

In order to gauge the variation of each individual around his own threshold, the intra-individual variability of each case was calculated. In this statistical procedure, the factors entering into the test performance of one individual, such as the difference between ascending and descending determinations, are taken into account, and the individual's variance at each of the testing periods is computed. The variances thus obtained were treated by analysis of variance. The results reveal that there are no statistically significant differences in the mean intra-individual variability between the operatees and controls at any of the three testing periods.

**Correlational Analysis.** Using data obtained with 32 patients at the preoperative test period the scores on seventy-two tests, including the CFF, were intercorrelated. There was not a single correlation between CFF and any other score which reached $+0.45$ (.01 level of significance). Five correlation values between $+0.35$ and $+0.40$ (.05 level of significance) were secured but none of the five were logically meaningful nor did they shed light on possible relationships. The CFF seemed to be a most independent variable, one which showed no evidence of entering into any relationship such as that which Halstead formed when he entered the CFF into a Power factor.

When the individual changes in CFF following operation were examined, it was found that 9 operatees exceeded or equalled the largest decrease shown by any control patient at R1, and that 7 of the 9 still exceeded or equalled at the R2 testing. No operatee showed an increase in CFF equal to that shown by any control patient. When the patients were ranked in order of amount of decrease, the correlation between the R1 and R2 testing periods is $+0.81$, indicating that the direction of change shown tends to be consistent at the two testing periods. The operatees exhibit a relatively consistent change following operation, namely a decreased CFF. The change in CFF at R1 and R2 was subjected to correlational analysis together with the background factors of age, I.Q., years of schooling, weight of cortical tissue excised, and social recovery rating. No one of the correlations approached statistical significance. In a similar way the CFF changes at R2 were correlated with the changes shown in other psychologic test variables. The correlation with changes on anxiety scores was $+0.04$, with symptoms $+0.30$, Porteus M.A. $+0.42$, and complex performance test $-0.14$. None of these correlations indicated a substantial relationship.

Was this decrease associated with the removal of certain areas? Inspection of table 66 indicates that there is no clear association between area removed and the amount of decrease exhibited.

Further examination of the individual records showed that 9 operatees and only 3 control patients showed a loss in CFF from O to R1 followed by a small gain between R1 and R2. Eight of the 9 were the same individuals who exceeded or equalled the controls at R1, and 7 of the 8 were the same as those who equalled or exceeded at R2. The remaining patients in the operatee group showed patterns of change which were similar to the control group patterns, in that most patients exhibited an increase in CFF from O to R2.

TABLE 66.   DECREASING RANK ORDER OF OPERATEES IN AMOUNT OF CHANGE IN CFF PRODUCED BY OPERATION, WITH PORTIONS OF THE FRONTAL CORTEX ABLATED OR INVOLVED AND THE OBTAINED CFF FOR EACH TESTING PERIOD

| Patient No. | Areas involved | CFF | | | |
|---|---|---|---|---|---|
| | | 0 | R1 | R2 | R4 |
| 49 | 10, 11[a], 46[a] | 26.2 | 22.5 | 22.1 | 24.1 |
| 4 | 46 | 26.5 | 22.7 | 23.6 | 24.1 |
| 7 | 8, 9[a], 10[a] | 26.3 | 23.6 | 23.5 | 23.6 |
| 40 | 24[a] | 28.6 | 25.6 | 26.1 | 25.0 |
| 21 | 10 | 24.9 | 20.1 | 22.6 | 22.6 |
| 38 | 6[b], 8[b], 9[b], 10[b] | 23.9 | 20.1 | 21.6 | 20.4 |
| 6 | 6[a], 8[a] | 24.0 | 20.5 | 21.9 | 21.5 |
| 3 | 6[a], 9[a] | 23.2 | 20.1 | 21.8 | 21.4 |
| 8 | 8[a], 9[a], 10[a], 46[a] | 22.4 | 21.4 | 22.3 | 22.7 |
| 25 | 8, 9, 10[a], 46 | 24.2 | 22.9 | 24.6 | 22.5 |
| 32 | 10[a], 44[a], 45, 46[a] | 22.2 | 22.1 | 22.7 | 23.1 |
| 31 | 9 | 20.6 | 19.4 | 21.5 | 20.4 |
| 2 | 6[a], 8 | 22.9 | 24.1 | 23.9 | 21.7 |
| 36 | 10, 11, 45, 46, 47 | 21.7 | 20.6 | 22.7 | 22.7 |
| 13 | 9[a], 10[a], 45, 46 | 19.4 | 17.3 | 20.5 | 21.2 |
| 27 | 6[a], 8[a], 9[a], 10[a] | 19.0 | 21.6 | 21.3 | 21.3 |
| 19 | 45[a] | 17.5 | 19.4 | 20.6 | 21.1 |

[a] Partial excision of area.
[b] Venous ligation affecting area.

This decrease in CFF from O to R1 with some slight increase to R2 was shown by patients 3, 4, 6, 7, 8, 21, 38, 40, and 49. The mean of the preoperative CFF for these 9 patients was 25.0; of the remaining 8 operatees it was 20.9; of the control group it was 21.2. At R2 these means were respectively 22.9, 22.2, and 19.9. Seemingly the operatees who had high preoperative CFFs suffered a reduction while those who were originally at the lower end of the distribution were but slightly changed. It would be interesting to know whether this reduction occurs only in individuals with high CCFs but we must wait for further investigation to clarify the point.

Of the 9 patients listed above, only patients 6, 8, and 40 failed to show social improvement after the operation. That is, 6 of the 9 were improved socially by the operation. The patients who improved and failed to show either of these CFF changes were patients 25 and 27.

## DISCUSSION AND CONCLUSIONS

In the light of these findings we may now examine the questions asked at the beginning of the study: "Will there be an alteration in CFF following frontal lobe topectomy?" and, "Will CFF variability be decreased by the operation?"

In examining group data there was no over-all decrease in CFF among all operatees nor was there a general decrease in the intra-individual variability at R1 or R2.

Nine of the 17 operatees showed a decreased CFF following operation. This decrease was most marked in those who had an originally high CFF. This loss was greatest three weeks postoperatively, and was in several instances slightly regained four months postoperatively. Six of the 9 who showed this change also showed clear social improvement from their psychoses.

The CFF with this group was a most independent variable. It failed to correlate with any of the scores on other psychologic tests before operation. The changes in CFF following operation were not regularly or consistently related to the changes which occurred in other psychologic tests. The changes in CFF were not related to the particular area or areas of cortical tissue removed, nor to the amount of tissue excised. The CFF changes were not related to any of the biochemical, hematological, or electroencephalographic changes. In brief, there was no regular association between CFF changes and any other psychologic or physiologic variable at our disposal. One particular sort of CFF change tended to be associated with social improvement.

Thus we find that not all operatees show alterations in CFF but that those who had a relatively high CFF before operation showed a clear decrease postoperatively. We did not find a decreased intra-individual variability in CFF as Halstead ('47) reported. We were unable to find evidence that CFF belonged in some combination with other psychologic test results which Halstead combined into a Power factor.

As mentioned above, Poppelreuter ('17), on the basis of tachistoscopic investigation of visual perception in brain-injured patients, reported a decreased efficiency in performance which has been called by Morgan ('43) a reduction in visual attention. We are not inclined to consider that the change which we found could be properly called one of attention, although it was a decrease in visual efficiency.

The meaning or significance of our findings is not clear. Further investigation must be conducted before we will be able to assess the meaning of this tendency for a decreased CFF to follow brain operation.

# Chapter 20

# Affectivity*

MORTIMER GARRISON, JR.

---

"The human brain possesses an extreme prefrontal cortex which is scarcely represented at all in lower mammals and nowhere approaches the human development. This region is in especially intimate relation with the thalamus through the so-called anterior peduncle of the thalamus, probably by both descending and ascending fibers. Keeping in mind that the thalamus appears to be the organ par excellence of affective experience, this thalamofrontal connection may provide for the addition within the prefrontal field of affective impulses of thalamic origin. The emotional drive which is so powerful a component of much intentionally directed effort is here knit into the cortical process in the field where motor patterns are in process of fabrication. Affective experience thus cooperates with cognitive experience in shaping the course of action and giving the response its dynamic power and volitional motivation. This is a very attractive hypothesis, though, it must be admitted, not adequately supported anatomically or physiologically." (Herrick, '26.)

Herrick ('26) has given the essence of the opinion of many investigators, namely that changes in emotional reactions do or should follow destruction of frontal lobe tissue or the severing of the connections between the thalamus and the frontal cortex. That such phenomena do occur is supported by the review of the extensive literature on unilateral and bilateral prefrontal lobectomy reported by Freeman and Watts ('42). These authors conclude:

". . . . That a great deal more has been learned about the functioning of the brain without the frontal lobes than has been learned about the function of the frontal lobes themselves. Practically every individual who has studied these patients sees them from a different angle and evolves a more or less different hypothesis concerning the function of the part removed . . . It is our intention to show that under certain circumstances an individual can think more clearly and more productively with less brain in actual operation." (p. 74.)

In effort to ameliorate the psychologic effects of mental disease, Freeman and Watts have developed an operation known as prefrontal lobotomy. They argue that this operation produces minimal effect in terms of the destruction of cortical cells and maintain that, since association fibers between those cells which are most directly affected by the operation are not severed, these cells may still function by means of their intimate connections with other undamaged cortical cells. They report clinical success with this method particularly in the cases of involutional depressions and obsessive tension states.

* This chapter was submitted in partial fulfillment of the requirements for the degree of Doctor of Philosophy in the Faculty of Pure Science, Columbia University.

The symptoms which they regard as being most directly affected are those of introversion and preoccupation which are connected with the affective tension states. Various somatic complaints such as indigestion, palpitation, and particularly hypochondriasis have tended to disappear after operation. They report ". . . that hallucinations and delusions, so characteristic of certain 'functional' mental disorders, become attenuated and tend to disappear following prefrontal lobotomy." (p. 288.) They report that of the symptoms following prefrontal lobotomy probably only a series of symptoms headed by tactlessness and procrastination are specifically frontal in origin. They state: "There is lacking, more or less, the need on the part of the patient to push forward to new accomplishments, on the one hand, and to restrain himself, on the other, from responding to the immediate stimulus." (p. 288.)

One of the most complete studies upon personality changes after removal of cortical tissue was that of Rylander ('39). He studied patients who had undergone unilateral frontal lobectomy usually for the removal of a tumor. He made an intensive study of the patients after operation attempting to relate his findings to the preoperative personality of these patients. He concluded that changes in the emotional sphere were most common and emphasized the relation between the premorbid personality and constitution.

The conclusions of Freeman and Watts with respect to emotional changes are supported by Hutton ('47) and Kisker ('45) and other investigators. There is a loss of emotional tension, of anxiety concerning the future, and a decrease in complaints and a corresponding leveling of over-all emotional reactions. Hofstatter, Smolik, and Busch ('45) report a series of operations performed so as to sever the orbital areas from the rest of the brain and hold that there is indication that these areas have a primary role in the regulation of emotion. They report improvement in depression with agitation, a case of chronic manic state, and a decrease in somatic complaints in 2 neurasthenics after operation. Of their schizophrenic patients, they report that the hebephrenic becomes more extraverted, interested, and active; the catatonic patient loses his impulsiveness and negativism; while the paranoid patient loses his intense interest in his delusions.

Freeman and Watts ('44) hold that social improvement in mental patients following prefrontal lobotomy is accomplished through the reduction of the emotional attitude towards the self as projected into the future. They suggest that the frontal lobes are the integrative center for "consciousness of the self" and that the interruption of the thalamofrontal radiation reduces the emotion attached to the patient's image of himself so that he becomes indifferent to the opinions of others, and is unable to generate his previous tensions and anxieties.

Robinson ('46) stated that symptoms appeared to be alleviated, that there was a change from introversion to extraversion, and that there was a decrease in self-consciousness in 9 schizophrenics who were followed during their postoperative course. These changes, she believes are the expression of a defect in prolonged attention. Brickner ('36), after intensive study of his famous case, concluded that a defect in the ability to synthesize accounted for the observed changes in personality.

Hebb ('45) concluded that there has been no clear demonstration of the effects of clean surgical removal of frontal areas upon behavior. He does not think conclusions are justified at this point because of the lack of proper experimental designs and comparability of cases. Cobb ('44) is in accord with Hebb and holds that although the frontal lobes have a relation to personality there has been no real evidence adduced for localization. He considers the widespread topography and multiplicity of pathways involved are prerequisite for the effective function of the frontal lobes. Jefferson ('37) suggests that the brain must function intellectually and emotionally as a whole. He reported cases in which unilateral removal of one or the other frontal lobe was done. He states: "Those [patients] who showed no mental alteration before the operation were unaffected by partial removal of the anatomical frontal lobes, . . .

those who had mental symptoms were much better after the lobe had been excised."
He suggested that the volume of tissue remaining functional was important in determining the postoperative course.

### PROBLEM AND SUBJECTS

The problem for this study was to determine what changes were produced
by topectomy in (1) anxiety, (2) symptoms or complaints, and in (3) blocking
or frustration experimentally produced; and to show relations between such
changes produced and other variables such as social improvement, areas excised, amount of tissue excised, and the preoperative personality of the patients.

TABLE 67.  PREOPERATIVE STATUS OF PATIENTS IN THE OPERATEE AND
CONTROL GROUPS WHOSE RESULTS HAVE BEEN UTILIZED IN THE PRESENT
STUDY

|  | Operatees | Controls |
|---|---|---|
| Number | 16 | 10 |
| Male | 11 | 6 |
| Female | 5 | 4 |
| Age—average | 44.9 | 46.5 |
| Age—range | 29–61 | 25–59 |
| Education—average years | 9.3 | 9.0 |
| Education—range in years | 6–19 | 4–19 |
| Wechsler-Bellevue I.Q.—average | 102.1 | 106.3 |
| Wechsler-Bellevue I.Q.—range | 89–131 | 75–121 |

Every attempt was made to obtain representative data on all of this group
of patients one month before operation or anesthesia and four months after
operation or anesthesia. Such data were obtained on 16 operatees and 10 controls. Because of the nature of the material this number varies somewhat
within the measures reported in this study. The status of the patients utilized
in this study as regards sex, age, preoperative Wechsler-Bellevue I.Q., and
education is shown in table 67.

### EXPERIMENTAL PROCEDURE

As the literature indicates, surgical interference with the cortex of the
frontal lobes is apt to bring about affective changes in the personality of the
patient. In some but not all patients these changes are said to be a lessening
in anxiety and physical complaints and in the way in which emotional reactions take place.

The attempt was made to obtain evidence, both by allowing the patient to
express his anxieties and complaints (through the Anxiety and Complaint
Inventories) and from his emotional reactions to a situation likely to arouse
them (through the Mirror Drawing Experiment). In both cases there was adequate opportunity for the experimenter to note the observable reactions in
his appraisal of the patients.

The utility of the testing methods about to be described, particularly the inventories, is dependent upon the cooperation of the patient and his willingness to express himself in such a way as to reflect his state. From the standpoint of comparability, an attempt was made to give each patient the opportunity to react to the same measures, and the scores for each patient were derived in the same fashion. The validity of these measures can only be assessed by comparison with the patient's ward behavior and the psychiatric estimates of the patient's condition. These factors have been taken into account and with very few exceptions the conclusion seems justified that these measures do represent with a fair degree of accuracy the patient's emotional reactivity.

**Anxiety and Complaint Inventories.** To obtain measures of such personality changes a list was made up of the common anxieties of the variety usually expressed by mental hospital patients. A similar list of common complaints was drawn up. These lists were designed to aid in making up inventories in such a manner as to reflect the symptomatology associated with those diagnostic categories said to be alleviated by surgery. The questions were to reflect actual physical complaints and anxieties as well as those which might represent the effect of some more general anxiety or hypochondriacal state. As a result the questions ranged from the anxiety connected with looking down from a tall building through that connected with the future or with disturbing dreams. The complaints ranged from headaches, heart spells, and backaches to difficulty in concentrating, dizzy spells, and queer pains. Both the Anxiety and Complaint Inventories (tables 68, 69) consisted of thirty items. In order to obtain a standard report from each patient as well as an estimation of the intensity of these anxieties and complaints, each inventory was accompanied by a card with definitions of the possible answers. That for the Anxiety Inventory consisted of six steps ranging from "not at all . . ." to "extremely . . ." and that for the Complaints consisted of five steps ranging from "never" to "everyday." As will be noted in the instructions to the patient below, an attempt was made to anchor the answers to the Anxiety Inventory at each end in a described situation. The answers to the Complaint Inventory represented a report of the frequency of occurrence of each complaint.

The instructions to the patient for the Anxiety Inventory were as follows:
"Read the statements on this card." (Present response card.) "Fine. Now I am going to ask you some questions about things which make you feel afraid or anxious. For each question I ask, I want you to pick out one answer on this card that comes closest to showing how you really feel.
"Before we begin, I want to explain what the first answer means. How would you feel if you were on an elevator, high up in a building, when all of a sudden the cable broke and you realized that in about one second the elevator was going to crash down to the bottom? You would feel terribly afraid and anxious if that happened, isn't that true? A feeling like that we call 'extremely afraid or anxious' and I want you to use that answer for things that *actually do* make you feel as afraid or as anxious as you would feel if you were in that elevator. For things that you don't feel at all afraid or anxious about, use the last answer at the bottom: 'Not at all afraid or anxious.' This one ('very slightly') would be for something that makes you feel very slightly afraid or anxious—like the way you would feel if you saw a small child who had a snowball in his hand and he said he was going to throw the snowball at you, but you knew that he was too young to be able to throw it very hard. That would make you feel just the least bit anxious or afraid and that is what this particular answer means.
"You can use any answer on this list for the questions I ask you, depending

on how much each particular thing makes you feel afraid or anxious. Always pick the one answer that comes closest to showing how afraid or anxious you really feel."

The following instructions were used with the Complaint Inventory:

"Read the statements on this card." (Present response card.) "Now I am going to ask you a number of questions about how you have been feeling during the past two weeks and I would like you to use these answers. Pick out the one answer for each question which comes closest to showing how often each thing has occurred during the past two weeks."

TABLE 68. THE ANXIETY INVENTORY

*"How Afraid or Anxious Do You Usually Feel When:"*

1. You look down from a tall building.
2. You have unpleasant dreams at night.
3. You think about the personal problems you have.
4. You are introduced to an attractive woman—man (use opposite sex).
5. You think about the possibility that you might get cancer.
6. You think about having sexual intercourse.
7. You think about your being married.
8. You wake up in the morning.
9. You have to sit in a small room with the door shut.
10. You think about your father.
11. You think about the fact that you will die someday.
12. You think about the possibility that you might become insane.
13. You think about the opinion other people have of you.
14. You think of the responsibilities you will have when you leave the hospital.
15. You think about being operated upon.
16. You remember the sexual experiences you have had in the past.
17. You think about whether you are able to control yourself at times.
18. You think about God.
19. You think about your mother.
20. You think about your future.
21. You think about your hatred for some people.
22. You think about the things that you did which were morally wrong.
23. You think of how much better other people can do some things than you.
24. You remember the failures you have had in your life.
25. You feel that someone is exerting a strong influence on you over which you have no control.
26. You think that you could like a man (same sex) more than a woman.
27. You think about wishing harm or death would come to some people you know.
28. You remember the things which you have done which were queer or strange.
29. You think of going blind.
30. You think about your health at the present time.

*Scoring Card for the Anxiety Inventory*

(The weights were not printed on the card given to the patient)

*Extremely* afraid or anxious—like the feeling you would have if you were in an elevator which was going to crash down. (Weight 6)

*Very* afraid or anxious. (5)

*Fairly much* afraid or anxious. (4)

*Somewhat* afraid or anxious. (3)

*Slightly* afraid or anxious. (2)

*Very slightly* afraid or anxious—like the feeling you would have if a little child threatened to throw a snowball at you. (1)

*Not at all* afraid or anxious. (0)

The subcategories were derived from the Full Anxiety Inventory as follows:

1. Questions relating to Self-Referred Anxiety.
    1. You look down from a tall building.
    2. You have unpleasant dreams at night.
    3. You think about the personal problems you have.
    11. You think about the fact that you will die someday.
    12. You think about the possibility that you might become insane.
    17. You think about whether you are able to control yourself at times.
    20. You think about your future.
    22. You think about the things that you did which were morally wrong.
    24. You remember the failures you have had in your life.
    28. You remember the things which you have done which were queer or strange.

2. Questions relating to Externalized Anxiety.
    10. You think about your father.
    13. You think about the opinion other people have of you.
    14. You think of the responsibilities you will have when you leave the hospital.
    19. You think about your mother.
    27. You think about wishing harm or death would come to some people you know.

3. Questions of a Mixed nature.
    5. You think about the possibility that you might get cancer.
    6. You think about having sexual intercourse.
    7. You think about your being married.
    8. You wake up in the morning.
    9. You have to sit in a small room with the door shut.
    15. You think about being operated upon.
    16. You remember the sexual experiences you have had in the past.
    18. You think about God.
    23. You think of how much better other people can do some things than you.
    25. You feel that someone is exerting a strong influence on you over which you have no control.
    29. You think of going blind.
    30. You think about your health at the present time.

4. Questions related to Self-Consciousness (these may overlap the other subcategories).
    3. You think about the personal problems you have.
    7. You think about your being married.
    8. You wake up in the morning.
    11. You think about the fact that you will die someday.
    13. You think about the opinion other people have of you.
    14. You think of the responsibilities you will have when you leave the hospital.
    16. You remember the sexual experiences you have had in the past.
    17. You think about whether you are able to control yourself at times.
    20. You think about your future.
    21. You think about your hatred for some people.
    22. You think about the things that you did which were morally wrong.
    23. You think of how much better other people can do some things than you.
    24. You remember the failures you have had in your life.
    27. You think about wishing harm or death would come to some people you know.
    28. You remember the things which you have done which were queer or strange.

TABLE 69.   THE COMPLAINT INVENTORY

*"During the Past Two Weeks, How Often Have You:"*

1. Had dizzy spells.
2. Felt that someone was talking to you even though you could not see the person.
3. Had to throw up.
4. Felt that you were going to die.
5. Suffered from constipation.
6. Had bad or disturbing dreams.
7. Had spells in which you felt your heart pound.
8. Had backaches.
9. Had queer, unpleasant feelings in some part of your body.
10. Lost your temper.
11. Suffered from headaches.
12. Had difficulty in concentrating.
13. Had a hard time falling asleep at night.
14. Had trouble speaking as fast and as clearly as you used to.
15. Had trouble in keeping your balance while walking.
16. Felt that your future was hopeless.
17. Felt compelled to do some little act over and over again.
18. Felt that your family had not treated you well.
19. Felt that certain people were plotting against your welfare.
20. Felt that you were well enough to leave here.
21. Read the newspaper.
22. Felt like having sexual relations.
23. Had wet dreams during the night.
24. Had severe pains in some part of your body.
25. Felt sad or blue.
26. Been disgusted at the sight of food.
27. Felt a ringing or buzzing in your ears.
28. Experienced a terrible fear of some ordinarily harmless object or situation.
29. Wished you were dead.
30. Had the feeling that certain places look unfamiliar to you, even though you have seen them before.

*Response Card*
(The weights were not on the card handed to the patient)

Everyday (5).
Almost everyday (4).
About twice a week (3).
Rarely—only once or twice during the past two weeks (2).
Never—not at all during the past two weeks (1).

The subcategories of the Complaint Inventory were as follows:

1. Questions concerning Physical Complaints.
   1. Had dizzy spells.
   3. Had to throw up.
   5. Suffered from constipation.
   7. Had spells in which you felt your heart pound.
   8. Had backaches.
   9. Had queer, unpleasant feelings in some part of your body.
   11. Suffered from headaches.
   24. Had severe pains in some part of your body.

2. Questions dealing with Mental Complaints.
    2. Felt that someone was talking to you even though you could not see the person.
    6. Had bad or disturbing dreams.
    10. Lost your temper.
    12. Had difficulty in concentrating.
    16. Felt that your future was hopeless.
    17. Felt compelled to do some little act over and over again.
    25. Felt sad or blue.
    26. Been disgusted at the sight of food.
    28. Experienced a terrible fear of some ordinarily harmless object or situation.
    29. Wished you were dead.

3. Questions of a Mixed Nature.
    4. Felt that you were doing to die.
    13. Had a hard time falling asleep at night.
    14. Had trouble speaking as fast and as clearly as you used to.
    15. Had trouble in keeping your balance while walking.
    18. Felt that your family has not treated you well.
    19. Felt that certain people were plotting against your welfare.
    27. Felt a ringing or buzzing in your ears.

Following these instructions, the questions were then read to the patients by the experimenter. He was able to note any comment made by the patient and was in a position to inquire about any particular anxiety or complaint. In addition to such observations the weights given each answer were recorded. The weights for the Anxiety Inventory ranged from 0 for "not at all" to 6 for "extremely" anxious. Those for the Complaint Inventory ranged from 1 for "never" to 5 for "everyday." The various items were put into question form as the experimenter prefaced each item (in the case of the Anxieties) with "How afraid or anxious do you usually feel . . . ," and "During the past two weeks, how often have you . . ." (in the case of the Complaints).

The possible range for the Anxiety Inventory was 0 to 180. The highest score which was actually obtained was 127. The possible range for the Complaint Inventory was 30 to 150. The highest obtained score was 99.

The questions used for the full inventory were a mixture which, it was hoped, would furnish leads as to different kinds of anxieties and complaints. The questions on the Anxiety Inventory were sorted out into ten items constituting a category of Self-Referred Anxiety, 5 of Externalized Anxiety, 12 of Mixed Anxiety, and 15 of Self-Conscious Anxiety (table 68). In a like manner the Complaint Inventory was divided into Mental Complaints (ten items), Physical (eight items), and Mixed (seven items). The questions included under Self-Conscious Anxiety may also appear in the above anxiety categories.

**Mirror Drawing. Experiment.** In order to obtain an indication of emotional expression from the patient's behavior, two scores were derived from the Mirror Drawing Experiment. The subject in this experiment is required to trace a star pattern and is dependent upon a mirror for observing his progress, direct vision being precluded by a screen. This experiment is regarded as a learning task involving interference with old habits. As used in the Columbia-Greystone battery, the patient was given a total of fourteen trials: two trials without the mirror, ten trials with the mirror, and two final trials without the mirror. Notes were taken of the subject's reactions and his comments.

Blocking and Frustration scores were obtained from this experiment. If there was an interruption in the performance as shown by the tracing, an interruption in which for a period of time no progress was made in the tracing of the pattern, the interruption was called a block, or blocking. This blocking may or may not be associated with the expression of emotion. The evidence of blocking was scored by counting the number of instances that it occurred during the first seven trials with the mirror both pre- and postoperatively. The number of trials to be used in determining this score was arrived at empirically since it was found that most of our patients completed at least seven trials and showed a tendency to improved performance in later trials which rendered them useless for this score.

The Frustration score was a rating derived from the behavior of the patients while completing these seven trials. The rating scale had the following steps:

0—No frustration exhibited.
1—Comments, curses, complains but continues task.
2—Stops working but resumes voluntarily without urging.
3—Stops, continues after urging.
4—Stops, refuses to continue in spite of urging.
5—Stops, with violent reactions of refusal.

## RESULTS

### GROUP DATA

In table 70 are shown the means, standard deviations, differences, and statistical measures for each of these measuring devices so that one may compare the group of operatees with the control patients.

The examination of the group results on the Anxiety Inventory may be briefly stated as follows:

1. The patients who were operated upon had a much higher mean and standard deviation on their scores before operation than did the control patients before anesthesia. The effect of the operation was to decrease the mean of the operatee group. That of the control group increased following anesthesia though not to a degree which made the two groups equivalent.

2. When questions dealing with the subcategories, namely Self-Referred, Externalized, Mixed, and Self-Conscious Anxieties, were separately and similarly examined, there was no evidence that one kind of anxiety rather than another changed (with the possible exception of Externalized Anxiety) so far as the groups were concerned.

3. The operatee group started with more expression of anxiety and lost about one quarter of their anxiety score, while the control group started with fewer expressed anxieties and gained an additional 28 percent in score during the four-month period.

The group results obtained from the Complaint Inventory may be summarized as follows:

1. On the Full Inventory and all three subgroupings, the operatee group expressed a greater number of complaints before operation than did the controls before anesthesia. The groups were most similar in the expression of Mental and Mixed Complaints.

2. After operation or anesthesia the groups were very similar in the average number of their complaints. The operatee group decreased; the control group showed little change.

TABLE 70.  MEANS, STANDARD DEVIATIONS, DIFFERENCES, AND PERCENT OF CHANGE FOR THE OPERATEE AND CONTROL GROUPS ON THE MEASURES USED IN THIS STUDY

| | N | Preoperative | | Postoperative | | Diff. | % of 0 mean |
|---|---|---|---|---|---|---|---|
| | | Mean | Sigma | Mean | Sigma | | |
| Anxiety-Full Inventory | | | | | | | |
| Operatees................. | 16 | 55.9 | 33.6 | 42.9 | 31.6 | −13.0 | −23 |
| Controls.................. | 9 | 14.7 | 8.2 | 18.8 | 17.5 | + 4.1 | +28 |
| Self-Referred Anxiety | | | | | | | |
| Operatees............... | 16 | 22.6 | 11.8 | 17.2 | 11.6 | − 5.4 | −24 |
| Controls................ | 9 | 5.4 | 5.3 | 8.7 | 8.3 | + 3.3 | +61 |
| Externalized Anxiety | | | | | | | |
| Operatees............... | 16 | 7.3 | 6.3 | 7.5 | 6.3 | + 0.2 | + 3 |
| Controls................ | 9 | 1.9 | 3.3 | 2.1 | 2.7 | + 0.2 | +11 |
| Mixed Anxiety | | | | | | | |
| Operatees............... | 16 | 20.6 | 14.9 | 15.4 | 12.9 | − 5.3 | −26 |
| Controls................ | 9 | 7.3 | 6.7 | 8.0 | 6.5 | + 0.7 | +10 |
| Self-Consciousness (from Anxiety Inventory) | | | | | | | |
| Operatees............... | 16 | 24.7 | 16.4 | 19.6 | 17.3 | − 5.1 | −21 |
| Controls................ | 9 | 5.6 | 7.6 | 8.0 | 6.5 | + 2.4 | +43 |
| Complaints—Full Inventory | | | | | | | |
| Operatees............... | 15 | 64.1 | 20.3 | 52.9 | 13.6 | −11.2 | −18 |
| Controls................ | 10 | 50.6 | 14.2 | 51.2 | 12.6 | + 0.6 | + 1 |
| Physical Complaints | | | | | | | |
| Operatees............... | 15 | 16.6 | 8.0 | 12.5 | 5.6 | − 4.3 | −26 |
| Controls................ | 10 | 12.2 | 2.2 | 12.1 | 2.9 | − 0.1 | − 1 |
| Mental Complaints | | | | | | | |
| Operatees............... | 15 | 23.1 | 8.6 | 16.4 | 4.6 | − 6.7 | −29 |
| Controls................ | 10 | 15.4 | 5.5 | 15.0 | 4.6 | − 0.4 | − 3 |
| Mixed Complaints | | | | | | | |
| Operatees............... | 15 | 13.9 | 5.0 | 11.3 | 3.9 | − 2.6 | −19 |
| Controls................ | 10 | 10.5 | 3.3 | 11.2 | 4.1 | + 0.7 | + 7 |
| Blocking on Mirror Drawing | | | | | | | |
| Operatees............... | 16 | 8.7 | 3.7 | 4.2 | 4.1 | − 4.5 | −52 |
| Controls................ | 10 | 8.9 | 2.1 | 4.4 | 4.1 | − 4.5 | −51 |
| Frustration Rating on Mirror Drawing | | | | | | | |
| Operatees............... | 16 | 1.8 | 1.7 | 1.6 | 1.0 | − 0.2 | −12 |
| Controls................ | 10 | 1.9 | 1.6 | 1.4 | 0.9 | − 0.5 | −26 |

3. The operatee group showed a mean decrease in the Full Scale which represented 17 percent of the preoperative mean. This decrease was mainly in Mental and Physical Complaints with little change in the Mixed Complaints.

The group results with respect to Blocking and Frustration may be summarized as follows:

1. The operatee and control groups were similar in both Blocking and Frustration before and after operation or anesthesia.

2. Both groups showed a tendency to decrease in Blocking and Frustration after operation or anesthesia.

There are several points brought out by these group comparisons which will bear further comment. The original scores of the operatee group clearly indicate that its members stood apart from the rest of the patients studied. Since members of the operatee and control groups were not matched originally with respect to Anxieties and Complaints, this study is of necessity based on the changes made by the operatees using the control group as an indicator of the direction of change that might have been expected on the repetition of such inventories after four months.

The control group showed changes in the direction of increased scores on Anxieties and Complaints at the end of four months; the operatees decreased. There is no doubt that one of the effects of the operation was an over-all decrease in Anxieties and Complaint scores.

The rank-order correlation between the original scores and the postoperative scores gives an indication of whether or not the operation tended to affect the individuals in a similar or dissimilar fashion. The figures are:

| | | | |
|---|---|---|---|
| Full Anxiety | +.67 | Full Complaint Inventory | +.54 |
| Self-Referred Anxieties | +.65 | Mental Complaints | +.40 |
| Externalized Anxiety | +.78 | Physical Complaints | +.73 |
| Self-Consciousness | +.79 | Mixed Complaints | +.52 |
| Mixed Anxiety | +.68 | Blocking | .00 |
| | | Frustration | −.17 |

The anxiety measures show the Self-Referred Anxiety was most disrupted, i.e. was the least reliable in a statistical sense. Mental Complaints were most affected of the complaint subcategories and Blocking and Frustration were completely changed. This point will be considered later in light of the examination of the individual records.

The group data certainly show that there were clear-cut tendencies for decrease in Anxiety scores, particularly Self-Referred Anxiety, together with a decrease in complaints about one's mental status.

### INDIVIDUAL CASES

Since the group of operatees is small and since the psychologic functions under examination are known only through the subjective reporting of co-operative psychotic patients, the changes which were brought about by the operation can be more clearly understood by considering the individual cases.

Patient 2. Male; age, 46; I.Q., 107; improvement rating, 0*; areas excised, 6†, 8;

---

* The psychiatric rating of social improvement, which is given below with each case, was based on the following steps: 5—disturbed ward, 4—medium ward, 3—best ward with ground parole, 2—home with supervision, 1—home working or capable of work. The difference between the preoperative and postoperative ratings was weighted by adding points as follows: from a disturbed ward to ground parole, 1 point; from anywhere in the hospital to home, 1 point; from anywhere in the hospital to home working at reduced capacity, 1 point; from anywhere in the hospital to home working at old capacity, 1 point. Scores were provided in this manner for each patient's social improvement following operation. They ranged from −1 to 8.

† Indicates area partially excised.

‡ O and R2 as used here refer to the pre- and postoperative testing respectively. The O (original) testing was done one month before operation; the R2 (repeat), four months after operation.

§ No score available.

Anxiety score, O‡=0, R2=3; Complaint score, O=38, R2=36; Blocking score, O=10, R2=9; Frustration score, O=1, R2=1.

There was little psychologic change or general improvement in this patient after operation. He was somewhat incoherent and evasive in his answers at both test periods. His only change on the tests was the addition of one Self-Referred Anxiety.

Patient 3. Male; age 61; I.Q., 125; improvement rating, 2; areas excised, 6†, 9†; Anxiety score, O=5, R2=5; Complaint score, O=46, R2=49; Blocking score, O=16, R2=4; Frustration score, O=0, R2=3.

This patient was quiet and reserved at both test periods. He seemed to be withholding his own confidence and inclined to conceal any anxiety or complaint. After operation his general behavior was some, but not much more, outgoing.

Patient 4. Male; age, 55; I.Q., 92; improvement rating, 2; area excised, 46; Anxiety score, O=127, R2=99; Complaint scc e, O=97, R2=75; Blocking score, O=9, R2=10; Frustration score, O=3, R2=3.

This patient expressed complaints and anxieties which were all encompassed in a general pattern composed of (in the patient's words) "queer pains, not really headaches," "burning sensations, not really pains," "always got the same fear, worriment, fear, burning, all the time," "memories keep coming back to me." There was a marked decrease in the intensity of these complaints following operation accompanied by less preoccupation with personal problems. After operation the patient was generally friendly and agreeable and he was proud of his ability to joke though still expressing much of the same sort of complaints but without former affective surcharge.

Patient 6. Male; age, 33; I.Q., 92; improvement rating, 1; areas excised, 6†, 8†; Anxiety score, O=76, R2=79; Complaint score, O=68, R2=71; Blocking score, O=5, R2=1; Frustration score, O=4, R2=0.

This patient was given to silly, inappropriate emotional reactions before operation. His verbalizations were inadequate and bizarre. He became aroused during the preoperative questioning concerning complaints and it was impossible to complete the inventory adequately. No explanation could be obtained for the refusal. After operation, although there was little change in the test score, he was more even in mood and completed all tests.

Patient 7. Male; age, 40; I.Q., 93; improvement rating, 5; areas excised, 8, 9†, 10†; Anxiety score, O=54, R2=39; Complaint score, O=99, R2=39; Blocking score, O=17, R2=1; Frustration score, O=5, R2=0.

The marked feature in this record is a decrease in both Anxiety and Complaint scores. The patient had been depressed and tense before operation but after operation he was less self-centered, thinking of reintegration into society and affable in his relations with others.

Patient 8. Male; age, 29; I.Q., 90; improvement rating, 0; area excised, middle frontal gyrus; Anxiety score, O=66, R2=64; Complaint score, O=55, R2=57; Blocking score, O=11; R2=5; Frustration score, O=5, R2=1.

Preoperatively this patient appeared cooperative and interested in most of the material but was irritated by the inventories and exhibited considerable impulsiveness and psychomotor tension. This was particularly noted during the Complaint Inventory. He consistently complained about his symptoms and asked help from the psychologist both in his test performances and in relation to his personal problems. After operation there appeared to be a lessening of emotional tension but the feelings of inadequacy and inability to face decisions persisted.

Patient 13. Male; age, 43; I.Q., 96; improvement rating, 6; areas excised, 45, 46, 9†, 10†; Anxiety score, O=48, R2=14; Complaint score, O=91, R2=63; Blocking score, O=5, R2=0; Frustration score, O=0, R2=2.

This patient was morose before operation and had to be urged to give definite responses to the inventories. After operation the answers came more easily and the patient appeared to react normally affectively. He was very cooperative but had difficulty with some of the verbal material because of educational deficiencies.

Patient 18. Male; age, 39; I.Q., 127; improvement rating, −1; area excised, 11†; Anxiety score, O=40, R2=15; Complaint score, O=54, R2=50; Blocking score, O=x§, R2=x; Frustration score, O=x, R2=x.

Before and after operation this patient was compulsive in his test performance. He was very cooperative and agreeable but complained of "mental fatigue" which required rest periods. After operation he was more outgoing in his social relations although still quiet and ruminative unless spoken to. The immediate "lift" of the operation appeared to be fading so that when tested four months postoperatively the change in score was not marked. In this record no anxiety of more than a mild degree was expressed. Only two complaints were mentioned to any extent. These were "voices" and "queer pains."

Patient 19. Male; age, 50; I.Q., 102; improvement rating, 0; area excised, 45†; Anxiety score, O=74, R2=96; Complaint score, O=47, R2=46; Blocking score, O=7, R2=6; Frustration score, O=3, R2=2.

Overactivity, garrulousness, and a quarrelsome sort of elation characterized this patient before operation. His test performance was adequate and competent when he could be kept to the task and his conversation halted. After operation he was much quieter, calmer, and self-possessed so that he seemed retarded or depressed. There was no real evidence of emotional improvement from these psychologic scores.

Patient 21. Male; age, 42; I.Q., 104; improvement rating, 6; area excised, 10; Anxiety score, O=95, R2=17; Complaint score, O=x, R2=x; Blocking score, O=x, R2=x; Frustration score, O=x, R2=x.

This patient was a quiet, depressed, backward person who cooperated very well once his shell of complaints and preoccupation was broken. After operation he was quiet and reserved but less depressed. Although he still had complaints they were not as immediate or pressing. The reduction in the score on Anxiety is very representative.

Patient 25. Male; age, 58; I.Q., 89; improvement rating, 8; areas excised, 8, 9, 10†, 46; Anxiety score, O=55, R2=22; Complaint score, O=61, R2=46; Blocking score, O=10, R2=6; Frustration score, O=1, R2=1.

This patient was suffering from an agitated depression which cut through and colored all his test performances. He was preoccupied with fears of the future and guilt and remorse concerning the past. After operation there was a general decrease in the intensity of his fear and guilt. The same tendency to agitated sadness was present but greatly reduced so that it was possible for him to make a fairly adequate social adjustment.

Patient 31. Female; age, 51; I.Q., 96; improvement rating, 1; area excised, 9; Anxiety score, O=19, R2=77; Complaint score, O=44, R2=49; Blocking score, O=6, R2=0; Frustration score, O=1, R2=1.

This patient was suffering from an agitated depression. After operation the same complaints were expressed but were less charged with emotion. She was quieter and appeared to be better adjusted. However, her Anxiety and Complaint scores both increased. In the tests, she retained all of her old complaints and anxieties and added new ones. Her test results are not in accord with her general behavior.

Patient 32. Female; age, 41; I.Q., 131; improvement rating, 0; areas excised, 8†, 9, 10†; Anxiety score, O=46, R2=34; Complaint score, O=81, R2=51; Blocking score, O=6, R2=0; Frustration score, O=0, R2=1.

Despite marked mood swings this patient's record reflects generally good performance. She was markedly variable in mood and one did not know whether she would be depressed or elated from day to day. This was equally true following operation although there was a fair reduction in psychologic scores.

Patient 36. Female; age, 53; I.Q., 93; improvement rating, 0; areas excised, 10, 11, 46, 45, 47; Anxiety score, O=93, R2=61; Complaint score, O=83, R2=85, Blocking score, O=8, R2=13; Frustration score, O=2, R2=3.

Preoperatively this patient was depressed and likely to discuss her personal problems. She was fairly cooperative but became tense during some of the psychologic tests. After operation there appeared to be some lightening of this tension and a slight increase in her reaction to social stimuli but without marked change.

TABLE 71. DIFFERENCE SCORES FOR THE OPERATEES TOGETHER WITH I.Q., AREA EXCISED, AND THE SOCIAL IMPROVEMENT RATING

| Patient's No. | I.Q. | Area excised | Improvement Rating | Blocking | Frustration | Self-Consc. | Self-Referred Anxiety | External. Anxiety | Physical Complaints | Mental Complaints | Full Anxiety | Full Complaint |
|---|---|---|---|---|---|---|---|---|---|---|---|---|
| 2 | 107 | 8, 6ᵃ | 0 | − 1 | 0 | 0 | + 3 | 0 | 0 | 0 | + 3 | − 8 |
| 3 | 125 | 9ᵃ, 6ᵃ | 2 | −12 | +3 | − 2 | − 2 | 0 | 0 | − 2 | 0 | + 3 |
| 4 | 92 | 46 | 2 | + 1 | 0 | −18 | − 7 | − 8 | − 8 | −13 | −28 | −22 |
| 6 | 92 | 8ᵃ, 6ᵃ | 1 | + 1 | −4 | +10 | + 8 | + 1 | + 5 | + 1 | + 3 | + 3 |
| 7 | 93 | 8, 9ᵃ, 10ᵃ | 5 | −16 | −5 | −10 | −10 | + 3 | −24 | −23 | −15 | −60 |
| 8 | 90 | MFGᵇ | 0 | − 5 | −4 | + 8 | − 3 | + 7 | + 1 | 0 | − 2 | + 2 |
| 13 | 96 | 9ᵃ, 10ᵃ, 45, 46 | 6 | − 5 | +2 | −19 | −12 | + 1 | − 8 | −15 | −34 | −28 |
| 18 | 127 | 11ᵃ | −1 | x | x | −13 | −11 | − 2 | − 2 | 0 | −25 | − 4 |
| 19 | 102 | 45ᵃ | 0 | − 1 | −1 | +14 | + 3 | + 8 | 0 | − 1 | +22 | − 1 |
| 21 | 104 | 10 | 6 | x | x | −44 | −34 | − 6 | x | x | −78 | x |
| 25 | 89 | 8, 9, 10ᵃ, 46 | 8 | − 4 | 0 | −18 | −11 | − 5 | −11 | − 2 | −33 | −15 |
| 31 | 96 | 9 | 1 | − 6 | +1 | +27 | +17 | +11 | 0 | − 2 | +58 | + 5 |
| 32 | 131 | 8ᵃ, 9, 10ᵃ | 0 | − 6 | +1 | − 5 | − 9 | − 7 | − 4 | −14 | −12 | −30 |
| 36 | 93 | 10, 11, 45, 46, 47 | 0 | + 5 | +3 | − 6 | − 3 | 0 | − 1 | − 2 | −32 | + 2 |
| 38 | 106 | VTᶜ | 8 | + 1 | +1 | − 3 | − 7 | 0 | − 2 | − 4 | − 9 | − 2 |
| 40 | 91 | 24ᵃ | 0 | − 7 | +2 | x | x | x | x | x | x | x |
| 49 | 111 | 10, 11ᵃ, 46ᵃ | 5 | − 3 | +1 | − 2 | − 9 | 0 | − 7 | −13 | −14 | −15 |

ᵃ Part of area.
ᵇ MFG = middle frontal gyrus.
ᶜ VT = venous tie.

Patient 38. Female; age, 38; I.Q., 106; improvement rating, 8; no area excised, venous tie affecting areas 6, 8, 9, 10; Anxiety score, O=18, R2=9; Complaint score, O=39, R2=37; Blocking score, O=6, R2=1; Frustration score, O=0, R2=1.

This patient was not too communicative about her anxieties or complaints before operation as the record shows. Her mood varied between silliness and tears in an abrupt fashion. After operation she was helpful around the ward and when paroled home is said to have made an excellent adjustment. There was some lessening in affective tension which is reflected in the Anxiety and Complaint scores.

Patient 40. Female; age, 28; I.Q., 91; improvement rating, 0; area excised, 24†; Anxiety score, O=x, R2=x; Complaint score, O=x, R2=x; Blocking score, O=7, R2=0; Frustration score, O=1, R2=3.

Before operation this patient presented constant complaints and excuses for not doing the psychologic tests. This difficulty could generally be surmounted but her cooperation was never good. After operation she became very difficult to work with, refusing material with great evidence of emotional resistance and, as a result, much of the postoperative data was either unobtainable or scanty. She had previously complained of a variety of somatic disorders and following operation stated bitterly that the operation had been a mistake.

TABLE 72.  PERCENT OF OPERATEES SHOWING LOSS OR ZERO CHANGE RELATED TO AREAS, IMPROVEMENT, I.Q., AND AGE

| | No. of patients | Blocking | Frustration | Self-Consc. | Self-Anxiety | External. Anxiety | Physical Complaints | Mental Complaints | Full Anxiety | Full Complaint |
|---|---|---|---|---|---|---|---|---|---|---|
| **Area** | | | | | | | | | | |
| 8 | 5 | 80 | 80 | 80 | 60 | 60 | 80 | 80 | 60 | 80 |
| 9 | 6 | 100 | 33 | 83 | 83 | 50 | 100 | 100 | 83 | 67 |
| 10 | 7 | 83 | 33 | 100 | 100 | 71 | 100 | 100 | 100 | 83 |
| 46 | 5 | 60 | 40 | 100 | 100 | 80 | 100 | 100 | 100 | 80 |
| **Improvement rating** | | | | | | | | | | |
| 8 to 2 | 8 | 72 | 43 | 100 | 100 | 75 | 100 | 100 | 100 | 88 |
| +1, 0, −1 | 9 | 75 | 50 | 50 | 50 | 50 | 75 | 88 | 50 | 50 |
| **Intelligence quotient before operation** | | | | | | | | | | |
| below 95 | 7 | 57 | 72 | 67 | 83 | 50 | 67 | 83 | 83 | 50 |
| 95–104 | 4 | 100 | 33 | 50 | 50 | 25 | 100 | 100 | 50 | 67 |
| above 104 | 6 | 60 | 60 | 100 | 83 | 100 | 100 | 100 | 83 | 83 |
| **Age at time of operation** | | | | | | | | | | |
| below 40 | 4 | 75 | 50 | 33 | 67 | 33 | 33 | 67 | 67 | 83 |
| 40–49 | 7 | 80 | 40 | 100 | 86 | 72 | 100 | 100 | 86 | 100 |
| over 49 | 6 | 67 | 50 | 67 | 67 | 67 | 100 | 100 | 67 | 50 |

Patient 49. Female; age, 39; I.Q., 111; improvement rating, 5; area excised, 10, 11†, 46†; Anxiety score, O=73, R2=59; Complaint score, O=57, R2=42; Blocking score, O=12, R2=9; Frustration score, O=1, R2=2.

Before operation this patient was apathetic and communicative only in a schizophrenic fashion. After operation there was a decrease in Self-Referred Anxieties and Mental Complaints. She was not relieved of all of the mental symptoms but they did seem somewhat lessened.

In reading through these accounts the impression is clear that when there was a social recovery or a general improvement in the patient's condition following the operation, the Anxiety and Complaint scores also changed. To shed light on this point the change or difference in scores for these measures together with the I.Q., areas excised, and the social improvement rating have been tabulated in table 71. The figures in this table may be reassembled for comparison with any other variables at our disposal. Such regroupings indicated that the changes were not related to sex, or to the weight of brain tissue excised.

In table 72 figures given in table 71 have been retabulated with respect to whether, after operation, there was a loss or no difference in score shown by the patients. The frequency of losses and no differences was expressed in terms of percent of the subgroup involved. The tabulation has been set up in this way on the general assumption that zero differences were counted among the losses since the average change of the control patients was a gain in these measures. This tabulation presents the subgroups for area excised, social improvement, I.Q., and age.

Removal of area 8 produced no regular change. Area 9 gave a reduction in Blocking score in each of the 6 patients involved. This is the only uniform change in either of the Mirror Drawing indicators. The same 6 patients all decreased in Physical and Mental Complaints though the Mixed Complaints of patient 31 increased which held her Full Complaint score at +5 and hence not all patients having area 9 out can be said to have shown a clear decrease in Complaint scores. As pointed out in the case summary, patient 31 gave test results not in accord with her general status.

All 7 patients having area 10 removed showed a reduction in scores on Anxieties and Complaints except patient 7 on Externalized Anxieties and patient 36 on the Full Complaint Inventory. Patient 7 increased three points on Externalized Anxiety and patient 32, two points on the Full Complaint Inventory.

Three of the 5 patients who had area 46 excised decreased in Complaints. The exceptions were patients 13 and 36. Unfortunately we do not have scores on enough patients in whom area 6, 11, 45, 44, or 47 was excised to base comparisons. However, there is very strong reason to believe that the removal of areas 9, 10, and 46, either alone or in some combination, resulted in a decrease in the Anxieties and Complaints of these psychotic patients.

Inspection of the figures with respect to Social Improvement shows that the decrease in Blocking and Frustration scores is not related to social improvement. All patients in this group who showed real social improvement had a decrease in score on Self-Consciousness, Self-Referred Anxieties, Physical and Mental Complaints and the Full Anxiety Inventory. Two patients who improved, 7 and 13, gave increases of three points and 1 point on Externalized Anxieties while patient 3 also gave an increase of three points on the Full Complaint Inventory. The 9 operatees who failed to improve usually show as many increases as decreases in Anxiety and Complaint scores.

When the patients are grouped for intelligence into low (less than 95 I.Q), average (95 to 104 I.Q.), and good (over 105 I.Q.), it is apparent that all but one operatee (2) with an I.Q. over 104 showed decreased scores for Complaints or Anxiety. All 4 operatees with average I.Q. (95 to 104) showed a loss in Blocking score.

Similar grouping for age into those less than forty years of age, those forty to forty-nine, and those over fifty shows that there was a tendency for those in the forties to show decreases in Anxiety and Complaint scores more frequently than did members of the younger or older groups.

## SUMMARY OF RESULTS

The investigation of the changes shown by this small group of 17 operatees cannot yield positive conclusions since no comparable control group was available. *The summary statements which follow are expressions of tendency to change and no more.*

*Mirror Drawing Blocking* was decreased when area 9 was excised in patients of average intelligence.

*Mirror Drawing Frustration* tends to increase when Blocking decreases. Changes in Frustration were not regularly associated with any of the criteria we have considered.

*Self-Consciousness and Self-Referred Anxiety* were decreased when areas 10 and 46 were removed. In this group the decrease in Self-Consciousness occurred in all patients with I.Q.s over 104 who were in their forties (one exception). This decrease was uniformly associated with good social improvement.

*Externalized Anxiety* decreased scores were not uniformly associated with any of these variables save that of having an I.Q. over 104.

*Physical Complaint* scores were reduced in all of these patients who had areas 8, 9, and/or 10 removed. This reduction was uniformly associated with an I.Q. over 95, an age over forty, and social improvement.

*Mental Complaint* scores were reduced in all of these patients who had areas 9, 10, and/or 46 excised. This reduction was uniformly associated with an I.Q. over 95, an age over forty, and social improvement.

The *Full Anxiety Inventory* scores decreased in all patients from whom areas 10 and 46 were removed. This decrease was associated with social improvement.

The *Full Complaint Inventory* scores decreased in patients who were in the forty to forty-nine age group.

### DISCUSSION

As pointed out in the opening paragraphs of this study, the claims which have been made as to the change in affective functions attendant on frontal lobe damage are most sweeping and most contradictory. The descriptions range from total change in personality with great emotional instability, through mild depression, childishness, and emotional superficiality to no alteration at all. From the literature one can only conclude that the effect of injury, of pathologic invasion, of surgical excision, and of the cutting of tracts leading to and from the frontal brain areas produces no regular changes in all conditions or in all patients.

The change in affective mental life brought about by prefrontal lobotomy (psychosurgery) in psychotic and neurotic patients is unquestionable in one fourth to one third of such patients. This change is clearly and unmistakably evident, even to an untrained observer. But it is most difficult to characterize. Freeman and Watts ('42) have termed it loss of painful or pathologic consciousness of self together with a diminishing of prolonged, painful, emotional turmoil. This change does not always follow lobotomy and the explanation for either the success or the failure is essentially unknown.

In this study symmetrical bilateral excision of various areas of the frontal lobes was done in 24 mental patients. Of the operatees who were paroled home, 11 were still home and making a good adjustment six months after operation. This is our best criterion of the effectiveness of the operation.

The Anxiety and Complaint Inventories which were employed contained items which the patients themselves considered self-descriptive, which items were in good accord with the previous histories of these patients. Representative data were obtained from 8 of the 11 improved patients before and after operation.

There was a clear decrease in the scores of these 8 when they were re-examined four months after operation. The decrease was most evident in the material relating to Self-Referred Anxiety, Self-Conscious Anxiety, and Mental Complaints. There was also a fair decrease in Physical Complaints and some, but not much, decrease in Externalized Anxieties. Examination of the test results obtained four months postoperatively on the 3 patients who did improve but on whom no preoperative data are available showed that their average scores corresponded very closely on each inventory and subinventory to the average scores of the 8 on whom full records had been obtained. It may be concluded that the Anxiety and Complaint Inventories give a fair and reasonably accurate picture of certain of the changes which were brought about by the operation.

But what of the patients who failed to recover, or at least, were not paroled, or if paroled, were very soon returned to the hospital? The Anxiety and Complaint Inventory scores of patients 32, 36, and 18 decreased. Despite the decrease in Anxiety and Complaints shown by patient 32 it is questionable as to whether or not these may be ascribed to the operation because of the variable moods of the patient. Patient 36 decreased in Anxiety and increased in Complaints and seemed to have less contact with reality after operation. Patient 18 appeared to have a transitory improvement following operation which was probably not maintained.

The Blocking and Frustration scores drawn from the Mirror Drawing Experiment were included in this study since it was hoped that they would provide indices of emotional organization and control. They failed to give clear-cut results. There was a tendency for patients who improved, judged either as social improvement or in terms of decreased Anxiety and Complaint scores, to show a decreased frequency of Blocking and an increase in Frustration rating. In a sense that goes with the clinical picture. The improved patients seemed to show greater interest in external affairs which might cut down Blocking. The patients were less preoccupied with their own inner problems, less reserved, and hence more outwardly expressive of the frustration felt in this experiment. Whether or not this is the correct explanation is difficult to say.

What is the essence of the affective change brought about by topectomy? H. E. King (chapter 14) found no permanent change in the intelligence measures or I.Q. in these patients. W. R. King (chapter 16) found no consistent evidence of loss in the abstract attitude in Goldstein's sense. H. E. King found no permanent loss in the ability to perform on the Continuous Performance Task and hence no evidence for a loss in sustained attention. It might, therefore, be concluded as Freeman and Watts have done, that the change is a diminution of painful self-consciousness and self-referred complaints, and anxieties. These anxieties and complaints are not lost but they are moved from the center to the edge of attention.

It is not apparent from these data whether or not this loss in self-conscious anxiety is identical with the connotations given this phrase by Freeman and Watts. As seen in the patient's behavior, there appears to have been a reduction in the press or flow of complaints and the discussion of personal problems. The patient who before operation appeared to be tense and agitated, who presented a problem to the psychologist because of his deep, withdrawn, depression; after operation, retained his concern for his personal problems but was more accessible and more likely to put his troubles aside to deal with the psychologic tests. Such a change may be characterized as a reduction in emotional tension, or as affective stabilization.

## Summary

The effect of topectomy on the affective mental life of these 17 psychotic patients may be summarized as follows: Bilateral removal of Brodmann's areas 9, 10, and 46 in patients who were over forty years of age, who had I.Q.s of over 105, and in whom there was free verbal expression of anxiety and complaints of mental troubles, resulted in a decrease in the Anxiety and Complaints which decrease was associated with social improvement or recovery from mental illness. This change is one of affective stabilization which results in a loss of psychomotor tension and of the painful preoccupation and self-centered concern with present and past personal problems, thus allowing the patient to react more readily to his environment.

# Chapter 21

# Rorschach Test

JOSEPH ZUBIN

---

THE nature of the Rorschach test as it was used is such that the test results cannot be treated adequately in a statistical manner. We shall, therefore, limit the statistical treatment to a minimum and present only the individual case interpretations before and after operation.

Each record was scored for all of the generally accepted Rorschach factors. In general, Klopfer and Kelley's ('42) scoring system was adhered to because of the finer nuances which this system permits. For classification of location, the D (large details) and Dd (small details) were scored according to Beck's norms, and the F+ and F− scoring also follows Beck ('44). Form responses which were not found in Beck's norms were simply scored as F without a suffix.

The first step in the analysis was to determine the relationships between the Rorschach factors and the other variables in the psychologic battery. In order to limit the number of correlations to a manageable number, certain groupings of factors had to be undertaken. The grouping was guided by the number of responses found for each factor in our cases as well as by the psychologic characteristics of the factor in question. The factors dealing with location of the responses were divided into two groups, the whole responses being placed in one category and all the other types of locations being placed in the second category. The determinants were classified into three groups: form responses (F+, F− and F), color responses (C, FC and CF), and movement responses (m, FM and M). The total number of responses (R) and the measures of reaction time (RT) were treated in the usual manner.

## CORRELATIONAL ANALYSIS

The Rorschach factors themselves showed the following intercorrelations. In each instance use was made not of the absolute frequency of response but of relative frequency in order to compensate for the high degree of variability in the total number of responses from patient to patient. The two location categories (W and non-W) showed a correlation of −.92 between themselves but did not correlate significantly with any of the other Rorschach factors. The determinants showed negative correlations of −.40 between F and M and −.61 between F and C. Reaction time to the first response on each card correlated negatively with C (−.45) and with F (−.61) but negligibly with all the other factors.

Since there were some sixty additional test scores available on each of the patients, the correlations of the Rorschach factors with the other test scores were computed. The results indicated that the number of responses, R, was significantly correlated with intelligence and learning measures. The location categories did not show significant relationships with any of the other tests. The proportion of Form responses (F) showed a negative correlation ($-.47$) with a measure of learning variability (Paired Associate Semi-meaningful). The proportion of Movement responses (M) was correlated .37 with the Wechsler-Bellevue Comprehension subtest. The average Reaction Time to the first response to each card was found to be correlated negatively with the intelligence test scores and learning.

### INDIVIDUAL ANALYSIS

The analysis of each individual record together with the tabulation of scores is presented in the following pages. Since all of the patients included in this study were chronic mental patients, the diagnostic features of the Rorschach test were not our primary concern, nor did we try to get a full personality evaluation of the patient since the psychiatric interview and the case history gave sufficient data for making the personality evaluation more directly. Our chief purpose in giving the Rorschach test was to determine whether or not any changes occurred between the two givings of the test. To this end, formal analysis of the scoring and subjective analyses of the meaning of the scores were undertaken to determine the areas of change and little or no attention was paid to the invariant area of personality in each case. Only those data which demonstrate these changes will be presented and only those aspects of the personality which they reflect will be discussed.*

At the beginning of each of the following case analyses there is a statement of the preoperative and postoperative (R2) scoring of each analysis. The symbols are the conventional ones of Klopfer and of Beck. They are used as follows. R=total number of responses: *Locations*, W=whole blot; W*=intended use of whole blot but part or parts omitted; D=large detail or portion of blot; Dd=small details or portions of blot; S=white space. *Determinants*, M=figures in human-like action; FM=animals in animal-like action; m=abstract or inanimate movement; K=shading as diffusion; k=shading as three dimensional projected on two dimensional; FK=shading as three dimensional in perspective; Fc=shading as surface appearance or texture; c=shading as texture; C'=Achromatic surface color; FC=definite form with bright color; CF=bright color with indefinite form; C=color only; F=form; F+ or F−=form level (Beck's tables.) *Content:* H=human figures; Hd=parts of human figures, not anatomical; A=animal figures; Ad=parts of living animals; At=human anatomy; Obj=all kinds of man-made objects; Na=nature; Geo=geographical concepts; Pl= plants; Pop=popular; Rej=rejected card; RT uncol=reaction time in seconds to uncolored cards; RT color=reaction time in seconds to colored cards.

Superior, lower-case italic a following an area number means that only part of the area thus designated was excised (example area 6ᵃ).

Case 1 (Control): Original test: R 51, W 9, W* 5, D 35, M 4, FM 3, m 3, K 1, F+F 25, F− 7, Fc 6, cC' 0, FC 1, CF 1, HHd 18, AAd 19, At 3, Obj 8, Clouds 1, Other 2, Pop 4, RT uncol 185, RT color 1.

Postoperative R2: R 38, W 8, W* 1, D 24, S 1, Dd 4, M 2, FM 0, m 0, K 1, F+F 30, F− 1, FC 0, cC' 2, FC 2, CF 0, HHd 16, AAd 12, At 3, Obj 4, Clouds 1, Other 2, Pop 4, RT uncol 144, RT color 119.

* The following interpretations are made according to conventional Rorschach procedure. It does not necessarily follow that the author is invariably convinced of their objective or subjective validity.

The underlying trend was basic aggression and hostility which were kept in check either by the anxieties which the overt expression of these tensions were likely to arouse or by some other inhibitory process. The tendency to see mutilated figures gave rise to a good number of bizarre responses indicative of a schizophrenic process. No change occurred from the first test to the second test in this regard. Depressive schizophrenic trends were a little more evidenced in the post-test. At the time of the first test the mood was predominantly one of elation with free-floating anxiety. The subject was more stimulated by colored than by the uncolored cards and this differential was especially marked in the retest indicating an increase in his extratensive trend. He was generally slower in his responses to the second test, but he still reacted more quickly to the colored than the uncolored cards. His aggression also increased as shown by the increase in the number of dismembered human beings reported. In general this patient changed in his degree of control on the retest, showing less control over his affective life but greater restriction on his intellectual or inner strivings.

Case 2 (Area 6$^a$, 8): Preoperative: R 18, W 5, W* 1, D 12, Dd 0, M 3, FM 2, F+F 12, F— 0, Fc 0, FC 0, CF 1, HHd 6, AAd 10, At 0, Obj 1, Other 1, Pop 6, Rej 1, RT uncol 182, RT color 105. Postoperative R2: R 25, W 5, W* 2, D 16, Dd 2, M 3, FM 0, F+F 16, F— 3, Fc 1, FC 1, CF 1, HHd 6, AAd 12, At 1, Obj 4, Other 2, Pop 5, Rej 0, RT uncol 54, RT color 75.

Before operation this patient was highly constricted and rigid. He was totally unreceptive to emotional stimulation and what little emotional feeling he experienced usually led to impulsive behavior. After operation his personality became more dilated, and he was more productive. His capacity to control his emotional outbursts increased and a certain degree of tactfulness and sensitivity to the needs of others became apparent. This gain, however, was not without its negative aspects. By reducing the degree of rigidity which he exhibited preoperatively, his degree of control lessened also and a certain deficiency in dealing adequately and realistically with his environment became evident.

Case 3 (Area 6$^a$, 9$^a$): Preoperative: R 11, W 2, D 9, M 1, FM 1, F+F 9, F— 0, HHd 5, AAd 4, At 1, Obj 1, Pop 3, Rej 2, RT uncol 121, RT color 144. Postoperative R2: R 8, W 1, D 7, M 0, FM 0, F+F 6, F— 2, HHd 2, AAd 6, At 0, Obj 0, Pop 2, Rej 2, RT uncol 88, RT color 45.

Despite this patient's initially limited imagination and limited contact with reality, he had a few redeeming features such as the response of a fairy-like figure in the last card. This imaginative touch was wiped out by the operation, when he seemed very much more limited and lacking in imagination and in contact. He was highly stereotyped in his reactions, compulsive, and less capable of appreciating reality. Before operation the neurotic affective features were more prominent; after operation depressive features predominated.

Case 4 (Area 46): Preoperative: R 19, W 4, W* 0, D 13, Dd 2, M 1, K 1, F+F 16, C' 1, HHd 8, AAd 9, Na 1, Clouds 1, Pop 3, RT uncol 145, RT color 206. Postoperative R2: R 18, W 3, W* 1, D 10, Dd 4, M 3, K 0, F+F 14, C' 1, HHd 11, AAd 7, Na 0, Clouds 0, Pop 3, RT uncol 70, RT color 173.

This patient exhibited considerable amount of anxiety, both before and after the operation but there was a slight reduction in the postoperative test permitting him to express some of his inner feelings and imagination to better advantage. In his preoperative as well as in the postoperative test he appeared to have the capacity for being an outgoing individual but in his actual life attainment he was quite withdrawn. This conflict between his essentially outgoing nature and the need for withdrawal produced by his anxieties was one of his basic conflicts. The operation seemed to have lessened this struggle somewhat and he was more at ease with himself.

Case 5 (Control): Original test: R 13, W 7, W* 2, D 4, M 1, FM 1, F+F 8, F— 3, HHd 2, AAd 5, At 5, Pl 1, Pop 3, RT uncol 240, RT color 285.

Postoperative R2: R 11, W 7, W* 1, D 3, M 1, FM 1, F+F 5, F— 4, HHd 3, AAd 5, At 2, Pl 1, Pop 4, RT uncol 159, RT color 267.

This patient was a schizophrenic with no relieving features and with no apparent changes between tests. Perseveration and poverty of ideas and response were the most outstanding characteristics. Insecurity about the adequacy of his response seemed to be the underlying theme throughout his performance.

Case 6 (Area 6ᵃ, 8ᵃ): Preoperative: R 11, W 8, W* 1, D 2, M 1, k 0, F+F 6, F— 0, Fc 1, FC 1, CF 1, C 1, HHd 1, AAd 4, At 2, Obj 1, Geo 2, Color 1, Pop 4, RT uncol 124, RT color 185.

Postoperative R2: R 14, W 10, W* 2, D 2, M 1, k 1, F+F 6, F— 3, Fc 1, FC 1, CF 1, HHd 2, AAd 7, At 3, Obj 1, Geo 1, Color 0, Pop 5, RT uncol 87, RT color 71.

This patient was an unproductive schizophrenic with hollow ambition unsupported by ability, very few movement responses, but an inclination towards outgoingness which remained unaltered by the operation. The additional F— responses after operation indicated an inability to adjust to the reality of the task and at the same time some loss of control over his intellectual functioning.

Case 7 (Area 8, 9ᵃ, 10ᵃ): Preoperative: R 41, W 7, W* 0, D 34, Dd 0, M 5, FM 3, m 1, k 1, K 0, FK 6, F+F 22, F— 1, C′ 0, FC 1, C 1, HHd 8, AAd 19, At 1, Obj 6, Pl 0, Na 3, Geo 0, Clouds 4, Others 0, Pop 6, RT uncol 112, RT color 157.

Postoperative R2: R 35, W 2, W* 2, D 29, Dd 2, M 3, FM 2, m 0, k 1, K 1, FK 0, F+F 21, F— 2, C′ 4, FC 1, C 0, HHd 11, AAd 14, At 1, Obj 2, Pl 2, Na 1, Geo 2, Clouds 1, Others 1, Pop 3, RT uncol 57, RT color 65.

Before operation this patient was compulsive and self-conscious, given to introspective moods and to impulsiveness and in general was more responsive to his own cravings and urges than to social interaction. After operation he became even less sensitive to promptings from without, less introspective but more prone to uncontrolled free-floating anxiety. Impulsiveness declined but there was an increase in the tendency toward depression. Although his outward behavior was more marked by withdrawal, his instinctive trends were not so marked in that direction. It is thus possible that the operation may have set his instinctual drives into opposition against his assumed role in society. By awakening dormant extratensive drives, the patient was less capable of adjusting to the intratensive role he had previously adopted.

Case 8 (Areas 8ᵃ, 9ᵃ, 10ᵃ, 46ᵃ): Preoperative: R 13, W 1, W* 1, D 10, Dd 1, M 1, F+F 12, F— 0, Fc 0, C′ 0, HHd 7, AAd 5, Obj 1, Pop 2, Rej 3, RT uncol 129, RT color 115.

Postoperative R2: R 20, W 2, W* 1, D 16, Dd 1, M 1, F+F 16, F— 1, Fc 1, C′ 1, HHd 7, AAd 12, Obj 1, Pop 3, Rej 0, RT uncol 59, RT color 48.

This individual was highly constricted and rather limited both before and after operation showing very little internal fantasy life and very little outgoingness. However, after operation he improved somewhat in his outgoingness, became a little more tactful and a little more responsive to external stimulation although not always in a controlled manner. He showed somewhat better mental efficiency at the expense of a good deal of stereotypy. He became more sociable and more courteous without an increase in content. The striking thing in his record was that after operation he became more cooperative and less inhibited by his fears and anxieties to the point that he refused none of the cards, while before operation he refused three cards. One of the cards which he rejected was card VI (sex symbols) but after operation he was capable of responding to this card. The actual content of his responses remained practically the same in the retest, but they emerged in a much clearer fashion without being shrouded by the "veil" which characterized his pre-treatment responses; for example, in card III the answer in the pre-test was: "Two figures, two human figures, hands here but they're not shape of hands covered with mitts. They are not doing any work. They are not playing. They have hands down. I don't know what this is." In the post-test the response was: "Two humans with boxing gloves on." There seemed to be more forthrightness and security in his responses to the second giving of the test. These gains were not without counterbalancing losses; he seemed less accurate in his evaluation of his environment (increase in F−).

Case 9 (Control): Original test: R 16, W 12, W* 0, D 4, M 2, FM 3, F+F 6, F− 3, CF 2, HHd 2, AAd 9, At 5, Pop 3, RT uncol 55, RT color 68.

Postoperative R2: R 12, W 9, W* 2, D 1, M 0, FM 0, F+F 6, F− 6, CF 0, HHd 1, AAd 5, At 6, Pop 2, RT uncol 98, RT color 115.

This patient was a rather inhibited, limited individual initially and became even more so on retest. He lost whatever spontaneity and capacity that he had in the first test and became much more careless and inefficient in his evaluation of the outside world on the retest. His mental efficiency declined considerably and he seemed to be incapable of doing anything spontaneously because of the extreme rigidity which was set up and kept him bound to his stereotyped approach to life.

Case 11 (Control): Original test: R 24, W 8, W* 1, D 14, Dd 1, M 0, FM 5, m 1, F+F 12, F− 2, C′ 0, FC 1, CF 2, C 1, H 0, AAd 17, Obj 0, Pl 1, Na 2, Blood 1, Clouds 2, Color 1, Pop 6, RT uncol 87, RT color 90.

Postoperative R2: R 16, W 7, W* 1, D 7, Dd 1, M 1, FM 3, m 0, F+F 8, F− 1, C′ 1, FC 0, CF 2, C 0, H 1, AAd 7, Obj 1, Pl 4, Na 1, Blood 1, Clouds 1, Color 0, Pop 3, RT uncol 104, RT color 95.

This patient decreased in responsiveness on the retest and showed changes both for the better and worse. He showed greater interest in people in the second test but less control of his affective responsiveness and some indication of depressive tendencies. The degree of his stereotypy decreased. In general he was beset by neurotic conflicts as well as by underlying psychotic trends. He was quite impulsive and anxious at both test periods.

Case 12 (Control): Original test: R 32, W 2, W* 0, D 24, Dd 3, S 3, M 1, FM 2, F+F 23, F− 2, Fc 2, FC 1, CF 1, HHd 4, AAd 21, At 2, Obj 4, Pl 1, Pop 3, Rej 0, RT uncol 150, RT color 112.

Postoperative R2: R 17, W 6, W* 1, D 8, Dd 1, S 1, M 1, FM 0, F+F 12, F− 4, Fc 0, FC 0, CF 0, HHd 3, AAd 8, At 0, Obj 6, Pl 0, Pop 2, Rej 1, RT uncol 172, RT color 133.

In the original test this patient possessed a dilated personality, being capable of responding to both internal as well as external stimulation, but some immature tendencies were also apparent indicating either an infantile or a stereotyped approach to life. In the retest his personality was impoverished, losing in quantity as well as in the breadth of personality responsiveness. He became less capable of dealing with reality, rejected one card, and in general showed indications of poorer performance in the post-test. Whether this was owing to a loss of interest in the test, or whether it was attributable to an actual loss of zest and outgoingness could not be determined.

Case 13 (Area 9ᵃ, 10ᵃ, 45, 46): Preoperative: R 22, W 6, W* 1, D 11, Dd 4, S 0, M 6, FM 1, m 2, FK 1, F+F 8, F− 1, Fc 1, c 1, CF 1, HHd 10, AAd 4, Obj 2, Pl 1, Na 4, Fire 1, Pop 1, RT uncol 225, RT color 255.

Postoperative R2: R 18, W 4, W* 2, D 11, Dd 0, S 1, M 4, FM 2, m 0, FK 0, F+F 10, F− 0, Fc 2, c 0, CF 0, HHd 8, AAd 7, Obj 3, Pl 0, Na 0, Fire 0, Pop 5, RT uncol 95, RT color 108.

This patient changed markedly after operation. He showed a reduction in the amount of outgoingness and less preoccupation with the bizarre, a reduction in the tendency to be introspective and brooding, and less internal conflict. His fantasy life was now under better control but the little responsiveness for emotional stimulation from the outside which he originally possessed disappeared. Instead of being worrisome, introspective, and somewhat bizarre in his thinking, he became more restricted in his interests, less capable of emotional interplay with others but much more amenable to social contacts and to extra-hospital adjustment.

It is interesting to note that the actual responses did not change in their general essence. They did, however, change in the direction of greater definiteness and greater clarity and certainty and especially in loss of bizarreness. For example in card II, before operation: "Yes, it looks like a fire and people running forwards and Christ is coming in the center and the whole crowd is following, etc . . ." After operation: "These look like two persons; this, like a light-flame." (Inquiry—"Looks like they are scared—fire—persons, spread out arms.")

Case 14 (Control): Original test: R 6, W 3, W* 1, D 2, M 2, FM 1, F+F 1, F— 1, C 1, HHd 3, AAd 2, At 1, Obj o, Color 1, Pop 2, Rej 4, RT uncol 54, RT color 52.

Postoperative R2: R 9, W 3, W* 1, D 5, M 2, FM o, F+F 7, F— o, C o, HHd 5, AAd 3, At 1, Obj 1, Color o, Pop 2, Rej 1, RT uncol 126, RT color 115.

This patient presented a picture of either severe organic damage or of deterioration. He was a little more productive at retest but this increase was at the expense of withdrawing within his shell, limiting himself to only obvious, rigidly controlled responses. However, he was capable of responding to all but one of the cards in the second test after rejecting four cards during the first test. This would indicate that his degree of schizophrenic withdrawal varies considerably from time to time. Evidence for a depressive trend was afforded in the first test by the fact that he rejected the uncolored card and showed no differential reaction time to the colored cards.

Case 17 (Control): Original test: R 11, W 8, W* 2, D 1, M o, FM 1, F+F 3, F— 5, C′ 1, FC o, C 1, HHd 1, AAd 9, Color 1, Pop 2, Rej o, RT uncol 122, RT color 96.

Postoperative R2: R 13, W 6, W* 1, D 6, M 1, FM 2, F+F 6, F— 2, C′ o, FC 2, C o, HHd 4, AAd 9, Color o, Pop 3, Rej 1, RT uncol 43, RT color 84.

This patient was rather limited in his responsiveness, probably suffering from an organic condition, in addition to the schizophrenic process. Certain neurotic features became quite apparent on the retest and this made his performance more variegated. His contact with reality was on a surer footing on the retest, and he showed better capacity for affective relationships with others, and less impulsiveness. He also showed a greater interest in people and fewer indications of depressive moods. In general some spontaneous improvement in his mental status was quite apparent.

Case 18 (Area 11): Preoperative: R 59, W 9, W* 13, D 27, Dd 2, S 8, M 6, FM 6, m o, k 1, K 1, F+F 36, F— 3, Fc o, C′ o, FC 4, CF 1, C 1, HHd 9, AAd 12, Obj 33, Pl 3, Clouds 1, Color 1, Others 1, Pop 6, RT uncol 124, RT color 148.

Postoperative R2: R 6o, W 4, W* 17, D 23, Dd 7, S 9, M 3, FM 5, m 1, k 1, K o, F+F 37, F— 2, Fc 3, C′ 2, FC 6, CF o, C o, HHd 7, AAd 14, Obj 36, Pl 3, Clouds o, Color o, Others o, Pop 2, RT uncol 193, RT color 152.

A very meticulous, conscientious patient who had high ambition, intelligence, and drive but who apparently was incapable of bringing the conflict between his inner somewhat immature promptings and his high external goals to an even balance. As a result of this conflict between his high ideals and some of his inner promptings which he regarded as being below these ideals he was in a continuous state of apprehension and anxiety, and his achievement in life had been interfered with. He worked at tasks not so much to accomplish them as to get away from his inner conflicts. With regard to this tendency not much change occurs after operation except that he became a little more depressed and a little more sensitive to stimulation from without. At the same time he seemed to get more control over his emotional promptings and held them under better check. His interest was primarily in objects rather than in living things. He showed a rather rich variety of types of responses which indicated that he was capable of having an interest in a wide variety of topics. Intellectual acumen did not seem to have suffered very much after operation. Although he seemed to be making an effort to get into greater rapport with the outside world, he at the same time exhibited less communality in his responses. His neurotic anxiety lessened somewhat after operation but it was replaced by depressive tendencies which were more in keeping with his psychotic trend. It is clear that his perfectionistic tendencies showed no change after operation. He still concentrated on the interpretation of every single spot on the blot and tried to incorporate all of them in his responses.

Case 19 (Area 45$^a$): Preoperative: R 18, W 11, W* 2, D 5, Dd 0, M 3, FM 1, k 1, F+F 10, F— 1, Fc 1, C' 1, FC 0, H 5, AAd 6, At 0, Obj 4, Pl 1, Na 1, Other 1, Pop 4, RT uncol 56, RT color 123.

Postoperative R2: R 12, W 5, W* 2, D 4, Dd 1, M 2, FM 0, k 0, F+F 4, F— 1, Fc 2, C' 0, FC 3, H 2, AAd 4, At 1, Obj 4, Pl 1, Na 0, Other 0, Pop 3, RT uncol 49, RT color 68.

A rather constricted patient with neurotic trends which seemed to have lessened in the postoperative period, so rendering him a little more sociable and more interested in things outside himself. Postoperatively he seemed to come more into contact with reality by exhibiting more tact and more controlled affectivity, together with a loss in the factors indicating immaturity and anxiety. Original indications of depression disappeared at retest.

He was more anxious, more ambitious, and more colorful before operation, becoming less anxious, less ambitious, and more matter of fact on retest. He was more tactful and better capable of handling emotional stimulation after operation. There was originally some evidence of contamination in his responses indicative of a definite schizophrenic trend but these disappeared in the retest.

Case 21 (Area 10): Preoperative: R 24, W 5, W* 1, D 15, Dd 3, FM 0, K 1, F+F 19, c 0, FC 3, CF 1, HHd 4, AAd 15, At 1, Obj 2, Pl 0, Na 0, Blood 1, Clouds 1, Pop 5, RT uncol 105, RT color 47.

Postoperative: R2: R 15, W 4, W* 0, D 10, Dd 1, FM 3, K 1, F+F 8, c 1, FC 1, CF 1, HHd 1, AAd 11, At 1, Obj 0, Pl 1, Na 1, Blood 0, Clouds 0, Pop 5, RT uncol 45, RT color 73.

This patient presented a schizophrenic picture of rather meager internal life based upon a personality structure which originally showed very little receptivity to inner strivings or to external stimulation. After the operation his personality emerged as introversive in its instinctual trend but extroversive in his actual behavior. As a result, he could not be very productive even though he had capacities for integrating and synthesizing his activities; the internal conflict consumed his energies so that none were left with which to pursue his organized plans. He was stereotyped and became more so after operation and the little capacity that he had originally to analyze situations seemed to have been lost after operation. His responses were rather banal and crude. He changed from a depressive psychotic to one capable of neurotic shock and anxiety. His preoperative rigidity loosened up a bit after operation. He became less mature in his strivings and revealed after operation the true undeveloped immature nature of his introversive tendencies which had gone unrecognized heretofore. Whatever capacity he had to control his affect before operation diminished and a tendency for free-floating anxiety appeared. In general, he lost his preoperative psychotic features which were replaced by more manageable neurotic tendencies.

Case 23 (Control): Original test: R 15, W 2, W* 1, D 9, Dd 3, M 1, m 1, k 2, FK 1, F+F 7, F— 1, FC 2, HHd 5, AAd 4, Obj 3, Na 1, Geo 2, Pop 2, RT uncol 67, RT color 71.

Postoperative R2: R 24, W 3, W* 1, D 14, Dd 6, M 3, m 2, k 5, FK 1, F+F 9, F— 2, FC 2, HHd 9, AAd 5, Obj 4, Na 0, Geo 6, Pop 3, RT uncol 42, RT color 56.

This patient was a highly withdrawn individual who had led an encapsulated existence throughout life despite his tendency to permit certain emotional attachments under very highly controlled conditions. There was little change in this regard after operation and the only outstanding change was a slight tendency for showing more bizarre schizophrenic thought and behavior. He was incapable of carrying out organized activities because small minute details distracted his attention. His productivity level remains relatively unchanged on retest. As a whole it can be said that whatever changes occurred were of no great consequence.

Case 25 (Area 8, 9, 10ᵃ, 46): Preoperative: R 18, W 2, W* 1, D 12, Dd 2, S1, M 1, FM 1, F+F 14, F— 1, C' 1, FC 0, CF 0, C 0, HHd 10, AAd 8, Obj 0, Pl 0, Color 0, Pop 3, RT uncol 123, RT color 403.

Postoperative R2: R 25, W 3, W* 1, D 18, Dd 3, S 1, M 0, FM 0, F+F 20, F— 1, C' 1, FC 1, CF 1, C 1, HHd 4, AAd 10, Obj 9, Pl 1, Color 1, Pop 4, RT uncol 58, RT color 73.

This patient was rather a worrisome individual, responding only to his own inner strivings and not at all to promptings from the outside. After operation he ceased to be responsive to his inner cravings and desires, and was completely at the mercy of external forces which he was unable to control. He became less capable of responding to the totality of the situation when human beings or living things were involved although his general interest in people and life had increased. He was still as constricted and limited in his output as he was before except for the fact that he now had an extroversive trend instead of the introversive trend which dominated him before the operation. Although he was frankly psychotic preoperatively he manifested certain neurotic features which seemed to diminish in intensity in the postoperative test.

Case 26 (Control): Original test: R 16, W 2, W* 1, D 10, Dd 3, S 0, M 1, FM 0, F+F 13, F— 2, HHd 4, AAd 9, Obj 0, Pl 2, Na 1, Pop 2, Rej 1, RT uncol 160, RT color 142.

Postoperative R2: R 25, W 2, W* 1, D 19, Dd 2, S 1, M 6, FM 1, F+F 16, F— 2, HHd 11, AAd 13, Obj 1, Pl 0, Na 0, Pop 1, Rej 0, RT uncol 225, RT color 155.

This patient is a schizophrenic who exhibited a rather high degree of rigidity at first, but reduced it somewhat at retest. He also showed a rather strong introtensive trend and a total lack of capacity for responding to emotional stimulation from without. However, since he had no way of controlling his inner strivings he was at the mercy of his environment and his only way of counteracting was to withdraw to his internal fantasy. All external stimulation was translated in terms of egocentric internal responses which he was incapable of controlling. No change was observed in his personality in the retest.

Case 29 (Control): Original test: R 8, W 2, D 6, FM 1, F+F 4, F— 3, CF 0, HHd 1, A 3, At 4, Pop 2, Rej 3, RT uncol 491, RT color 486.

Postoperative R2: R 6, W 3, D 3, FM 1, F+F 3, F— 1, CF 1, HHd 1, A 2, At 3, Pop 2, Rej 5, RT uncol 230, RT color 308.

This patient was very limited in his output, lacking human empathy and having no interest in interpersonal relationships. He was instinctually more receptive to his inner strivings but tended to direct his energies in an extroversive direction. In this regard there was a little change between tests. He was quite rigid and incapable of complying with the test requirements to such an extent that he rejected three cards in the first test and five cards in the second test. The paucity of responses led to great difficulty in interpretation. In general little, if any, change occurred between tests.

Case 31 (Area 9): Preoperative: R 12, W 5, W* 1, D 6, S 0, M 1, FM 1, F+F 8, F— 0, FC 1, C 1, HHd 2, AAd 7, Obj 1, Blood 1, Other 1, Pop 4, Rej 0, RT uncol 36, RT color 49.

Postoperative R2: R 10, W 6, W* 1, D 2, S 1, M 1, FM 1, F+F 4, F— 4, FC 0, C 0, HHd 2, AAd 8, Obj 0, Blood 0, Other 0, Pop 5, Rej 1, RT uncol 101, RT color 84.

This patient was a rather limited, highly constricted individual with little or no spontaneity and very rigid in her approach to life. As a result of the operation, she lost whatever responsiveness she did have to emotional stimulation and became somewhat less capable of dealing with her environment because of the fuzzy appearance that the world presented to her after operation. Although she was capable of accepting some stimulation from within her own personality, there was nothing to counterbalance this stimulation from without nor to control it. The tendency to give crude, undifferentiated and popular responses was enhanced by the operation, characterizing her as a person who responded to her world only in the crudest unanalytical fashion. The degree of stereotypy also increased in the postoperative test.

Case 32 (Areas 8ᵃ, 9, 10ᵃ): Preoperative: R 71, W 31, W* 3, D 28, Dd 2, S 7, M 1, FM 5, m 2, k 3, FK 2, F+F 38, F— 3, Fc 6, C' 1, c 0, FC 5, CF 5, HHd 4, AAd 16, At 1, Obj 31, Pl 4, Na 5, Geo 6, Others 4, Pop 7, RT uncol 32, RT color 20.

Postoperative R2: R 34, W 12, W* 2, D 18, Dd 1, S 1, M 1, FM 5, m 0, k 0, FK 0, F+F 22, F— 2, Fc 1, C' 0, c 1, FC 2, CF 0, HHd 3, AAd 12, At 1, Obj 12, Pl 0, Na 2, Geo 3, Other 0, Pop 10, RT uncol 62, RT color 50.

Before operation this patient exhibited a rather high level of responsiveness to the outside world characterized by a rather infantile level of inner fantasy and strivings. She paid for this infantile indulgence by having moments of conflict regarding her role in life. On the other hand, she was capable of handling her impulsive emotional outbursts on a rather adequate level, although at some cost to herself in the form of anxiety and conflict. She possessed a considerable amount of tact and a capacity to control her sensuous responsiveness. She was basically an introversive individual but in actual life she tried to play the role of an extroversive individual. Despite certain infantile traits she was capable of controlling her emotional responsiveness and capable of exhibiting considerable tact and capacity to understand her own feelings as well as the feelings of others before operation. After operation, although she still remained egocentric internally, she no longer had the advantages that she presented before. She had lost some of her tact and some of her introspectiveness. Stimulation from the outside did not cause her now as much difficulty as previously since her general level of reactivity had declined.

Case 34 (Control): Original test: R 42, W 8, W* 2, D 24, Dd 6, S 2, M 3, FM 4, K 1, F+F 22, F— 2, Fc 2, c 1, FC 4, CF 2, C 1, HHd 7, AAd 20, At 0, Obj 8, Pl 0, Na 4, Geo 0, Cloud 2, Color 1, Other 0, Pop 7, RT uncol 60, RT color 19.

Postoperative R2: R 34, W 5, W* 1, D 23, Dd 4, S 1, M 3, FM 2, K 2, F+F 13, F— 4, Fc 3, c 1, FC 4, CF 2, C 0, HHd 4, AAd 16, At 1, Obj 7, Pl 1, Na 1, Geo 1, Cloud 2, Color 0, Pop 7, RT uncol 37, RT color 28.

This patient was basically introversive but had adopted an extroversive type of adjustment. This was achieved at the expense of a certain amount of free-floating anxiety, which led to an intellectualization of her personality difficulties. There was very little change in the retest except for a slight reduction in impulsiveness and in immaturity of inner strivings and urges. There was, on the other hand, some reduction in the clarity with which reality was perceived.

Case 35 (Control): Original test: R 12, W 5, W* 1, D 6, S 0, FM 1, F+F 9, F— 1, Fc 0, FC 1, HHd 1, AAd 8, At 3, Obj 0, Pop 3, Rej 1, RT uncol 22, RT color 39.

Postoperative R2: R 16, W 3, W* 0, D 12, S 1, FM 2, F+F 10, F— 2, Fc 2, FC 0, HHd 1, AAd 9, At 2, Obj 4, Pop 3, Rej 0, RT uncol 128, RT color 125.

This patient was a rather unimaginative, colorless individual, unresponsive to her own strivings as well as to external stimulation. On both tests she was rigid and constricted. There was a poverty of ideas which was unchanged. On retest there was a slower reaction time and a loss in receptivity to emotional stimulation for which was substituted a capacity for tactful dealing with the environment.

Case 36 (Areas 10, 11, 45, 46, 47): Pre-operative: R 28, W 8, W* 1, D 17, Dd 1, S 1, M 3, FM 1, m 1, FK 3, F+F 13, F— 2, Fc 1, C′ 0, FC 4, CF 0, HHd 5, A 6, At 2, Obj 9, Pl 1, Na 5, Fire 0, Pop 2, RT uncol 25, RT color 14.

Postoperative R2: R 24, W 3, W* 1, D 19, Dd 0, S 1, M 2, FM 4, m 0, FK 0, F+F 10, F— 0, Fc 1, C′ 1, FC 5, CF 1, HHd 3, A 10, At 0, Obj 8, Pl 2, Na 0, Fire 1, Pop 4, RT uncol 18, RT color 14.

This patient possessed a high degree of responsiveness to both her own inner promptings as well as to stimulation from without. She showed signs of inner conflict accompanied by a definite tendency towards introspection. This capacity for resorting to introspection to alleviate her conflicts did not succeed too well since she had to resort to loss of contact with reality in order to resolve the conflicts, and definite indication of anxiety also emerged. After operation she lost her introspective tendencies and was somewhat less rigid but only by sacrificing some degree of maturity in thought and action, since the majority of her inner strivings were reduced to an immature level. She was also less capable of organizing her environment into larger units but the organization that she did effect was a little more tied to reality, and more practical in nature than it was before operation. In general, her receptivity to promptings or strivings from within as well as her receptivity to stimulation from without was not on as mature a level as it was before operation, She showed better contact with reality and responded in a manner indicative of greater communality with her fellows.

Case 38 (Venous ligation involving areas 6, 8, 9, 10): Preoperative: R 13, W 4, W* 0, D 7, Dd 0, S 2, M 2, FM 2, K 0, FK 1, F+F 7, F— 1, c 0, FC 0, C 0, HHd 5, AAd 8, At 0, Obj 0, Na 0, Color 0, Pop 2, Rej 1, RT uncol 485, RT color 178.

Postoperative R2: R 33, W 6, W* 2, D 13, Dd 6, S 6, M 1, FM 2, K 1, FK 1, F+F 18, F— 5, c 1, FC 3, C 1, HHd 14, AAd 12, At 1, Obj 2, Na 2, Color 1, Pop 2, Rej 0, RT uncol 99, RT color 99.

Before operation this patient was somewhat limited in output, giving only thirteen responses. This low level of responsiveness indicated a withdrawn, though practical-minded individual with definite resistances and oppositional trends limiting her productivity. After operation, the oppositional tendencies were still apparent but she became much more responsive, more than doubling her number of responses. She tended to become absorbed in insignificant aspects of her environment and became more communicative about these insignificant aspects of her life. The increase in responsiveness occurred largely in the realm of anxiety-reflecting responses and in outgoingness. This increase in outgoingness was very marked and is generally well under control except for one impulsive outburst. The increase in responses also brought about a much higher degree of rigidity and some indication of free-floating anxiety, as well as a softer focus in her perceptual capacities and ability to understand her environment. At the same time an increase in the number of responses which indicated a capacity to deal with emotional stimulation arose and an indication of some tendency towards depressive responsiveness also occurred. In general the operation brought the patient out of her preoperative shell, but did so at the expense of less intellectual control and increase in anxiety and depressive moods.

Case 39 (Control): Original test: R 18, W 8, W* 1, D 8, Dd 1, M 2, FM 2, F+F 9, F— 1, Fc 1, FC 1, CF 1, C 1, HHd 3, AAd 10, At 3, Obj 0, Pl 1, Clouds 1, Pop 6, RT uncol 44, RT color 33.

Postoperative: R2: R 23, W 5, W* 1, D 16, Dd 1, M 3, FM 0, F+F 18, F— 0, Fc 0, FC 0, CF 0, C 1, HHd 7, AAd 12, At 0, Obj 3, Pl 0, Clouds 0, Pop 1, RT uncol 156, RT color 154.

This patient was inclined to view her environment in a rather crude undifferentiated manner on the first test with relatively little attention paid to practical matters. Her strivings and inner promptings were similarly on an immature level but she showed some capacity for emotional adjustment and tactfulness, although there were indications of impulsive behavior as well. Her interest in human beings was at a low ebb and she showed several evasive responses and several indicating anxiety. On retest considerable improvement became apparent. She became more practical in her outlook, more accurate in the perception of reality, more mature in her strivings, but she suffered some loss in capacity to control her emotional stimulation. The indications of anxiety disappeared, but her responses became less popular and more individualistic indicating a trend away from the usual and expected. In general, this patient improved considerably between the tests.

Case 40 (Area 24ᵃ): Preoperative: R 28, W 7, W* 1, D 19, Dd 1, S 0, M 5, FM 2, F+F 11, F— 3, Fc 1, C 0, FC 2, CF 2, C 2, HHd 10, A 5, At 4, Obj 5, Na 1, Geo 1, Fire 1, Blood 1, Other 0, Pop 3, Rej 0, RT uncol 156, RT color 41.

Postoperative R2: R 12, W 2, W* 0, D 8, Dd 1, S 1, M 0, FM 0, F+F 10, F— 0, Fc 0, c 1, FC 0, CF 0, C 1, HHd 4, A 2, At 0, Obj 3, Na 0, Geo 0, Fire 0, Blood 1, Other 1, Pop 1, Rej 1, RT uncol 79, RT color 223.

Preoperatively this patient was quite communicative, giving twenty-nine responses and exhibited a rather practical-minded approach to life. She was receptive toward her own striving and prompting and was capable of responding adequately to emotional stimulation from without. Some indications of evasiveness and anxiety were apparent and a certain dysphoric tendency and depression prevented her from sizing up reality adequately. After operation her responsiveness decreased to less than half of her former performance, her inner urges and promptings were completely repressed but she no longer suffered from inability to evaluate reality correctly. She lost all her capacity for emotional responsiveness excepting on the impulsive level. She became more suspicious and negativistic and showed neurotic color shock instead of the original depressive tendencies. She found difficulty in controlling her emotions and would have been happier to be completely withdrawn within her own shell. She did not find it possible to trust people at all times because she could not understand them which gave rise to this alternating attitude of suspiciousness versus trust. It is doubtful whether the postoperative test is representative of her personality. Accepting these data on their face value, it appeared that the operation reduced her mental life considerably. In fact the operation impoverished it to such a point that there was hardly anything left except the clinging to formal ways of responding. Only one uncontrolled texture response and one uncontrolled pure-color response were given, which indicated helplessness in the face of external stimulation.

Case 42 (Area 11): Preoperative: R 20, W 6, D 9, Dd 4, S 1, F+F 9, F— 4, Fc 2, c 1, C' 1, FC 1, CF 1, C 1, Hd 1, AAd 4, At 7, Obj 3, Pl 1, Na 2, Blood 1, Color 1, Pop 1, RT uncol 57, RT color 54.

Postoperative R2: R 13, W 11, D 2, Dd 0, S 0, F+F 3, F— 9, Fc 0, c 0, C' 1, FC 0, CF 0, C 0, Hd 0, AAd 3, At 8, Obj 0, Pl 1, Na 1, Blood 0, Color 0, Pop 0, RT uncol 71, RT col 100.

This patient was quite communicative preoperatively giving twenty responses. She exhibited considerable interest in the significant aspects of the blots and was somewhat negativistic. She rejected her own inner strivings but showed considerable capacity for tact and for outgoingness. She was quite rigid and showed a lack of capacity for interpreting her environment correctly. Also present were a considerable amount of impulsiveness and a dysphoric affect. After operation her responsiveness dropped to nearly half of what it was before operation. Most of her responses indicated a rather crude unintegrated approach. Her contact with reality dropped to an even lower level and she became much more rigid. Her capacity for tact vanished and so did her tendency to dysphoric moods as well as her impulsiveness. The content of her responses was still primarily anatomical and did not represent even as wide a variety of content as she had before operation.

Case 47 (Area 44): Preoperative: R 9, W 3, W* 0, D 6, FM 0, F+F 2, F— 1, c 0, C' 1, FC 1, CF 2, C 2, H 1, AAd 3, At 1, Obj 1, Na 1, Color 1, Other 1, Pop 0, Rej 3, RT uncol 96, RT color 74.

Postoperative R2: R 12, W 6, W* 1, D 5, FM 1, F+F 6, F— 1, c 1, C' 0, FC 0, CF 1, C 2, H 1, AAd 6, At 0, Obj 3, Na 1, Color 1, Other 0, Pop 1, Rej 1, RT uncol 85, RT color 110.

This patient was so low in productivity that either functional deterioration or organic defect was suspected. She inhibited her inner strivings completely but did permit herself to respond to external stimulation, although generally in an uncontrolled impulsive manner. After operation she lost control over her responsiveness, gave more commonplace responses but became more dilated in her expression of personality trends. By decreasing her rigid control, she increased her capacity for responding impulsively and permitted expression of her less mature inner promptings. This general reduction in maturity indicates a definite worsening of personality functioning. The data are so meager that these statements must remain tentative.

Case 49 (Area 10, 11$^a$, 46$^a$): Preoperative: R 17, W 9, W* 1, D 7, S 0, M 1, FM 2, k 1, FK 1, F+F 8, F— 1, Fc 1, FC 1, CF 1, HHd 1, AAd 8, At 1, Obj 2, Pl 2, Na 0, Geo 2, Pop 2, RT uncol 187, RT color 157.

Postoperative R2: R 17, W 4, W* 5, D 7, S 1, M 1, FM 1, k 0, FK 0, F+F 11, F— 1, Fc 0, FC 1, CF 2, HHd 1, AAd 7, At 0, Obj 3, Pl 4, Na 1, Geo 1, Pop 4, RT uncol 75, RT color 75.

Before operation this patient tended to inhibit her own inner strivings and urges and permitted only the less mature ones to emerge. She was quite introspective and brooding and tended to intellectualize her anxieties. She was tactful in her interpersonal interactions and possessed fairly good control of her emotional responsiveness. Because of her shut-in life she exhibited very little interest in people and tended to be somewhat negativistic. She changed very little in total responsiveness after operation but altered her style of response becoming more constricted and utilizing less of the categories available to her, especially those which indicate free-floating anxiety as well as introspection arising from anxiety sources. In place of this rather manifold type of response which characterized her preoperatively, she was, after operation, capable of responding only with the rather noncommittal form of responses. The operation apparently robbed her of a certain amount of colorfulness even though it reduced her anxiety level. She exhibits still less interest in people after operation and is a little more noncommittal in the type of material with which she chooses to respond. The operation resulted in greater constriction with a slight decrease in the capacity to analyze the blots in terms of their details. The patient was capable of seeing less human details after operation. There was a strong drive to give organized whole responses extremely out of keeping with the barrenness of the subject's mental content, indicating hollow contentless ambition but this tendency was reduced by the operation.

## SUMMARY

An examination of the Rorschach records of the patients subjected to operation indicated that some of the subjects have been altered in their personality trends while others remained unchanged. No definite pattern of changes emerged. Furthermore, the control patients frequently showed the same types of changes observed in the operatee group.

In view of these considerations a statistical analysis was attempted of the individual Rorschach factors before and after operation. In this analysis each Rorschach factor was dealt with separately, and no groupings were made as was done for obtaining the correlations reported above. The most pronounced change was found to occur in reaction time. In this measure the operatees showed a greater decline than was observed in the control group. In the other factors no statistically significant findings emerged. Some trends, however, were noted. The factors which showed a tendency to decrease in the operatee group after operation are: R, W, M, m, k, FK. The factors that tended to increase after operation are W* and F—. The factors that tended to show a decrease were those that are said to be primarily associated with anxiety, ambitiousness, conflict, and introspection. The factors that tended to show an increase are those which are thought to have to do with lessening of ambition and lowering of standards of accuracy.

## Chapter 22

# Other Tests

ROBERT M. BEECHLEY AND RALPH RUST
with the collaboration of
KATHRYN ALBERT, IHLER GRIMMELMANN, VIOLET HAMWI,
VIRGINIA KIRK, AND ESTELLE RAPPORT

---

I N ADDITION to the tests and experiments reported in previous chapters there is an additional group of tests which was used and which can be more briefly summarized. These tests fall into four categories: Immediate Memory Tests, Visual Perception Experiments, Sustained Attention Tests, and a group of Concept Formation Tests.

### BENTON VISUAL RETENTION TEST

The Benton Visual Retention Test (Benton, '45) is a performance test of immediate memory, requiring the patient to draw a geometrical figure which he has looked at for ten seconds. The test consists of seven simple geometrical designs, graded in difficulty from one figure to three complex figures on one card. Each drawing is scored as correct or incorrect, the maximum score being 7.

On total scores for the three administrations of the test there were no statistically significant differences in performance between the operatee and control groups. Two designs (no. 4 and 5) differentiated between the two groups, with the operatees doing better on these two designs than did the controls. On each separate design, the operatee group showed a trend towards better performance. This test showed no impairment of immediate memory following operation.

### MEMORY FOR OBJECTS

The Memory for Objects is a test of visual memory span (see fig. 101). A large card, containing pictures of different objects, was exposed for ten seconds, and then the patient was asked to name as many of the pictured objects as he could. The score was the total number of objects recalled.

A second large card, containing all the pictures on the first card plus additional objects, was next shown to the patient. He was asked to pick out those pictures which he recognized as having seen before on the first card. The score was the total number of pictures correctly recognized.

The recall memory span increased in both groups on retesting. No significant differences in this respect were found between the control and operatee groups,

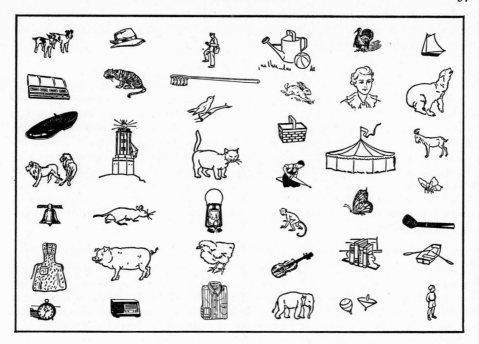

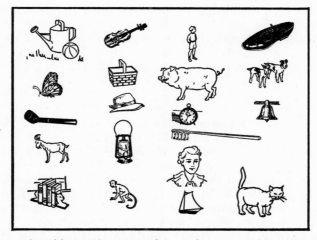

FIG. 101. Memory for objects. The top card is used for recognition; the bottom card for memory.

although the operatees tended to benefit more from the practice effect. The memory span as measured by the recognition method increased significantly in the operatee group while showing no steady improvement in the control group.

An analysis of the tests of immediate and incidental memory indicated that as far as recall was concerned no advantage accrued to the operatees. In recognition, the operatees excelled the controls on some tests and on others they showed a greater variability in performance, some gained considerably while others lost.

### Aphasia and Lateral Dominance

Eisenson's ('46) test for aphasia, agnosia, and apraxia and Harris' ('46) test of lateral dominance were given before and after operation or anesthesia. There was no evidence of any aphasic phenomenon as indicated by this test in either operatees or controls in preoperative or preanesthesia and postoperative or postanesthesia testing. The records of the operatees with area 44 (Broca's area) removed were particularly carefully studied for signs of aphasia and none were found.

There was no evidence of changes in cerebral dominance in operatees or control patients from preoperative or preanesthesia to postoperative or postanesthesia testing.

### Levy Movement Cards

The Levy Movement Cards (Rust, '48) gauge the capacity of an individual to perceive movement in a stationary semi-structured visual field. It was an outgrowth of the method of testing the limits for the perception of movement in the Rorschach test. Since this test provided objective scores for the evaluation of the movement response, it was hoped that it might reveal changes in this capacity following operation.

A comparison of the operatee and control groups indicated that both groups tended to benefit somewhat from the practice effect but the operatee group tended to benefit more, showing an increase in the number of movement responses. This was not statistically significant, but it was quite marked in the patients with area 9 removed. The gain in these patients was significantly greater than in the other operatees and than in the control group.

### Rubin Figures

The Rubin ('21) Figures Test measures the capacity to reverse an ambiguous perspective. It consists of two cards (white on black and black on white) containing contours drawn to represent either a goblet or two facing human profiles, equally well. The score on this test consisted of whether the patient could see first one and then the other representation by himself, or of how much help he needed and whether or not he could reverse at all. Although no group differences were found there was a definite difference in the acceptability of demonstration (figures pointed out to those who otherwise could not see them at all) in favor of the operatee group following operation.

### Bolles Progressive Completion Test

The Bolles Progressive Completion Test (Lynn, Levine, and Hewson, '45) is a test of perceptual closure. A series of cards were displayed to the patient. On each card were drawn portions, but not all, of a picture. In a series the first card contained a few elements of the picture, a second which contained these same elements with more added, and so on until the complete picture was assembled on the sixth card. There were seven different pictures with a series of six cards for each picture. These were displayed to the patient one at a time, and he was asked what he thought the pattern on each card represented. The score consisted of the card upon which the correct answer was given.

There were no differences in the group performance of the operatee and control groups on this test. The scores did not increase, and the operation seemed to have no effect on this type of closure situation.

### SUBTRACTION AND ADDITION TESTS

The Continuous Subtraction Test and the Addition Test were included in an effort to obtain some measure of ability to carry on sustained mental work. The literature on frontal lobe functions includes mention of impairment of ability to give prolonged attention, to concentrate, to give sustained effort, and similar attributes. Robinson ('46) has recently formulated the basic loss following lobotomy as being one of deliberativeness, defined as prolonged attention.

In the Subtraction Test the patient was required to count backward by threes from 100 to 1. The scores were time in seconds required to complete the task, and errors, each single failure to subtract three being counted as one error. Initially the operatee group was much slower than the control so that changes which occurred were not readily interpreted in light of control-group performance. On the Addition Test the patient was required to add 180 pairs of single numbers as rapidly as possible. The score was time in seconds required to complete the task. The operatee group was slightly superior to the control at O but became progressively worse at $R_1$ and $R_2$, while the control group improved progressively but the differences between the groups were not statistically significant.

Although Addition and the Anxiety Inventory score did not correlate before operation, the decreases in both for postoperative patients correlated $+0.58$, suggesting the possibility that the increase in speed of addition may be a function of decrease in anxiety. A comparison of the increases in speed in the operatee and the control groups indicated that although the operatees showed a much greater increase it was not statistically significant. The reason for the lack of significance is to be attributed to the contrary trends found among the operatees, some gaining markedly in speed and others showing only moderate gains. In the control group the gains were much more uniform.

The claims made for these two tests in the literature were not fully substantiated although the Subtraction Test did show changes in variability which are attributable to the effects of the operation.

### CAPPS HOMOGRAPH TEST

The Capps Homograph Test (Capps, '39) consists of a series of simple words which have more than one meaning. The patient was required to give as many different meanings for each word as he could. The total number of different meanings exclusive of the first was taken as the score and it was regarded as a measure of verbal flexibility. The control group benefited from the practice effect afforded by the repetition of the test while the operatee group did not show as much improvement and differed significantly from the control group in this respect. Some of the operatees showed losses at $R_1$ followed by gains at $R_2$ similar to that found on the Porteus Test.

An examination of the individual gains and losses in the operatee group in relation to improvement indicated that of the 13 operatees who were regarded as socially improved 9 showed gains on the shift score. In the unimproved patients the number losing was balanced by the number gaining. The control group did not show this relationship to improvement. With regard to areas, those patients who had areas 45 and 46 excised showed a significant loss as compared with members of the control group or with other operatees. It may be concluded that the topectomy operation interfered with verbal flexibility on the Capps Homograph Test and that the operations in which areas 45 and 46 are involved were productive of the greatest interference.

### Albert Test

The Albert Test* consists of a series of twenty-seven sets of five small toys. Each set presents a pattern of relationship which includes four of the objects but not the fifth and the task of the patient is to select the odd object.

The operatees increased while the control group decreased slightly in the postoperative or postanesthesia testings. The difference was not statistically significant. The patients with areas 45 and 46 excised showed a significant increase over the control group as well as over the gains in the other operatees.

### Double Alternation Experiment

In the Double Alternation technique used in animal experimentation the animal finds food first twice on the right and then twice on the left. This has been considered as evidence of ideational learning. Nichols and Hunt ('40) applied a more difficult adaptation of this task to a patient with extensive frontal lobe damage and found him unable to master the problem, although normal subjects solved it easily.

The Nichols and Hunt problem, with some variation, was applied to the patients of the Greystone Project. Playing cards were dealt face down in a row, the ace of spades appearing twice on one end and twice on the other. The patient was instructed to turn up the ace with as few turns as possible. His problem was to learn the "system" or pattern of alternation. If he failed in this, a simpler task was tried, or if he solved it the examiner would pass to a more difficult one, all the tasks involving such a "system" of generalization. A score consisted of the number of deals required to arrive at the use of the proper system, either verbalized or repeated successful solutions.

Performance and results on this test showed that the operatees did not experience the type of disability at this task reported by Nichols and Hunt. The only operatee to deviate in any recognizable fashion was patient 6 who showed a decrease.

### Levine Simultaneous Concept Test

The Levine Simultaneous Concept Test (Lynn, Levine, and Hewson, '45) consists of a graded series of tasks in which the patient is required to keep in mind simultaneously two, three, and four concepts on the basis of which objects are to be classified. The test consists of two equivalent parts—a pic-

* This test is an adaptation of methods outlined by Raven ('41-43) and Penrose ('44) .

torial test in which the objects are presented pictorially and a verbal test in which the names of the objects are used. This test gave inconclusive results because the objects constituting the test were interpreted in various ways by the different patients so that no consistent scoring system could be devised.

## HUMOR TEST

Because of the reports in the literature that *witzelsucht* often accompanies frontal lobotomy a series of jokes and humorous cartoons were collected and presented to the patients with instructions to rate them for goodness. This technique failed to yield any consistent results.

*Chapter 23*

# Test Results One Year After Operation

CARNEY LANDIS

with the collaboration of

MORTIMER GARRISON Jr., VIOLET HAMWI, ANNE KENNARD STAUFFER, HENRY EUGENE KING, AND KATHLEEN MARY YOUNG

O N MAY 13-16, 1948, approximately one year after the period of operations, 29 of the 32 patients on whom the majority of the psychologic tests had been carried out were re-examined. The Porteus, Weigl, Capps, Flicker, Anxiety, and Complaint procedures were applied since these particular tests were those which showed the clearest evidence of change at some one or more of the test periods after operation. It will be recalled that the original group of 24 patients was operated upon in May-June, 1947, and that in October, 1947, 7 control patients and 1 patient from the operatee group were subjected to prefrontal lobotomy. This second operation further reduced the number of control patients available for statistical comparisons. In light of this, most of the comparisons which have been made with respect to the one-year-after data were based on the previous performance of each individual patient concerned. As in previous chapters the original preoperative test period is designated as O, the three-week postoperative as R1, the three-month postoperative as R2, the eight-month postoperative as R3, and the one-year postoperative as R4.

## PORTEUS MAZES

In most patients the immediate effect of the operation was a reduction of one year or more in mental age (chapter 14). Eight months after operation this loss had been regained so that the average M.A. of the control and operatee groups was no longer statistically significantly different. The average mental age for each group for each test period is given in table 73. From the figures given in this table it is apparent that after a year's time no difference in average M.A. remains.

Five of the 6 patients who showed the greatest drop in M.A. three weeks postoperatively made excellent social recoveries. The original average M.A. of these 5 at each test period was O = 13.5; R1 = 11.4; R2 = 13.2; R3 = 14.6; and R4 = 15.0. Patient 4 was out of the hospital at the end of the year although he had not previously been rated by the psychiatrist as showing social improvement. His five test scores were 11.0, 9.0, 11.5, 15.0, and 13.0. In other words he showed the drop in M.A. which in other patients had gone with subsequent social recovery. The only patient who was out of the hospital at the end of one year who did not show the drop in M.A. after operation was patient 49. Her scores were 14.5, 16.5, 14.5, 17.0, and 17.5.

Patients 2, 6, and 40 also showed drops of more than one year in M.A. after operation but failed to make social recoveries. The operations (areas 6 and 8, and 24) were not those which produced an amelioration in any patient. Patient 40 (area 24) is the only patient in the series who failed to recover her initial M.A. at some test period after operation. Her scores were $O = 14.5$, $R1 = 6.5$, $R3 = 7.0$, and $R4 = 10.0$.

TABLE 73.  AVERAGE MENTAL AGE FOR EACH TEST PERIOD OF PORTEUS
MAZES

|  | 0 | R1 | R2 | R3 | R4 |
|---|---|---|---|---|---|
| Operatees..................... | 13.2 | 12.0 | 13.3 | 13.5 | 14.3 |
| Controls...................... | 13.2 | 14.1 | 15.0 | 14.4 | 14.2 |

In summary, the Porteus Maze reflects a pattern of performance which is usually associated with social recovery following topectomy. With one exception, neither topectomy nor lobotomy produced a loss in M.A. which lasted throughout the period of a year.

## WEIGL TEST

This test and the results obtained with it were described in chapter 15. The mean scores given in table 57, together with the one-year-after average, provide the data given in table 74.

Statistical analysis indicated that none of the differences between these means were significant.

TABLE 74.  MEAN SCORES ON WEIGL TEST

|  | 0 | R1 | R2 | R4 |
|---|---|---|---|---|
| Operatees............................... | 7.76 | 8.71 | 8.47 | 8.72 |
| Controls............................... | 8.00 | 8.46 | 8.69 | 8.30 |

The tabulations provided in chapter 16, table 59 indicated that patients 4, 24, 25, and 36 had been able to shift attitude in the sorting on this test before operation, but at both R1 and R2 testing after operation were unable to shift. Patients 24, 25, and 36 were able to shift on the test one year after operation but patient 4 was still unable to shift without coaching. (As table 59 shows patient 4 did not show any other evidence of loss of the abstract attitude.) Among the control group, patient 17 showed the same pattern of test response to the Weigl that patient 4 did, namely ability to shift at O and inability to shift at R1, R2, and R4.

The year-after retest indicated that any loss of abstract attitude which the

Weigl Test might have indicated, particularly in respect to area 46, did not persist in 3 of 4 cases. Topectomy did not bring about a permanent loss in the ability to shift attitude, as indicated by this test.

### CAPPS HOMOGRAPH TEST

The average Capps scores for the different test periods are given in table 75.

As mentioned in chapter 22 the drop in the average score following operation is statistically significant. Eleven of 19 operatees showed a decreased score at R1 and in six instances the original score had not been regained in one year's time. The more significant loss which was associated with removal of areas 45 and 46 at R2 did not continue to R4, nor was the loss so clearly associated with social improvement at the year's end. There seems no doubt but that the operation itself—not the recovery from psychosis—did cause a decrease in the ability to make verbal shifts and that in 6 of the 24 cases this loss persisted over a year's time. The test itself deserves greater standardization and further application.

TABLE 75.  AVERAGE CAPPS SCORES FOR DIFFERENT TEST PERIODS

|  | *0* | *R1* | *R2* | *R4* |
|---|---|---|---|---|
| Operatees | 15.8 | 14.6 | 16.9 | 16.4 |
| Controls | 17.2 | 19.1 | 22.2 | 21.4 |

### CRITICAL FLICKER FREQUENCY

Like the Porteus Maze and the Capps, the Critical Flicker Frequency (CFF) showed a decrease in threshold determinations when determined three weeks postoperatively which was partly regained by the three-month postoperative test period (chapter 19).

At the end of one year 7 patients showed some decrease from their three-month postoperative scores, 6 patients showed increases, and 2 remained the same. No increase or decrease was particularly noteworthy.

Evidently the loss in CFF is to be attributed to the immediate effect of the operation and is usually recovered in a three-month period.

### ANXIETY AND COMPLAINT INVENTORIES

The scores on the Anxiety and Complaint Inventories and their subscales at the various test periods are given in table 76.

As was pointed out in chapter 20 the operatee and control groups were not matched on Anxiety or Complaint scores at any test period, so that the only value of the comparison was the indication of the direction of change shown by the control group. The control patients showed a fewer number of Anxieties and Complaints at the end of one year than at any previous test period. This was attributed to such factors as greater familiarity with the examiners, the test procedure, and the significance of taking part in the program. It might also have been owing in part to the fact that 3 of the 7 available control patients had also had lobotomy operations.

The score on the Anxiety Inventory and its parts was lower at R4 than at any previous test period. In part this was attributable to a definite attitude shown by those operatees who had been paroled from the hospital. They strove to impress the examiner with the fact that mentally they were "all right," and that they were endeavoring to say nothing which might indicate that they might better be returned for a further stay in the hospital.

TABLE 76.  SCORES ON ANXIETY AND COMPLAINT INVENTORIES AND THEIR SUBSCALES

|  | 0 | R1 | R2 | R4 |
|---|---|---|---|---|
| Full Scale Anxiety |  |  |  |  |
| Operatees | 55.9 | 41.4 | 42.9 | 31.8 |
| Controls | 14.7 | 17.9 | 18.8 | 10.8* |
| Self-Conscious Anxiety |  |  |  |  |
| Operatees | 24.7 |  | 19.6 | 13.3 |
| Controls | 5.6 |  | 8.0 | 2.0* |
| Self-Referred Anxiety |  |  |  |  |
| Operatees | 22.6 |  | 17.2 | 13.2 |
| Controls | 5.4 |  | 8.7 | 3.7* |
| Full Scale Complaints |  |  |  |  |
| Operatees | 64.1 | 54.2 | 52.9 | 52.8 |
| Controls | 50.6 | 54.7 | 51.2 | 41.8* |
| Mental Symptoms |  |  |  |  |
| Operatees | 23.1 |  | 16.4 | 16.3 |
| Controls | 15.3 |  | 15.3 | 11.6* |

* Based on 7 of original 10 controls.

On the Complaint Inventory and its derived mental-symptom scale the R4 score was practically the same as it had been at R1 and R2. The drop in score on Complaints followed immediately after the operation (R1) in contrast to Anxiety which seemingly decreased more gradually over the entire year.

SUMMARY

The repetition at the end of one year of certain of the tests which had been found to have changed scores after the operation (or the amelioration from psychosis) showed the following points of general interest:

1. The effect on Porteus, Weigl, Capps, and Flicker was shown most clearly and distinctly three weeks after operation and was followed by a return to pre-operative level during several succeeding months. No one of the changes resulted in a permanent loss. The change can be directly attributed to the effect of the operation. The change was, more often than not, associated with an amelioration from psychosis and social recovery.

2. Anxiety diminished clearly and constantly during the course of the post-operative year. Complaints dropped rather sharply immediately following operation and were then maintained on the new lower level for the remainder of the year.

## Chapter 24

# Psychologic Changes Following Topectomy

### CARNEY LANDIS

WHICH effects or changes which were found should be attributed to the recovery from mental illness without the topectomy? Were the effects or changes which occurred due to the intensive study and interest which was given to this particular group of patients? Where can we clearly say that the operation was the primary cause of the change?

All patients in this study received the same general care except that half were subjected to operation. Of the control patients 3 improved and were paroled home from the hospital. All 3 of these had shown evidence of improvement before the operations were started. None of the patients who were operated upon seemed to be improving before operation. There is no evidence that any changes occurred which can be attributed to the "total push" of the entire investigation which affected the operatees to a greater or less degree than they affected the controls. There were very few differences between the groups in psychologic test scores before operation. There were a few differences both three weeks and four months after operation. In those specific instances where changes did take place the data were very closely examined to see if the change could be attributed to recovery from psychosis rather than attributing the changes to the operation.

It is most remarkable, in view of most previous claims about the great importance of the frontal lobes to the mental life of the individual, that so few changes were found. We gave thirty-five different tests before operation; we repeated most of them three weeks after operation and all of them four months after operation. From the thirty-five tests we derived 135 different scores of performance from the tests. Nine times out of ten neither the average or the variability of the operatee group differed significantly from that of the control group.

The Wechsler-Bellevue Intelligence Test, either in its entirety or in the analysis of the twelve subtests which make it up, was unchanged. The sorting tests which indicate the ability to generalize or to abstract were not significantly changed. Word Association, Time Judgment, Mirror Drawing, Continuous-Problem Task, all learning scores, and most memory scores were all unaltered. Eight of the ten scales to evaluate personality based on the Levy Movement Cards were unchanged. Most of the Rorschach scores were unchanged.

The list of tests or indicators which showed real changes which might be attributed to the effect of the operation is both short and puzzling. There was a change in 30 percent of operatees in their ability to do the Porteus Maze Test. This change amounted to a loss of about one year of mental age three weeks after operation, which loss was regained by eight months after operation. There was a decrease in the Critical Flicker Fusion threshold shown by most but not all operatees, which decrease was more marked three weeks after operation than it was four months after operation. On Continuous Subtraction, the variability of the operatee group was increased over that of the control group. Certain of the patients, following operation, showed an improved efficiency in memory considered either as recall or recognition. The outstanding alteration brought about by the operation was the decrease in Self-Referred and Self-Conscious Anxiety and in Mental and Physical Complaints. These changes in Anxiety and Complaints seemed to constitute a highly specific alteration and one which was closely allied to social recovery. This loss in Anxiety and in Complaints may be the basis for the changes we obtained in the other tests. The evidence must be considered in detail.

The examination of all of our test results showed that no general factor of mental operation was significantly altered. The factors of intelligence, speed, power, memory, attention, ability to abstract, verbal facility, or imagination were not altered by a general decrease or increase. The changes which did take place were in rather specific performances which were, so far as we could tell, interrelated principally in that they were associated with social recovery.

This leads us to the next perplexing point. Some of the operatees improved; what were the essential psychologic changes going with this improvement? When the operatees were presented to the hospital parole board four months after operation 20 of the 24 were recommended for parole. Of those paroled a majority seem to have made a good social and work adjustment outside of the hospital. In other words, they showed a remission from their mental illness. Which psychologic test scores reflect this change? The change in the Porteus, Capps, and in Flicker Fusion might be thought of as an interference in efficiency due to injury and that this interference tends to disappear or decrease with the passage of time. The changes in Word Association reaction time may result from diminished self-preoccupation and greater responsiveness to the test. Even the changes in memory scores, particularly recall and recognition, could be thought of as greater responsiveness to the task. The greatest changes were the marked loss of painful self-consciousness and mental complaints which was the alteration which the patients themselves recognized and considered important. The behavior of the patients at each testing period illustrates the same point. When first seen, many of the patients were preoccupied and harassed by their own troubles. Often it was with difficulty that the psychologist broke through this shell of self-preoccupation in getting the patient to set aside his troubles for the moment in order to do the required psychologic tasks. After operation, particularly four months after operation, those operatees who were improved were not particularly preoccupied with themselves or their troubles. Cooperation was easily secured. The results on the majority of the test scores were not significantly different from those of the original scores, but the patient was somewhat more cooperative and amiable in going about the task before him. In any event it is simplest to conclude tentatively that the operation somehow reduced emotional tension. This reduction seems to have given rise to most of the changes in psychologic test scores as well as the social improvement.

Another line of evidence may now be brought forward. In 133 out of 135 test comparisons the differences between R1 and O scores and between R2 and O scores of the operatees equalled or exceeded the highest or lowest score made by any control patient and this in spite of the fact that few of the mean or variability scores for the groups were significantly different. The operatees had a greater spread or range of scores.

TABLE 77.  PERCENTAGE OF MARKED GAIN, LOSS, AND CHANGE FOR ALL PSYCHOLOGIC TESTS COMBINED

| Group | Number of patients | Three weeks postoperative | | | Four months postoperative | | |
|---|---|---|---|---|---|---|---|
| | | Percent of gain | Percent of loss | Percent of change | Percent of gain | Percent of loss | Percent of change |
| Controls................ | 13 | .05 | .08 | .13 | .07 | .06 | .13 |
| Operatees.............. | 19 | .14 | .17 | .31 | .15 | .13 | .28 |
| Area excised | | | | | | | |
| 6................... | 2 | .16 | .23 | .39 | .12 | .17 | .29 |
| 8................... | 5 | .16 | .23 | .39 | .14 | .15 | .29 |
| 9................... | 6 | .16 | .21 | .38 | .15 | .14 | .28 |
| 10.................. | 4 | .16 | .13 | .29 | .17 | .13 | .29 |
| 46.................. | 4 | .13 | .21 | .34 | .14 | .15 | .29 |
| 45.................. | 2 | .13 | .16 | .29 | .13 | .16 | .29 |
| 11.................. | 3 | .12 | .09 | .21 | .10 | .12 | .22 |
| Improvement rating | | | | | | | |
| 8 to 4............... | 9 | .16 | .17 | .33 | .17 | .12 | .29 |
| 2 or 1............... | 4 | .12 | .21 | .33 | .12 | .13 | .25 |
| 0 or −1............. | 19 | .08 | .09 | .17 | .08 | .09 | .17 |
| Gross amount of cortical damage | | | | | | | |
| Most............... | 2 | .20 | .14 | .34 | .16 | .14 | .29 |
| Medium............ | 10 | .14 | .19 | .33 | .15 | .13 | .28 |
| Least.............. | 6 | .10 | .15 | .25 | .13 | .14 | .27 |

Those changes which equalled or exceeded the highest or lowest score made by any control patient have been referred to in the previous chapters as *marked deviations*. Comparisons made in these terms are open to statistical criticism. They do provide evidence of direction of change and when considered together with other evidence assume meaning. The changes in scores made by each of the 32 patients on whom psychologic tests were available were assembled in such a fashion that the difference scores for each individual were entered on a single sheet together with other relevant data about that patient. Since different patients took a differing number of tests the number of marked deviations which were increases and the number which were decreases were divided by the number of tests done by each patient so giving a quotient or percentage. This provides a "percent of gain," a "percent of loss" and when the two are added together a "percent of change." Table 77 and figure 102 give a summary of the percent of gains, losses, and changes for both the three-week and four-month postoperative testing periods. The table gives separately the figures for operatee and control patients: for the areas excised, for the improvement rating, and for the gross amount of cortical damage.

The figures in the table justify the following statements:

1. The percent of gain and loss for controls is practically the same at $R_1$ and $R_2$. (That there is a percent of gain, loss, or change for the control group rests on the fact that the marked deviations *equalled* as well as exceeded the most extreme score of the controls. Subtracting out the control percentage at the top of the column for each figure in the column would give the percent of operatees who exceeded all controls.)

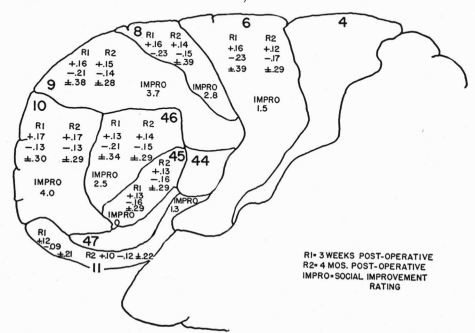

FIG. 102. Net changes in all psychologic tests, showing the percentage of operatees who equal or exceed the scores made by any control.

2. For the operatee group there was a decrease in the percent of loss, $R_1$ minus O (17 percent) to $R_2$ minus O (13 percent), indicating that the immediate losses following operation are partly regained.

3. For areas excised the gains are the same for areas 6, 8, 9, and 10 (16 percent) and for 45, 46, and 11 (13 percent) at $R_1$. At $R_2$ the gains are greatest with area 10 and least with area 11.

4. The losses at $R_1$ are most marked with areas 6, 8, 9, and 46 and least with area 11. At $R_2$ the losses have stabilized and are usually slightly more than are the gains. Area 6 has the most loss and area 11 the least.

5. The percent of change (gains plus losses) at $R_1$ decreases regularly from 39 percent for area 6 to 21 percent for area 11. At $R_2$ the percent of change is remarkably similar (29 percent) for all areas save 11.

6. Patients who made good social improvement had more gains and fewer losses at both $R_1$ and $R_2$ than those who improved slightly or those who failed to improve. At $R_2$ this is most marked in that good social improvement had twice as many gains or losses as did those patients who failed to improve.

7. Based on the cytologic evidence (chapter 5) Dr. Mettler provided us with an estimate of the amount of cortical damage. At R1 the 2 patients with most damage had a larger percent of gains and a smaller percent of losses than those patients with medium or little damage. This distinction disappears at R2 at which time there is little evidence that the gross amount of damage differentially affects the marked changes in psychologic test performance.

It will be remembered that these percentages represent quotients obtained from all of a wide variety of test scores obtained from this group of 32 patients, and that they represent only the changes which we have called marked deviations. The point now arises: Were some kinds or groups of tests more responsible for these deviations than other kinds of tests? An answer to this question might have been obtained by the application of some statistical method such as factor analysis or multiple correlational analysis. Zubin has previously indicated (chapter 13) why these methods were not applied. We made a very close inspectional scrutiny of both the individual and group changes but were unable to discern any general relationships existing between the marked deviations. We are of the opinion that the changes have little in common.

This portion of the analysis of results indicates that marked changes were brought about in all tests: that there were slightly more gains than losses and that the changes were probably stabilized in the four months after operation. Other than a general relationship to loss of anxiety no common factor existed among these changes.

Turning for a moment to two practical questions, we may consider prognosis and amelioration in terms of psychologic test results or scores. It was conceivable that some one of the tests or some score on some of the tests or some combination of scores on the tests given before operation would provide an indication of the chances that marked improvement would be brought about by the operation. We correlated sixty-seven tests arrays secured before operation with the social improvement rating and failed to secure even one coefficient of correlation which reached the level of statistical significance, let alone a level of prediction value.

The second question is that of a scale which would indicate the amount of improvement brought about by the operation and furnish an objective standard on which to judge the changes which take place in a patient, which changes may lead to his parole from the hospital. From the O and R2 scores on Anxiety, Complaints, Addition, Subtraction, Flicker, Capps, Wechsler-Bellevue, and Verbal Directions it was possible to work out statistical combinations which correlate with social improvement ratings. The actual combination of such test results into a new index would be possible and may be attempted in some future study.

## CONCLUSIONS

Psychologic and psychometric changes do take place in patients in whom there have been a bilateral symmetrical removal of specified anatomical areas from the frontal lobes. These changes are relatively independent of such background variables such as age, intellect, sex, or years of hospitalization.

No patient in this group of 19 operatees which we have studied had a real or permanent impairment of mental function brought about by the operation, which could be demonstrated in any way by our exhaustive psychologic test battery. In individual patients specific losses in the form of marked decreases in scores did occur but these losses were, so far as we could tell, more than compensated for by other marked gains and hence did not lead to impairment.

There was no real loss in memory, learning, or intellectual functions brought about by any of the topectomy operations. There was a real valid gain in some recall and recognition memory scores in many of the patients which gain was usually associated with the social recovery of the patient.

Impairment or loss of a categorical attitude (the ability to perform mental abstractions or generalizations) could not be regularly demonstrated. Isolated instances of decreases in the sorting test scores or inability to shift on one test but not another were found. Actually we failed to find a single instance of an over-all, clear-cut loss in the abstract attitude.

There was no permanent loss or gain in intelligence test scores. There was a transient loss in the mental age score on the Porteus Maze Test which was gained back in four months by the patients who had made a social recovery. In only one patient (40, area 24) was the Porteus loss not regained in eight months.

The threshold for Critical Flicker Frequency was markedly decreased in 9 patients, 7 of whom made good social recoveries. Other patients who improved did not show this specific change.

The ability to estimate and reproduce time intervals of five, ten, and fifteen seconds was not altered in any constant fashion by any of the operations.

There were tendencies shown by various tests which are indicative of a greater loss in psychologic test efficiency three weeks after operation when areas 6 and 8 are involved. This loss is usually partly regained during the four months after operation.

There was a marked decrease in the scores on the inventories for Anxiety, particularly Self-Referred Anxiety and Self-Conscious Anxiety and for Mental Complaints. There was a smaller decrease in Externalized Anxieties and in Physical Complaints. These changes were closely associated with social recovery. Indeed these changes are those to which the patients attributed their own improvement. In this particular group, the patients over forty years of age, with I.Q.s over 105, who had areas 9, 10 and 46 removed, always showed decreases in Anxiety and Complaint scores.

Ablation of areas 9, 10, and 46 produced more gains than losses and the gains are associated with social recovery. Ablation of area 11 produced little or no change. Ablation of area 44 was not associated with any loss in speech or verbal function.

Excision of areas 9, 10, and 46 in psychotic patients is followed by a loss in Self-Conscious Anxiety and in Complaints which loss is not shown in any uniform fashion by patients who did not have these areas excised. The excision of areas 6 and 8 alone or in combination with 9 or 46 resulted in more losses than gains and may have negated or complicated part of the gains attendant on 9, 10, 46 removals. In most part the changes in psychologic test performance are easiest understood in terms of increased efficiency due to loss of emotional tension. There remains a certain portion of the changes which we have found which conceivably are somehow related to the nonlanguage or performance loss probably coming from excision of 6, 8, and perhaps 9. This loss may be that which Halstead ('47) termed "impairment of biological intelligence."

The topectomy operation is a therapeutic procedure in the same way that removal of part of the thyroid gland is a therapeutic procedure for goiter. In each instance there results a decrease in emotional tension, and when successful, a better life adjustment. Removal of areas 9, 10, 46 of the frontal lobes permits the restabilization and orderly balance of psychologic functions in mental patients who have much self-referred anxiety together with many mental and physical complaints.

# Psychiatry, Neurology, Pathology

# Chapter 25

# Psychiatry

ROBERT G. HEATH, JOHN J. WEBER, AND ARCHIE CRANDELL

## Introduction

THE psychiatric material will be presented in five sections, in the following order:

1. Abstracts of the case histories of all the patients.

2. Improvement. Methods of evaluating improvement are discussed and charts are presented correlating improvement with area removed.

3. Correlation of factors in patients' backgrounds with improvements.

4. Presentation of Payne Whitney-Phipps behavior charts with a discussion of the recorded changes.

5. A summary correlating and interpreting the effect of frontal lobe surgery on psychotic behavior.

## Abstracts of Case Histories

The abstracts will not be presented in numerical order, but are arranged according to the following outline.

I. *Control group:*
    A. Patients who changed without operation. Cases will be arranged so that the one with greatest improvement is presented first, the one with least improvement last (34, 39, 15, 9).
    B. Control patients who did not improve.
    C. Control patients who were later lobotomized (11, 20, 5, 23, 28, 46).
II. *Operatee group:*
    A. Those who definitely showed specific change as the result of operation.
        1. Lasting improvement (4, 7, 8, 13, 21, 22, 25, 36, 49).
        2. Temporary improvement (3, 27, 33).
    B. Patients in whom improvement was questionably related to operation (38 and 42).
    C. Patients unchanged by operation.

There are diagrams of the approximate cortical sites removed in each patient included in chapter 3.

### PATIENTS WHO CHANGED WITHOUT OPERATION

**Patient 34.** *Age:* 33. *Sex:* female. *Marital status:* single. *Occupation:* shop steward. *Religion:* Protestant. *Informants:* mother and brother. *Diagnosis:* schizophrenia, paranoid type.

*Presenting Picture.* The patient was excited and delusional when transferred to Greystone in March, 1946.

*Present Illness.* In January, 1946, the patient began to complain that the girls working with her would not speak to her and her employer telephoned her home to report that the patient was not well, although he gave no details. She stopped working and at the same time began to complain of headaches and vibrations in her head. When she became seclusive, somewhat overtalkative, and overactive, a physician was called who recommended that she be hospitalized.

*Previous Personality Disorders.* There had been no personality disorders prior to the present illness.

*Family History.* The patient's father was an American-born carpenter who died of pneumonia in 1937. Her mother, aged sixty-one years, was in good health. The patient was always especially close to her mother although she maintained a good relationship with her father during his lifetime. (She did not show any emotion on her father's death but one month later she "broke down and went to pieces.") There were two younger brothers, one of whom was married shortly before the patient was hospitalized. The marriage was strongly opposed by the patient's mother.

*Personal History.* Delivery and early development were said to be normal. The patient was born in New Jersey in January, 1913, and had the usual childhood diseases but no serious illnesses. Menarche was at eleven years and menses were always regular but usually were accompanied by irritability and complaints of headache and flushing. The patient began school at seven and left in the ninth grade at the age of sixteen to work as a telephone operator. Later she operated an elevator and for nine years before her admission she was a machine operator and shop steward. She was conscientious as a student as well as in her work.

*Personality.* Before her illness the patient was shy and a poor mixer. She was never interested in men or dates and never discussed the possibility of marriage. Her mother was always able to influence her thinking and the patient was dependent on her mother's decisions in such things as choosing clothes and making other purchases. She was meticulous in caring for her clothes, and took great pains to arrange them in what she considered the correct order.

*Hospital Course.* On admission the patient was requiring restraint and was resistive to all nursing care. After electroshock treatment was started she soon quieted and became cooperative and neat although ideas of reference were still present. Her condition varied subsequently from marked excitability to withdrawal and preoccupation. She described vibrations in her head and voices but did not describe the content of her auditory hallucinations. At one period she made active homosexual advances to other patients. A parole application was denied and she was transferred to the project.

*Mental Status.* The patient was neatly groomed, cooperative, and pleasant throughout the interview. The speed of mental activity was not unusual, affective responses were appropriate, and neither elation nor depression was manifest. The outstanding finding was the presence of auditory hallucinations. The subject described "pleasant, whispering voices" and "mechanical sounds." She said that she had masturbated without orgasm as a child but had never had intercourse. An attempted seduction at an early age was also discussed as well as her feeling of being discriminated against by her mother in favor of her younger brother. The sensorium was clear, orientation was good, and partial insight into the illness was manifest.

*Follow-Up Notes.* During the earlier part of the postoperative period the patient remained pleasant and cooperative; she was on ground parole. No abnormal behavior traits were noted.

At the time of interview on August 28, 1947, the patient was spending much time on home visits. She was making a satisfactory social adjustment and no longer had hallucinations although she remained somewhat preoccupied and shallow.

On January 17, 1948, she was working as a sales clerk in a department store and had the top sales record of her department. She had no complaints except that occasionally she became tired in the afternoon. No signs of psychosis were found at this time and she appeared to have made a recovery to the pre-illness level.

Improvement was maintained until May 8, 1948, although she was unable to come to the hospital for a follow-up examination on that date.

**Patient 39.** *Age:* 44. *Sex:* female. *Marital status:* widowed. *Occupation:* clerical worker. *Religion:* Hebrew. *Informants:* husband, father. *Diagnosis:* manic-depressive psychosis, manic.

*Presenting Picture.* The patient was first admitted to Greystone in November, 1924, with a history of violence and assaultiveness, delusions, and auditory hallucinations.

*Present Illness.* Two months after the birth of her son (July, 1924) she became talkative, confused, and unable to care for her child. She became irritable, expansive, and threatened to kill her husband. She said her milk was poisoned and that she was Cain's daughter and therefore superior. She washed her hands and cleaned her fingernails frequently. In October she was taken to a private sanitarium where she said someone was trying to hypnotize her and where she seriously injured a nurse, making it necessary that she be transferred to Greystone.

*Previous Personality Disorders.* There was no history of previous personality disorders.

*Family History.* The patient's father was Russian born and is a retired tailor who now has cardiac disease. He remarried after his wife committed suicide in 1916 when she learned she had a carcinoma. The patient was the second of four children by the first marriage. There were also three half-siblings in the family.

*Personal History.* The patient was born in New Jersey in December, 1902, and supposedly had a normal birth and childhood development. She began school at five years of age and graduated from elementary school at thirteen and one-half with an excellent record (winning prizes and skipping grades). As a child she preferred reading to playing with other children. She showed no emotion at her mother's death. Menses began at thirteen and were never painful or irregular. After graduation the patient attended a business school for nine months and then did clerical work for three different companies before her marriage. At nineteen she had a tonsillectomy and this was followed by a period, of six months' duration, of complaints of weakness and moderate depression. She had no male friends before her marriage and never went on dates until she met her husband. When her husband kissed her before marriage she would often weep and become excited but after their marriage in 1923 she was "passionate," demanding nightly intercourse. Her husband was a dry goods-store owner whom she had known for one year before marriage.

*Personality.* The patient was described as opinionated and easily excited.

*Hospital Course.* The admission in 1924 was marked chiefly by overactivity and overtalkativeness although there were periods during which the patient was noted to be dull, apathetic, and indifferent. Late in 1924, she was treated conservatively for acute glomerulonephritis and late in 1925 she began a gradual upward trend with improved memory and orientation. Assaultiveness ceased and in December she was paroled. She returned to work and made a good adjustment despite many legal battles instituted by the patient in order to compel her husband to support her. In October, 1941, she was readmitted with a picture closely resembling the original one. Insulin and electroshock treatments were given followed by marked improvement. The patient was paroled in March, 1942. Her adjustment at home was marginal throughout the parole period and she was readmitted in December, 1943, when she was once more overtalkative, exhibitionistic, abusive, and showed flight of ideas and memory impairment. This condition persisted until her transfer to this project except for a short period of quieting after insulin and metrazol treatment in September, 1944. Her husband died in 1945 but the patient did not appear to understand the news when it was given her.

*Mental Status.* The patient was neat. She was quiet as the interview began but rapidly became overactive and overproductive as it progressed. There was abundant affective display in the form of forced laughter. Her talk was rambling and she was markedly distractible. Her mood appeared to be one of euphoria or superficial elation. She discussed feelings of not being wanted at home and gave these as the reasons for her marriage, which she now regretted. Much hostility was expressed against her husband, accompanied by gleeful laughter. No delusions or hallucinations were elicited. She was well oriented; her memory was intact. She did not consider herself mentally ill.

*Follow-Up Notes.* In the two to three weeks preceding the interview of July 4, 1947, the patient's motor activity, ideation, and emotional responses slowed to within a normal range. At the time of interview she discussed at length her realization that her husband was dead, a fact which she had been told one and one-half years previously but which she had not absorbed until recently. Her judgment was good at this time.

Improvement was maintained over the period from September 9, 1947, to January 17, 1948, and the patient was paroled. She returned to part-time work and made a good social adjustment although she could be described as somewhat hypomanic and it was felt that her adjustment was precarious. She remained garrulous, rather demanding, and was preoccupied with the idea of remarrying although she denied any interest in sex.

On May 8, 1948, there were indications that the patient had remained hypomanic. She was scattered and overproductive. It was felt that re-hospitalization would soon be required.

**Patient 15.** *Age:* 55. *Sex:* male. *Marital status:* widower. *Occupation:* bartender, laborer. *Religion:* Roman Catholic. *Informants:* friend, social worker, physician, stepson. *Diagnosis:* schizophrenia, hebephrenic type.

*Presenting Picture.* The patient was admitted to Greystone Park in April, 1937, and was described at that time as depressed, confused, hypochondriacal, and disoriented.

*Present Illness.* About two months before admission, the patient expressed ideas that people on the street were laughing at him and interpreted trivial remarks as ridicule directed against himself. Sleep became poor and he spent many nights in restless walking. After expressing feelings that he had nothing to live for, he was hospitalized by his friend in a general hospital where he said that he wished he were dead and that he believed he was going to be electrocuted. No suicidal attempt was ever made, however. After physical examination had been completed he was transferred to Greystone.

*Previous Personality Disorders.* The patient's adjustment was precarious throughout his adult life. Following severely traumatic experiences in the Polish army during World War I he remained excitable and irritable. Later he over-reacted to a robbery at his place of business and to his wife's death.

*Family History.* Little is known of the patient's family. His father was a farmer in Poland, his mother a peasant woman who died of cancer when the patient was nine years old. There were supposedly four or five older children, all of whom remained in Poland. No information could be obtained on psychoses or constitutional illness in the family.

*Personal History.* The patient was born in March, 1892, in Poland. Nothing is known of his childhood history except that he left school at the age of fourteen, worked on his father's farm and in Polish factories, and then came to the United States at the age of twenty-one. He remained only a short time and then returned to Poland where he fought in World War I and was wounded in the thigh. He supposedly took part in much action and one of the informants, who knew the patient at that time, says that the patient was one of seven survivors in a machine-gun squad of eighty-eight men. After an honorable discharge he came to the United States again in 1920 and was employed as a button maker until 1931, and was subsequently a bartender. In 1928 he married a Polish woman who had been married twice before. There were no children of this union but his wife had a son by her first marriage. Reports on the married life conflict. According to the least biased observers, the wife was regarded as mentally ill most of her life; she was dull, nagging, constantly finding fault, and periodically caused public disturbances; the patient handled her with unfailing kindness and gentleness. The stepson, on the other hand, describes the patient as a gambler, stingy, resentful of his wife's son, and a man who constantly aggravated his wife's condition to produce frequent quarrels. The wife died a cardiorenal death one month after admission to Greystone in 1934 where a diagnosis was made of psychosis with somatic disease. Subsequently the patient made frequent visits to his wife's grave and appeared to lose interest in his surroundings.

*Personality.* The patient was described as worrisome and reserved, especially with women. In his youth he liked to gamble at cards but was never interested in sports or politics. Although he belonged to several Polish social clubs, he was apparently interested only in the card-playing opportunities they afforded. A willing and industrious worker, he was frequently imposed upon but rarely objected or showed anger. Although he had many friends, he could be sharp and critical at times and was supposedly often "misunderstood." He drank beer and whisky socially but was never observed to be intoxicated. His general health was good but he often complained of "gas on the stomach" and avoided certain foods.

*Hospital Course.* Following admission in 1937 the patient was confused and restless but usually cooperated well. He complained that people on the street and at work called him "dopey, a murderer, killer, robber, and Jello," and that they accused him of performing fellatio. At times he was agitated and fearful and would wring his hands. He also said that he received messages to the effect that he was crazy. No definitive treatment was given, although he received hydrotherapy and colonics. Throughout his hospital stay his condition changed only in the direction of increased seclusiveness and preoccupation.

*Mental Status.* Examination in 1947 was not productive. The patient was a small, thin man who looked frightened and usually sat in a corner of the ward. When questioned he answered in a weak voice, frequently wept, and turned his head from side to side as though responding to auditory hallucinations. He was markedly underproductive and affect was shallow except for fear. He was oriented for place and said that he was "here because I must be crazy" but would not elaborate except to say with a smile, "I'm here a long time." He denied auditory hallucinations and to other questions replied only with a confused "I don't know." Other aspects of the formal mental examination could not be tested.

*Follow-Up Notes.* Following a severe pneumonia in May, 1947, the patient showed no immediate change in his condition. On the interview of June 13, 1947, he showed evidence of auditory hallucinations as well as much preoccupation and blocking. He complained of "weakness of the bones" and said, "People say bad words about me. They get mad with me."

At the time of the interview of August 26, 1947, the patient had improved somewhat. His replies were still brief but he no longer expressed paranoid delusions and he was less preoccupied and seclusive. He was spending much time cleaning and working around the ward and it was apparent that he had changed for the better, although insight was lacking and judgment was poor.

The patient was paroled in October, 1947, and went to work setting up pins in a bowling alley and doing other menial jobs for a Polish recreation club.

On January 17, 1948, he appeared somewhat bewildered but expressed satisfaction with his job and being once more outside the hospital. He had no activities other than his work. Little emotion was expressed but he answered questions very briefly though coherently. Recent memory, recall, and orientation for the date were all deficient. The only thought content elicited was a preoccupation with the death of his wife and two brothers who he said were killed in the Polish army and no paranoid trend, delusions, or hallucinations were described. His employer told the examiner that the patient did his job well but had no outside interests and no ambitions.

At this time the picture appeared to be a complicated one, involving schizophrenia in a man of originally modest intellect who was perhaps showing signs of organic brain disease.

On May 8, 1948, the patient's condition was not different from that of the previous interview. He described a simple hallucination which consisted of his wife's voice repeating his name over and over as he lay in bed at night.

**Patient 9.** *Age:* 44. *Sex:* male. *Marital status:* single. *Occupation:* baker. *Religion:* Lutheran. *Informant:* brother. *Diagnosis:* schizophrenia, paranoid type.

*Presenting Picture.* The patient first entered Greystone Park in August, 1940, at which time he alternated between periods of depression with retardation and periods of violence, during which he expressed ideas of persecution. Grandiose delusions were present and he had hallucinations in the auditory sphere.

*Present Illness.* Symptoms began in June, 1940, with complaints of headache and a noticeable loss of initiative. The patient became irritable when forced to stop work by his brother; he brooded, and refused to listen to the family's advice that he see a physician. His behavior became unpredictable and it was noticed that he avoided people, was no longer able to sit through a meal or a movie, and spent much time on long, restless walks. He expressed the belief that he was guided by the sun, that he was responsible for the whole universe, and that the world would soon come to an end because he had ruined it. His diet was eccentric and he refused food when it was offered to him though he never expressed a belief that it was poisoned. Sleep was poor but there were no evidences at home of suicidal or violent tendencies. On the advice of a nurse, the patient was admitted to another hospital where he remained one week before coming to Greystone.

*Previous Personality Disorders.* In 1928 the patient was hospitalized in a New York State institution for about eighteen months, following an unsuccessful courtship. Details of the illness are not known. Supposedly a second illness occurred in 1933 or 1934 while the patient was in the Far East, but this history was not definitely established.

*Family History.* The German-Austrian grandparents were poorly described. The patient's father (aged seventy-two) was living in Germany. He was a shoemaker who was hard working and was said to have been kindly, though a disciplinarian. The mother, who died in Austria in 1931 (aged fifty-four), appeared as a more important figure, described as quiet but ambitious and a good business manager. She supposedly instilled in her children a burning ambition to get ahead. The patient was the fourth of nine children, the first of whom died in infancy. All except the informant (next younger) were living in Germany. All except the patient and the youngest brother were satisfactorily married, some with children, and were supposedly well adjusted. Their occupations included shoemaker, housewife, domestic, and mailman.

*Personal History.* The patient was born in Germany in December, 1902. There was little information on the patient's infancy and adolescence. The brother stated, however, that the children were seriously warned by their father of the great harm that would come of masturbation and said, "I don't think (the patient) did much masturbating as a result." The boys were also warned against girls because of venereal diseases but the informant stated, "we were brought up in the rural districts of Germany so sex was not strange to us." The patient said that home life was pleasant and he began to make social and sexual contacts at the age of eighteen or nineteen with intercourse on one occasion at the age of twenty-two or twenty-three. In 1927 he left Germany after attending baker's school and traveled extensively, working as a baker in various parts of the world. While in the United States he developed a mental illness, previously referred to, and was subsequently deported back to Germany. In 1931 he was sent to China by an English firm and while there he supposedly lived with a Chinese woman. Another breakdown is said to have occurred during these years. In 1939 he returned to the United States to work in his brother's bakery and remained there until his admission to Greystone. According to the patient there were no sexual contacts from 1939 on.

*Personality.* The patient was described as ambitious and "almost too aggressive," a strict self-disciplinarian. Supposedly friendly, he liked company, including that of women. A common-sense businessman, he held good jobs although his earnings were meager. Financially cautious, he was not considered miserly. He was a serious, rather worrisome person who was nervous and excitable but seldom held grudges. Always interested in sports, he was an amateur boxer in his youth. He was interested in politics, liked to study history and geography, and was religious without being a zealot.

*Hospital Course.* Following admission in 1940 he was uncooperative and restraint was necessary at times. On the ward he was restless, appeared confused, and often attempted to slip out of the doors. In August, 1941, electroshock treatment was tried but soon discontinued because the patient developed induration of the buttocks. There was a good response to this treatment, however, and he rapidly became more cooperative, was permitted visits home, and was paroled in November, 1941. After four months of satisfactory adjustment, he suddenly developed insomnia, wept, and became fearful and depressed. Saying that he had to see if the moon was up, he plunged his hand through a windowpane and was then readmitted to the hospital where he was once more uncooperative, resistive, and agitated. In September, 1942, shock treatment was started again and he received nine insulin comas with improvement for a few days, followed by relapse. Electroshock was tried again with good results for a few months, followed by return to his former behavior and in July, 1943, another course of eight electroshocks was given with good results. He became once more friendly and cooperative and was recommended for parole in October, 1943. His outside adjustment was adequate until September, 1944, when he had to be returned in a disturbed and agitated state. More electroshock permitted a parole in December, 1944, but three months later he was inefficient on the job and in July, 1945, was readmitted in an agitated state, pacing up and down repeating over and over, "God bless you!" and expressing persecutory delusions. In this condition he was transferred to the special ward of this investigation.

*Mental Status.* On examination (1947) he was cooperative and friendly, smiled, and shook hands with the interviewer. Speech was not unusual but his affect was flattened throughout the interview. He complained of neither elevation nor depression of mood and denied any fluctuation. He was defensive throughout, repeating his desire for release. After his confidence had been won to some extent he admitted that he was suspicious, though no delusions or hallucinations could be elicited. According to the patient, his hospitalization was an injustice, as had been his 1928 hospitalization. Sensorium was clear and he was oriented in all spheres but no insight into the fact of his illness was present and his judgment was poor.

*Follow-Up Notes.* On May 30, 1947, at the time operations were being carried out, this man showed more seclusive and preoccupied behavior, refusing to answer questions, although he seemed to be responding more to hallucinations. He mumbled constantly in German.

During the examination on June 13, 1947, the patient appeared frightened and confused, responded constantly in German to voices which he denied were present. When asked about them, however, he turned his head to talk to them. He was preoccupied with "mistakes" he believed he had made and showed omnipotent trends. "Should I blame myself for creating the world and heaven?" he asked. Some insight was present but this was fleeting.

Shortly after this interview the patient became more agitated and, for administrative reasons, it was necessary to transfer him to another ward where he was given two electroshock treatments. Thereafter he became silly, distractible, and somewhat euphoric. Objectively the hallucinations disappeared but he remained suspicious.

On September 2, 1947, the patient's condition was unchanged. Orientation was intact but insight was not present and judgment was faulty.

At the time of the interview on January 18, 1948, the patient was paroled and was working with his brother. He looked thin, tense, preoccupied, and somewhat dazed. There was little affect and he smiled inappropriately. Talk was rambling and disjointed but no delusional or hallucinatory material could be elicited. Apparently his social participation in life had been narrow. Insight was lacking and both recent and remote memory were impaired. It was recommended that he be returned to the hospital but the suggestion was resisted by the patient's brother who felt capable of caring for him.

The patient was returned to the hospital in February, 1948, after he became unmanageable at home. At the time of interview on May 7, 1948, he was preoccupied and had hallucinations but was no longer agitated.

### CONTROL PATIENTS WHO DID NOT IMPROVE

**Patient 1.** *Age:* 55. *Sex:* male. *Marital status:* single. *Occupation:* electrician. *Religion:* Protestant. *Informants:* Parents and sister. *Diagnosis:* schizophrenia, catatonic type.

*Presenting Picture.* The patient was admitted to Greystone in September, 1938, when he became disturbed and delusional while awaiting a herniorrhaphy in a general hospital.

*Present Illness.* In August, 1938, he became more expansive than usual and made elaborate and expensive plans to celebrate the golden wedding anniversary of his parents. After complaining of poor sleep for a week he entered a hospital to have a hernia repair performed and subsequently became so complaining and obstreperous that restraint was necessary and operation had to be deferred. He told of seeing religious writings on the walls of his room and made frequent references to God. The transfer to Greystone was made on the pretext that further x-ray examinations were necessary; the patient later resented this subterfuge.

*Previous Personality Disorders.* In 1915 (when twenty-three years of age) the patient was found lying rigid and mute in the coalbin of his parents' home. Following a four-month hospitalization he remained well for six months and then became sleepless, seclusive, and irritable and was returned to the hospital where he again improved after four months. Similar episodes occurred in 1922 but hospitalization was not required. Between attacks he had insight into the fact that he had been mentally ill.

*Family History.* The paternal grandmother was mentally ill for several months before her death (at the age of sixty-seven) following a cerebrovascular accident. Other grandparents were of Scotch-Irish-English stock and lived well-adjusted lives until they died in advanced years. The father was a New Jersey-born baker, described as friendly and sociable, who died in 1943 at the age of eighty-four. The mother was quick-tempered, a hard-working woman, who died in 1939 at seventy-eight years of age. There were four children: (1) a boy who died in infancy, (2) the patient, (3) a girl who has remained single and now suffers from migraine, (4) a girl who married and a short time later (1931) died in childbirth. The father was domineering in his treatment of the patient, while the mother was critical and irritable. There were many quarrels between the patient and his older sister but he was much attached to his younger sister and was upset by her death. He was also disturbed by his mother's death but showed no reaction to that of his father, which took place while he was in the hospital.

*Personal History.* The patient was born in Massachusetts in February, 1892. The delivery was normal. Development was not unusual and he had the usual childhood diseases. No information is available on his reaction to the birth of his sisters. He started attendance at school at six years of age and finished elementary school without failures and without distinction. Subsequently he completed a course as an electrician, worked for an electrical company for one year, and then went into business for himself. He was never successful because his business judgment was poor and he worked only sporadically. According to the patient, masturbation began when he was twenty-five years of age and was accompanied by so much guilt that he consulted a mental hygiene clinic. He showed no interest in girls throughout his life, had had no sex education from his parents, and had never had intercourse. He did not smoke or drink alcohol. His mental illnesses have already been mentioned. In 1928, during his father's critical illness, the patient took on responsibility for the home and did well until the father recovered at which time the patient reverted to his usual pattern of irresponsibility and seclusiveness.

*Personality.* Outstanding in this man was his shyness and inability to handle people socially as well as his variability in work habits and emotional expression. He always attended church regularly and was interested in cathedrals, monuments, and the like. Intelligence was at least average and his reading habits were serious for a man of his background (he enjoyed Shakespeare, books on astronomy, and similar works).

*Hospital Course.* On admission in 1938 the patient was exalted and said that he had been reborn six years before and would soon become sexually active since he would reach adolescence. This picture quieted rapidly and within a year he was paroled to his home, where he remained passive and preoccupied until March, 1940, when he suddenly became violent. After a brief quiet period in the hospital he showed destructive and assaultive tendencies, setting fire to a building and attempting to kick a door in. Subsequently he remained preoccupied and quiet until transferred to this project. Eight electroshock treatments were administered in 1941 with no effect.

*Mental Status.* The patient came into the room carrying a huge bag filled with books and said he had been reading up on Dr. I. Q. so he could overcome his inferiority complex. He was well dressed and cooperative but showed little emotion. Answers were coherent and the progress of speech was not unusual. The content of thought centered around his "inferiority complex" and sexual-religious problems. He described flashes of light which were present during his first illness and visions of religious persecution which were present at the same time. During that period he also felt he was "omniscient," as he believes God is. He also discussed the family constellation at some length. No hallucinations were elicited during this interview. Insight was partial and orientation was good, sensorium clear, judgment fair.

*Follow-Up Notes.* Examinations were made on June 11, 1947, August 19, 1947, and January 17, 1948. There was no over-all change in behavior although there seemed to be a slight improvement at the time of the first examination when the patient appeared to respond to the amount of attention which was available on the ward. The later interviews were marked by statements of "depression" and suicidal thoughts and the patient expressed the wish that he could have had the same operation that was performed on the other patients. In other respects there was no improvement or worsening of the picture. Six months after the operative period this patient remained at his former level of adjustment.

The one-year examination was made on May 7, 1948. At that time the patient was at the end of a period of marked excitement which had lasted three weeks. During the excited period he had taken off his clothes to go for a swim in the reservoir and had been overactive and aggressive on the wards.

**Patient 10.** *Age:* 44. *Sex:* male. *Marital status:* single. *Occupation:* baker's helper. *Religion:* Hebrew. *Informants:* father and brother. *Diagnosis:* schizophrenia, hebephrenic type.

*Presenting Picture.* When admitted to Greystone in October, 1928, this patient was assaultive, irrational, and had hallucinations in the auditory sphere.

*Present Illness.* About one month before admission he began to express fears concerning the future and complained of restlessness, insomnia, and loss of appetite. He was much concerned about a girl whom he wanted to marry and stayed up late at night to see her. When she refused him he gave a ring to a dance-hall girl he met in New York; this relationship was broken up by the family. When he became incoherent in his speech he was taken to a general hospital where he said that he believed that his family was trying to get rid of him. Here he attacked the attendants and was unmanageable so a transfer to Greystone was arranged.

*Previous Personality Disorders.*    There was no history of previous personality disorders.

*Family History.*    The patient's father was a Polish-born baker who died in 1931. The mother, also Polish born, was described as "nervous." The patient was the second of eight children. An older sister is married, two younger brothers are lawyers, and the standard of achievement for the other children was higher than the patient's own accomplishment. The patient was always closely attached to his mother and envied his brothers because they were able to go to college while he had to stay at home and help support the family.

*Personal History.*    Born in Poland in December, 1903, he was brought to the United States when only a few months old. He walked and talked at one year of age; development was not unusual except for a severe attack of pneumonia when he was eleven years old. He was constipated throughout his life and took many patent laxatives. He began school at five and left high school (at the age of eighteen) in his last year in order to give financial help to the family. For seven years before he became ill he worked in the bakery with his father and made deliveries. He was dissatisfied with the work but was conscientious about it as he was with everything he did. A good mixer, he always preferred the company of men to that of women and he was very careful in his selection of the few girls he dated. Little is known of his sex life since he was "secretive" about it and confided in no one.

*Personality.*    The description given was that of an active and ambitious man who was nevertheless sensitive to criticism and shy. He was strongly attached to his family but resentful of the obligations placed on him. A notable trait was his need for order and neatness in the home and in his personal dress.

*Hospital Course.*    Following his hospitalization in 1928 the patient was paroled for a short time but he deteriorated at home and was returned to the hospital in May, 1932, when he was evasive, agitated, had hallucinations, and believed that he had been doped. Subsequently he expressed ideas of being influenced by ultraviolet rays which caused hair to grow all over his body and he expressed ideas of persecution. After quieting somewhat he was recommended for parole in August, 1932, but his adjustment at home was inadequate and he was returned to the hospital after three months. Progressive deterioration in his behavior became apparent from that point on and his course was consistently downhill despite frequent parole visits which were granted at the family's request. Insulin and metrazol treatment was given in 1940 and electroshock in 1941 to no avail.

*Mental Status.*    The patient's appearance was slovenly and he smiled and laughed inappropriately throughout the interview. He made many dramatic gestures and was easily distracted. Talk was in a low monotone with occasional perseveration and neologism formation. His affect was one of superficial euphoria. It was not possible to make contact with him in order to question him and he babbled continuously in disjointed phrases. It was obvious that he had hallucinations and responded to auditory hallucinations. He said, "I wouldn't be too stuck up on myself without a little bit here and a little bit there. I didn't finish high school but I was really sincere. I've got it! We'll satisfy her with—we have something, anyway." "This is a nice chair. They give you a kiss sometimes—not up your ass—a nice kiss—on the baby's mouth." He was able to give his own name but was not oriented for time or situation.

*Follow-Up Notes.*    On interviews on August 25, 1947, January 18, 1948, and May 7, 1948, this patient's behavior remained entirely unchanged. He continued to be silly, confused, manneristic, and to have hallucinations. At various times he ate the ends of burnt matches, drank his own urine, carried out ritualistic acts, and made symbolic gestures. His thought content remained disjointed and ununderstandable; neologisms were frequent. There was no change in his ability to make judgments and he remained disoriented.

**Patient 12.** *Age:* 57. *Sex:* male. *Marital status:* married. *Occupation:* upholsterer. *Religion:* Protestant. *Informant:* wife. *Diagnosis:* schizophrenia, paranoid
type.

*Presenting Picture.* On admission in November, 1940, the patient was grandiose
and expressed persecutory ideas and ideas of influence.

*Present Illness.* Four months before admission the patient began to express ideas
that people were watching and following him. He began to stare into space for long
periods of time. Occasionally he wept and otherwise appeared depressed. Sleep was
poor and he was retarded though able to continue at his job. Two days before admission he hit himself on the forehead with a hatchet. Sutures were required and after
the wound had been repaired the patient returned to his home. The next day he
attempted to strike his wife with a hammer and he was thereupon admitted to
Greystone.

*Previous Personality Disorders.* There was no history of previous personality disorders.

*Family History.* The patient's German-born father was a glassmaker and was
described as talkative and outgoing. He died in 1937 at the age of seventy-two. The
patient's mother died of childbirth at about the age of thirty. A stepmother was
still living (age sixty-two) at the time of the patient's admission to the hospital. She
was described as sociable and well adjusted. The patient was the third of six children,
all boys except the oldest sibling. There were supposedly two children by the second
marriage, both of whom died in infancy. There is little information on the patient's
relationship to his siblings. They are all financially more successful than he and are
all married and have families.

*Personal History.* Little is known of the patient's early life. He had a supposedly
normal birth in Germany in April, 1890. In 1902 he came to the United States and
worked as an upholsterer. Later he started his own business but was never successful.
He was somewhat handicapped physically by the residua of an automobile accident,
occurring in about 1910, resulting in a midthoracic fracture requiring hospitalization
for two years. In 1913 he married a Hungarian-born woman two years his junior.
There were no children but the marriage was said to have been a happy one. Sexual
intercourse occurred two to three times weekly but the patient's sexual urge dropped
considerably shortly before the onset of his illness. He accepted the fact that his wife
was unable to have children and never made any effort to find out why she did not
conceive. He was a social drinker and a moderate smoker.

*Personality.* The patient's intelligence and judgment were good and he supposedly
made fast friends. He was described as being ambitious, frugal, and somewhat stubborn, however, and his interests were confined largely to technical books, his garden,
and his home. His social life was definitely limited and he always leaned heavily on
his wife in this regard.

*Hospital Course.* On admission in November, 1940, the patient appeared retarded,
depressed, and anxious. In January, 1941, he was operated on for an inguinal hernia.
In February he had shown improvement, some insight was present, and he was released
on parole in March. His subsequent adjustment was adequate and in December, 1941,
he weathered an automobile accident in which both he and his wife were severely
injured. In March, 1944, he again became retarded and preoccupied; shock treatment
was given in April, 1944, with apparent improvement. However, he attempted to cut
his throat with a razor one month later and was readmitted to Greystone. The picture
was much as it had been on his previous admission. After gradual improvement without specific treatment he was paroled in June, 1944, and readmitted in May, 1945,
when he was markedly grandiose and agitated. He was paroled for four months in
October, 1945, having made a spontaneous improvement. While on parole in April,
1946, he attempted to cut his throat. He was returned to the hospital where he was
continuously a patient until his transfer to this project.

*Mental Status.* The patient was cooperative, neatly dressed, and talked spontaneously and overproductively. His mood was one of euphoria and he showed considerable

affect, most of it inappropriate to the content of thought. Content consisted of persecutory and grandiose delusions and ideas of influence; for example, he stated: "The shooting is supposed to have stopped. It has with real bullets but they still shoot. The shots go through walls without making a hole and into my heart. I'm the Prince of Peace. I am the living Son of God. I didn't commit suicide only once; I did it many times." He made many references to God, Hitler (spelled backwards), MacArthur, neon-rays penetrating his brain, and so on. His sensorium was clear and he was well oriented to time and place.

*Follow-Up Notes.* On June 13, 1947, it was noted that during the postoperative period there had been considerable fluctuation in this patient's behavior. Generally he was less euphoric, less overactive, and quieter. During these periods he read a great deal, displayed appropriate affect, and discussed his paranoid delusions with the comment that they might be "imaginary." He said he had a breakdown caused by "tension" which was "pulling him apart." At other times he was overactive and omnipotent, describing himself as the son of Pope Pius, or similar personage.

At the time of interview on September 2, 1947, the patient was better oriented but paroxysms of confusion and overactivity still occurred occasionally. At times he was well enough to be given ground parole but at others it was necessary that he be kept on a disturbed ward. He was preoccupied with his breasts and his testicles. Auditory hallucinations were denied during the interview. There was a tendency to reminisce about the distant past and recent memory was impaired, suggesting that some organic brain disease was present.

On the interview of January 18, 1948, little change from his state during the previous interview was noted. He was cooperative and quiet and did not overtly express delusions or hallucinations. However, he believed it possible that radium rays could be affecting him and he still considered Hitler as a magical savior and protector. There was no insight. Recent recall was impaired and calculations were done poorly.

On May 7, 1948, at the end of a one-year follow-up period, the patient was gay and grandiose.

**Patient 14.** *Age:* 47. *Sex:* male. *Marital status:* married. *Occupation:* physician. *Religion:* Presbyterian. *Informant:* wife. *Diagnosis:* schizophrenia, hebephrenic type.

*Presenting Picture.* The patient was first admitted to Greystone in December, 1939, when he was described as excited and irrational.

*Present Illness.* Before the onset of symptoms he had been in charge of a 160-bed hospital for a few days and had had large responsibilities. One week before admission he became irritable and complained of insomnia. A few days later he made several allegorical allusions in a telephone conversation with his wife, and the next day his fellow physicians telephoned his wife that he was ill. He was reluctant to be hospitalized at first, but accepted the idea without actual physical resistance, and was admitted to Greystone the same night.

*Previous Personality Disorders.* This patient's first mental illness occurred in November, 1932, following a period of intense study, and concurrent with the birth of his first child. His wife left with the infant to stay six months with relatives in the West and was not at home during this hospitalization, which lasted five months. Details of the symptomatology are not known, except that the illness began with irritability and the patient was depressed and discouraged for a few months after his release in May, 1933. Recovery was apparently completed with time, however, and he remained well until October, 1936, when he became overactive, irritable, and sleepless after carrying a large private practice. He was voluntarily hospitalized for seven months and was apparently well again when released in May, 1937.

*Family History.* The patient's father was a Nova Scotia-born superintendent of schools who died in 1936 at an advanced age, and who was described as intelligent, cheerful, and socially active. His mother was Canadian born and ten years younger than her husband. She was a serious woman who set high standards of performance for her five children, the patient being next to the youngest in age. The children apparently got along well with one another and with the parents, but they did not maintain family ties after growing up. The father was described as being "strict."

*Personal History.* The patient's wife could give no information on his early life beyond the fact that he was born in Nova Scotia on May 22, 1900. He began school at five and did well. At the age of ten he was badly "stunned" for several hours after a fall downstairs. When he was eleven years old his parents moved to the state of Washington, eventually becoming citizens of the United States. During adolescence he was very much interested in sports and apparently did well at them. He was warned by a Sunday school superintendent that sexual thoughts were sinful and stated that, as a result, he suffered great guilt feelings over any sexual desires and had no intercourse before marriage. (After marriage intercourse occurred only once in two or three months.)

Following graduation from high school at the age of sixteen, the patient attended college for three years and medical school for two, during which period he worked very hard and labored under many economic difficulties. After medical school he interned in a general hospital and then served obstetric and psychiatric residencies of unknown durations. In 1927 he married the informant, who was one year older than himself and the daughter of a physician. He worked for three years as a mill physician from 1929 to 1932, when he resigned because of his illness. (See "Previous Personality Disorders.") After his illness he began practice in another town and in May, 1938, he moved to New Jersey where he accepted a post in an industrial hospital.

*Personality.* The patient was described as a hard-working, philosophical man who had many interests but who took little time out for recreation. He was a moderate smoker and drinker.

*Hospital Course.* After admission he was cooperative, but appeared confused. He was generally cheerful, but restless and at times silly. He frequently expressed grandiose delusions, centering chiefly about medical subjects, and believed he was the rightful discoverer of the therapeutic value of liver extract, that he had discovered the cause of epileptic convulsions, and so on. After a few months he began to strike and annoy other patients and was secluded. Shock treatment (metrazol and insulin) was begun, but he had a prolonged and severe coma (of three days) following his seventh insulin treatment and further shock was discontinued at that time. A memory deficiency was treated with vitamin E, with concurrent improvement. In December, 1940, he was paroled, but at home he slept excessively and, while staying at his brother's ranch in March, 1941, he regressed to his former condition and was readmitted to Greystone in September, 1941. No more shock treatment was attempted because of his reaction to the first series. Until he was recommended for this project he was at times retarded, at other times excited and had to be restrained, but there was no indication of spontaneous improvement.

*Mental Status.* Throughout the interview the patient chain-smoked, made smacking noises with his lips, and tic-like movements of his mouth. He was much slowed in his psychomotor activity and slightly underproductive. He appeared neither elated nor depressed and his lack of affective response to the material discussed was outstanding. He talked of many apparently unimportant details in his early life and also his earlier illnesses, for which he showed no insight. He described his lack of sexual initiative, which he interpreted as being due to his wife's lack of interest. Both parents were described as having been kind to him. No delusions or hallucinations could be elicited at that time and he felt that he was ready for discharge. There was a complete amnesia for the period in which he was committed, and his judgment and orientation for time and situation were faulty.

*Follow-Up Notes.* This patient was interviewed on July 4, 1947, August 25, 1947, January 17, 1948, and May 7, 1948. Throughout the follow-up period he remained seclusive, expressionless, and underproductive. His only activities consisted of reading and bumming cigarettes from passing strangers. He remained conspicuous for his lack of affective response.

*Patient 16. Age:* 50. *Sex:* male. *Marital status:* single. *Occupation:* clerk. *Religion:* unknown. *Informants:* maternal aunt and uncle. *Diagnosis:* schizophrenia, hebephrenic type, possible organic brain disease.

*Presenting Picture.* On admission in May, 1938, the patient was fearful, resistive, and required restraint.

*Present Illness.* About three weeks before admission this patient began complaining about his throat and said that if it did not improve he would "go out of his head." A local physician offered no specific treatment or diagnosis and the patient became seclusive and began taking long walks. His appetite diminished, he appeared depressed, and feared that he would have to be hospitalized. On one occasion he said that the police were after him and shortly thereafter he was found sitting on the bathroom windowsill, from which he fell without injury when his aunt attempted to restrain him. On the same day he began to strike his head against a wall and, after he had exhausted himself, he was taken to a general hospital for commitment.

*Previous Personality Disorders.* There was no history of previous personality disorders.

*Family History.* The patient's mother was German born and was described as easygoing and sociable. She died during childbirth in 1900. His father was born in the United States, of German stock, and had been a milkman before his remarriage after his first wife's death. The father drank to excess, especially when nagged by his second wife, who objected to his being unemployed frequently. The stepmother died of pneumonia three years before the patient's admission. She was described as "an irritable woman." An older sibling was hospitalized for six months at Greystone and discharged to another hospital early in 1934 with a diagnosis of manic-depressive psychosis, depressed. The patient was next to the oldest child; the third child was stillborn. He had a half sister who died following an accidental fall twelve years prior to the patient's admission. One paternal uncle committed suicide.

*Personal History.* The patient was born in New Jersey, June 8, 1897. He weighed $8\frac{1}{2}$ to 9 pounds at birth, delivery and development were supposedly normal. He had whooping cough and measles as a child and enuresis was present until he was eleven to twelve years old. His mother's death occurred when he was about three years of age. From that time until he was nine or ten he lived with his paternal grandmother with whom he was supposedly happy. However, when his father remarried he went to live with his stepmother and father. After a year, during which he was neglected and rejected by his stepmother, on his father's request his grandparents consented to take care of him and his brother.

In 1918 he had pneumonia and influenza. He began to stutter at the age of six, when he entered school. He did poorly in school though he never repeated any grades. He left school at thirteen to work as an expressman; later he drove a truck for his uncle. In 1932 the uncle lost his business and thereafter the patient did odd jobs until he was hospitalized. In November, 1933, he was operated upon for a peptic ulcer, and subsequently had drainage for six months with associated complaints of gas and belching.

*Personality.* The personality description was that of a man of below-average intelligence who was trusting, dependent on his older relatives, shy, worrisome, and unconfiding. He was socially ill-at-ease, rarely went out with girls, and never expressed any interest in marriage.

*Hospital Course.* On admission to the hospital the patient was fearful, resistive, and seclusive. He spoke unintelligibly at times and warned the staff that he had a dreadful disease which was catching. He was generally oriented, but memory was only fair. During his hospital stay he was retarded, appeared depressed, and frequently complained of constipation and "kidney trouble" which he attributed to smoking and drinking beer. He was cooperative, but uninterested in occupational therapy and ward work. He consistently denied hallucinations, but on at least one occasion it was the physician's impression that he was responding to auditory hallucinations. He made occasional home visits. Although partial insight into his condition was always present, he remained confused on detailed information, especially for time. In April, 1940, he attempted to cut his throat with a tin cup and when discovered he explained that he was going to shave. No shock treatment was given during his hospitalization.

*Mental Status.* Examination was difficult and unsatisfactory because of marked stammering and retardation accompanied by perplexity and blocking. The patient was neatly dressed and attempted to cooperate, but it was difficult to break through his retardation and speech difficulty, and he responded only to direct commands or questions. He appeared somewhat apprehensive, but there was little affective display, and he seemed neither elated nor depressed. The thought content was meager and related only to the questions asked him and consisted of such statements as that he was "all right," when asked how he was, and that he would like to get out to "help people at home." He gave his age as thirty-five (actually he was fifty), his length of stay as one year (it was actually nine years), and gave the year as 1946 (it was 1947). He identified the institution as "Parkrest Home, ain't it?" No delusions, hallucinations, or projective tendencies were elicited. It was felt that the picture could be most easily explained on a schizophrenic basis, but that an underlying organic brain disease was also a definite possibility.

*Follow-Up Notes.* Prior to the interview of June 13, 1947, this patient had not changed appreciably until a few days preceding this examination when he became mute and more deeply preoccupied. His only activity at the time of examination consisted in whistling occasionally and, aside from turning his eyes as the examiner walked about the room, he did not respond to his environment.

On the interview of August 26, 1947, he would once more reply to direct questions but he remained severely preoccupied. At times he laughed inappropriately as though in response to voices.

On both January 17, and May 7, 1948, he was again entirely mute and unresponsive, occasionally breaking out in inappropriate and unprovoked laughter.

**Patient 17.** *Age:* 60. *Sex:* male. *Marital status:* married. *Occupation:* salesman. *Religion:* Catholic. *Informants:* son and wife. *Diagnosis:* schizophrenia, paranoid type.

*Presenting Picture.* About November, 1933, this subject became unusually quiet, appeared depressed, began to lose weight, and expressed the belief that someone was looking for him for something he had done. He soon stopped working and would no longer leave the house. At the same time he complained of weakness in his legs, pains in his head, and began to pray a great deal. When he acquired a bottle of Lysol, the patient's family had him admitted to a mental hospital, even though he denied a suicidal intent. In the hospital he said he was "between two fires" (two hospitals) and he wondered if a nearby priest would "press charges against him." After three days he was admitted to Greystone.

*Previous Personality Disorders.* The patient was admitted to a New York State hospital in November, 1904, paroled in September, 1906, and discharged in November, 1907, as recovered. His diagnosis was dementia praecox. A second illness and hospitalization supposedly occurred before his marriage, but no details were available.

*Family History.* The family history was scanty. The patient's father died in 1933 at about the age of seventy in a New York State hospital where he had been for one month before his death. The father had had no previous mental illnesses. The patient's mother died of natural causes in 1926 at about the age of sixty. There were two male siblings, one of whom was said to be "nervous" and in the Army. The other was in the Southwest and had not been heard of for some time. Two maternal uncles were said to have died of alcoholism.

*Personal History.* The patient was born in New York of Irish-English parents on August 1, 1887, and was a healthy child as far as is known. He received a grammar-school education and then held various short-term jobs until 1916 when he began selling adding machines. This continued to be his occupation until he was hospitalized.

Before his marriage he was a heavy drinker and it was stated that he had had syphilis at seventeen to eighteen years of age, for which he was not treated. (Physical and laboratory examinations revealed no indication of syphilis.) He offered chronic complaints of pain in the abdomen for many years and often complained of constipation. In 1910 he married a Polish girl, two years his junior, without telling this girl of his previous illness. He had four children, two boys and two girls, born between 1912 and 1926. All are apparently in good health. The patient got along well with his wife and children, but he was never affectionate, although he appeared to favor his second son to some extent.

*Personality.* According to his son, the patient fluctuated widely in his relations with his family, being at times sociable and at other times irritable and upredictable. He was generally suspicious of other people, made few friends, and had no hobbies or recreation. His wife referred to episodes of drunkenness during which he threatened the children and indicated that he had not been mentally well during his entire married life.

*Hospital Course.* When admitted in 1934 the patient was haggard, emaciated, and appeared to be under a great deal of tension. He expressed persecutory delusions at first and was agitated, but in a short time he became retarded, mute, and appeared to be responding to auditory hallucinations. Until 1939 he spent much time in seclusion because he was destructive, resistive, and assaultive; but by December, 1939, he had quieted down and was transferred to a less disturbed ward. During the following three years his behavior varied from the extremes of restlessness with auditory hallucinations and delusions to seclusiveness and reticence. About 1941 he became more in contact with his surroundings, but at that time he began to offer many somatic complaints. He received no shock treatment.

*Mental Status.* The patient was a small, neatly dressed man whose voice was hoarse and who was overtalkative and especially garrulous when discussing his somatic complaints, such as epigastric pain and flatulence. (X-ray examination revealed a duodenal-ulcer deformity.) Affect was displayed appropriate to the thought content. The thought content consisted of rambling and apparently unconnected references to his former job, his wife, his position in the hospital, the nurses, and his financial condition. He admitted his former illness, but denied having had hallucinations at any time during his illness. He had many suspicious complaints against nurses and attendants, and implied that the nurses were somehow interested in him as a potential husband. His judgment was poor, but he was well oriented.

*Follow-Up Notes.* The patient was interviewed on July 4, 1947, and August 26, 1947. Following the initial examination, the patient's behavior fluctuated somewhat but he remained restless, overactive, and overtalkative, resulting in marked hoarseness. He displayed marked hostility toward the nurses, accusing them of alcoholism and sexual indiscretions, and he expressed persecutory delusions involving the other patients in sexual acts. He also expressed the belief that another patient had syphilis and that "people who smoke would commit murder," all of these productions being delivered with much hostility. Hallucinations were still denied. On the interview of September 2, 1947, the patient's behavior was found to have continued as during the previous interview and, in addition, he was performing symbolic writing in the air and was responding to auditory hallucinations.

No deviation from the previous status was apparent during interviews on October 20, 1947, January 17, 1948, and May 7, 1948.

**Patient 26.** *Age:* 35. *Sex:* male. *Marital status:* divorced. *Occupation:* laborer. *Religion:* Catholic. *Informants:* brother, mother, sister-in-law. *Diagnosis:* schizophrenia, hebephrenic type.

*Presenting Picture.* When the patient was committed in June, 1944, he was described as overactive and assaultive.

*Present Illness.* In January, 1944, the patient began to complain of weakness and to weep occasionally because his wife had been attentive to other men. Shortly thereafter he gave up his job and his wife left him, taking their child with her. The patient came to live with his family and saw his wife only to give her money. He began to drink heavily and became abusive to women, calling them all (including his mother), by his wife's name. He talked continually about sexual relations, but would not go out with any women. At times he had violent outbursts of behavior resembling temper tantrums in which he threw things on the floor, tore up the table-cloth, and performed other similar acts. A two-week hospitalization quieted him some-what, but soon after his release he put his hand through the windowpane of a bar after he was refused a drink. Commitment was forceful even though the patient had recognized for some time that he was not well.

*Previous Personality Disorders.* No history of previous personality disorders was obtained.

*Family History.* The patient's parents were Italian born and came to the United States together while in their twenties. His father was a wholesale importer of groceries who was a diabetic and died in 1933 after an operation. The father liked to play the role of host at home, but was strict with the children, even selecting their companions. The mother rarely disagreed with her husband and was apparently dominated by him. The patient was the seventh of eight children, the youngest of whom died of diabetes at the age of twenty-six. Two of the brothers are lawyers, one sister is a librarian, and the general level of family achievement is above that of the patient. According to his older brother, the patient was especially favored by an older sister and both parents tried to keep him "infantile."

*Personal History.* The patient was born in New Jersey in March, 1912. The delivery was normal. His early development was not remarkable. The economic con-dition of the home was satisfactory. He finished the first year of high school and had one year of night school, but left when eighteen to work in the wholesale grocery business. After his father's death he was in the numbers' racket for five years, then worked six months as a navy guard, and was then employed as a laborer until the onset of his illness. In February, 1941, he married a woman of German descent (age unknown). He had one child, a girl, born in 1942. Charging that the patient drank to excess and gambled, his wife sued for divorce one month before he was admitted to the hospital and the divorce was granted uncontested, with custody of the child going to his wife's mother. The patient was drinking to excess at that time.

*Personality.* The patient was described as being "happy-go-lucky," enjoying the company of everyone and ingratiating himself with everyone. He had great ambitions to make money, but never wanted to work and was always trying to get ahead "the easy way." He was supposedly devoted to his wife and always defended and indulged her. Nothing could be learned of his sexual habits.

*Hospital Course.* Following his admission in June, 1944, flight of ideas, hallucina-tions, and overactivity were noted. Electroshock and insulin coma treatments were begun in July, 1944, at which time he was described as quiet, listless, and despondent. During treatment he refused to accept the fact that his wife had instituted divorce proceedings, but at the end of the treatment he no longer had hallucinations, he was sleeping well, and was friendly and sociable, although he appeared somewhat con-fused. He was paroled in January, 1945, and adjusted satisfactorily at home for six months, until he again became assaultive, insulting to women, and somewhat depressed. He was readmitted and shock treatments (insulin and electric) were started for a second time in August, 1945. He did not improve this time and subsequent months of inactivity led to the recommendation that he be transferred to this project.

*Mental Status.* The patient was personally tidy, but his facial expression was one of preoccupation, and he frequently grinned and turned his head in response to auditory hallucinations. He made many restless movements and he often hit his nose with his hand and moved his arm down his side as though he were brushing an imaginary figure away. There was little emotional display, except occasional irritation in response to the hallucinations. The thought content reflected a strong preoccupation with sex, such as, "I always wanted a woman to do it and not a man," and "I wanted a mate." He had great difficulty in describing his hallucinations, saying that they were not voices but "a noise that goes through you—a detective or something like that I guess." He referred to certain ideas as originating in other people, but was not able to describe them. He indicated that he had had some homosexual experiences and that he had felt inadequate in sexual relations with his wife. His interpretation of his hospitalization was that it was caused by drinking too much. Orientation was good.

*Follow-Up Notes.*   On June 25, 1947, the patient's condition remained as described in the "Mental Status." He continued to talk of sexual matters, and was especially preoccupied with the idea of anal rape.

Before the interview of September 2, 1947, he had been transferred to a more disturbed ward because he had been making sexual advances to women on the ward. At the time of this examination he was once more seclusive and preoccupied and he continued to respond to auditory hallucinations.

On January 17, 1948, and May 7, 1948, the patient's status had not changed from that of September 2, 1947.

**Patient 29.**  *Age:* 20.  *Sex:* male.  *Marital status:* single.  *Occupation:* none. *Religion:* Hebrew.  *Informant:* father.  *Diagnosis:* schizophrenia, catatonic type.

*Presenting Picture.*   The patient was admitted to Greystone in May, 1945, with a history of assaultiveness and unpredictable behavior.

*Present Illness.*   About four years before admission (at the age of thirteen and one-half) the patient's table manners began to deteriorate, he frequently argued with his mother, and was destructive about the house. He became seclusive and was taken out of school on the advice of a physician and sent to Florida for a month, where he attached himself closely to his father and avoided boys his own age. Shock treatment was recommended but not carried out, and he was then hospitalized in a state institution for fifteen months. He was then paroled and discharged one year later, after improving without specific treatment, though he was still irritable and difficult to manage. Twelve electroshock treatments were administered privately without improvement and the patient was sent to a rest home for two months. After a three-month period of working in the store of a relative he stopped work and again became unmanageable and destructive. Shock treatment was started once more and he was hospitalized privately for seven weeks. He continued to be assaultive and destructive, however, and was admitted to Greystone.

*Previous Personality Disorders.*   Prior to the present illness no personality disorders had been manifest.

*Family History.*   The patient's father was a Russian-born plumber. His mother was born in the United States of Polish-Russian parents; she was in good health and a full-time housekeeper. The patient was six years older than his only brother, who was supposedly in good health. The patient's mother was never able to discipline him and he always turned to his father for help or comfort when he was frightened.

*Personal History.*   The patient was born in New Jersey in September, 1927. Delivery was normal. He walked and talked "at an early age" and supposedly had a normal development. Scarlet fever without sequelae was the only serious illness. As a small boy he had many nightmares and was often frightened. At such times he would sleep with his father. He started school at five and a half and left, when he was fourteen, in his first year of high school. His school record was excellent until the onset of his illness and he was considered unusually intelligent by his teachers. With boys his own age he was domineering, but nothing was known of his attitude toward girls. He was always easily hurt by criticism from his father, but rarely obeyed his mother. When angry he would throw things, slam doors, and break windows.

*Personality.*   The personality is described under "Personal History."

*Hospital Course.*   After admission the patient was cooperative and compliant. He said that during his previous illness he had heard voices calling him bad names and threatening to kill him, but that these had been replaced by a single voice. His judgment and memory were defective. In the succeeding months he injured himself many times, on one occasion stating that he did this in response to a voice. He appeared preoccupied most of the time and was described as displaying little emotion. As of September, 1946, he had undergone a total of eighty-nine insulin comas, forty-nine electroshock treatments, and twenty-one metrazol treatments given in two separate series, with temporary improvement only after the first series. At this time he described auditory hallucinations, ideas of reference, as well as homosexual and heterosexual experiences in which he had taken part before his admission. Subsequently he continued to be destructive and disturbed until transferred to the project.

*Mental Status.* The patient appeared dull and preoccupied. There was some slowing of psychomotor activity. Affect was flattened and occasionally inappropriate. At this time no definite delusional material was elicited. He denied that he was having hallucinations, but admitted to hearing voices in the past. His behavior at this time did not suggest that he was having hallucinations. He was helpful on the ward but very seclusive. Orientation and memory were good. He had no insight into his illness and judgment was faulty.

*Follow-Up Notes.* On the interview of June 25, 1947, the patient remained seclusive, retarded, and unspontaneous. Tic-like sucking movements were present and his productions were no different from those recorded in his initial interview.

Before the interview of September 2, 1947, the patient had been transferred to a more disturbed ward, but he was once more retarded at this time. He described auditory hallucinations once more and was preoccupied with thoughts of masturbation.

On January 17, 1948, the patient's condition had not changed appreciably from that of the previous interview, except that he denied hallucinations at this time.

An increase in retardation was noted at the May 8, 1948, examination, with other features of the illness remaining unchanged.

**Patient 30.** *Age:* 45. *Sex:* male. *Marital status:* separated. *Occupation:* laborer. *Religion:* Protestant. *Informant:* father. *Diagnosis:* schizophrenia, hebephrenic type.

*Presenting Picture.* The patient was transferred to Greystone from the county jail with a history of irrational, excitable, and destructive behavior.

*Present Illness.* Until the present admission the patient was working as a laborer and handyman and was doing jobs which made few demands on him. His illness began with expressions of hostility against his brother and against all policemen (his brother was a policeman). He became excited, broke windows in his home, and was forcibly taken to the hospital in November, 1932.

*Previous Personality Disorders.* In 1917 the patient returned from a hike in a dazed and confused state after one week's absence, and was unable to account for his activities. He recovered spontaneously. In July, 1919, he was admitted to Greystone after an acute onset of confusion and excitement. He was released in October of the same year and readmitted in October, 1923, when he became irritable, seclusive, and uncommunicative. He had episodes of weeping and subsequently developed hallucinations and became excited and destructive. This hospitalization lasted six months.

*Family History.* Very little information concerning the family was available. The patient's Irish father died after complaining for several years of dizziness, unsteadiness of gait, and a marked speech defect. His mother was hospitalized for a psychosis associated with the menopause in January, 1923, dying in June of the same year. Five brothers and three sisters are living, of whom one brother was hospitalized for a mental illness in 1932.

*Personal History.* The patient was born in New Jersey in December, 1901, and was said to have had a normal birth and development. He graduated from elementary school in 1917 without any failures. Thereafter he worked in a mill, drove a delivery wagon, and did other more menial jobs between his illnesses. His work record was marked by frequent changes of job, as well as by the interruptions due to illness. He married sometime after 1934, but lived with his wife for only three months.

Subsequently his wife bore two children, but they were not fathered by the patient.

*Personality.*   The patient was described as being friendly but shiftless and unstable. Outstanding was his close attachment to his mother while she lived.

*Hospital Course.*   During his earlier admissions the patient was usually overactive, excited, and destructive. The present admission was marked by excitement at times, depression at other times. Early in this hospitalization and again in 1937 auditory hallucinations were prominent, consisting of voices which called him bad names. In the latter period he became hostile toward women and on several occasions he was assaultive.

*Mental Status.*   The patient was untidy and partially disrobed. His expression was vacuous for the most part, except for an occasional inappropriate grin, and he was emotionally flattened. He was retarded and inattentive and did not speak spontaneously. The mental content was evaluated on the basis of direct questions, which had frequently to be repeated, and consisted of self-condemnation (without corresponding affect), without delusions or hallucinations. He was correctly oriented and memory was good, but no insight was present.

*Follow-Up Notes.*   The patient was interviewed on June 25, 1947, August 26, 1947, and May 8, 1948. Throughout the follow-up period he showed little change, except in the direction of increased preoccupation and unresponsiveness. Occasionally he shouted impulsively but usually he sat quietly in bizarre positions, laughing and smiling inappropriately and speaking in nonsense syllables unless he were questioned, when he answered briefly though usually appropriately. He remained well oriented and his memory continued good.

**Patient 35.**   *Age:* 59.   *Sex:* female.   *Marital status:* divorced.   *Occupation:* dressmaker.   *Religion:* Protestant.   *Informants:* aunt, uncle.   *Diagnosis:* psychopathic personality with schizoid features.

*Presenting Picture.*   The patient was admitted voluntarily in November, 1940. She had many somatic complaints and was vaguely suspicious.

*Present Illness.*   About one year before admission the patient began to have many somatic complaints and began to weep occasionally. She was "suspicious" of anyone other than her aunt. Her complaints were quite diffuse: pain in the arms, legs, knees, and ankles; headache; vomiting. It was noted that she talked about her complaints in great detail to any visitors at her home. She was hospitalized twice without relief. Six months before admission she felt that people were talking about her and one week before admission she was forgetful and unable to work without assistance.

*Previous Personality Disorders.*   There was an unsubstantiated history of admission to Greystone in 1926, her stay lasting three months. No record of such an admission could be found.

*Family History.*   Information on the patient's family was scanty. Her father drank excessively and died at fifty-two after falling from a cliff. Her mother, who had been married before, died in her forties when the patient was seven years old. The patient was the oldest of two daughters by the mother's second marriage. There were also four half-siblings, three of whom died in infancy. A paternal great-aunt drank heavily and was also said to be a morphine addict. The patient's daughter was at Greystone in 1944-1945 and discharged in 1946; the diagnosis was dementia praecox. One year later this daughter was in good health, according to her husband.

*Personal History.*   The facts on the patient's early development were also limited. She was born in New Jersey in July, 1888, and moved about the state until 1916. From that time until 1930 her whereabouts was unknown. After her mother's death she lived with an aunt until she was twelve years old when the aunt also died. She left school at thirteen while in the fourth grade, and worked subsequently as a domestic servant until her marriage, three years later, to a jeweler. She had two children by this union which ended in divorce proceedings which were instituted by the husband. Thereafter the patient ran a boarding house, worked in an arsenal, and as a seamstress. Before being hospitalized she had complained for many years of leukorrhea, constipation, asthma, hay fever, migraine, and various injuries. She had an operation for the relief of a stomach ulcer twenty-five years before admission, another laparotomy four years before, and she had had seven or eight induced abortions.

*Personality.* The patient was always talkative, quick-tempered, selfish, and revengeful. She did not attempt to maintain any contact with her children although she preferred her son to her daughter. She did not take responsibilities seriously and was described as having a "happy-go-lucky" disposition.

*Hospital Course.* Following her admission in 1940 the patient was garrulous, rambling, and circumstantial. She wept easily and talked of suicide at times. She frequently complained that her uncle had made sexual advances toward her and often expressed fears about her son's safety. In May, 1941, she was removed from the hospital at her aunt's request to be readmitted voluntarily in April, 1946, when she complained of diarrhea and inability to move her legs. The picture was otherwise as it had been previously. In July, 1946, she was again paroled to be admitted again in October after an impulsive suicidal attempt the month before in which she attempted to cut her wrists. Some depression was present on admission but her subsequent course was one of constant complaining and rambling accounts of her various "illnesses." At no time was she uncooperative but parole could not be recommended in the absence of a suitable relative to assume responsibility for her.

*Mental Status.* The patient was spending most of her time on the ward sewing or knitting and was garrulous with anyone who engaged her in conversation. She was overproductive and, though her mood was not unusual, she displayed an abundance of affect in discussing her somatic complaints and the way she felt she had been treated by various members of her family. The thought content centered about her numerous somatic complaints and her feelings that her husband and daughter had somehow been "against her." When questioned about her excessive use of alcohol and her sexual life she became markedly defensive and denied that there had been anything unusual in these spheres of behavior. She was correctly oriented and there was no disturbance of the sensorium but she had no insight into her complaints.

*Follow-Up Notes.* The patient was interviewed on the following dates: June 25, 1947, September 2, 1947, January 17, 1948, and May 7, 1948. Her condition showed no essential change throughout the follow-up period. She continued to offer many somatic complaints and to be demanding of special attention. At times she wept petulantly when refused attention but for the most part she was content to remain a hospital patient and gave no indication of desire to leave the hospital environment. At no time could her behavior be classified as psychotic.

**Patient 37.** *Age:* 38. *Sex:* female. *Marital status:* married. *Occupation:* none. *Religion:* Hebrew. *Informant:* husband. *Diagnosis:* schizophrenia, hebephrenic type.

*Presenting Picture.* The patient was admitted in September, 1944, with a history of depression and persecutory delusions.

*Present Illness.* In July, 1944, the patient began to express fears of Nazi persecution, to neglect her housework, and withdraw from her husband. She bought many newspapers in an attempt to discover who was looking for her and insisted that her clothesline be taken down since it might be used by the Nazis to hang a member of her family. She refused intercourse with her husband without explanation, and suspected that someone was attempting to poison her. Commitment was arranged through the police.

*Previous Personality Disorders.* While in Paris from 1935-1940 the patient's behavior was seclusive and at times she appeared to have hallucinations. In 1942 a psychiatric picture began to develop which was almost identical with that of the present illness. After electroshock treatment in August, 1943, she improved greatly and was able to function adequately until the onset of this illness.

*Family History.* The patient's father was born wealthy and was occupied as a butter-and-egg dealer in Poland before he died in 1928 of diabetes and cardiac disease. The patient's mother was German born and was living in good health in Denmark. The patient was the third girl born and had one brother, two years younger than herself. One sister married a broker in the United States, one married a physician in Denmark, and the patient's brother went to Palestine when he was unable to complete his medical studies in Germany; all are in good health.

*Personal History.* The patient was born in Saarbrücken in May, 1909. Nothing is known of her early development except that she was overindulged as a child, always had her own maid, and never had to learn housework. Religious training in childhood was strict. She began school at six and finished the equivalent of high school at sixteen. Thereafter she went to business school for a year although she never worked. She was a good student in all of her classes. In 1927 she married the informant and in 1933 a son was born. In April, 1941, the patient and her husband and son left Germany for the United States where the husband secured a job selling hosiery from house to house.

*Personality.* The description given was that of a self-centered woman who considered herself superior to everyone around her. She was sexually demanding and socially very much dependent on her husband. For many years before her illness she was suspicious that strangers were spying on her.

*Hospital Course.* In November, 1944, insulin and electroshock treatment was started. This was continued until April, 1945, by which time the patient was quiet except when visited by her husband. She remained silly, shallow, and unreasonable in her demands, however. It was difficult to interpret her psychopathologic state because of the language difficulty. During 1945-1946 she underwent a gradual regression, becoming seclusive and assaultive toward other patients. She stated that the Germans were going to make a "bad woman" of her and, in spite of the difficulties of communication, it was felt that she was delusional and subject to hallucinations.

*Mental Status.* At times the patient was excited and assaultive on the ward. When interviewed she was disheveled and carelessly dressed. She sat quietly, grinning throughout the interview and apparently reacting to hallucinations. Any affective reaction was silly and inappropriate but it was impossible to evaluate either her mood or thought content because of her constant incoherent babbling, which consisted chiefly of garbled German. She answered direct questions in English only to reply that she felt "good" and that she was single.

*Follow-Up Notes.* The patient was interviewed on the following dates: July 4, 1947, September 2, 1947, January 18, 1948, and May 7, 1948. Throughout the follow-up period she remained out of contact and unapproachable, even when spoken to in her native tongue. There was no significant change in the behavioral picture in any of the interviews.

**Patient 41.** *Age:* 46. *Sex:* female. *Marital status:* married. *Occupation:* waitress. *Religion:* Catholic. *Informant:* husband. *Diagnosis:* schizophrenia, hebephrenic type.

*Presenting Picture.* In December, 1936, the patient was transferred to Greystone from an observation ward where it was observed that she had religious delusions and hallucinations.

*Present Illness.* In November, 1936, after the extraction of a tooth under gas anesthesia, the patient began to accuse her husband of being unfaithful and of having homosexual experiences with his brother. Subsequently she began to pray excessively and said that she and a certain priest were destined to save the world. These ideas were accompanied by increased motor activity although the patient continued to perform her household duties well. She was admitted to a local hospital where she had a vision of her sister as a saint, and other religious and mystical experiences. Sexual material was also present. After ten days she was transferred to Greystone.

*Previous Personality Disorders.* There was no history of previous personality disorders.

*Family History.* The patient's father was a farmer who died in Ireland in 1930, aged seventy-five years. He was described as "quick-tempered." Her mother was twenty years younger than her father. The mother also remained in Ireland. She was described as "quiet, reserved, and level-headed." The patient was the youngest of three daughters. Both sisters died in young adulthood of tuberculosis.

*Personal History.* The patient was born in Ireland in March, 1901. There is no information on her early life. Menses began when she was thirteen years of age and were usually accompanied by cramps. After completing public school in Ireland the patient entered a convent in England where she remained for one year until she decided she had made the wrong choice. She then entered training as a nurse but gave that up and came to the United States in 1922 at the invitation of her sister. She worked as a children's nurse for one and one-half years, then as a factory supervisor for four years until her marriage in 1928. Her husband was a maintenance mechanic and the couple had no children although no contraceptive measures were taken, and no medical reason for infertility was found in either partner.

*Personality.* The patient was described as timid, easily hurt, and dependent on her husband for emotional support. She preferred the company of women older than herself and was not interested in social life outside of her home. Although she attended church regularly, she was not unusually religious before her illness.

*Hospital Course.* Following her admission in 1936 the patient was overactive, noisy, incoherent, and partially disoriented. She was silly, confused, and at times assaultive. The following sample of speech was recorded in April, 1937: "Pat—Mary—Kelly—Anne—Frank—I am in hell. Pat—black—Father M. vote for Roosevelt over the waves. Going to save for the Lindbergh baby." The patient lost 20 pounds in weight although physical disease could not be demonstrated. In November, 1938, she had eleven metrazol-induced convulsions followed by only transient improvement. Her condition thereafter remained unchanged until February, 1942, when she became mute and impulsive, and assaultiveness returned. In this condition she was transferred to the project.

*Mental Status.* Throughout the interview the patient preferred to sit hunched over in her chair, her hands folded in her lap, although she occasionally moved about the room in response to a direct request. Her facial expression was empty and she was untidy. She was mute, deeply preoccupied, and almost completely unresponsive to her environment. Her only responses were answers to the questions: "Are you tired?" ("no") and "Do you enjoy eating?" ("yes").

*Follow-Up Notes.* The patient was interviewed on the following dates: July 4, 1947, September 9, 1947, January 18, 1948, and May 7, 1948. Throughout the follow-up period she remained preoccupied and essentially mute. On a few occasions she replied with a short, inappropriate phrase to direct questions.

**Patient 45.** *Age:* 41. *Sex:* female. *Marital status:* married. *Occupation:* farm worker. *Religion:* Greek Orthodox. *Informant:* husband. *Diagnosis:* schizophrenia, hebephrenic type.

*Presenting Picture.* The patient was admitted to Greystone in May, 1942, because of depression and paranoid ideas.

*Present Illness.* In February, 1941, the patient expressed ideas of reference to her husband and said that a neighbor was trying to take her away from her husband. She was hospitalized in New York and then removed to a state hospital where she was given electroshock treatment followed by great improvement. In October, 1941, she was paroled, remaining well until two weeks before admission to Greystone when she expressed ideas that people did not like her or her husband. Her appetite diminished and she became forgetful. The last day at home she began to weep and she shouted that she no longer cared for the children.

*Previous Personality Disorders.* There was no history of personality disorders prior to the present illness.

*Family History.* The patient's father was a Greek laborer who died in 1933 at the age of seventy. Her mother is still living in Greece; no information was obtained concerning her. The patient was the fourth of five children and all the other siblings were reported to be in good health.

*Personal History.* The patient was born in Greece in July, 1906. No information was available on her early development. She had six years of schooling up to 1932 at which time she came to the United States to do farm work. In the same year she married a cook who was also born in Greece. There were three children, the youngest being severely anemic and requiring periodic blood transfusions. The marriage was compatible and the patient appeared to have made a good adjustment to the United States although she never learned to speak English well.

*Personality.* The patient was devoted to her home, children, and husband. She was always faithful in church attendance.

*Hospital Course.* For one year after admission the patient was kept on a disturbed ward and was noted to be excited, uncooperative, depressed, assaultive, and to have hallucinations. Insulin and electroshock treatments were started in May, 1943, following which she became cooperative, quiet, and no longer delusional or subject to hallucinations. It was noted, however, that she tended to exaggerate physical complaints. She was paroled but remained home only six months. The return of her symptoms was gradual. After nine months on a disturbed ward, shock treatment of the same type was again resumed but improvement was slight and the patient was returned to the disturbed ward where she remained until she was transferred to the project.

*Mental Status.* The patient was tidy and well dressed but she approached the examiner suspiciously; her perplexed appearance was outstanding. She was markedly underproductive. Her emotional responses were flat except for an occasional inappropriate smile. Much of her talk was in Greek and her English was often not understandable. She indicated that she was hearing the voices of members of her own family. Only after many repetitions of the question did she give the name of the hospital correctly.

*Follow-Up Notes.* This patient was interviewed on July 4, 1947, September 9, 1947, January 18, 1948, and May 7, 1948. There was no change in her condition throughout the follow-up period. At each interview she was preoccupied, suspicious, disoriented, and showed evidence of having hallucinations.

**Patient 48.** *Age:* 26. *Sex:* female. *Marital status:* single. *Occupation:* N.Y.A. worker. *Religion:* Protestant. *Informants*: mother and aunt. *Diagnosis*: schizophrenia, hebephrenic type.

*Presenting Picture.* The patient was admitted to Greystone in June, 1941, with a history of bizarre and destructive behavior.

*Present Illness.* In June, 1941, she suddenly became seclusive and began to laugh inappropriately. Frequently she waved a handkerchief out the window, offering no explanation. The following day she broke a window after a physician had been called to examine her. In the observation ward she was denudative.

*Previous Personality Disorders.* The patient first became suddenly ill in September, 1938. She was cared for at home even though she was subject to hallucinations and delusions and showed considerable regression for a period of about six weeks. Another sudden onset occurred in September, 1940. At this time she again had delusions and hallucinations and was socially unpredictable, but once more her mother refused hospitalization. She supposedly recovered in April, 1941, after treatment at a neurologic clinic and remained well until the present illness.

*Family History.* The patient's father was an English-born bookkeeper who died after a "stroke" in 1940. He was described as "sociable and talkative." The patient "grieved a great deal" after her father's death. Her mother was born in New York and was in good health except for asthma and hay fever. The patient was the oldest of three children and the only girl. All of the children were unmarried.

*Personal History.* The patient was born in New Jersey in October, 1921. She was a full-term baby with normal delivery. She began to walk and talk at nine months and one year respectively. Menses began when she was thirteen and, concurrently, she contracted "malaria" for which she was treated for three months. In childhood, there were several instances of falls or blows to the head, the vagina, and other portions of the body without known sequelae. She started school at six but was not a good student and she gave up school in the eighth grade. For a short time before her illness she worked for the National Youth Administration. Her mother was overprotective of the patient and gave her no sexual instruction.

*Personality.* The personality description indicated that the patient was a sensitive, rather withdrawn girl who was very dependent on her family.

*Hospital Course.* Early in her hospital stay the patient was at times assaultive and at times affectionate and loving toward the personnel. She was usually overactive and confused, frequently expressing persecutory delusions. After seven months, parole was granted at the request of her mother although no major improvement had occurred. After two months at home, during which constant care was required, she returned to the hospital. For the past five years there has been little change although episodes of relative quiet have been interspersed with periods of excitement and assaultiveness.

*Mental Status.* The patient was passively cooperative but showed no initiative or spontaneity. During the interview she responded to direct questions at times. She was in poor contact; her mood was flat and marked by inappropriate laughter and giggling. She described auditory and visual hallucinations. Her thought content centered about incest and other sexual themes. She stated that she had been married to her father, uncle, and brother, had had children, and that she was her mother's rival. She also described masturbation fears, and discoursed at length on her preoccupations with religious denominations. She was disoriented for time and place and her sensorium was cloudy.

*Follow-Up Notes.* The patient was interviewed on July 4, 1947, September 9, 1947, January 18, 1948, and May 7, 1948. She showed no significant change throughout the follow-up period. She continued to have hallucinations, her delusions were unaffected, and she remained disoriented. Affectively she continued to be flat.

### CONTROL PATIENTS WHO WERE SUBJECTED TO LOBOTOMY

**Patient 11.** *Age:* 44. *Sex:* male. *Marital status:* married. *Occupation:* laborer. *Religion:* Roman Catholic. *Informants:* wife and sister. *Diagnosis:* schizophrenia, paranoid type.

*Presenting Picture.* On admission to Greystone in January, 1943, the patient was agitated and suicidal. Delusions of persecution and auditory hallucinations were present.

*Present Illness.* About two weeks before admission he expressed ideas that the men in his shop were talking about him. He was restless, sleepless, and his appetite became poor. At times he was irritable, appeared discouraged, and had spells of weeping, and he expressed a wish to be dead. He was found unconscious after attempting suicide by gas. He was taken to a general hospital where he expressed ideas that he was being influenced and that his food was being poisoned. After attempting to choke himself with a sheet he was transferred to Greystone.

*Previous Personality Disorders.* There was no history of previous personality disorders.

*Family History.* The patient's father was an Italian-born laborer who came to the United States at the age of fifty and died in 1944 at the age of eighty-eight. The patient was always fond of his father who was said to be a quiet and considerate man. When his father died the patient had a relapse of his illness. The patient's mother was also Italian born and died in 1945 at the age of seventy-eight. She was a friendly but reserved woman whose only interests were in her home and children. There were six children of whom the patient was fourth oldest. One brother was four years older than the patient; the other siblings were girls. All were married, had large families, and were apparently in good health.

*Personal History.* The patient was born in New York in August, 1903. Nothing is known about his early development except that he had whooping cough as a child. He completed grammar school at the age of fourteen and then worked in a silk mill for five or six years. He worked as a plumber's helper for a short time but after his marriage, in 1925, he returned to the silk mill for two or three years. During the depression he was unemployed for seven or eight years. For two years before his admission he worked as a laborer for an aircraft company. His wife is three years older than he, a devout Catholic, and supposedly well adjusted. The couple had three children, born 1925, 1927, and 1931, all of whom were well; there were three "miscarriages." Sexual relations occurred two or three times weekly. The patient had a herniorrhaphy in 1939, "rheumatic fever" in 1942, and he was treated intermittently for a peptic ulcer during the two years prior to his admission to the hospital. He began to smoke somewhat to excess before his admission, but previously he had been a moderate smoker and had not used alcohol at all.

*Personality.* The picture given was that of a man who was energetic and ambitious in his work but who had little social life and very few friends. He was usually kind-hearted and good humored at home but could be stubborn and argumentative at times.

*Hospital Course.* Following his admission in January, 1943, the patient was co-operative but suspicious and he expressed persecutory ideas. Following treatment with colonic irrigations and hydrotherapy he quieted down. In June, 1943, he was paroled to his home where he made a satisfactory adjustment until early 1944. At that time he reacted strongly to the death of his father and he developed auditory hallucinations during an attack of influenza. He received electroshock and insulin therapy in the spring of 1944, followed by much improvement. He was again paroled for a year. In November of 1945, however, he was returned to the hospital because he had become destructive and was once more having hallucinations and expressing persecutory ideas. Shock therapy (thirty-three insulin comas and twenty-nine electro-shock convulsions) was given without effect; he remained noisy and threatening and continued to have hallucinations and delusions until he was transferred to this project.

*Mental Status.* The patient appeared carefree and pleasant. He smiled frequently as he spontaneously poured out his many complaints. He displayed much affect, particularly as he discussed his paranoid delusions, but his affect was not always appropriate to the disturbing ideational content. Productions centered around these paranoid ideas and included statements that he was dead, that a kidnapping had brought him to the hospital, that a paralyzing electrical ray was somehow being applied to his body, and similar assertions. He described auditory hallucinations but did not identify them nor the specific content of the hallucinations. Consciousness was not clouded and he was well oriented.

*Follow-Up Notes.* On interviews made on June 13, 1947, August 25, 1947, and October 20, 1947, no significant change from the patient's preanesthesia behavior was noted. Any variation was in the direction of increased irritability and brief periods of rage.

On October 31, 1947, a bilateral prefrontal lobotomy was performed.

On November 3, 1947, the patient was alert and active in bed. He was oriented for place but did not recognize the examiner nor was he able to understand why the bandage was on his head. His former irritability was lacking, a delusional system could not be elicited, and he was cooperative. The day after this interview he was assisting other patients and the nurses in the performance of their duties on the ward.

On November 7, 1947, he was distractible and his delusional system was still present though it was difficult to elicit it, in contrast to his readiness to talk about it pre-operatively. His behavior was unpredictable, being at times cooperative and at other times irritable and threatening. Performance on simple tests involving memory and calculation was also unpredictable.

The patient was again interviewed on January 17, 1948. At this time he had made visits home but had no definite plans for a future job. He was pleasant, cooperative, and smiling. Most outstanding was the diminished affective response and there was no longer agitation or pacing of the floor. His delusional material had not changed but he seemed no longer concerned about the electrical stimulation, the voices, or other illusions to which he was being subjected. He was aware that he had been operated upon but did not know why. Recent and remote memory, orientation, and calculation were good but there was no insight; he seemed to feel no concern about himself beyond the immediate fact that he wanted to get out of the hospital.

At the time of the interview on May 7, 1948, seven months after lobotomy, the patient was working daily but beneath his former capacity. He was making an acceptable social adjustment, although he was superficial and easily distracted. The delusional material was still present; hallucinations persisted, although they no longer concerned him and this lack of concern and carefree attitude about all things was an outstanding feature of his condition. His wife indicated that his behavior was similar to that before he became ill except that he tended to lose his temper if crossed, so that the family had learned not to argue with him. Sexual activity was about the same as before the illness began.

**Patient 20.** *Age:* 28. *Sex:* male. *Marital status:* single. *Occupation:* farmer. *Religion:* Roman Catholic. *Informant:* father. *Diagnosis:* schizophrenia, hebephrenic type.

*Presenting Picture.* When admitted to Greystone Park in March, 1942, the patient appeared dull and apathetic, heard accusing voices and was self-deprecatory.

*Present Illness.* He entered the Army early in 1941, expecting to serve for one year, and got along well until January, 1942. Having spent a Christmas furlough at home, he returned to camp and within two weeks his father received a letter from the patient asking forgiveness for all the trouble he had caused. When his father visited him, the patient did not appear particularly disturbed but the doctors at the Army hospital stated that he believed he was in love with a local waitress (whom he had never taken out) and that other men in camp were getting him in trouble. After a disability discharge from the Army he was admitted to Greystone.

*Previous Personality Disorders.* There was no history of previous personality disorders.

*Family History.* No information was obtained concerning the Polish-born grandparents. The father, aged fifty-five, is a truck farmer who came to the United States from Poland in 1900. In good health and apparently well adjusted, he feels that his son's illness is a reflection of the boy's "laziness." The mother, aged forty-nine, is also Polish born. She has been overprotective and was described as being "the kind of person who always likes to please." There is one married brother, aged thirty-two, who was preferred by the father and who dominated the patient until he was seventeen years old, at which time there was a verbal "battle" which freed the patient of his older brother. The brother is now a partner in the family farm.

*Personal History.* The patient was born in New York State in July, 1919, weighing 8 pounds at birth. He walked when fifteen months of age and talked at eighteen months. Except for the usual childhood diseases he was well. He began school when he was five years old and he left in his second year of high school (at fifteen) to help out on the farm where he remained until he was drafted in January, 1941. He liked sports and did moderately well at them with the exceptions of football and hunting. (On the only occasion when he killed a rabbit he was much upset at having taken a life.) At one time he expressed an interest in aviation but this was abandoned in the face of family objection, particularly from his mother who objected to it as a dangerous occupation. He was always outshone by his brother who learned more easily and. was a successful Army captain, in contrast to the patient's record. The patient's father feels that he absorbed the pacifist ideas which were common in the years after World War I and felt betrayed when events led to a second world war.

*Personality.* Of at least average intelligence, the patient was described as being "a retiring sort," always appearing calm and unruffled. He was excessively conscientious and self-critical, always overly neat. Like his father, he did not attend church, though he had received a church education. He was never concerned with his own health but always worried about the health of his father and brother. Nothing was known of his sexual activities and he never discussed the subject with his father.

*Hospital Course.* After admission the patient was correctly oriented but agitated, restless, and assaultive at times. He admitted hearing the voices of men talking about him, said he had been in trouble with his officers and had thought he loved a girl, but this was all past. He spoke of writing threatening letters to his father (a statement which was not true, according to the father) and said his trouble was caused by masturbation. Maternal incest and homosexual thoughts were also prominent. After nineteen insulin comas and fourteen electroshock treatments, he quieted down but was slow and indolent. He was paroled in August, 1942, and worked (poorly) on the farm until November, 1943, when he was readmitted to the hospital. In March, 1944, another course of insulin and electroshock therapy was given attended with little improvement, although the patient was again paroled for a short time. Several parole visits followed during which he was able to adjust only by virtue of his mother's protectiveness. In June, 1946, while in the hospital, he became impulsive, broke windows, struck people, and said he was afraid he would attack his "sister" (non-existent) sexually. He feared he would soon die or be hurt by other boys and heard the voices of famous people as well as other voices calling him bad names. Electroshock treatments were again started but soon discontinued because he became fearful and apprehensive. He was transferred to this project.

*Mental Status.* When interviewed in 1947 the patient was apathetic, listless, underproductive, and somewhat resentful of being questioned. He was only partially oriented, his memory was fair, and insight and judgment were poor. He stated that his nervous system was "on the blink" and that people talked about him. The thought content was largely sexual and revolved about masturbation, a waitress he had known while in the Army, a widow whom he had once visited, and fears that he would sexually attack his father's sisters if he were to see them in bed.

During the operative control period this patient showed no change. He remained slow, apathetic, and preoccupied.

On October 31, 1947, a bilateral prefrontal lobotomy was performed.

*Follow-Up Notes.* On the interview of November 3, 1947, it was noted that immediately after operation, the patient was disoriented for time, gave correctly the name of the institution and its function, but did not remember his physicians. He did not know he had been operated on and said his head was bandaged because he was sick in bed. All of his responses were slow and repetitive; he had to be restrained to prevent picking at his bandages.

On November 7, 1947, the patient remained preoccupied, resistive to procedures, and slovenly (though he was not incontinent). He yawned frequently, speech and movements were slow, and he showed no emotion. Auditory hallucinations were still present as unrecognized people who said ". . . encouraging things, like 'Keep smiling.'" He had to be reminded to use his handkerchief since apparently the value of the article did not occur to him spontaneously. The date was given as "mid-July, 1919" (his birthday). When asked the nature of the institution, he no longer responded to questioning, no matter how direct.

At the time of the January 18, 1948, interview the patient was making home visits. He was still slow and lacking spontaneity, but this was somewhat less marked than on previous examinations. His speech was less monotonous and occasionally he smiled. Auditory hallucinations were denied though he described them vaguely as having occurred earlier. The sexual content was no longer present. He stated that he continued to masturbate, had occasional wet dreams, and had more interest in girls, but there was an obvious lack of drive behind these statements. Orientation was good, memory fair, and he appeared unable to plan for the future. When asked if he had been sick, he replied, "I probably was."

The patient was interviewed again on May 8, 1948. He had returned to his home in January and was working well on his family's farm. Speech and movements were slow. He was emotionally flat and was still preoccupied with masturbation and other sexual ideas. Auditory hallucinations which were reassuring to him were present. His mother pointed out that he remained suspicious and shy, forgetful, and dependent on his parents. They also remarked on his lack of ambition and planning beyond a day-to-day basis.

**Patient 5.** *Age:* 35. *Sex:* male. *Marital status:* married. *Occupation:* welder. *Religion:* Roman Catholic. *Informants:* brother and wife. *Diagnosis:* schizophrenia, hebephrenic type.

*Presenting Picture.* On admission to Greystone in February, 1945, the patient was agitated, depressed, and suspicious. He expressed persecutory delusions.

*Present Illness.* The patient's illness developed slowly, beginning apparently at the age of eighteen years (1930) when he accused his brother-in-law (a co-worker) of interfering with his advancement on the job. During the following eight years he was noticeably suspicious of his fellow employees. Beginning in 1938, while working in a roller-bearing plant, he expressed ideas that others were retarding his advancement and conspiring against him. In 1942 he was advised to take a rest. A year later he was dismissed because of his unjust accusations against other workers. Other jobs then followed with similar consequences. Before admission he accused his wife of infidelity, was suspicious of everyone, expressed passive ideas of influence, was apprehensive, and lost interest in sex. Eight weeks before admission he began to have frequent crying spells but expressed no suicidal ideas.

*Previous Personality Disorders.* There was no history of previous personality disorders.

*Family History.* No significant mental illness was described in the grandparents. The patient's father was a New Jersey-born Coast Guardsman who was "sociable but quick-tempered." The mother was a retiring, quiet, serious woman who was ineffectual and who had few friends. The patient was the youngest of six children. The two oldest siblings died of influenza and tuberculosis, the first death occurring when the patient was six and the second when he was twelve years old. The other offspring were satisfactorily married and apparently well at the time of the patient's admission. All members of the family were unusually thin. When the patient was nine his mother and father separated and later were divorced because the father was interested in "another woman." The patient was bitter about this as a child. His mother subsequently "babied" him; he was always much devoted to her, considering her opinion above that of his wife in later years.

*Personal History.* Born in New Jersey in February, 1912, the patient's delivery was not unusual and his development was supposedly without incident. He had measles and mumps as a child but no enuresis, night terrors, or convulsions. His reaction to the deaths of siblings is not known (see "Family History"). In school he was often a truant. He was a poor student; he failed several times and left in the seventh grade (aged fourteen) to work in a shoe factory. Symptoms of mental illness began four years later (see "Present Illness"). At twenty-four he married a Catholic girl five years his junior who was a schoolteacher. She encouraged him to better himself and he learned welding at her suggestion. After six months of marriage, however, she left him and sued for divorce, supposedly without any explanation. The patient's family expected this and were not surprised at the turn of events. Thereafter his work record was unstable and he drank somewhat more than usual ("4 to 6 glasses of beer a day"). In May, 1944, he married again. Following this marriage he drank somewhat less. His second wife was a woman he had known for three years. She was a passive, highly dependent woman. The subsequent course of events has been covered under "Present Illness."

*Personality.* As a child the patient was always quiet, restrained, and reticent. Early in the onset of symptoms he became stubborn and suspicious. He was ambitious and energetic as a boy but this was short-lived, disappearing after he began to work. He had few friends but enjoyed the movies, bowling, and playing shuffle-board.

*Hospital Course.* Following his admission in February, 1945, the patient was cooperative to treatment with hydrotherapy and colonics, but, when no improvement was forthcoming after a month, electroshock and insulin treatments were started. Thereafter he was friendly, pleasant, calm, and no longer delusional. In September he was paroled to his wife and adjusted well to their child, born while the patient was still hospitalized. Improvement was not maintained, however, and by February, 1946, he had again developed paranoid delusions and was jealous of his child. In March he was returned to the hospital where his condition remained unchanged. He was transferred to this project as a seclusive and underproductive patient.

*Mental Status.* The patient was retarded and preoccupied, his facial expression being one of confusion or perplexity. He rarely spoke spontaneously and answered direct questions only briefly and incompletely. His voice was monotonous and affect was flat. The mental content was limited to a few subjects; there were large areas of amnesia. He did not remember his first marriage nor the names of many places where he had worked. Characteristic statements include: "I had a breakdown a year ago. That's why I'm here." "I can't accuse anyone without seeing them. I don't remember that anyone has ever done anything to me. I keep writing to my doctor to let me go home." He reacted with perplexity when asked if his wife were unfaithful. The sensorium was clouded though he was correctly oriented. Insight and judgment were both poor.

*Follow-Up Notes.* The patient was interviewed on June 12, August 19, and October 10, 1947. During the control period covered by these dates, he showed little change except in the direction of some increase in preoccupation and retardation.

On October 30, 1947, a bilateral prefrontal lobotomy was performed. Thereafter he went through a stormy postoperative course.

On November 7, 1947, the first day after his febrile reaction had subsided, his attention was poor, he was disoriented for time, place, and situation, and all responses were slow and incomplete. He was incontinent in respect to urination.

Gradual improvement took place and when seen on January 17, 1948, he was more spontaneous, less flat, and emotional expression was more appropriate though it could not be considered adequate. He still sat rigidly and with some suggestion of posturing, but his stream of mental activity had increased slightly and he occasionally smiled. He was interested in his child and other patients who had returned to the hospital for a check-up. Sexual desire was present on visits home but he achieved orgasm only by external contact with his wife and not by actual penetration. Calculation and memory were satisfactory but there was no insight and judgment was still poor.

The patient did not return at the time of the one-year examination (eight months after lobotomy). Later developments revealed that this was because his psychotic symptoms had recurred. He was readmitted to the hospital early in June, 1948, but after a few weeks again showed some improvement and was reconsidered for parole.

**Patient 23.** *Age:* 39. *Sex:* male. *Marital status:* divorced. *Occupation:* mailman. *Religion:* no church affiliation. *Informants:* wife and mother. *Diagnosis:* schizophrenia, paranoid type.

*Presenting Picture.* When admitted to Greystone in June, 1942, the patient was agitated, depressed at times, and showed fixed delusions.

*Present Illness.* About one and a half years before admission he began to feel that other workers in the post office were against him and at the same time the quality of his work fell off, resulting in frequent reprimands, which he felt were unjustified. He had devoted an excessive amount of time to a fraternal order and was about to be made master of the lodge, but was forced to resign from office at this time because he was unable to remember the rituals. He obtained a leave of absence from his job, but did not improve during the vacation. He went on a trip and during this he lost all sexual desire. On his return, he was unsuccessful in a one-day trial at the post office and was not allowed to continue working. Since he was unable to support his family, his wife went to live with her sister, and the patient returned to his mother. He brooded about the separation, but did not express suicidal tendencies, though he talked about the "futility" of life. On June 3, 1942, his wife had him committed for observation. While in the observation ward he said that his baby had somehow changed, that electric currents were coming into his house, and he expressed much interest in mental telepathy. One week later he was committed to Greystone.

*Previous Personality Disorders.* There was no history of previous personality disorders.

*Family History.* The patient's American-born father died of intestinal obstruction in 1928, at the age of forty-eight. He was an assistant postmaster and was described as reserved and sensitive. The patient's mother was born in 1885 and is still living, though she suffers from arthritis. She developed some disorder of her thyroid while pregnant with the patient, and had cardiac difficulties after his birth. The patient is the oldest of six boys, one of whom was described as very nervous and irritable and another of whom has a history of an ocular tic as well as "St. Vitus' dance" in childhood.

*Personal History.* The patient was born in New Jersey in August, 1908. Delivery was difficult and instruments were used, which left their mark on his head throughout early childhood. He weighed 9 pounds and 10 ounces at birth, began to talk at twelve months, and to walk at fourteen months. At seven years of age he had diphtheria, followed by a paralysis of both legs which was treated for two months at the Neurological Institute in New York. He gradually regained full use of both legs. Several months later he had an uneventful recovery following an appendectomy. About five years of age he began kindergarten and he did well throughout his school career. While in high school he was restricted in activity because of a "heart condition," but subsequent examinations revealed no pathologic basis for the diagnosis. After the patient graduated from high school he worked in the stock exchange for one year. He then received a civil service appointment as a mail carrier and worked for fourteen years at this job until his hospitalization. In August, 1929, he married a girl two years his junior. There was one child (girl), but his wife secured a divorce in 1945. She was supposedly socially ambitious and presented a financial strain to the patient. He was described as "normal" sexually until the onset of his illness, when sexual desire began to decrease leading to a complete absence of sexual interest at the height of his symptoms.

*Personality.* The patient was of better than average intelligence and enjoyed reading "deep" books and writing poetry. He was sensitive to criticism and found it difficult to make friends. His interests were centered about his home, but he was dissatisfied with his job and the economic status of the family, though he was indecisive about planning any moves. After a lapse of religious interest at the age of seventeen there was a revival of such interest beginning at the age of thirty.

*Hospital Course.* On admission in 1942 the patient described ideas of food poisoning and persecution, but denied all statements in his commitment papers. He was paroled with supervision in July, but returned in October, 1942, because his persecutory ideas had increased. Insulin and electroshock treatment was started in April, 1943, following which he improved but remained suspicious. Parole was granted in October, 1943. He remained on extended parole until October, 1945, when he was discharged as recovered.

He was readmitted in January, 1946, at which time he was voluble, overproductive, scattered, and was subject to hallucinations and delusions. His persecutory system involved himself as an agent of the F.B.I. and he somehow felt that he was being persecuted and subjected to alien control by means of electricity and telepathy. He made use of an extensive vocabulary and cloaked his delusions in a pseudoscientific vocabulary, using such terms as "psychosomosis" and "encasements." A large sexual element was also present in his system of delusions. There was no change in his condition and he was therefore referred to this project.

*Mental Status.* At the time of this examination the patient was moderately over-active but neatly dressed and productive on the ward (cleaning, assisting attendants). He was euphoric and affect was dissociated from the thought content. Frank delusions and auditory hallucinations were expressed; visual hallucinations were also suspected. "Something fishy is going on here . . . we are missing medical current from a nurse . . . I have the institution under arrest by the intelligence department" are samples of statements made. At times the patient held his hands over his ears and said he was tuning in on the wave lengths of other patients; there were many examples of ideas of alien control. His sensorium, memory, and orientation were in good order, but there was no insight.

*Follow-Up Notes.* The patient was interviewed on June 25, and August 25, 1947. There was little change over this period. He continued to write notes in which he disbarred doctors and nurses from practice; excessive cleanliness of a compulsive type appeared; and he became more grandiose (giving himself titles connected with the Department of Intelligence, F.B.I., Bureau of Weights and Measures, American Tele-phone and Telegraph, and the Soviet Union).

By the time of the interview on October 20, 1947, the grandiosity was well estab-lished and the patient's attitude toward the doctors whom he had disbarred was a condescending one. He was preoccupied with the oral cavity and genitalia. Intellect and orientation were well preserved, but judgment and insight remained seriously impaired.

On October 29, 1947, a bilateral prefrontal lobotomy was performed.

The patient remained stuporous until October 31, 1947, and when questioned in the morning no evidence of his old delusional systems or hallucinations was present. By evening, however, the old material was once more present.

Evidence of delusions and hallucinations was obtained in the examinations made November 3, and November 7, 1947, as on previous examinations. These were usually extracted only on direct questioning, however, and were not volunteered. The patient was suspicious, resistive, and petulant. Many of his responses were inappropriate. His intellectual performance in response to test questions was spotty and answers fre-quently involved condensation with material from the previous question, or material of his own preoccupations.

The patient was interviewed on January 18, March 14, and May 8, 1948. His condi-tion remained quite static throughout this period. There was perhaps some diminution of affective response (although he had very little before operation). He lost interest in current events and was no longer oriented for time even with the aid of a calendar. He was capable of simple jobs around the hospital, however, and was not a problem in management.

**Patient 28.** *Age:* 27. *Sex:* male. *Marital status:* single. *Occupation:* laborer. *Religion:* Catholic. *Informants:* mother and half-brother. *Diagnosis:* schizophrenia, hebephrenic type.

*Presenting Picture.* On admission to Greystone in September, 1944, the patient was untidy, excited, and paranoid.

*Present Illness.* About one year before admission he became irritable and much concerned about his health. He quit his job, became seclusive, and fought with one of his half-brothers. Occasionally he helped with housework but usually he sat staring out of the window. For a time he was overcareful about turning off the gas and warned his brothers to drive their car carefully. For two months he received injections at a local clinic without relief, and subsequently his dress became slovenly, and at times he wore women's clothes. In the month before admission he became confused and expressed fears that someone would choke him. Although suspicious he was not threatening nor did he express suicidal thoughts. After a period in an observation ward he was admitted to Greystone.

*Previous Personality Disorders.* There was no history of personality disorders prior to the present illness.

*Family History.* The patient's father was an Italian-born shoemaker and bricklayer who drank excessively until 1937, when he stopped abruptly. His mother was also Italian born. She had had a previous marriage and ten children by her first husband, four of whom are still living. The family's economic condition was always marginal. One half-brother had an illness diagnosed as "psychosis with epidemic encephalitis, emotional instability" before his death at Greystone in 1936. Another had surgical treatment as a baby for "water on his spine," and is now largely illiterate. Another was given a medical discharge after a "nervous breakdown" following seven months of Army service. The patient's only brother, six years younger, is deaf in one ear.

*Personal History.* The patient was born in New Jersey in September, 1920, weighing 9 to 10 pounds at birth. He began to walk at fifteen months, to talk at eighteen to twenty-four months. His development was not unusual. When he began school he was slow to learn and did poorly in his school work, though he was conscientious. At the age of fifteen he left the seventh grade to go to work. He worked on a road gang for two years, in a woolen mill for a year and a half, and for a printing company for a shorter time, until he was called up for an Army physical examination. The Army doctor rejected him for "neurosis," and he then worked in a defense plant, and for a pharmaceutical house until nine months before admission. No definite information was obtained about his sexual life, although one of the informants implied that he had had heterosexual experiences.

*Personality.* The personality descriptions given were conflicting in some spheres, but the general picture was one of a conscientious, obedient man who was below average in intelligence and cautious about making friends.

*Hospital Course.* For four months after admission the patient was excited, confused, and subject to delusions and hallucinations. Electroshock and insulin therapy were given at this time and the patient gradually improved with disappearance of the auditory hallucinations and a return of personal neatness. In March, 1945, he was recommended for parole and made a borderline adjustment for five months, after which his old delusions and hallucinations returned, and he was readmitted for electroshock treatment. After treatment he improved for a month, and then deteriorated to his former state. Blocking of speech became more pronounced and he was again restless and subject to delusions and hallucinations. In this condition he was transferred to the project.

*Mental Status.* The patient was retarded and untidy, his buttons open, and his trousers soiled with urine. He was cooperative but could not maintain his attention. He stammered and in addition there were long periods of blocking in his speech. No emotional reaction of any sort was displayed throughout the interview. The content of thought could be obtained only by direct questioning, and the answers were disconnected and illogical: "I accidentally wet my trousers. I had to go to the toilet bad. I feel good." "I was dying. I ain't crazy." "After I got the electric—the machine treatment—" "My mother took me there. I used to be in the other crazy building. I was crying and sorry." He said there was something wrong with his ears, but denied auditory hallucinations, although he was obviously responding to them. His sensorium was cloudy but he was oriented for time and place.

*Follow-Up Notes.* The only change noted on examination on June 25, 1947, was the presence of compulsive rituals in sitting down, lining up his toes perpendicularly, and in similar performances.

The patient had improved somewhat when the August 26, 1947, interview was recorded, in that incontinence was no longer present and he was helpful on the ward, serving other patients and helping to clean the floors. There was less blocking. He was more spontaneous, but he remained preoccupied and spent much time staring into space.

The patient's condition on October 20, 1947, was much as described in the previous interview.

On November 1, 1947, a bilateral prefrontal lobotomy was performed.

On November 3, 1947, the patient responded when pressed for answers, but was quite drowsy. He was correctly oriented and passively cooperative, but there was no change in the mental content.

On November 11, 1947, the patient was now incontinent in respect to urination and sat most of the time slumped over the table with his head in his hands. He did not swallow food, blocking and stammering were increased, and he was once more untidy in his dress.

At the time of interview on January 18, 1948, he remained slovenly, stammering, blocking, and unproductive. No delusions, hallucinations, or paranoid content could be elicited, however, and he was working on the ward and cleaning in the hospital cafeteria. He had no insight into the fact of his illness, and said that he wanted to go home to work "because you have to live."

By March 14, 1948, the patient was doing odd jobs around the hospital, though he was still retarded in speech, thought, and movement. His level of adjustment was a simple one, however, and he had no interests beyond doing his repetitive tasks and listening "to whatever they put on the radio."

On May 7, 1948, it was noted that the patient was very retarded, markedly underproductive, disoriented for time, and was no longer capable of working around the hospital.

**Patient 46.** *Age:* 29. *Sex:* female. *Marital status:* single. *Occupation:* telephone operator. *Religion:* Catholic. *Informants:* parents and sister. *Diagnosis:* schizophrenia, hebephrenic type.

*Presenting Picture.* The patient was admitted to Greystone in February, 1939, at which time she expressed persecutory delusions and was felt to be suicidal.

*Present Illness.* About two months before admission the patient told her family that a man had attempted to rape her but the incident was not confirmed. Subsequently she was apprehensive and markedly suspicious. She expressed many sexual fears. Early in February she became preoccupied with religious topics and she feared her food was being poisoned. Suicidal impulses were suspected and she was admitted to an observation ward.

*Previous Personality Disorders.* There was no history of previous personality disorders.

*Family History.* The patient's father was Italian born, an iceman who lost his business and went on relief for seven years during the depression. Like his wife, who was also Italian born, he was in good health when the patient was admitted. The patient was the fourth of ten children, one of whom was described as "nervous."

*Personal History.* The patient was born in New Jersey in August, 1918. Delivery was not unusual, she began to talk at eleven months and to walk at one year. "Two or three" convulsions were reported at ten months. Menses began when she was fourteen and were usually associated with cramps early in the cycle. The patient started school at six and finished the third year of high school at sixteen. Thereafter she worked for a few months in a garment factory, remained home one year, and then worked as a presser and clerk in a dry cleaning company until her admission. She had few dates but was apparently interested in a local musician whom she saw frequently until he left town in August, 1938. She appeared to be disappointed when he did not write to her as he had promised.

*Personality.* The personality description was of little value except that it indicated the patient was overly sensitive to criticism and easily angered.

*Hospital Course.* On admission the patient was silly and at times assaultive. She heard voices accusing her of "dirty" things. Insulin and metrazol treatments were started six months after admission and, at her family's request, she was placed on parole even though she remained impulsive and evasive. She was discharged from parole at the end of a year and subsequently went to work as a telephone operator until her readmission in 1945. At that time persecutory delusions were noted and she was assaultive and having hallucinations. Over a two-year period she remained seclusive and uncooperative.

*Mental Status.* The patient was overactive, untidy, and uncooperative on the ward. She was reluctant in coming to the interview and refused a chair which was offered. Instead of sitting down she crawled about the floor on her abdomen, tasted dust from the furniture, and made gestures as though indicating an invisible companion. Although she giggled and moved her lips as though speaking, she was markedly unproductive, and responded irrelevantly to only a few questions.

*Follow-Up Notes.* The patient was interviewed on July 4, September 9, and October 20, 1947. She remained mute, unresponsive, and continued to assume postures during this period.

On October 30, 1947, a bilateral prefrontal lobotomy was performed.

Postoperative interviews took place on the following dates: October 31, November 3, and November 7, 1947. During this period the patient's behavior fluctuated markedly from one day to the next and even during a single interview. At times she answered questions relevantly and was cooperative. At other times she was noisy, difficult to manage, and obviously responded to hallucinations. It was felt that she showed a slight improvement in that she was occasionally able to make contact with the examiner but she remained highly labile emotionally and extremely distractible.

On January 17, 1948, she was negativistic, resistive, and mute. It was not possible to make any contact with her.

At the final interview on May 7, 1948, the patient greeted the examiner (not by name) but sat with her head bowed and was mute for the rest of the interview.

### PATIENTS WHO SHOWED LASTING IMPROVEMENT FOLLOWING TOPECTOMY

**Patient 4.** *Age:* 55. *Sex:* male. *Marital status:* single. *Occupation:* porter. *Religion:* Roman Catholic. *Informant:* sister. *Diagnosis:* schizophrenia, paranoid type.

*Presenting Picture.* When admitted to Greystone in September, 1946, the patient appeared anxious, depressed, and retarded and expressed many somatic complaints as well as suicidal intentions.

*Present Illness.* About one year before admission the patient had many complaints which were referred to hemorrhoids and his prostate gland. He was unable to eat, lost 26 pounds in weight in a few months, felt that people were staring at him and that certain people were able to put electric shocks through his head. He lost interest in outside activities, remained at home, and expressed impulses to throw himself into the river and to jump from moving vehicles. After requesting help from the local police he was admitted to Greystone.

*Previous Personality Disorders.* In 1934 he was jailed for alcoholism and, after his release, was fearful of people and markedly hypochondriacal. After a one-month stay in a mental institution he was discharged but he remained seclusive and wept frequently, often expressing suicidal thoughts. This symptomatology was interrupted one year later when he made a marked improvement following the death of his stepfather.

*Family History.* The patient's Italian-born father was described as "strict" and an alcoholic. The father worked in a silk mill until his death (at the age of thirty-seven) following a kidney disorder. The mother was also Italian born and supposedly overindulged the patient. In 1946 she was senile and forgetful. The patient was the oldest of two children, his sister being six years younger. She was married and was described by the interviewer as "obviously neurotic." Five years after the father's death, the patient's mother married an Italian artist who was described as nervous, irritable, and only a fair provider. The patient got along with him but never accepted him as a father.

*Personal History.* Little information was available on the patient's early years following his birth in Massachusetts in September, 1892, beyond the fact that he had a tonsillectomy and much trouble with his ears as a young child. He entered school at the age of six, completed the sixth grade but was a poor student and was often a truant. His reactions to his sister's birth (when he was six), his father's death (when the patient was nine), and his mother's remarriage (when he was fourteen) are not known. After leaving school the patient continued to live at home, working at odd jobs and playing baseball and other sports with boys in the neighborhood. He was uninterested in girls and attended church only occasionally. Nothing is known of his activities from adolescence to the age of forty-two when he began to drink himself into a state of daily intoxication. He stopped work and became abusive to his family at times, leading to his arrest and hospitalization. Following his stepfather's death he became more stable, worked in shipyards, and was drafted into the Army for the last six months of the war. Thereafter he worked at odd jobs until he was hospitalized in 1946.

*Personality.*　The personality description was of limited value. Outstanding were his lifelong hypochondriacal tendencies, the great pride which he took in his clothes, and personal neatness and cleanliness.

*Hospital Course.*　Following his admission in 1946 the patient remained seclusive and retarded. He expressed ruminative and obsessive ideas, chiefly of a sexual nature, although he was able to do minor chores on the ward. Electroshock treatment was begun in October, 1946, and, after twenty-three treatments, he appeared to improve temporarily but soon relapsed and his obsessive thoughts became even more prominent than they were before treatment.

*Mental Status.*　Although the patient appeared depressed and retarded, he was markedly overproductive in his speech. As he discussed his various sexual fears he was agitated and sometimes expressed suicidal ideas. Content was centered about various sexual topics which were repeated at length throughout the interview. Ideas of influence and visual hallucinations were implied in some of his productions: "I think always of a man and a penis. If a man moves his tongue I think something is going to happen, that I can't resist it." "When I was drinking and I went into a men's room, I got a shock in my leg. I see dead people all around the neighborhood. Everyone who has died comes to me. I see faces of dead people on the wall. I always get visions of policemen chasing me, too." At other times he talked of fellatio, masturbation and anal intercourse, incest, menstruation, and suicide, the latter in connection with aiming a revolver. He said he began drinking because of these thoughts and the agitation accompanying them and that his ruminations were made worse by shock treatments. He was well oriented but insight and judgment were poor. No auditory hallucinations were elicited.

*Operation.*　On May 19, 1947, area 46 and a slight amount of area 10 were removed bilaterally.

*Follow-Up Notes.*　On May 26, 1947, one week after operation, the patient offered fewer somatic complaints but the sexual content was unchanged although the emotional intensity was less. This improvement was not stable, however, for on May 28, 1947, he once more offered many somatic complaints in association with considerable affect, although agitation was still less marked than it had been preoperatively.

In the interviews of May 30, and June 11, 1947, no change was found from the findings of the previous examination.

On August 19, 1947, the patient was less agitated and tense, well oriented, more interested in outside activities, and capable of doing more work on the ward. He appeared less depressed than he had been preoperatively although he was still concerned with the same somatic and obsessional material.

On January 17, 1948, approximately seven months after operation, he was sociable, pleasant, and cooperative though still overproductive and rambling. The thought content had not changed but the patient's emotional reactions were less intense than before operation. He stated: "I still get depressed and I still get fears but they are not as bad. I am trying to forget everything but they still come up." He spoke of being threatened (at the age of thirteen) with a gun by a boy's father after he had seriously injured the boy with a frozen snowball (cf. "Mental Status"). He had had sexual intercourse once (with premature ejaculation) and nocturnal emissions at least twice since leaving the hospital. He had not looked for work but was content to live at home and make an occasional dollar doing odd jobs, but this was not the result of any increased lack of foresight and he anticipated finding satisfactory work.

On May 7, 1948, one year after operation, the thought content continued unchanged except that the patient expressed less fear of penises. He continued to react with emotion to his other obsessive ideas. His physical condition had improved and he was working regularly for the sanitation department of his home town.

**Patient 7.** *Age:* 40. *Sex:* male. *Marital status:* married. *Occupation:* machinist. *Religion:* Roman Catholic. *Informant:* wife. *Diagnosis:* schizophrenia, paranoid type.

*Presenting Picture.* The patient was admitted to Greystone in December, 1942, after stabbing himself in the chest. He was agitated, depressed, and had many somatic complaints.

*Present Illness.* Following a herniorrhaphy in September, 1942, the patient complained of insomnia, nervousness, and fatigue. He became depressed and self-critical after his mother's death in October. Thereafter he no longer did his work well, had episodes of weeping, complained of pain in his ear and burning sensations in his rectum. In November he stabbed himself below the clavicle with a pair of clipping shears and, after a short stay in a general hospital, he was admitted to Greystone.

*Previous Personality Disorders.* There was no history of personality disorders prior to the present illness.

*Family History.* The patient's father was described as "a tough Irishman" who was a dock worker until he retired. The Irish-born mother died in the United States in 1942 of cardiac disease. Information on the patient's siblings is sketchy but there were at least seven children, the patient being fourth in the order of birth, the three eldest being girls. A younger brother supposedly recovered after a mental illness which came on while he was with the Army in the Pacific. Four children supposedly died in infancy. According to the informant the patient's siblings had little to do with one another and were always jealous of one another's successes.

*Personal History.* The patient was born in New Jersey about 1907. No details were available on his early life. After attending grammar school he attended a technical school for two years and then worked as a machinist. He had an undescended testicle about which he was quite sensitive and as a child he would not go in swimming with other boys for this reason. At the age of thirty-one he married a woman who died four months later of uremia; two years later he married the informant, a Presbyterian who had been divorced. The marriage was supposedly a happy one but in the course of the patient's hospitalization it became apparent that the wife was a demanding, suspicious woman who considered herself a martyr to the patient's illness. The patient was a moderate drinker and smoker and his sexual activities were characterized only as "normal."

*Personality.* Apparently outstanding were this man's shyness and sensitivity. He made few friends although he was well liked at work. For relaxation he enjoyed reading technical books, dining out, and going to the movies. He supposedly worried over small matters and usually confided in his wife about them.

*Hospital Course.* After admission the patient was fairly cooperative, was well oriented, his memory was good, and no hallucinations were evident. However, he was underproductive, apprehensive, agitated, and depressed. Three weeks after admission he again stabbed himself in the supraclavicular region, this time with a fork. One week later (January, 1943) shock therapy was instituted; in all twelve insulin comas and fifteen electroshock convulsions were induced. The patient improved during treatment. He was paroled in March, 1943, but complaints soon began again, centering about his legs and anus. He lacked confidence at work, began drinking to excess, and returned to the hospital in November where another course of treatment (twenty-three insulin comas, eight electroshock convulsions) produced less improvement. Beginning in July, 1944, he received an additional eleven insulin comas and eighteen electro-shocks followed by improvement which lasted only a few months. (After the later courses of treatment suspiciousness, hypochondriasis, and ideas of reference were prominent.) The patient made other parole visits home, on one occasion (1945-1946) working for a year, but he continued to be threatening and a suicidal risk and was subsequently recommended for this project.

*Mental Status.*   At the time the mental status was appraised the patient's behavior on the ward varied from cooperative helpfulness to agitated and irritable destructive-ness. He was neat in his personal appearance but changed rapidly in his expression of emotion and thought. At times he appeared depressed and self-pitying; at other times suspicious, evasive, and irritable or slightly elated. He sometimes smiled inap-propriately. He was overproductive. His thought content centered chiefly about his somatic preoccupations (largely anal) and the precipitating stress of his mother's death. He also expressed considerable resentment against his wife and discussed his concern about having masturbated. He expressed veiled ideas that doctors somehow influenced and controlled him. His attitude toward the forthcoming operation was that of a potential martyr who was willing to do anything to help others. Orientation was intact and there was no insight into the psychotic nature of his symptoms.

*Operation.*   On May 22, 1947, areas 8, 9, and 10 were removed bilaterally.

*Follow-Up Notes.*   The patient was examined on May 26, June 5, and June 20, 1947. In the first four weeks after operation he spent much time in bed and was generally seclusive, suspicious, tense, and somewhat negativistic. The mental content and affect were not different from those found preoperatively though he did not describe his anal and genital preoccupations in the first postoperative week unless he were asked about them. A facial tic (which was present preoperatively) had not changed. The patient said, "I hope to God I'm not (insane). I was sent here from ——————. They sent me because I was so restless from the pain and they couldn't find any cause for the pain. If I go before the [lunacy] Commission and nothing organic is found, then I'd be in a spot. Why am I being held here? Is it of a mental nature or what?"

On August 25, 1947, the patient was more pleasant and cooperative, less irritable, and he offered fewer somatic complaints. Affect was not always appropriate, however, and he complained of "tension" in his body. He had considerable insight into the psychogenic nature of many symptoms and his judgment was somewhat improved.

On January 18, 1948, nearly eight months after operation, the patient was working at home and living with his wife. He had lost one job but was not concerned about it since other men had been discharged at the same time and he had obtained another job as a machinist without any trouble. He remained somewhat suspicious but his somatic complaints were no longer present and when asked about them he said, "I have no pains. Occasionally there is a little quiver according to the weather. There are no fears that I know of." He had had sexual intercourse infrequently because his wife discouraged it and he had many complaints about her attitude toward him since he felt that she asked too many questions, did not give him enough responsi-bility, and kept their relations uncertain by frequent discussions of divorce. Accord-ing to the patient's wife his adjustment was good on the job and with other members of his family. She insisted that he abused her and had done so for many years but that she would consider a divorce only if he asked for it. The wife herself displayed many overt psychotic symptoms, she was flighty and suspicious, insisting that the room was wired by dictaphones and that this was a plot against her. The patient could not be persuaded that he should not live with her.

On May 7, 1948, one year after operation, the patient was objectively free of tension and his affective responses were appropriate. He was easily distracted by his environment. His attitude toward his wife was carefree; he planned to go back to her even though she had returned him to the hospital a few weeks before, charging that he had assaulted her while drunk. (The facts were never established, but the patient was not intoxicated when admitted and he denied that he had struck his wife.) Despite his defective judgment, it was the examiner's opinion that the patient was capable of a satisfactory adjustment if his wife's handling of him could be controlled and he was returned to parole on May 16, 1948. Almost immediately he found employment as a machinist.

**Patient 8.** *Age:* 29. *Sex:* male. *Marital status:* single. *Occupation:* janitor and short-order cook. *Religion:* Roman Catholic. *Informant:* maternal step-grandmother. *Diagnosis:* schizophrenia, paranoid type.

*Presenting Picture.* The patient first entered Greystone Park in May, 1944, at which time he was anxious, depressed, confused, and expressed vague ideas of persecution as well as hypochondriacal and phobic ideas.

*Present Illness.* Symptoms began in March or April, 1944, while the patient was working in a hotel. He became dissatisfied with his work and complained about it. There were periods when he talked excessively and others when he refused to talk at all. He subsequently went to a resort to look for a new job and five weeks prior to admission telephoned the informant in an excited state, saying that he was having trouble with his landlady and his job, that he was mixed up, dizzy, and could not see things properly. The informant suggested that he contact his father since she was about to leave town and the patient was subsequently admitted to Greystone.

*Previous Personality Disorders.* In 1940 it was noticed by the family that the patient perspired profusely, preferred to be alone, and appeared to be depressed. At times he said he would be better off dead. In February, 1942, he was admitted to a New York City hospital where he had applied for admission after debating suicide by drowning. In March, 1942, he spent a short time in a New York State hospital where his sister arranged his release after a diagnosis of psychoneurosis, anxiety state, had been made.

*Family History.* The patient's English-born father died in 1945 (at the age of fifty-three). A shipyard worker, he was said to have been even-tempered but a heavy drinker and to have paid little attention to his son after the patient's mother died. The mother died in 1927 after childbirth and was described only as a "charming person." Following four stillbirths and a child who died in infancy, a daughter was born, two years older than the patient. She became a nun and a nurse and views her brother's illness as a disgrace, the knowledge of which must be kept from their friends at all costs. A maternal aunt died in Greystone; the diagnosis was "dementia praecox, hebephrenic type." A paternal half-aunt and half-uncle were described as "nervous and emotional." No family history of mental deficiency, suicide, drug addiction, or criminal tendencies was elicited.

*Personal History.* Born in New Jersey in June, 1918, the patient had a supposedly normal delivery, was full term, and weighed 8½ pounds. Walking and talking were not unusual. Convulsions, night terrors, and enuresis were denied. After the usual childhood diseases he had pneumonia at the age of six, requiring surgical treatment for empyema. Later he sustained head and leg injuries when he was struck by an automobile. He began school at the age of six and graduated from grammar school at sixteen. When the patient was nine he went to live with his father, following his mother's death. The informant obtained court custody of the patient two years later because his father had been drinking excessively and the boy was without parental guidance. Masturbation began when the patient was twelve or thirteen and supposedly continued through adulthood. After grammar school he enrolled as a Jesuit novice but failed in his second year. At that time he complained about his stomach and left the seminary to work in a lunchroom. Subsequently he enlisted in the Navy and was discharged three weeks later because of "nervousness." His activities thereafter are not known in detail but during the time before his Greystone admission he was hospitalized at two mental institutions (see above) and had jobs as a caretaker, dyer, and short-order cook between hospitalizations, though his adjustment was borderline throughout.

*Personality.* A good description of personality is not available. It is apparent that the patient received little affection as a child. He was quick-tempered but affectionate and always apologetic. Ambitious and inclined to be selfish, he worried over trivialities and was pessimistic in his outlook on life. He was a poor social mixer and uninterested in women but before his admission read many books dealing with sexual matters. Supposedly there was much bitterness toward his father and his father's family and the informant also believed that he brooded about masturbation.

*Hospital Course.* Following admission to Greystone in May, 1944, he was described as cooperative but depressed and apprehensive. He did not have hallucinations. Shock treatment was begun in November (electric shock and insulin comas) when he was preoccupied and seclusive. After a period of self-assertion and argumentativeness he quieted and in August, 1945, he was paroled to his father. In November, 1945, his father died and thereafter he became excitable and confused and was readmitted to the hospital. Following another course of electric shock he quieted but homosexual tendencies were noted. In the fall of 1946 he was started on electric shock treatment again because of excitement and ideas of reference. In this condition he was transferred to the project.

*Mental Status.* When interviewed in 1947 the patient was eager to discuss his condition but appeared confused and overproductive. At times he ran his words together and the progression of ideas was erratic. Anxiety and apprehension were apparent as well as some depression. His thought content centered about homosexuality and masturbation; he was much disturbed by homosexual thoughts he had had at the seminary and in the hospital and admitted such experiences had actually occurred in the hospital. He said, "Facts of suicide and religion were all mixed up. The fears of masturbation keep coming to my mind. I know it will make me dopey and lead to softening of the brain—paresis." He stated he had had no heterosexual experiences for religious reasons. The sensorium was clear, he was well oriented, and memory was good. He was aware that he was ill but it was felt a delusional system was present. Hallucinations were denied.

*Operation.* On May 16, 1947, the middle frontal gyrus (parts of Brodmann's areas 8, 9, 10, and 46) was removed bilaterally.

*Follow-Up Notes.* On May 26, 1947, a somewhat faraway look was present and mental activity appeared to be slowed. Most apparent was the lack of anxiety even when sexual perversions were discussed. In discussing such matters in detail the patient said that he didn't understand why they once bothered him. That his attitudes had not changed was indicated by his statement that he believed extramarital relations wrong because a girl should be a virgin when she married but he placed emphasis on the fact that he was no longer concerned with sexual matters. No delusional content was elicited.

On May 28, two days later, the patient was irritable and excited, still apparently dazed. He blamed his agitation on the noise made by other patients and offered many complaints about the running of the institution. Two stitches were required to repair his hand which he thrust through the window after complaining of the noise although only one quiet patient was in the room at the time.

On the following day, May 29, his complaints continued though he stressed that he didn't "worry about the sex stuff any more." He showed hostility toward the women whom he said were favored, complained that attendants were always making notes, and said he wanted to "get out of this joint and into a veteran's hospital."

On June 11 the patient was still irritable on the ward and eager to get out of the hospital. He stated that he was tense but this had no relation to sexual thoughts, about which he was not concerned. He stated: "I have inferior feelings about what I'll do when I get out." The sensorium was clear and he was well oriented. Talk of suicide was present.

From June 11 to August 19, 1947, the patient was outgoing, spontaneous, and working on the ward. He was greedy, however, and accumulated small items such as foodstuffs. Something of a "show-off," he manifested an obvious sexual interest in women. "Why did Dr.— ask me if I desired men sexually? Where did he get such ideas? I don't consider it serious because I like women better." "I was masturbating and felt I wasn't worthy of the vows of chastity." "Thoughts that depressed me before operation come back into my mind but they don't bother me now." "Socially I feel different. I'm at ease when I'm around people."

At the time of the interview on January 17, 1948, the patient had developed seizures (ten in all) and was taking phenobarbital. He was working in the doctors' kitchen and in the cow barns. Superficially he was cooperative but labile affect was present in abundance and was readily discharged. No body concern was present but he was extremely resentful. "I feel like blowing up. People ask questions and I don't know how much to tell them." "If I had to come back to this ward I'd commit suicide. I've been in three places and I can't lead a normal life." "Dr.— asked me about my sexual feelings. I feel like telling him to go to hell. I swear frequently." Although he said he was treated satisfactorily and he had none of his old complaints, he was close to rage reaction at all times. He was busy complaining about the difficulties of the present but was not projecting well into the future. No dreams were reported but he said that he masturbated and thought of women. Orientation was good but calculation was slow, as it had always been.

On May 7, 1948, one year after operation, this patient's condition had not changed from that described in January.

**Patient 13.** *Age:* 43. *Sex:* male. *Marital status:* separated. *Occupation:* waiter. *Religion:* Catholic. *Informant:* wife. *Diagnosis:* schizophrenia, paranoid type.

*Presenting Picture.* When committed to Greystone in October, 1944, the patient was described as violent, incoherent, depressed, and suicidal.

*Present Illness.* In 1942 he became concerned about his work, his home, and children. He refused to leave the house in the evening and complained of fatigue and insomnia. There was no marked change until June, 1944, when the manager of the restaurant in which he worked called the informant and said that the patient was confused and unable to add up the customers' checks properly. Suicidal attempts were made in August and September and he became fearful that someone was following him in order to shoot him. He remained depressed during September, expressing feelings of futility. In October he was involved in an accidental fire and was taken to a general hospital for treatment. There he was resistive and had to be restrained and after one week he was transferred to Greystone.

*Previous Personality Disorders.* There was no history of personality disorders prior to the present illness.

*Family History.* The patient's German father was a cabinet-maker, supposedly alive at the time World War II began. He was described as being gentle, good-hearted, and quiet. The patient's mother, who was similarly characterized, died in 1927 of appendicitis. His oldest brother (born in 1900) came to the United States and became a preacher. A second brother lived in the United States until 1937, returning to Germany at that time. The patient was the next child and he was followed by two girls, both of whom remained in Germany where they married. He was especially attached to his younger sister and his mother, although he got along well with all members of the family.

*Personal History.* Information on his early life is lacking except that he was born in Germany in May, 1904, that he became undernourished in the aftermath of World War I and had to be sent to a rehabilitation camp for twelve weeks. There was a history of childhood and adult "epilepsy," including attacks in 1931 and 1933 when he complained of "a funny feeling around the heart" and was "unable to control himself" but did not lose consciousness.

After eight years of schooling he went to sea where he began to learn the trade of ship's carpenter. At the age of sixteen he was struck in the right frontal area with a hammer and thereafter complained intermittently of pain in that location. At nineteen he sustained a head injury in a shipwreck and was taken 80 miles to port in an unconscious state. In 1926 (at the age of twenty-two) he emigrated to the United States where he worked as a waiter for fifteen years before becoming ill. He married the informant in 1930. She was Hungarian born, a Catholic, and one year older than the patient. Seven years later he was converted to her religion. A girl was born in 1940 and another in 1942, at which time he began to develop symptoms.

*Personality.* The description was that of a man slow to grasp ideas but who was devoted to his family (especially his children) and who took his responsibilities very seriously. He was always sensitive, seclusive, and stubborn.

*Hospital Course.* Following commitment in October, 1944, the patient presented a picture of severe depression with a suicidal trend alternating with periods of excitement and persecutory delusions. Insulin and electroshock therapy were started in May, 1945. He became more friendly and cooperative following treatments but continued to be "tense and worried." He was paroled during the summer but in October he was depressed, wept frequently, and had paranoid ideas about his family and neighbors. It was at this time he learned that his wife had been living with another man during his hospitalization and following his discovery, the wife took the children to another state and the patient moved to his brother's home where his condition worsened, necessitating his return to Greystone in July, 1946. Because of his depression and paranoid projections, combined shock therapy was resumed at that time with the result that his ward adjustment improved but he remained tense and apprehensive. He was unable to accept the fact that his wife had divorced him. Depression and persecutory delusions worsened and he was transferred to the project.

*Mental Status.* The patient was neatly dressed and sat rigidly in his chair without changing his position or his facial expression, which was one of sadness. Occasionally he wept. The mood was one of depression but this did not affect his verbal productiveness. The content consisted of rambling protestations that he was loyal to his wife, to the National Guard, and to the country. There were poorly organized delusions that people were talking about him and "torturing" him. There were frequent references to his mother and father. He said, "If mother were here I would be safe." No hallucinations were definitely described. He appeared somewhat confused but was roughly oriented for time and correctly so for person and situation. Judgment was poor and insight faulty.

*Operation.* On May 20, 1947, areas 45, 46, and parts of areas 9 and 10 were removed bilaterally.

*Follow-Up Notes.* On May 26, 1947, the patient still appeared somewhat confused and a question of organic involvement was raised by the examiner. No delusions or persecutory ideas were present. The patient discussed the situation with regard to his wife quite rationally, saying that he would have nothing more to do with her. Depression was no longer present and he interpreted the events before operation as being "like a dream."

On May 30, 1947, his condition was essentially as it had been on the previous interview except that he stated that he would be willing to take his wife back.

On June 17, 1947, he was meek, eager to please, and unsure of himself but in good spirits. His talk was rambling, however, and he frequently referred to his desire to be back with his wife and children and to his experiences at sea and in the National Guard. Various persecutory ideas were brought up during the lengthy examination but these were poorly organized and did not appear to disturb him greatly. Insight into the nature of his illness was slight and there was almost complete amnesia for the period of his psychosis. Judgment within the limited field of the inquiry was satisfactory. Outstanding was the lack of concern and absence of tension which before operation had accompanied the persecutory ideas.

The picture on August 25, 1947, was essentially unchanged from that of June 17, with mild confusion, superficiality, and repetitive discussion of the subject matter brought out at that time.

At the time of interview on January 17, 1948, the patient had been working for four months as a caretaker and furnace man for a Lutheran welfare organization which was satisfied with his services. His condition and content of thought were as previously described and the paranoid nucleus was still present. He stated, however, that his beliefs were not upsetting to him and that he never talked to people other than his physicians about them.

The patient was again interviewed on May 7, 1948. Two seizures had occurred in January and another in April but the patient did not appear to be disturbed by them. He remained slightly euphoric. His thought content continued as before. The church continued to be pleased with his work.

**Patient 21.** *Age:* 42. *Sex:* male. *Marital status:* single. *Occupation:* butcher. *Religion:* Methodist. *Informant:* father. *Diagnosis:* manic-depressive psychosis, depressed phase.

*Presenting Picture.* The patient was committed to Greystone Park Hospital in November, 1926, after threatening members of his family. He was overactive, overtalkative, and boastful.

*Present Illness.* In January, 1926, the patient left his job as a butcher, saying that he was tired and, after six weeks' rest, announced that he was going to make $500 per week in the trucking business and was going to become a star singer in radio. In October he was arrested for vagrancy by the New York police after he had gone to Manhattan to look for a radio job. Returning home, he continued boasting of his abilities which by now extended to all trades. He wandered about the house in the early morning hours, his personal habits became slovenly, and appetite and sleep were poor. He insisted on taking various household appliances apart "in order to keep busy." Later in October he threatened that he would "lick everyone in the house." He was admitted to Greystone after a short stay in jail.

*Previous Personality Disorders.* There was no history of previous personality disorders.

*Family History.* No mental illness is reported in the patient's grandparents or other members of the family. His father was born in New York, was a shipping clerk, and died of cancer of the liver in February, 1947, at the age of sixty-nine. The patient's mother was born in Brooklyn and is still living at the age of sixty-four. Eight children were born after five miscarriages. One boy and one girl are older than the patient and three boys and two girls younger than the patient. All siblings are described as being in good health except for one sister who is said to be "nervous." They are employed as clerks, bookkeepers, typists, etc. The patient was always considered the "odd one" of the family because he was never tractable or amenable to discipline.

*Personal History.* The patient was born in Brooklyn in January, 1905; delivery was normal. He was slow in walking (two years of age), speaking, and learning. Enuresis, convulsions, and nightmares were denied. He entered kindergarten at five but disliked school and was often in trouble. At seven an operation was performed to relieve a strabismus which had been present from birth. At eight he cut his scalp slightly in a fall. His testicles remained undescended at this time and he supposedly suffered from "bladder trouble" as well. Following graduation from elementary school at fourteen he worked as an errand boy and later as office boy for an electrical concern but was discharged because of personal untidiness. He lost a similar job the following year and then worked sporadically as a plumber and butcher. During adolescence his friends were boys considered to be ruffians by the family and the patient spent much time in gambling and attending sporting events, all of which gave rise to friction at home. He spent much time in the company of a married woman to whom the family objected.

*Personality.* The patient was described as being of average intelligence but unable to apply himself to his job. Much given to joking and horseplay, he was slow to anger but sometimes violent when his anger was aroused. At home he resented any restraint, confided sometimes in his mother but never in his father. He was personally popular with a "fast" crowd but was always careless in his personal appearance. He was always talkative and outgoing and apparently advantage was often taken of him in his attempts to gain the approval of his friends. A moderate smoker, he began to drink heavily only six months before he was hospitalized. His father believed that he masturbated throughout his early years but little more was known of his sexual habits.

*Hospital Course.* Following admission in 1926 the patient remained overactive and boastful for a few months. He said he left home because he was abused by his father and that he suffered a "nervous breakdown" because he was unable to control his sexual impulses. Without specific treatment he gradually improved and was paroled to his parents in the spring of 1927. He adjusted satisfactorily thereafter and worked as a butcher until October, 1932, when he was readmitted. Thereafter, except for brief visits, he remained continually hospitalized. At times he was tractable and agreeable, at other times assaultive, noisy, and quarrelsome. His old boastfulness was frequently noted. When seen in surgical consultation for correction of his undescended testicles he was antagonistic and surgery was deferred, as it had been on his first admission. He often described his father as domineering and overbearing and said that he would like to institutionalize his father. Some paranoid coloring was present at times but that was never a leading feature of his illness. Throughout both hospitalizations he was personally clean and tidy. In 1933 he showed signs of depression more frequently and he had intervals of poor concentration and loss of interest, interspersed with periods of overactivity and profanity. On several occasions it was necessary to remove foreign bodies from his ears and he received many minor injuries and abrasions. No definite treatment was ever given but he received hydrotherapy and colonic irrigations. Although no definite cycle was established, depression became more constant and in this condition, with many somatic complaints, he was transferred to the project. At one period, about two years before the project began, he rapidly gained almost 100 pounds in weight.

*Mental Status.* The patient appeared depressed and psychomotor activity was reduced. Belching occurred frequently throughout the interview and he complained of insomnia, constipation, and pains in the lower back. Affect was appropriate to the depressive and hypochondriacal content. Otherwise thought content was nonspecific; he talked of "memories of Sunday school when I was young" and events which had taken place in Greystone during his stay at the hospital. Sensorium was clear; he was well oriented and realized that he was depressed. No paranoid content could be found.

*Operation.* On May 20, 1947, Brodmann's area 10 was removed bilaterally with slight infringement on area 46.

*Follow-Up Notes.* On May 26, 1947, the patient appeared more depressed than before operation, slept excessively, and was incontinent. He complained of lack of energy and perseverated on simple sentences. There was almost no spontaneous speech.

On May 29, there was little change from the previous note except that he spontaneously got out of bed and, in a dazed, perplexed way, staggered into the next room. He willingly submitted to being led back to bed.

On June 5, he no longer appeared depressed and subjectively felt that his depression had lifted. He was working about the ward, cooperative, occasionally joking. Somatic complaints were still present, however, and judgment was only fair, although he was well oriented and had some insight into the nature of his illness.

On August 25, three months after operation, the patient was making a good adjustment though he occasionally was petulant and complaining. Somatic complaints were no longer prominent. He said, "I no longer dwell on the past. Other patients here still think of their fears and emotions. Those thoughts don't bother me any more." "I feel very good now. I hope I don't get that depressed feeling again. I want to get back to work." He stated that before his hospitalization he had had intercourse once or twice a week ("when I had money") but now, although he has an occasional wet dream, he has less sexual urge. He added: "Perhaps that is due to age."

On January 17, 1948, seven months after operation, the patient was working as a laboratory handyman and doing his job well. His social life was limited to an occasional movie and card games with his family. He had little interest in women though he mentioned the possibility that he might marry an early sweetheart "if she is still single." His sleep and appetite were good. He had no difficulty subjectively or objectively in concentrating and no memory impairment. He stated: "When I read, I know what I'm reading and I grasp it, but the whole picture isn't there," but was unable to elaborate further. He felt that the operation had "knocked the depression out" of him. Dreams still occurred. (In one he dreamed of being strangled and woke screaming. His only association was a similar incident which occurred while he was a patient.) He stated that he still wept in the movies when the action was sad. Because of bickering at home, particularly with his sisters, he was considering moving out and living alone in New York. However, he was unsure of taking such a step, saying that he was rather frightened because "you can't walk out of a place like this (Greystone) where you have been confined for fifteen years and then forget about it in a day. Nobody can do that, no matter who he is." In his everyday contacts he was inclined to be garrulous and unable to take a mild hint (for example, that the interview was to be terminated). He was easily hurt by small slights. Some somatic preoccupations were still present but were described only if they were specifically asked for (fatigue, clicking sounds in the ears). A complaint of frequency was found to have an organic basis in prostatic obstruction; the patient reacted to this news with considerable annoyance, saying, "I kept telling them there was something wrong but they said it was all in my head." That some insight into dynamics was present is indicated by his statement that he became ill because he was "brought up to be too conscientious; you can't help the way your family brings you up." At another time he described his father as a domineering man who was unloved in the family and maintained his position only by fear.

On May 8, 1948, the patient's behavior had not changed from that described in January, 1948. He continued to be a conscientious and imaginative worker but sensitive to personal criticism.

**Patient 22.** *Age:* 50. *Sex:* male. *Marital status:* married. *Occupation:* weaver. *Religion:* Catholic. *Informants:* wife and sister. *Diagnosis:* schizophrenia, paranoid type.

*Presenting Picture.* On admission to Greystone in February, 1944, the patient was under the influence of sedatives and was confused, noisy, and resistive.

*Present Illness.* In 1940 he began to drink to excess and to associate with "bad company." In July, 1942, he was arrested in a tavern after making derogatory remarks about the United States Government and was investigated by the F.B.I. Following his release from jail he was often fearful that F.B.I. agents were watching him and often remarked that he "wanted to be free again." There was no worsening of his condition until a few weeks before admission when he lost interest in his surroundings, had periods of weeping and laughing, and expressed suicidal thoughts. Simultaneously he interpreted newspaper stories as being printed expressly to frighten him; he feared that everyone was against him and that someone was trying to harm him at night. He got into arguments and fights at work and believed his food was being poisoned. After a few days in an observation ward he was admitted to Greystone.

*Previous Personality Disorders.* There was no history of previous personality disorders.

*Family History.* Both parents were Austrian born. The patient's father was described as a "good-natured" man who worked as a part-time gas-station attendant. His mother had had asthma, bronchitis, and eczema of the hand for many years and was described as "irritable." The patient was the oldest of three children, a sister being three years younger and a brother six years younger. He feared his father, who supposedly had disciplined him strictly as a child while his mother "spoiled" him.

He got along well with his sister, but there was no information on his relationship with his brother.

*Personal History.*  The patient was born in Austria in February, 1897. He was a normal, full-term baby, and walked and talked "at an early age." As a child he lived for some time with his paternal grandmother and slept in the same room with her. After he became ill he often remarked that his grandmother was the only one who ever "understood" him.

He graduated from public school at fourteen and became a printer's apprentice, but gave this up after he developed "lead poisoning." In 1913 he came to the United States where he learned weaving, living in various towns in the Northeast until he came to New Jersey. In 1915 he struck his head against a swimming pool while diving and complained of severe headaches for two weeks thereafter, but did not seek medical attention. His medical history was not otherwise remarkable, except that at times he developed a dermatosis of one leg which could be controlled by diet. He occasionally became intoxicated and at such times became argumentative with strangers, but intoxication was never a problem to his family. In 1926 he married an Austrian woman five years his junior. She was pregnant at the time of their marriage, and this resulted in the birth of a girl who is now married and a clerical worker. A son was born in 1930. Both children and the patient's wife are in good health, except that the wife has occasional "migraine" attacks. When first married, the patient liked to "have a good time" while his wife was more interested in her home. In later years he liked to read books and listen to the radio at home and his wife found him affectionate and easy to get along with. He sought intercourse about once weekly.

*Personality.*  The personality description was that of an industrious man who did not take his responsibilities heavily. He was uncritically generous with money and sensitive to the criticisms and opinions of others. He did not make friends easily and many people "did not understand him."

*Hospital Course.*  On admission in February, 1944, the patient was noisy and resistive. He expressed pro-Nazi and paranoid ideas. During the first few months he broke windows, saying, "The actors made me do it." He feared that he was being poisoned and spied upon, and interpreted radio programs as somehow applying to him. In June he was started on insulin shock treatment and in a few weeks he became more friendly and cooperative, sleep and appetite improved, and his persecutory delusions disappeared and were interpreted as "stuff that came from (his) head." He was paroled in September, 1944, and discharged one year later. His adjustment was good until August, 1946, when he became somewhat agitated and thereafter there was a gradual return of his old paranoid material with considerable agitation. In November, 1946, he was readmitted, and in the spring of 1947 he was transferred to the project.

*Mental Status.*  At the time of examination this patient was assaultive and hostile toward other patients. At times he was destructive on the ward and often hurled loose objects. He was suspicious of the physician who examined him, spitting in his face and insisting that he was not a doctor. There was an abundance of hostile affect which was generally appropriate to his thought content, and he also appeared to be mildly depressed. He was overproductive and expressed many persecutory delusions, though no hallucinations could be elicited. Although he said that he was being persecuted and that the doctors were trying to harm him, he would not elaborate on his statements, and attempts to press him for information led only to threats against the physician. There was no insight into the fact of his illness, but his sensorium was clear and his orientation good.

*Operation.*  On May 19, 1947, areas 9, 10, and 46 were removed bilaterally.

*Follow-Up Notes.*  On May 26, 1947, one week after operation, it was noted that no depression was apparent, but the patient still remained assaultive at times, and he continued to be resistive, suspicious, and to have delusions.

On May 30, 1947, his persecutory trend was less marked, he cooperated for a neurologic examination, and stated that he felt "happier." However, his day-to-day behavior on the ward fluctuated markedly; at times he was uncooperative and insulting.

On June 2, 1947, he was extremely uncooperative, spitting toward the examiner and refusing examination.

On June 12, 1947, the picture was unusual in that irritability was marked and associated with distractability and overtalkativeness. The patient stated: "Nobody believes what is said. Who is boss in this hospital? Tell me and I will talk with him as long as he likes! He can examine me, he can take my clothing off—everything! He can even play with this little thing here (he points to his penis). I'm not ashamed of my body. He can put a scar on a man's head. Someone gave permission for this. I don't know what it's all about."

The patient was again interviewed on August 26, 1947. After a period of improvement during which he was on ground parole, the patient went home on visit August 3, 1947, but when he suggested retiring at 7:30 p.m. his wife objected and said that he should stay up later, leading to an argument. He was returned to the hospital less than twenty-four hours after his visit had begun. At the time of this interview he was cooperative and helpful on the ward and pleasant with the examiner. The persecutory trends noted on previous examinations were not present, although he expressed aggravation with his wife, who had not told him of his mother's death until he went home, and who treated him as a person stigmatized by his illness. Affective responses were appropriate to the situation.

On January 17, 1948, he was still on ground parole, delusions were not present, but he appeared dejected and his mood was one of moderate depression. He gave a garbled story of picayune arguments with his wife, which led to his return to the hospital, and led into an account of his past life. Orientation and memory were intact, and he recognized his earlier behavior was abnormal, although he attributed his behavior to the situations which he had encountered.

On May 7, 1948, the patient was on ground parole and presented no problem to the hospital. He was well oriented, his memory was good, and he was cooperative. The confused and rambling speech noted on the previous interview was no longer present. Affective responses and the mental content were not unusual, although the former were rather superficial. He was, however, unable to consider any course of action which would not include a return to his wife. His wife would not permit his family to remove the patient and this patient's parole was thus blocked by a woman whom the staff doctors considered "extremely unstable."

On June 27, 1948, the patient's improvement continued and he was paroled from the hospital.

**Patient 25.** *Age:* 58. *Sex:* male. *Marital status:* married. *Occupation:* newspaper mailer. *Religion:* Protestant. *Informants:* youngest brother, woman friend. *Diagnosis:* involutional psychosis, depressed type; possible organic brain disease.

*Presenting Picture.* In August, 1945, the patient was transferred to Greystone from a general hospital. He was agitated, depressed, and suicidal.

*Present Illness.* Two months before admission the patient began to complain of insomnia and fatigue. Subsequently he became restless and fearful that he might have heart disease. He consulted several physicians who reassured him about his physical condition. One month before admission his fears worsened and depression became apparent. One week before admission he wept occasionally, threatened suicide, and was fearful that he was going to die.

*Previous Personality Disorders.* There was no history of previous personality disorders.

*Family History.* The patient's father was an Irish-born leather worker who was described as "the boss" of the family but good natured and hard working. The patient's mother was also Irish born. She had a pleasant disposition and was a good homemaker. She died at the age of sixty-eight of a "stroke" and her husband died at forty-eight of unknown causes. There were nine children, all boys, of whom the patient was the next youngest. One brother was said to drink to excess, though he had a good work record as a truck driver. One died at twenty-three (possibly tuberculosis), another at forty of "dropsy," and another at fifty-eight of unknown causes. Little could be learned of the relationship between the brothers, and apparently they saw one another infrequently in later life.

*Personal History.* The exact date of the patient's birth is not known (about 1889), and no information was available on his early development. He went as far as the seventh grade, then became a truck driver and, as a young man, moved to Boston where he married. His wife was of Irish extraction and a few years his junior. After two months he returned to New Jersey and his wife refused to accompany him. Subsequently he lost all contact with her and did not contribute to her support, although he made no attempt to secure a legal separation. For fifteen years before his illness he worked as a newspaper mailer, a job which he "hated," although he made no attempt to change jobs. He had few affairs with women, but for twenty years he associated steadily with the co-informant with whom he had intercourse about once a year. Until the onset of his illness he was a moderate smoker and drank very infrequently.

*Personality.* He was always a retiring, quiet, conscientious man who was particularly solicitous of his mother. He was never well informed on what was going on in the world and his friends were similarly dull and unsociable. His chief recreation was attending movies. He appeared to be dependent on the co-informant, whom he admired because she was more aggressive than he.

*Hospital Course.* Following his admission in August, 1945, the patient was agitated, depressed, and constantly expressed fears of dying. Beginning in November, 1945, he received electroshock treatment and thereafter was friendly and took part in hospital activities. His depression lifted. He was paroled in February, 1946, adjusting well until July, 1946, when he again became depressed and fearful. He fractured his scapula in a fall (suicide attempt?) and during his second admission restraint was frequently necessary because of his marked agitation. In this condition he was transferred to the project.

*Mental Status.* The patient's facial expression was dramatically wide-eyed. He was overactive, tense, and impulsive in his movements. He paced excitedly throughout the interview. There was a marked pressure of speech, which was at times almost explosive. He was circumstantial, rambling, and repetitious, and the content was confined to self-deprecatory ideas and somatic delusions, all delivered with intense feeling directed toward himself: "Doc, I have a dropped stomach. I went to the toilet four times in the last ten months. I am a wild man. Look at them arms. They just aren't there. I'm not bound for this earth. This Sunday I won't be here. I'll be dead." He was obviously depressed, though he did not describe his mood as such. He referred to changes or absence of various organs, including stomach, bowels, eyes, jaw, nose, and arms, and expressed ideas of unworthiness. Sensorium was clear and he was correctly oriented, but judgment was grossly inadequate.

*Operation.* On May 26, 1947, areas 8, 9, and 46 and part of 10 were removed bilaterally.

*Follow-Up Notes.* On the interviews of May 28, and May 30, 1947, the patient was restless, still in bed, and seldom spoke spontaneously. When questioned he responded with the same material he had shown preoperatively, though with less affect.

On June 5, 1947, he complained of lack of energy. His stream of mental activity was slow. No evidence of agitation was present, but he was forgetful and frequently repeated himself.

During the interview of June 25, 1947, the patient had a rather vacuous appearance and was relaxed. He was no longer agitated, no longer a management problem, and was sleeping well, but he remained garrulous. Thought content was unchanged, but there was a shift in emphasis and the previous delusions were less fixed or had disappeared entirely. Much of his talk involved rambling discourses into the past, i.e. incidents involving his mother, or brothers. He was disoriented for time, but not for place; he was unable to remember the names of attendants and physicians who saw him regularly. Judgment remained poor.

On August 26, 1947, no delusions could be elicited. The patient was sociable, pleasant, and relaxed. Outstanding, however, was his tendency to ramble into events of the past and his poor memory, particularly for recent events, which was interpreted as indicative of organic deterioration which probably preceded operation.

On January 17, 1948, he had returned to his old job of newspaper mailer and was making an adequate social adjustment in spite of his rambling thought and memory defect which had not changed. His woman friend was interviewed at this time; she stated that he had spontaneously gotten his old job back, that he was saving money, and was socially exactly as he was before becoming ill. His sexual interests had not changed. She noted no new defects in memory or intelligence, attributing his poor performance to his lack of education.

On May 8, 1948, one year after operation, the patient was making a good work adjustment. His memory had improved since January and rambling accounts of events in the remote past were less frequent.

**Patient 36.** *Age:* 53. *Sex:* female. *Marital status:* separated. *Occupation:* housewife. *Religion:* Protestant. *Informants:* son, male friend. *Diagnosis:* schizophrenia, paranoid type.

*Presenting Picture.* The patient was transferred to Greystone in April, 1945, from an observation ward when she was described as confused and subject to delusions and hallucinations.

*Present Illness.* About six months before admission the patient's husband requested a divorce, upsetting the patient considerably. Sometime after this encounter she began to think people were following her, that voices were calling her names and saying that her house was dirty. She believed her food was being poisoned and that she was being watched as she wrote to her son. As her agitation increased she lost weight, became unmanageable, and was admitted to the observation ward of a hospital.

*Previous Personality Disorders.* No personality disorders were noted prior to the present illness.

*Family History.* The patient's parents were both Pennsylvania born, of German farmers. Both died natural deaths about 1937 and both were described as "easy going, friendly farmers." The patient was the second of three girls in a family of five children. Nothing is known about the other siblings except that one boy remained on the farm and received little education. The patient always spoke affectionately of her parents in later years.

*Personal History.* The patient was born in Pennsylvania in October, 1894; she lived in the town of her birth until eighteen when she moved to New Jersey. Nothing was known of her early development. She left school while in the sixth grade in order to work on the farm. In 1914 she married a man four years her senior who is now employed by the telephone company. A son was born in 1918 and in 1927 the patient separated from her husband, because of his infidelity and alcoholism. She supposedly refused a divorce for fear that she would lose alimony payments. The patient supported her son by working in various factories. She was a hard worker who managed her affairs economically. Three years before admission she had a hysterectomy; there was also a history of one induced abortion. There was no history of sexual relations after the patient left her husband, although the patient herself alluded to such incidents.

*Personality.* The patient was described as a trusting, sociable woman who was well liked by her neighbors. Her attachment to her son was marked, however, and she resented any girls in whom he was interested although she seemed to accept his marriage easily.

*Hospital Course.* On admission the patient expressed persecutory ideas. Olfactory as well as auditory hallucinations were present. She complained of electric currents and said her body was being tampered with. Without obvious improvement she was paroled in July, 1945, remaining at home until December of that year although she continued to have hallucinations, to express delusions, and to be mildly depressed. On her return in December electroshock treatment was given followed by general quieting. She was paroled in February, 1946, but returned in June with the same content as described previously. Agitation was also remarked upon. Again she quieted spontaneously in a short time but soon after parole she was returned to the hospital. After December, 1946, her condition remained unchanged. Ambulatory shock treatments were occasionally necessary because of agitation.

*Mental Status.* On the ward the patient was mildly agitated, insomniac, and appeared perplexed. The mood was one of mild depression. She displayed considerable (but not entirely appropriate) affect attached to self-deprecation and paranoid ideas. Voices were described which were accusatory and informed her that her son was also a patient and in danger of mutilation. She made frequent references to disease of her body such as cancer, and genital pus and blood. Her delusional system was loosely organized, involving a plot and vague representations of persons unknown. It was accompanied by self-deprecation concerning her past. The sensorium was clear.

*Operation.* On June 3, 1947, areas 10, 11, 45, 46, and 47 were removed bilaterally.

*Follow-Up Notes.* On June 4, 1947, one day after operation, the patient was responsive but the mental content had not changed.

On July 4, 1947, agitation was diminished and affective responses were not unusual. Delusions were no longer present. Somatic complaints were discussed logically. The patient poured forth resentment against several of her (female) neighbors but discussed her husband's behavior with greater restraint than on previous occasions. Her appetite was now good, she was correctly oriented, and judgment was much improved.

On September 9, 1947, the changes described on the previous note were not maintained. The patient was preoccupied, seclusive, and emotionally flattened. She described hallucinations once more and stated that her son was being held prisoner across the street. Somatic delusions had not reappeared though she continued to express numerous somatic preoccupations.

In interviews made on October 30, 1947, January 17, 1948, and May 7, 1948, the patient was no longer found to be seclusive or agitated but her delusional and hallucinatory material was present in full force on each occasion, including a return of somatic delusions. She was tried unsuccessfully on a home visit at the beginning of this period. Affect during this time was well modulated and appropriate to the thought content and the patient was no longer a problem in management.

**Patient 49.** *Age:* 39. *Sex:* female. *Marital status:* single. *Occupation:* none. *Religion:* Protestant. *Informants:* mother, sister. *Diagnosis:* schizophrenia, paranoid type.

*Presenting Picture.* The patient was admitted to Greystone in July, 1933, when she became suspicious and assaultive.

*Present Illness.* In June, 1933, the patient began to weep and became excited, saying that her old sickness had returned. She walked aimlessly, worked compulsively about the house, and became profane. Her appetite and weight were diminished. She accused her family of talking about her and tried to strike her sister. On a physician's advice it was decided to send her to a hospital from which she was transferred to Greystone a day later.

*Previous Personality Disorders.* This patient first became ill in 1924 when she was "melancholy" for a short time and, after a short remission, became excitable and had to be removed from school. A febrile illness in 1925 was accompanied by a delirium lasting two or three weeks. In 1926 she ran away from home during an excited period. In 1928 she was again ill. In 1930-31 she was hospitalized in a Swiss sanitarium where she made a spontaneous recovery, returning then to the United States. At the end of six months she again became ill and for the following six months she was once more a patient in Switzerland.

*Family History.* The patient's father was Swiss born. He was an ineffectual man who came to the United States after he lost his money. The mother was also Swiss and the more dynamic figure in the family. The patient was the third of four children, one sister being younger. The patient received more attention as a child than did her siblings since she was frequently ill. Two maternal cousins and a paternal great-aunt were hospitalized for mental illnesses.

*Personal History.* The patient was born in Switzerland in 1908. Her birth and early development were not unusual. As a child she had scarlet fever, diphtheria, several operations on her throat, and was anemic. Menses began when she was twelve to thirteen years of age and were always regular and without pain. She started school at six and finished the second year of high school, when her family took her out of school because the patient had developed "mental symptoms" on three occasions when she was about to start a new term. She was never able to work but took courses in sewing, cooking, and porcelain painting. She never showed any interest in men and was excessively modest.

*Personality.* The patient was overly critical of herself and others—a perfectionist who tended to be preoccupied and shy. She was agreeable when with people but did not go out of her way to make friends, she insisted that things had to be just right, and fretted more than other people in the house. She definitely wanted the approval of others. There was always a childlike dependence upon her sister and other members of the family.

*Hospital Course.* Upon admission, the patient alternated between excitement and retardation but soon managed to make a fair adjustment on the ward. After a year she was paroled even though delusional, at the request of her mother. Adjustment at home was marginal for six months, after which she became very excited and was actively subject to hallucinations so that return to the hospital was necessary. During the next two years hallucinations and excitement gradually disappeared although delusions remained. The patient was again paroled for nine months. Adjustment at home was barely marginal. She returned to the hospital, again excited and having hallucinations. The excitement lessened and at times she was quite cooperative, although delusions and hallucinations persisted. Six and a half years elapsed following the last parole before she was transferred to the project. She received no shock treatment.

*Mental Status.* When seen in April, 1947, the patient was suspicious and preoccupied but neatly dressed. She was reluctant to answer questions but spontaneously was quite productive. Affect was appropriate to the persecutory delusions in that she spoke hatefully and appeared angry. Content of speech reflected persecutory delusions and an attitude of martyrdom. She admitted past hallucinations but denied them at this time. She described herself as being confused. Some insight was indicated in the remark. "I hate it here, but I get sick as soon as I go outside; my memory goes bad." She felt people used her by driving her to work and also that she had been doped and used as a prostitute by doctors in the hospital. Orientation was good; sensorium clear; insight was limited—she realized that the voices she heard were imaginary but delusions were fixed.

After the first patients were operated upon, the patient became very disturbed and auditory hallucinations returned and persisted through the period of operation.

*Operation.* On June 5, 1947, area 10 and parts of areas 11 and 46 were removed bilaterally.

*Follow-Up Notes.* For two weeks following operation the patient was quiet and cooperative although delusions persisted. On the interview of July 4, 1947, she was again agitated and persecutory ideas were expressed.

On September 9, 1947, she was greatly improved, cooperative, and cheerful. She took an active part in ward activities and had ground parole. There was considerable insight into her persecutory delusions. She described her illness as something past, adding, "I'm looking forward to going home."

On January 17, 1948, the patient had resided at home for four months and was making a good adjustment; there was no irritability or insomnia. She had gained considerable weight. She looked a little apprehensive and affect was somewhat flattened. She complained of lacking confidence and said that her memory was not too good. There was insight in that she recognized past ideas as delusional. Planning ability was unimpaired. She remembered a novel she had read the week before. Some doubts were expressed about the permanence of her cure "because there were so many illnesses in the past." She planned to take a job for the first time in her life. The next week she began work as a maid in the home of one of us.

At the beginning she was not efficient on the job, often appeared preoccupied, and showed little initiative. At all times, however, she was pleasant and conscientious. She liked the children. Her cooking during the first two weeks was not good in that she did not time things well. In this respect she rapidly improved. She socialized poorly in the community and neighbors regarded her as a rather ineffective, shy person. The patient said she was self-conscious over having spent so much time in mental institutions. No defects in planning were apparent. She enjoyed her day off; she spent it at the movies or went shopping with her sister, on whom she continued to be very dependent. She was very interested in current events; listened to the radio, read the newspapers, and quite rationally discussed the international crisis. Her efficiency improved considerably during the four months she worked on this job.

Just one year following operation she suffered a partial, temporary relapse. One of the children sustained a concussion which upset her considerably. She became frightened, developed insomnia which lasted only two nights, expressed the desire to be closer to her sister, and soon lost her appetite. When seen during the one-year examinations, she was irritable and tense. She did express some mild persecutory ideas making statements such as: "I've been cheated." When interviewed she showed some insight but was quite depressed. This episode lasted about two weeks and was followed by prompt remission. She then secured another job, again as a domestic, but with a family who had fewer children and where there was less responsibility.

### PATIENTS WHO SHOWED TEMPORARY IMPROVEMENT FOLLOWING TOPECTOMY

**Patient 3.** *Age:* 61. *Sex:* male. *Marital status:* married. *Occupation:* accountant. *Religion:* Protestant. *Informant:* wife. *Diagnosis:* involutional psychosis, mixed.

*Presenting Picture.* The patient was admitted to Greystone in July, 1940, when he was delusional, agitated, depressed, and threatening suicide.

*Present Illness.* In 1936 he began to assume unnecessary responsibility for the firm which employed him and had short periods of depression in which he worried about business conditions. At such times he was heard sobbing in the bathroom; he reacted with weeping to the mildest personal suggestion. In 1938 he began to sleep poorly though his appetite was not affected. He began to scold and swear at his wife and was generally irritable. He became unusually religious and also threatened suicide— without attempting to carry out his threats. Early in 1939 he gave up his job and soon thereafter overactivity and excitement became more prominent in the picture. He insisted he was going to write a lucrative story for the stage and began spending a great deal of money. In April, 1940, he registered at an expensive New York hotel and was arrested in the early morning hours while running nude around the halls. Before his admission to Greystone he thought people were watching him and believed he was going to operate and deliver a baby. He told his wife that he would have to kill her, his children, and grandchildren though he regretted doing it and he felt that the hospital was a jail to which he was permanently confined for having committed a crime.

*Previous Personality Disorders.* There were no personality disorders prior to the present illness.

*Family History.* The grandparents were all United States born, of Scottish and English ancestry. The maternal grandmother became mentally ill after her husband died a prisoner in the Civil War. The father was a sociable, even-tempered calico worker who died of a heart attack in 1936, at the age of eighty-one. The mother, five years younger, was quiet and seclusive and supposedly was psychotic before and after the patient's birth. She was overprotective toward the patient and her accidental death in 1928 was a great blow to the patient. One sister, seven years older than the patient, died in a mental institution in 1939 following enucleation of an eye.

*Personal History.* No details were available on the patient's early development following his birth in New Jersey in 1886. He talked little until he began school at the age of six. After completing the first year of high school he went to business school for one year and then took a job as clerk in a dye factory, eventually working up to the position of accountant and treasurer of the company. At twenty-two he was seriously ill with typhoid fever and at thirty-six underwent an operation for hemorrhoids. He maintained a close relationship with his family, was a moderate drinker but a heavy smoker. He attended church regularly. At the age of twenty-four he married a pleasant and understanding woman one and one-half years his junior. Two children were born, both well adjusted, successful, and happily married at the present time. The patient's economic condition was always good though he suffered financial losses from time to time.

*Personality.* Outstanding in the pre-illness picture was the man's meticulousness, perfectionism, and conscientiousness. He was unaggressive though popular with other people and "took his job much too seriously."

*Hospital Course.* Following his admission in July, 1940, this patient was suspicious and antagonistic, self-deprecatory, and expressed an attitude of hopelessness. In August, shock treatment (sixteen insulin comas and eleven metrazol convulsions) was started but he became confused and incoherent so treatment was discontinued. Subsequently his mood was one of despair. He asked when his ears were to be cut off. In November he was given nine metrazol convulsions without much effect and he continued to have ideas of reference and to believe that he was responsible for the world's troubles. Although he made occasional home visits and was able to work in the hospital in a minor clerical capacity there was no significant improvement in subsequent years and he was therefore recommended for this project.

*Mental Status.* The patient showed psychomotor retardation. His facial expression was one of sadness and suspicion. Affect was often inappropriate to the content of speech, however, and he smiled as he talked of his guilt and the sorrow he had caused the world. He complained of tightness across the head, visual difficulties, and of mathematical problems which were constantly on his mind. He stated: "I have always been given more than I gave. My parents always did more for me than I deserved. My father was not severe enough with me, he was too good to me." Auditory hallucinations were described in the form of dreamlike voices but no definite content was ascribed to them and they were not connected with the patient's marked feelings of guilt. Suspiciousness was marked and on one occasion he said that "people here are watched through television." Memory and orientation were not affected but judgment was impaired.

*Operation.* On May 15, 1947, the caudal part of area 9, part of area 8, and part of area 6 were removed bilaterally.

*Follow-Up Notes.* On May 16, 1947, the day after operation, the patient was alert, somewhat restless, spontaneous, and his memory was good. He was well oriented. He knew that he had been operated on the day before and was able to give many details about his illness. When asked if he felt he had sinned, he chuckled and answered that it was a part of his illness. He expressed confidence in his own abilities and a desire to return to work.

On May 26, 1947, mild compulsive behavior was noticed. The patient appeared somewhat slower and less confident than he was immediately after operation.

During the interview of June 11, 1947, it was apparent that the patient had once again become depressed and suspicious. He was apathetic and ideas that he was being observed by television were once more present. Guilt feelings were again prominent but there were no accusatory voices at this time.

On August 19, 1947, the picture had not changed except for the presence of auditory hallucinations. The patient was not as depressed as he was preoperatively but it was apparent that he had not maintained the level of improvement which was achieved immediately after operation.

On January 17, 1948, seven months after operation, the patient was living at home, spending his time doing various household tasks. He was somewhat brighter, friendly, and more spontaneous than he was on previous occasions; paranoid trends and hallucinations were no longer present and his depression was not marked. However, he complained that he lacked confidence, was unable to look for work because he did not want to admit his illness, and he felt that he lacked his pre-illness drive. There was no sexual urge. His wife was much encouraged by the absence of periods of excitement and weeping which had characterized his behavior before he was hospitalized but stressed his lack of confidence, his oversensitivity to personal criticism, and his failure to show signs of affection (such as kissing her before retiring). She pointed out, however, that his memory for figures was still excellent, that he spontaneously offered to do many jobs around the house, and that he participated with enthusiasm on festive occasions such as Christmas.

In March, the depression became more intense and some confusion developed, necessitating return to the hospital.

The one-year follow-up interview (May 7, 1948) found the patient retarded and somewhat depressed but paranoid features were less evident. He continued to have little drive to work and no sexual interest, although he was well read on current affairs and his intellectual performance was not impaired.

**Patient 27.** *Age:* 34. *Sex:* male. *Marital status:* single. *Occupation:* none. *Religion:* Hebrew. *Informants:* father, mother, sister, physician. *Diagnosis:* schizophrenia, hebephrenic type.

*Presenting Picture.* When admitted to Greystone in July, 1939, the patient was confused, excited, delusional, and hallucinating.

*Present Illness.* About four years before admission the patient became irritable, somewhat suspicious, and refused to work because it was "beneath him." During the year preceding admission his suspiciousness increased and he became "depressed." During this period he was married for a short time, but an annulment was secured and he later said that the annulment papers were made out to prove that he was mentally ill. For two months before he entered the hospital he slept and ate poorly, and expressed ideas of reference. He read many medical books and discussed sex, particularly homosexuality, at some length. Shortly before admission he was jailed for disorderly conduct. When he was taken to the family physician he refused to talk, saying that a dictaphone was hidden in the office, and he was referred to another physician for admission to Greystone.

*Previous Personality Disorders.* No personality disorders were noted prior to the present illness.

*Family History.* The patient's father was a Polish-born tailor who was forty-nine years old at the time of the patient's admission and suffered diabetes. The patient's mother was ten years older than his father; she also was Polish. The patient was the second of five children. The oldest sister (married to a carpenter) and her husband were both under treatment for syphilis at the time of the patient's admission. All the other children were unmarried. Relationships among the parents and siblings were supposedly harmonious.

*Personal History.* The patient was born in New Jersey in October, 1913; he was a full-term, normal baby, weighing 10 pounds at birth. He walked when a year and a half old and talked at two years. In addition to the usual childhood diseases there was a history of scarlet fever at the age of eight. At five years of age he began school, where he was an excellent student, graduating from high school at sixteen, and subsequently attending normal school for a year and a half before he decided against a teaching career. Subsequently he enrolled in a college journalism course, then worked as a shipping clerk, a grocery store clerk, and tailor's helper. Abruptly in 1938 he married a Jewish girl whom he had been out with only a few times. The couple lived together week ends for two months, but the bride secured an annulment one week before the patient's admission because he was impotent. His family stated that he had often brooded about "being thrown over by girls," and during his infrequent visits to prostitutes he had never had intercourse, being satisfied merely to lie on the bed with the girl.

*Personality.*   The patient was described as stubborn, sensitive to criticism, and as having a poor sense of humor, although he was intelligent and had a good memory. He enjoyed reading, particularly medical and legal books.

*Hospital Course.*   After a year on a disturbed ward, during which time the patient was delusional and hallucinating, insulin treatment was started but was stopped, after sixteen comas, on his mother's insistence because he received a minor injury in a fight with another patient. He improved slowly until November, 1940, when he was paroled and then discharged one year later. He held one job for a year, others for shorter periods, but by February, 1944, he was again restless, weeping, and having hallucinations, and he was returned to the hospital. In January, 1945, he was again paroled, only to be returned in May of the same year. In October, insulin and electroshock treatment was administered with temporary improvement followed by immediate relapse to his previous condition of assaultiveness, retardation, and confusion with hallucinations.

*Mental Status.*   The patient was hypokinetic and appeared preoccupied. At times he laughed suddenly and inappropriately, but without force, and he was disinterested in his environment. His talk was slow, his voice flat; the progression of talk was disjointed and distractible. Affect was flattened and lacking in lability. Auditory hallucinations were described as coming from the same room and the content of these productions involved women and sexual relations. Visual hallucinations were also suspected. The patient was not oriented for time or place; his sensorium was cloudy. Insight was lacking and judgment obviously faulty.

*Operation.*   On May 27, 1947, partial removal of areas 6, 8, 9, and 10 (superior frontal gyrus) was carried out bilaterally.

*Follow-Up Notes.*   During the period of interviews of May 28, and June 2, 1947, the patient was unresponsive, though capable of eating.

On June 25, 1947, the picture was essentially as it had been before operation. The patient was impulsively overactive at times, retarded and seclusive at other times. Hallucinations and the sexual content continued as before.

On August 26, 1947, he was more in contact with his surroundings and answered questions more freely, but he remained disoriented; hallucinations and preoccupations remained the same and judgment continued to be poor.

On January 17, 1948, the patient had improved sufficiently to be paroled, and he was making $100 per week as a salesman despite lack of conscientiousness. His lunch hour was prolonged and he often reported late in the morning. He was no longer subject to delusions or hallucinations. He was cheerful and pleasant with the examiner and with other patients whom he had not seen for some time. His affective responses were still flattened but more appropriate than on previous interviews. Some suspiciousness remained, however; his train of thought was rambling and unconnected at times, and he remained preoccupied with sexual relations, impotency, and the like. At the same time he told how he planned to woo and win many girls. Orientation, calculation, and memory were good, but judgment was faulty. (He asked to be excused from an appointment to see the psychiatrist because he was attending another college and didn't want to run the risk of not graduating by visiting Columbia.) In short, his thinking remained schizophrenic, but the more obvious psychotic manifestations were no longer present.

In March, 1948, the patient became confused and excited after a visit to Greystone, during which time he made dates with several of the female patients, and was picked up by the police while trying to get into City Hall on Easter Sunday morning.

At the time of the interview on May 8, 1948, the patient was hospitalized on a disturbed ward, where he was mute and unresponsive. He sat passively, smoking a cigarette and occasionally sucking or biting his thumb, trying to insert his fingers into his nostrils or down his throat, and indicating his epigastrium with his other hand. He responded to no stimuli on the ward, except to the presence of student nurses whom he sometimes tried to examine sexually.

*Patient* 33. *Age:* 27. *Sex:* female. *Marital status:* single. *Occupation:* mill-worker. *Religion:* Catholic. *Informant:* father. *Diagnosis:* schizophrenia, catatonic type.

*Presenting Picture.* The patient was first admitted in January, 1944, with a history of bizarre behavior and confusion.

*Present Illness.* In December, 1943, the patient left her job, became seclusive, and began to play pointless pranks on her mother. (Menses had ceased several months before.) She hid clothing, threw food about the room, and demanded that the lights in the house be dimly lit. She was nearly mute and at times she wept. It was apparent that she was confused in her environment.

*Previous Personality Disorders.* There was no history of personality disorders prior to the present illness.

*Family History.* The patient's father was a Polish-born butcher; he was sociable and in good health. Her mother was also born in Poland, was ten years younger than her husband, and was described as "quiet." The patient was the oldest of four living children, the other siblings being in good health. One brother died with "convulsions" when eighteen months old; another of whooping cough at nineteen months of age. The family relationship was a harmonious one although the patient never confided in her siblings or her parents.

*Personal History.* The patient was born in New Jersey in June, 1920. Her birth and development were supposedly normal. Menses began when she was thirteen and were not accompanied by any emotional upset. She started school at six and completed high school at nineteen. Although she was always a serious student and a person who enjoyed reading, she did not do well in school and took five years to complete high school. During school years she helped her father in his business. After graduation she went to work as a machine operator in a textile mill. She had been interested in one boy and had seen him frequently over a six-month period until into the Army, but she did not react strongly to his leaving. For several years before her illness she was self-conscious about her weight and took reducing pills.

*Personality.* The picture given was that of a very shy, self-conscious girl whose friends were almost exclusively female and who clung to her home and mother for support.

*Hospital Course.* On admission in 1944 the patient appeared tense, confused, disoriented, and somewhat depressed. She was retarded in psychomotor activity and was evasive. The thought content on admission centered around her relationship to men whom she said she liked. It was felt that she was having hallucinations although she did not describe any hallucinatory experiences. In February, 1944, insulin and electroshock treatment was started. At the beginning of treatment she was noisy and having hallucinations but by July, 1944, she was considered ready for parole although she was shallow and had achieved no insight. At home she worked in a defense plant and made a marginal adjustment until February, 1946, when she was readmitted after she had lost her job and become assaultive, resistive, and negativistic. She was nearly mute at the time although she expressed some mild persecutory ideas. Electric shock treatment was given in April with a very brief period of improvement followed by relapse into disturbed and impulsive behavior. In this condition she was transferred to the project. At the time of operation she was mute.

*Mental Status.* The patient huddled in corners of the room usually in a knee-chest position. She appeared frightened; she was mute until an attempt was made to examine her, at which time she would scream loudly and become assaultive, biting, kicking, and scratching. She would then scramble under the bed or attempt to hide behind a dresser. Restraint was necessary in order to gain any cooperation for testing. Content could not be elicited. It was not possible to test memory or orientation.

*Operation.* On May 30, 1947, the inferior frontal gyrus (area 45 and parts of areas 10, 44, and 46) was ablated bilaterally.

*Follow-Up Notes.* On June 4, and 5, 1947, the patient was unresponsive.

On June 11, 1947, she did not speak spontaneously but under sodium amytal (6 grains) she was more alert, wept, and tried to speak. A motor aphasia was suspected.

On July 4, 1947, she was passively cooperative, reading, and feeding herself. Examination was made difficult by excessive salivation and the speech defect (see the neurologic evaluation p. 449), although she was able to make short replies. Her attention wandered and she was affectively flat. No complaints were elicited.

On August 26, 1947, affective responses were appropriate and the patient participated in all ward activities. The mental content was not unusual but speech continued as before. Orientation and judgment were good. When asked about her illness she said that she had been angry at her father and upset because her brothers were away.

On January 18, 1948, the patient was working in a textile mill and making an adjustment which she and her family found no different than her pre-illness behavior. She said that she would like to get married but had had no dates. Her speech difficulty continued unimproved.

Two days before the interview of May 8, 1948, the patient lost her job but she would not explain her dismissal except to say that other girls had been discharged at the same time. Her speech had not improved. She appeared more withdrawn although no other evidence of psychopathologic nature could be obtained. She referred many questions to her brother who felt that her difficulty in making herself understood was of great importance. He pointed out that she had spent much time in speech practice, after her discharge from the hospital, and that she had been discouraged when no results were forthcoming.

On May 15, 1948, the patient was returned to the hospital in a catatonic stupor. She had remained in bed for five days and refused to eat or talk.

### PATIENTS IN WHOM IMPROVEMENT WAS QUESTIONABLY RELATED TO OPERATION

**Patient 38.** *Age:* 38. *Sex:* female. *Marital status:* separated. *Occupation:* bookkeeper. *Religion:* Hebrew. *Informant:* sister. *Diagnosis:* manic-depressive psychosis, manic.

*Presenting Picture.* The first admission to Greystone was in October, 1942, when the patient was described as excitable, restless, overtalkative, and impulsive.

*Present Illness.* About two weeks before admission the patient became overactive, overtalkative, and concerned about her relations with her boy friend. She expressed fear about her heart and physical condition in general, and expressed resentment toward many people. Her conversation was rambling, her daily activities grew unpredictable, and sleep became difficult although her appetite was maintained. On one occasion she said that she could see her father's spirit in the mirror at midnight. She was committed after creating a disturbance in a bank.

*Previous Personality Disorders.* At sixteen the patient had a definite episode of overactivity which did not require hospitalization. At this time she was picked up by the police after being reprimanded by her father for associating indiscriminately with men. Subsequently she was committed to a Connecticut institution in a manic state and after her release she was apparently depressed for several weeks. Two other hospitalizations in Connecticut followed, each attack being manic followed by a short depression. The dates and lengths of illness are not known.

*Family History.* The patient's father was Russian born and a carpenter who died in 1939 of arteriosclerotic heart disease. He was a strict disciplinarian and was always resented by the patient. His wife was a first cousin, also Russian, and was described as "protective and easy to get along with." The patient was the fourth of five children.

The other four siblings were in good health and satisfactorily married. The patient always felt that her family criticized her excessively and her feelings toward her older sister were especially strong in this respect.

*Personal History.* The patient was a full-term baby. She was born in New Jersey in 1909. She enjoyed good health as a child except for minor childhood diseases, diphtheria at six (uneventful recovery), and "rheumatism" at twelve with a subsequent cardiac murmur. Menses began when she was thirteen. At sixteen she suffered a fractured pelvis in an automobile accident. There was a history of several months' treatment for syphilis beginning when she was fourteen (repeated blood Wassermanns were negative in this study). She began to associate indiscriminately with men at an early age and has always preferred male to female company. Her sexual activities were not known. Between hospitalizations in Connecticut she married but the marriage was stormy and the couple lived together only one and one-half years.

*Personality.* The patient was always "stubborn" and difficult to contact although she had a great need for group approval. She never confided in women and never formed close friendships with women nor did she ever have any special hobbies or interests.

*Hospital Course.* In January, 1942, insulin coma and electroshock treatments were begun and after three weeks of treatment the patient became less active and more sociable and manageable although she remained shallow and flighty. Following parole in March she obtained a job in a defense plant but she continued to be irresponsible in her affairs and was managed only with difficulty by her family. She was readmitted in July, 1945, after she created disturbances in various public places. On admission she was once more overactive, overtalkative, facetious, and preoccupied with men and marriage. No hallucinations or delusions were elicited. After several months she went into a retarded depression in which she was unproductive and preoccupied with the thought that she had been inadequately treated for syphilis. In this condition she was transferred to the project.

*Mental Status.* This patient was retarded and markedly underproductive, appearing frightened and depressed. Subjectively her mood was one of depression accompanied by self-deprecation and accusation. She accepted vaginal sensations as a sign of venereal disease despite the numerous negative reactions to tests, the results of which she knew. This was interpreted as punishment for premarital intercourse. Sensorium was clear, orientation intact, and insight meager.

*Follow-Up Notes.* During the week preceding the interview of May 26, 1947, the patient's behavior changed from depressed to manic, with overactivity, playful exhibitionism, and sexual preoccupation. At the time of the interview she denied her Jewish ancestry stating that she was Irish and adopted by her mother. She also insisted that her real mother was also a patient and identified various hospital patients in the role of sister rivals.

On June 2, 1947, a bilateral venous ligation was performed.

During the interview of June 4, 1947, the patient appeared to be more distractible and superficial than she was preoperatively.

By July 4, 1947, she had quieted considerably and was cooperative although she was still rambling and distractible. The thought content remained unchanged.

On August 28, 1947, considerable change was noted in this patient. Although garrulous and superficial, her attention was maintained and it was possible to get relevant answers. She was planning to return to her old job and was quite content with the arrangement. Syphilis was no longer a concern and she stated that she had never been promiscuous. (There was much evasion and giggling when sexual matters were discussed and it was not possible to get any details of her sexual adjustment, orgasm, etc.) In reviewing her marital situation she was noncommittal, preferring to handle the problem by ignoring it.

The patient was interviewed on January 17, 1948. She had been working four months as a typist, filing clerk, and bookkeeper at this time and was making a good adjustment although she remained slightly verbose, distractible, and overactive. She stated that she had no sexual urge although she was making regular dates, and that she was considering divorce although she was taking no steps to secure one.

On May 8, 1948, no change was noted as compared with the previous interview. The patient continued to make a good work adjustment despite her mildly hypomanic condition.

**Patient 42.** *Age:* 40. *Sex:* female. *Marital status:* married. *Occupation:* salesgirl. *Religion:* Catholic. *Informant:* father. *Diagnosis:* Manic-depressive psychosis, manic.

*Presenting Picture.* On admission to Greystone in July, 1928, the patient was restless, agitated, incoherent, and disoriented.

*Present Illness.* About six months before her first admission to Greystone the patient came into conflict with her family because she was devoting too much time to a young man who lived nearby. She became irritable, profane, gradually overtalkative, and unpredictable in her behavior. She was alternately playful and threatening. On one occasion she threatened to commit suicide by jumping through a window. The week before hospitalization she slept poorly, and sang and screamed at night.

*Previous Personality Disorders.* At the age of fifteen, following an attack of scarlet fever, the patient was severely depressed for three to four weeks. At that time paranoid content was also noted.

*Family History.* The patient's grandfather was a periodic alcoholic. Her father was a New York-born electrician who was a conscientious worker and a strict disciplinarian of the children. His wife was English born and was described as "moody and nervous." She died at the age of fifty-four when the patient was twenty-three years old. The patient was the third of four children and the only girl now living. An older sister died of septicemia at seventeen and the younger brother was described as "slightly nervous." The patient supposedly maintained a good relationship with all her siblings but was especially close to the sister who died.

*Personal History.* The patient was born in New York in November, 1906; the delivery was considered normal. She walked and talked at one and a half years of age and had the usual childhood diseases. At six she entered school, leaving after the first year of high school because she "disliked" learning. Thereafter she worked as a clerk until a few weeks before admission. The patient's menses began about the time of her sister's death. She reacted to her sister's death with marked grief, so severe that the family moved to a new location in order to distract her. She was socially popular, made many dates, and indulged in sexual intercourse on many occasions before her illness.

*Personality.* The patient was usually conscientious, jovial, talkative, and practical, but she often adopted a superior attitude toward her friends and was more of a disciplinary problem than were her siblings.

*Hospital Course.* There were four hospital admissions, each marked by overactivity or depression, sometimes with persecutory ideas. The patient improved in seven months after the first admission, was paroled, discharged, and made a satisfactory adjustment until 1934 despite the death of her mother during this interval. Her 1934 admission was marked by excitement and overactivity. Outstanding in the content was her hatred of men. After three and one-half months she again improved and was discharged. In 1937 she married a widower who had four children and two months later she became quarrelsome, wept frequently, and appeared depressed. At times she identified her husband with a priest from New York, at other times she denied being married, said there were bombs in the cellar, and threatened to kill one of her husband's children. On admission she was overactive, gay, and had hallucinations (hearing bell-like sounds). Thereafter she went through a period of depression, then leveled off and was paroled in September, 1940. Her last admission was in May, 1945, and again she was overactive and paranoid content was observed. The picture of excessive activity continued until she was transferred to this project.

*Mental Status.* On examination the patient was gay, flirtatious, and playful but personally neat. She frequently made sexual advances to the physician and to other patients passing in the hall. Distractibility was marked and a flight of ideas was present. Her emotional response was one of superficial gaiety and she often responded in this way inappropriately to discussions of subjects such as death. Her content of thought covered various relationships to her family, men, religion, and sex. She stated that she had had an abortion and indicated that she had never been capable of orgasm. A delusional trend appeared in her statements that she had "cancer all over" and that her "heart flew out but you can live without it." She was preoccupied with death and spoke about a previous suicidal attempt. The sensorium was clear and orientation was intact.

*Operation.*   On May 29, 1948, area 11 was removed bilaterally.

*Follow-Up Notes.*   In the interview of June 2, 1947, the patient continued to be gay, laughing, and silly.

By July 4, 1947, she was less overactive and more cooperative and friendly. She was less silly; delusions or hallucinations were not present. Her discussions of her marital and family background and sex were logically organized.

The patient was interviewed on September 9, 1947, and January 17, 1948. Improvement was maintained over this period although the patient remained somewhat euphoric. After she was paroled she acted as superintendent of sixteen apartments in her building as well as taking care of her own apartment. Her husband commented that she was "better than she ever was" although he described her sexually as being "like dead wood" but added that "she was never interested in it."

The patient had had four seizures on April 22, 1948, and returned to the hospital for a checkup and medication, remaining at Greystone for one week. She described a mild state of depression which was present for two weeks before the seizures but lifted quickly in the hospital. When interviewed on May 8, 1948, she presented a picture much like that seen in September-January and no depression was apparent, although she was somewhat flighty.

#### PATIENTS UNCHANGED FOLLOWING TOPECTOMY

**Patient 2.**   *Age:* 46.   *Sex:* male.   *Marital status:* married.   *Occupation:* blue-print sketcher.   *Religion:* Roman Catholic.   *Informant:* wife.   *Diagnosis:* schizophrenia, hebephrenic type.

*Presenting Picture.*   In November, 1938, the patient was admitted to Greystone when he became argumentative and assaultive because he believed people were talking about him.

*Present Illness.*   Early in October, 1938, he began to complain of headache and to fear that he would lose his job. In November he left his job for "a rest," believing that other employees were talking about him and looking at him strangely. He was preoccupied and restless, his appetite was poor, and he had numerous somatic complaints. After a week in a general hospital he was admitted to Greystone.

*Previous Personality Disorders.*   There had been no previous personality disorders.

*Family History.*   Little is known about the family beyond their Irish antecedence. The father was born in 1876 and was reputed to be a heavy drinker. The mother was about the same age as the father and was described as pleasant and sociable. The patient was the third of six children, all of whom were said to be in good health.

*Personal History.*   After a normal birth in Massachusetts in March, 1901, the patient's development was supposedly not unusual although no specific information could be obtained. The patient started to go to school when six years old and he did well enough to skip at least one grade. At the age of twelve he had an attack of pleurisy but otherwise there were no serious illnesses. At fifteen, while in his second or third year of high school, he falsified his age to join the Navy for three years and subsequently worked as a blue-print sketcher. His father died when the patient was twenty-one but the patient's reaction to this is not known. When he was twenty-three he moved to New Jersey and two years later married a woman his own age who was already pregnant at the time of the marriage. The marriage was supposedly a happy one. Six children were born between the years 1927 and 1940, all of whom were in good health.

*Personality.* According to his wife, the patient's pre-illness personality was not remarkable. He was described as intelligent, kind, easy to please, gentle, and interested in his home and family. No pre-illness tendency toward suspiciousness was noted.

*Hospital Course.* Following his admission in 1938 the patient was underproductive and retarded. He was suspicious and expressed ideas that he might be a pregnant woman and that he might be God or Jesus. Gradual improvement took place while he was receiving hydrotherapy and colonics. He was paroled in January, 1939, at which time he was able to attribute his previous symptoms to mental illness. Many somatic complaints were still present but he made an excellent adjustment at home, returned to his job, and seemed quite happy at the birth of a son in January, 1940. Readmission was necessary in February, 1941. At this time he was spasmodically over-active but usually quiet and cooperative on the ward. Occasionally he became excited and assaulted other patients.

*Mental Status.* During the examination the patient appeared to be under some tension. He made many random gestures but was cooperative, volunteered much information, and attempted to answer direct questions promptly. He was quiet for long periods but overproductive once speech was initiated. His mood was one of superficial well-being with euphoria being the outstanding quality. He frequently laughed quietly and often said that there was nothing wrong with him and that he had never felt better in his life. Talk was disjointed; he skipped from one subject to another without logical transition. The content of thought centered around war and his naval service, his belief that he was at Greystone on naval orders in order to await a call to active duty, and his preoccupations with the medical profession which he somehow compared to the oil industry. He insisted that he had never been married. The following is typical of his statements: "I couldn't have a record here under the medical law anyway. It's War laws. There are War laws and Peace laws. It's called oil field wampum laws, which is good medical talk anyway. Somebody wants to know just how your serums are made and what they look like." He was able to recall events from the recent and remote past and was correctly oriented except for his situation. Hallucinations were not elicited; insight and judgment were both poor.

*Operation.* On May 28, 1947, area 8 was removed bilaterally.

*Follow-Up Notes.* On May 30, 1947, two days after operation, the patient was alert but the only change noted was a decrease in the amount of spontaneous talk. At the time of interviews on June 25, and August 19, 1947, he had returned to his preoperative level with a return of spontaneous talk. Content and behavior were in no way altered except that he stated he was married (cf. "Mental Status") and that his wife visited him occasionally.

When seen about five months after operation, on October 25, 1947, the patient was still overproductive and inappropriate. Auditory hallucinations were present; for example, he said, "There are a man and a woman talking in the place, in a distant style, like in the talkies—you see what I mean? The trouble is there is no screen— you only hear the voices. When accustomed to it, it doesn't bother you." Content and general condition were otherwise as before.

On October 29, 1947, bilateral prefrontal lobotomy was performed. Following operation the patient was stuporous for only one day. He subsequently answered questions only by saying that he was "all right." He picked at his dressings con-tinuously and managed to remove several of them.

All spontaneous activity except for repetitious picking at the bandages was absent at the time of interview on November 7, 1947. The patient was indolent and un-responsive to directions though passively cooperative to procedures which were carried out on him. Orientation was not changed but he was unable to answer simple ques-tions of fact, unable to do simple calculation, and unable to give the point of the "Cowboy Story" even though he could recall the incidents of the story. He once again felt that he was single. Insight was lacking and judgment still poor.

On January 18, 1948, seven months after topectomy and three months after lobotomy, there was no significant change from the preoperative state except for some loss of spontaneity. The patient remained delusional and autistic in his thinking and judgment was still very poor.

The patient's condition still remained unchanged at the time of the interview on May 7, 1948.

**Patient 6.**  *Age:* 32.  *Sex:* male.  *Marital status:* single.  *Occupation:* shipping clerk.  *Religion:* Protestant.  *Informants:* mother and father.  *Diagnosis:* schizophrenia, hebephrenic type.

*Presenting Picture.*  On admission to Greystone in November, 1940, the patient was confused, incoherent, and severely preoccupied.

*Present Illness.*  In November, 1939, the patient was dismissed from his job as a crane operator and subsequently felt that he had been framed by fellow employees. Thereafter he complained of fatigue and a feeling that something had snapped in his head. After resting for a month he enlisted in the Army in January, 1940, and left for Honolulu one month later. Personality disturbances were noted by the family before he sailed and they were soon notified that he had been hospitalized. He was returned to his home in August where he was indolent and preoccupied with his fantasy life. Despite the family's efforts to stimulate him to social activity he continued to withdraw and, when a diagnosis of dementia praecox had been made by a local physician, he was admitted to Greystone after a month in a general hospital.

*Previous Personality Disorders.*  There were no personality disorders manifest prior to the present illness.

*Family History.*  The German-born grandparents were supposedly not unusual except that the maternal grandfather was "very domineering." The patient's father, a German-born bookkeeper, was also a strict disciplinarian who often scolded the patient for his disinterested attitude. The mother was three years younger than her husband, was American born and "cultured," a woman who always showed much concern for the patient. One son is a year older than the patient. He is a college graduate, a successful engineer, and the father of two children. One sister, four years younger than the patient, has a successful business career.

*Personal History.*  The patient weighed 6½ pounds when born in New Jersey in December, 1914. Delivery was not unusual. He walked and talked at seventeen months and had the usual childhood diseases. Enuresis and masturbation were not reported but a single convulsion was recalled as occurring when the patient was eleven months old by one informant and when he was eleven years old by another. Night terrors were reported as occurring when he was twelve years of age. He was often criticized as "a loafer and a bum" by his grandfather, with whom the children often spent the summer; the patient did not seem to object to these sharp words. He began school at the age of five and though he graduated from high school without failures he was always shy and never self-assertive. He made few friends and was "serious minded." He was given no sexual instruction and showed little sexual interest. After high school he attended business school for six months but gave it up for lack of interest and then worked four years in a glove concern where his father got him a job as shipping clerk. He drank periodically to excess at this time and complained often of nervousness and indigestion. In 1938 (at the age of twenty-four) he abruptly decided to study radio mechanics, but was greatly disappointed when he was unable to find employment in the field. Subsequently he worked briefly in an airplane factory, on a construction job, and then enlisted in the Army.

*Personality.*  Outstanding in his personality were his seclusiveness, shyness, and lack of aggression. He had a good memory but was easily discouraged and lacked the ability to follow through on a job when the going got tough. He was often scolded by his father for his indolence but never reacted outwardly to these reprimands. He often compared his own meager achievements with those of his more successful siblings.

*Hospital Course.* In the hospital the patient was at first seclusive and retarded. His memory was intact but he had no insight into his illness and judgment was poor. In January, 1941, treatment, consisting of forty-eight insulin comas and seventeen metrazol convulsions, was started and thereafter he was silly and emotionally shallow, complained that he was being hypnotized and that voices were "coming out of my eyes." In May he was paroled at his family's request though he was still having hallucinations. He made a borderline adjustment until October, 1945, when he was returned to the hospital in an excited and confused state. In the hospital he was very retarded and disoriented but no persecutory ideas or hallucinations were demonstrated. Shock treatment (sixty-eight insulin comas and twenty-five electroshocks) produced a general quieting effect but in ten months there was no further change and he was recommended for this project.

*Mental Status.* The patient's gait was slow and methodical. He appeared to be somewhat confused or dazed. There were long pauses in the middle of sentences; he sometimes blocked completely and giggled or smiled inappropriately. There was little emotional response during the interview and the affect was definitely flat. The thought content was discontinuous; he rambled from topic to topic without logical progression of ideas (e.g. "I am trying to hide. I feel fine." "My mind was O. K. I didn't have all the answers. I don't know how I made out." "I was making a good salary"). When asked about his sex life he replied, "I never overworked." He said that he heard voices: "I understand they're in the mind. They are my own thoughts. I'd like to keep them there. They are very pleasant." He was disoriented for time and place and his judgment was very poor.

*Operation.* On May 27, 1947, areas 6 and 8 were removed bilaterally. (Removal of area 6 was not complete.)

*Follow-Up Notes.* The patient was interviewed on May 28, and June 11, 1947. Immediately after operation he was confused, dazed, and lethargic. He continued to have hallucinations and was distractible and perseverative.

On July 4, 1947, auditory hallucinations were no longer elicited. The patient felt subjectively better. He remained intensely preoccupied, however, and his speech, judgment, and response to the environment continued to reflect this preoccupation.

During the interview of August 25, 1947, the patient was somewhat more spontaneous and passively cooperative. Auditory hallucinations were once more present, however, and the content of thought was disjointed. He blocked frequently and there was much inappropriate laughing and giggling.

On October 20, 1947, the only improvement noted in the patient's condition from that of August 25 was that he was more interested in ward activities and occasionally talked to the nurses and worked in the kitchen. In other respects he had not changed.

On October 27, 1947, a more complete excision of area 6 was carried out on the right.

On October 30, 1947, the third postoperative day, the patient was somnolent and incontinent but responded verbally and by movement to direct commands.

On November 3, 1947, there was little change from his condition as of October 30.

On November 7, 1947, and January 18, 1948, the patient's psychiatric condition showed little change from the preoperative status. Hallucinations were denied, but he remained preoccupied, inappropriate, irrelevant, and shallow. He was unconcerned about his partially paralyzed left arm.

On May 7, 1948, the patient's mental status remained unchanged. He giggled inappropriately, was confused, had delusions, and was subject to hallucinations in the auditory sphere.

**Patient 18.** *Age:* 39. *Sex:* male. *Marital status:* divorced. *Occupation:* physicist. *Religion:* Methodist. *Informant:* wife. *Diagnosis:* schizophrenia, hebephrenic type.

*Presenting Picture.* When admitted to Greystone in July, 1943, the patient was described as depressed, suspicious, irritable, and hypochondriacal.

*Present Illness.* The patient began to behave unusually in 1933, soon after his marriage, when he demanded that his mother-in-law not kiss her daughter and complained that she did not understand him. He remained "nervous," irritable, and easily upset, blaming his wife severely when their son was bumped by a car in 1938. The following year his wife was unsuccessful in trying to get him in to a physician, but in 1940 his job advisor persuaded him to go to a doctor because of his behavior on the job. The physician prescribed thyroid extract, which did no good, and the patient gradually became suspicious of other people and felt that his company was "using" him. He also complained of sore throat and abdominal pain, and was operated on for the latter. During his convalescence his conversation was "morbid." In the spring of 1942 he obtained a new job and appeared cheerful for a short time, but when he joined his wife on the birth of their third child he appeared depressed and displayed ideas of reference. Various events were interpreted as having hidden meaning and he believed someone was trying to break up his marriage. He avoided his co-workers and his behavior became generally unpredictable. After three visits to a local psychiatrist, hospitalization was advised and he was admitted to Greystone.

*Previous Personality Disorders.* There had been no previous personality disorders.

*Family History.* The patient's father (aged sixty-five) was in charge of an automobile accessories division in the South. The patient's mother was two years older than her husband and was a Southern-born schoolteacher. Both parents were described as "high-strung," and the patient's father was also hypochondriacal. One daughter, four years younger than the patient, was married to a defense worker and living with her parents. The family relationship was congenial, but the patient was indulged by his parents who were ambitious for him, especially in his scholastic work. A maternal uncle supposedly died by suicide.

*Personal History.* The patient was born in South Carolina in 1908. Delivery was normal; he was breast-fed for ten months and walked and talked at the usual ages. He began school at the age of six and proved a good student. At fourteen he had an appendectomy and herniorrhaphy, and at eighteen or nineteen was unconscious for one and a half hours after being struck by lightning. When twenty he graduated from college, and at twenty-two he obtained his Master's Degree while teaching part-time. He had frequent respiratory infections thereafter and complained of headaches, stomach upsets, and eyestrain on numerous occasions. In 1933 he married the informant and in 1936 received his Ph.D., working for eighteen months thereafter in a research laboratory. A son was born in 1936, a daughter in 1940, and a second son in 1942. All the children were well, though the oldest boy was described as "high-strung." All the children were wanted and he showed no favoritism, though his wife felt he was especially fond of their daughter. He sought intercourse several times a week during the early years of marriage and twice weekly thereafter, but about eighteen months before admission a disturbance of potency developed.

*Personality.* The patient was intelligent and learned easily, but was overconscientious and always easily worried. He rarely displayed anger, but his moods were highly labile. Financial affairs were left up to his wife. He was active in church affairs and had many hobbies, but did not make friends easily.

*Hospital Course.* On admission to Greystone in July, 1943, the patient was passively polite and his speech was rambling. Sensorium was clear, memory intact, and he was well oriented, but he was apprehensive, mildly depressed, and persecutory ideas were present. Compulsive behavior was noted and he admitted vague hallucinatory experiences. In August, 1943, insulin and electroshock treatments were started and he improved markedly for a few days, but then relapsed to his former behavior. In July, 1946, his wife applied for a divorce, and when informed of this he showed no reaction, though he was correctly oriented at that time.

*Mental Status.* The patient was neatly dressed and approached the interview pleasantly and cooperatively. He volunteered some information spontaneously, but was obviously preoccupied and sat in one position for long periods of time, staring out the window. He occasionally smiled appropriately, but his affect was generally flattened and his mood was one neither of elation nor depression. Voluntarily, however, he stated that he sometimes was depressed to the extent of anticipating suicide. The content of thought centered around his present condition (into which he had partial insight), as well as his auditory and visual hallucinations and persecutory delusions. He gave a lengthy biophysical description of electrical impulses which he was receiving, stating that some could be imaginary but not all since there could be a sound physical principle behind them. He also described visual impressions of various "grayish" shapes, and unusual auditory and gustatory sensations. The sensorium was clear and he was oriented for time and place.

*Operation.* On May 21, 1947, area 11 was partially removed bilaterally.

*Follow-Up Notes.* On the interviews of May 26, and May 28, 1947, the patient was quite cheerful, garrulous, and rambling in contrast to his preoperative seclusiveness. He was more interested in his environment than before operation and felt better subjectively, but his delusional and hallucinatory experiences remained unchanged.

A lengthy interview was held on June 19, 1947. At this time indications of spontaneity and activity were still present, along with some euphoria and inappropriateness of affective response. The patient's talk involved long and cumbersome, pseudo-intellectual sentences which at times were meaningless. Delusions and hallucinations were still present and judgment was poor. He did not appear to be aware of the fact that his wife had divorced him.

On August 25, 1947, he continued to express the belief that he was improving, but it was apparent that he had become more preoccupied and seclusive and was approaching his preoperative condition. Thought content remained unchanged.

On January 17, 1948, little change was noted from that of the interview in August, except that the degree of preoccupation had become even greater. The patient sat staring into space for long periods of time and was distracted with greater difficulty.

On May 7, 1948, one year after operation, he was on ground parole and had been granted the privilege of making visits outside the institution. He preferred to remain in the hospital, however. There was a marked lack of spontaneity and his old delusions and hallucinations remained. Memory and calculation were not impaired and he was well informed on current events, but he was disoriented for time.

**Patient 19.** *Age:* 50. *Sex:* male. *Marital status:* married. *Occupation:* candy-store owner. *Religion:* Lutheran. *Informants:* wife and brother. *Diagnosis:* schizophrenia with affective and psychopathic features.

*Presenting Picture.* The patient was admitted to Greystone Park in March, 1933, after five years of unpredictable and irresponsible behavior associated with expansiveness and irritability.

*Present Illness.* In 1927 the patient complained of being run down and took to bed for six weeks, remaining there without talking to anyone and refusing to take medications prescribed by his physician. By the spring of 1928 he was much improved but in 1930 he began leaving his family for long periods of time, offering no explanations for his activities. At times he ignored his business for weeks, gave away large sums of money, and bought merchandise which he could not afford. In 1931 he was under observation in the county jail and later at a city hospital, where he had to be restrained. Following his release from this hospital, his wife attempted to have a legal guardian appointed but the patient blocked this move with the help of a good lawyer. Subsequently he was disagreeable at home, stayed away much of the time, and ran up large taxi bills which he was unable to pay and which sometimes landed him in jail. At this time he was committed to Greystone Park Hospital.

*Previous Personality Disorders.* There were no previous personality disorders.

*Family History.* The patient's mother died in Germany of influenza in 1918. His father was still living in Germany in 1933 and was sixty-two years of age. He was reported to be mentally ill with a tendency to wander away from home. The patient was the oldest of eight children, five of whom remained in Germany and none of whom have been hospitalized for mental illness. A paternal uncle was hospitalized for three months in Germany because of symptoms resembling the patient's.

*Personal History.*   Born in Germany in 1897, the patient came to the United States when he was fourteen years old, at which time his education was stopped. No information was available on his early years. After working as a shopkeeper for several years, he opened his own confectionery store at the age of twenty-three. Two years later he married a woman his own age and subsequently was the father of two girls, one of whom was described as "nervous." In 1931 he was forced by his father-in-law to sell his store when his behavior became irresponsible.

*Personality.*   Supposedly of average intelligence, the patient was usually kind to his family but undemonstrative. Reticence was his outstanding characteristic and financial problems his chief preoccupation before illness. His moral standards were high but he was not a religious man. No sexual irregularities were described. In the hospital, the patient said he did not respect his wife because he and she had been intimate before marriage and he expressed considerable resentment against his father-in-law.

*Hospital Course.*   This man's course was marked by the same variability which had been present in the years before he was admitted. At times he was cooperative, easily managed, and recognized that his previous behavior was erratic. In September, 1933, he was paroled after six months in the hospital and remained at home for one year, though his behavior during that time was highly unpredictable. In May, 1934, he was readmitted for six months. During this time he expressed resentment toward his wife and was overtalkative and flighty. Without any improvement in his condition, he was once more paroled to his home at the family's request, remaining out of the hospital until January, 1940, when he was again admitted with the same behavior history as on previous admissions. He had been ordering expensive cars, writing bad checks, drinking to excess, and wandering about New York without letting his family know his whereabouts. In addition, some hypochondriacal complaints were present and he believed he was expectorating pus. Beginning in May, 1940, he was subjected to seventeen insulin comas followed by reduction of his overactivity, but within a year he was again overactive, assaultive, and often involved in fights with other patients. In September, 1945, he disappeared from the hospital and was found living in the nearby woods. Early in 1946 he was transferred to a disturbed ward where he remained until his transfer to this project.

*Mental Status.*   The patient appeared somewhat suspicious but came to the interview willingly. He spoke freely but was evasive and minimized his past abnormal behavior trends. Outstanding was his carefree attitude. He showed no emotion in lightly explaining away his sojourn in the nearby woods, saying in a silly fashion that he merely wanted to go camping. In describing his assaultiveness when on the disturbed ward, he said, "I had to defend myself. They put me in with a bunch of bad actors." He denied any aggressiveness on his part and insisted he had helped the attendants keep the other patients in their places.

He was well oriented. Memory and recall were intact but judgment was markedly impaired.

*Operation.*   On May 26, 1947, area 45 was partially removed bilaterally.

*Follow-Up Notes.*   On May 27, 1947, one day after operation, the patient was alert but his mental content remained the same as it had preoperatively.

On May 30, 1947, the patient was up and around the ward but appeared somewhat garrulous and there was evidence of persecutory trends. He stated: "They played tricks on me. I don't know who it was, but they're still here."

On June 2, 1947, approximately one week after operation, he was restless and talkative. He wore several pairs of trousers at a time, smoked cigars in a steady stream, was grandiose in his talk of making millions and making the examiner governor of the state.

The patient was again interviewed on June 24, 1947. By this time his emotional and motor activities had quieted considerably. He was well oriented and able to discuss his illness, though he was evasive about the reasons why he was hospitalized. When asked about his previous elation, he replied, "I was only kidding." After stating his wish to go home, he launched upon a lengthy description of his wife and her shortcomings, particularly her fear of pregnancy and her menstrual difficulties. Judgment was still faulty and he was not able to accept responsibility for his periods of overactivity. Instead they were attributed to chance arguments with policemen or he maintained that it was an "injustice" that he was hospitalized.

On August 25, 1947, three months after operation, he was cooperative, sociable, and sleeping well; his affective responses were appropriate, and his judgment was much improved. He stated that he wanted to return to work in his store, that he could now get along with his wife. He said, "We are getting along all right now. We argue but I am getting over my tendency to argue minor points. I want to make the best of things because of my two grown daughters." Some insight was present and, regarding the effects of operation, he said, "I now feel more contented and settled. I realize I was a little high-strung at times before."

Soon after this note was written the patient went home on a trial visit. After a short time he returned voluntarily to the hospital (without his wife's knowledge) and then escaped from the ward. Nearly two weeks later he was found hiding in a system of tunnels which connect the various buildings of Greystone Park Hospital.

On January 17, 1948, six months after operation, he was again interviewed and at this time he was cooperative and quiet. He smiled sheepishly when talking of his recent behavior but did not otherwise display emotion when talking of it. He said, "I wanted to go back to the hospital because I liked it here, so I left home. I was put on a ward I didn't like, so I took a walk into town." (No mention was made of his flight to the tunnels.) Insight was limited and judgment obviously poor but the extremes of overactive and depressive behavior were no longer present and no delusions or hallucinations were elicited.

On May 7, 1948, one year after operation, the patient's condition had not changed from that noted in January, 1948, and custodial care was still required.

**Patient 24.** *Age:* 41. *Sex:* male. *Marital status:* single. *Occupation:* baker. *Religion:* Catholic. *Informants:* mother, sisters, cousins. *Diagnosis:* schizophrenia, catatonic type.

*Presenting Picture.* When admitted to Greystone in January, 1933, the patient was described as disturbed, delusional, and a suicidal risk.

*Present Illness.* The onset of pathologic behavior was abrupt, leading to admission three days after the original symptoms appeared. A few days after he had been refused in a proposal of marriage he complained of being nauseated and asked to have someone accompany him in making his round of deliveries for a local bakery. That afternoon he was picked up by the authorities because he was acting "queerly." He was brought home by his family, but he refused to eat and retired early, saying that he was afraid. Early in the morning he awakened and began to scream, praying and talking to the Saints, pouring water over his head, and running naked around the house until a sedative was given by a local physician. His bizarre behavior continued for the next two days, culminating in a leap through his bedroom window, which led to his admission to the hospital.

*Previous Personality Disorders.* There were no previous personality disorders.

*Family History.* The patient's parents came to the United States from Italy in 1913, remaining aliens. His father was a janitor who led a very narrow social life and who was "quick-tempered." His mother was an amiable woman whose background was similar to her husband's. The patient was the oldest of six children (including an adopted daughter). One daughter (second eldest) became mentally ill in 1935 and was in a hospital at the time of the patient's admission. The fourth child, a boy, was hospitalized in an army hospital overseas for mental illness. There was little information on the family life, except that the patient got along well with all concerned and "never gave any trouble."

*Personal History.* The patient was born in Italy in August, 1906, weighing 10 pounds at birth. Delivery was normal. Development also was supposedly normal. The patient entered kindergarten at five in Italy and again at seven when he arrived in the United States. As a child he raised pigeons and played the violin, but he was never interested in athletics and had few childhood friends. In later years he expressed disapproval of "the way young men spend their spare time." At the age of fourteen he left the seventh grade to become a baker's helper, since his father was unemployed at the time. He was interested in only one girl whom he had courted for two years before she rejected him, prior to the onset of his illness.

*Personality.* The personality description as supplied was meager, but indicated an undemonstrative, unconfiding man who took pride in his high moral and ethical standards.

*Hospital Course.* On admission in January, 1933, the patient was overproductive, assaultive, noisy, and disoriented. He was maintained on a disturbed ward for three months, during which time he was the victim of hallucinations. By April, 1933, he had improved without specific treatment and was transferred to a private sanatorium from which he was paroled. He adjusted satisfactorily to work at home, but in November, 1934, he was readmitted with symptoms as before. In his delusions he identified himself with animals and talked at great length about extramarital sexual relations with women. Affect was always appropriate, though generally flattened. Metrazol convulsions were induced in October, 1938, but twenty-eight convulsions gave no improvement and the subject developed a catatonic-like stupor with coarse tremors of the extremities, rigidity, and mutism occurring intermittently in episodes lasting one to two weeks. Metrazol convulsions were induced in March, 1943, without effect.

*Mental Status.* The patient was lying in bed expressionless and supine with his head flexed on his chest. He followed movements with his eyes, but did not turn his head, and displayed a marked startle reaction but did not speak. His hands were held at his sides with thumbs flexed under the palms and protruding between the third and fourth fingers. A coarse, rhythmical, symmetrical tremor of the legs was present, which disappeared or diminished when the patient was distracted. On passive movement resistance was encountered which disappeared with distraction. After the intravenous administration of 5 grains of sodium amytal, the motor phenomena disappeared and the patient acquired a fixed grin. He sat in a chair, dressed himself, walked about the ward, and talked, although he said only a few words. As the interview progressed the tremor returned in the left leg. He was preoccupied with the number "4" and wrote it on a sheet of paper, but no other content could be elicited. His emotional responses under amytal consisted of silly laughing and giggling, apparently in response to auditory hallucinations.

*Operation.* On May 23, 1947, area 6 was partially ablated bilaterally.

*Follow-Up Notes.* The patient had not responded by June 2, 1947, but when seen on June 24 he was able to go to the bathroom by himself and was eating in the dining room with other patients. His muscular rigidity was much less, he was able to answer simple questions in one or two words, and he was oriented for time and place.

Early in August, 1947, the patient again went into a stupor which lasted until a few days before the examination on August 26. At this time he showed an occasional coarse tremor of the right arm and his stream of mental activity was retarded, but he answered questions well stating that he had been mentally sick but was feeling better, although he still heard voices. He referred to his mother as "the boss," but said that he liked her. His affective responses were flattened and inappropriate at times, and there were periods of preoccupation.

On October 27, 1947, the patient was once more mute and posturing.

On October 28, 1947, a more complete excision of area 6 was carried out on the left. Thereafter the patient's psychiatric condition did not change and, after an unsteady postoperative course, he died of pneumonia on November 19, 1947.

**Patient 31.** *Age:* 51. *Sex:* female. *Marital status:* married. *Occupation:* housewife. *Religion:* Catholic. *Informant:* husband. *Diagnosis:* involutional psychosis, paranoid type.

*Presenting Picture.* In June, 1941, the patient was admitted to Greystone from an observation ward where she was described as depressed, affected by delusions, and violent.

*Present Illness.* The illness began in 1935 when the patient blamed herself for the accidental drowning of her stepson. She subsequently became depressed and wept frequently. At the same time menses became irregular, she slept poorly, and became suspicious of her husband's activities. Further progress of her suspicious trend forced her husband to give up many activities during the next four years, and on several occasions she accused other women of extramarital relations with him. Menses stopped in 1939; she became more religious, increasingly fearful of her children's safety, had many physical complaints, and gradually developed generalized fears that people were plotting against her. After wandering half clothed in the streets and making a suicidal gesture, she was hospitalized for observation.

*Previous Personality Disorders.* No personality disorders had been noted prior to the present illness.

*Family History.* The patient's "high-strung and stubborn" father was a German-born marble polisher who died in 1929, at the age of seventy-two. Her mother was twelve years younger than her father and was still living. The patient was the third of four children. The youngest daughter was described as "extremely nervous," and two cousins had had serious mental illnesses. The patient had never had a good relationship with her mother, but always got along well with her father and mother-in-law.

*Personal History.* The patient's birth (September, 1896) and subsequent development in New York were supposedly normal. She had pneumonia with empyema when seven years of age. The onset of menses was not marked by any unusual reactions known to the informant. At thirteen she left the eighth grade to work as a domestic, and subsequently she worked as an operator in an embroidery factory. For ten years before her marriage she worked at a biscuit factory. At the age of twenty-five she married a widower, one year her senior, who was a police detective. He had a son by his first marriage. The couple had a son and daughter, the first child being born when the patient was twenty-eight and the second when she was thirty-four. The patient adopted her husband's religion and the marriage was apparently a happy one. She did not show favoritism among the children, though she worried excessively about all of them.

*Personality.* The patient's pre-illness personality was one marked by excitability, apprehension, suspicion, and jealousy. She was untrusting in many social situations, and unable to form close friendships.

*Hospital Course.* The hospital notes indicated only that the patient was cooperative after admission and that she attributed her illness to the "change of life." Three weeks after admission insulin coma and electroshock treatments were instituted, following which the patient improved and was paroled. She was discharged one year later as recovered. She was readmitted in November, 1945, and made a good adjustment on the ward, although she was depressed, restless, and at times disheveled. Insight and judgment remained defective. In 1947 she began working in the hospital cafeteria, but when she attempted to go home she was transferred to a less privileged ward. At this time she was seclusive, tense, agitated, and argumentative, but no longer had hallucinations or active delusions. In March, 1947, she lacerated her throat in a suicidal attempt.

*Mental Status.* On the ward this patient was agitated and appeared depressed. In the interview she was slightly overproductive, appeared anxious and depressed, and expressed feelings of helplessness. No hallucinations were elicited, but the thought content consisted of poorly organized, sexually colored, persecutory delusions directed against her and her daughter. She also expressed numerous fears about her children and suspicions about her husband's activity. Sensorium was clear and she was correctly oriented but lacking insight.

*Operation.* On May 29, 1947, area 9 was removed bilaterally.

*Follow-Up Notes.* The examinations made June 2, and June 5, 1947, revealed the absence of agitation so prominent before operation. The patient was responsive, though somewhat confused, and the old fears and delusions were no longer present. Ground parole was granted.

On June 25, 1947, she continued to be calm and pleasant, conversing with other patients, and reading. Her appetite and sleeping habits were good. Her mental content was similar to that before operation, but it was not disturbing to her, and she expressed her old fears as things which *might* happen rather than as events which had already occurred. Mild confusion still persisted.

On August 26, 1947, the patient continued to be calm and cooperative and was on ground parole. She remained confused, however, and the paranoid trend continued as before operation, though it was not accompanied by the former affect. She doubted that her son was really her own child and talked of various methods to test his genuineness.

After one day at home the patient was returned to the hospital by her husband because he felt her judgment in running the house was not adequate. When interviewed on January 18, 1948, the patient was correctly oriented and replied logically to questions. However, she believed that something had been "done" to her son and that he was not really her offspring, though she had not discussed it with him because, as she said, "I would not want to hurt him." Her affective responses were not unusual.

On May 7, 1948, affect remained appropriate, but the patient was rambling, circumstantial, and diffuse paranoid projections were present relating to the Catholic Church, the sexual behavior of teachers, her daughter, other patients, and her husband. She was correctly oriented. She was considerably agitated and was on a more disturbed ward.

**Patient 32.**  *Age:* 41.  *Sex:* female.  *Marital status:* married.  *Occupation:* secretary.  *Religion:* Protestant.  *Informant:* husband.  *Diagnosis:* manic-depressive psychosis, manic.

*Presenting Picture.*  The patient was first admitted to Greystone in January, 1935. At that time she was self-condemning and a suicidal risk.

*Present Illness.*  In January, 1935, she began to have terrifying dreams and stated that she was fighting against a recurrence of her former illness. She felt inadequate to take care of her child, wept, and complained of fatigue, nausea, and poor appetite. The onset of symptoms coincided with the period when her child was to have been returned to her care, after a lengthy period of care by the grandparents.

*Previous Personality Disorders.*  Late in 1933, after financial reverses in the family, the patient complained of fatigue and said that something terrible was going to happen. She was unable to sleep, had terrifying dreams, and feared that someone would take her baby away. After a six-months' hospitalization beginning in June, 1934, she was discharged as well.

*Family History.*  The patient's American-born parents were both living at the time of admission. Her father was a policeman. Neither parent had had any emotional illnesses. The patient had two older sisters, one a nurse, and the other the wife of a clerk, as well as a younger brother who was a clerk. All were in good health. Four maternal uncles were described as excessive drinkers.

*Personal History.*  The patient was born in a small town in Pennsylvania in June, 1906. The facts of her early development were not known. She began school at six and completed high school at seventeen, with a good school record. Menstruation began at sixteen and was regular but painful. After high school she attended business school, and then worked as a stenographer. She attended a school for missionaries for one year but then returned to secretarial work until her marriage in 1930 (at the age of twenty-four). Her husband was an electrical engineer, one year her junior.

During 1932-1933 the couple were separated for economic reasons but the marriage was successful until the onset of the illness. One (wanted) boy was born in March, 1933.

*Personality.* Outstanding traits appeared to be labile temper, extravagance, and financial irresponsibility. The patient was a neat housekeeper. She was very much interested in her religion and in household hobbies such as knitting and sewing.

*Hospital Course.* The 1935 admission was one marked chiefly by depression and retardation. The patient rejected her baby and expressed fears about him. Mild persecutory ideas were also present ("dope in the food") as well as terror dreams in which she killed her mother and child. The depression lifted in one month. She was paroled in two months and discharged after a year.

In April, 1941, the patient was readmitted with an interval history of a borderline depressive adjustment until she became pregnant in the spring of 1936. The following June she again became depressed and, after a brief private hospitalization, a second child was born by cesarean section and her tubes were tied. After several brief fluctuations of mood she was hospitalized at another state hospital for six months for a confused and depressed reaction which was treated with seventeen metrazol injections. She was well on her release and remained in equilibrium until December, 1940, when short episodes of depression and overactivity appeared. Suicidal thoughts were present at times but hallucinations were never noted. Her second Greystone admission was ended by parole in May, 1941, after lifting of the retardation and depression. She was readmitted in August, 1941, with similar symptoms and was again paroled in October, 1941, August, 1942, and on two occasions during 1943. In April, 1944, she was returned to the hospital and since that date she has remained a patient continuously except for a few short visits. Manic behavior was present in 1944 with irritability, overactivity, and frequent changes of interest.

*Mental Status.* On the ward the patient was gay and talkative, often dancing and joking with other patients. At times she became overactive, irritable, and destructive. She was distractible and elated when interviewed. Her thought content was marked by hostility directed against her mother and husband, feelings of inadequacy about caring for her children, and an immature appraisal of sex. No delusional trends or hallucinations could be elicited. She was well oriented, her sensorium was clear, and she had some insight into the nature of her illness.

*Operation.* On June 6, 1947, area 9 and part of areas 8 and 10 were removed bilaterally.

*Follow-Up Notes.* The patient was interviewed on June 27, 1947. After operation she was usually cooperative but she continued to be superficially gay, elated, irritable, and at times resistive. Affective responses did not appear to be changed. She continued to express resentment, particularly toward her husband and other men. She remained well oriented and there was no clinically observable impairment of intellect.

On August 28, 1947, any change noted was only slight and in the direction of decreased irritability and hostility.

On January 17, 1948, no further change was noted and it was felt that operation had made her neither worse nor better.

At the time of examination on May 7, 1948, the patient's behavior on the ward was occasionally sarcastic and noisy but she was not overactive when interviewed. Thought content included the previous material about her husband, men, and sex but in addition she said that she believed she was pregnant and she made several references to God and to faith. It appeared that a depressive element was present for the first time but any such change was slight. There was flight of ideas and the patient was quite overproductive.

**Patient 40.** *Age:* 29. *Sex:* female. *Marital status:* single. *Occupation:* salesgirl. *Religion:* Catholic, *Informants:* mother, brother. *Diagnosis:* schizophrenia, paranoid type.

*Presenting Picture.* The patient was described as being hypochondriacal and depressed when admitted in June, 1943.

*Present Illness.* About two months before admission the patient became inefficient in her work, made frequent errors, and complained of excessive fatigue. She became irritable, gave up her job, and complained of pain in her abdomen and throat. After consulting her family physician and a priest, she entered the hospital voluntarily.

*Previous Personality Disorders.* There were no indications of personality disorders prior to the present illness.

*Family History.* The patient's father was an Irish-born coal-miner who died at the age of seventy-five of "asthma." His wife was twenty years younger than he, a rather unintelligent, passive woman who was still living at the time of the patient's admission. The patient was the fifth of five children and the only girl. The oldest brother died in infancy but the other brothers were all married and in good mental health.

*Personal History.* The patient was born in New Jersey in July, 1918, weighing 8½ pounds at birth. She was a full-term baby. She walked and talked at fourteen months but was a feeding problem during her first year. Enuresis persisted until she was two to three years of age and recurred with the onset of her illness. As a child she had severe temper tantrums and was considered "high-strung." She obeyed only her father and preferred to be alone rather than to play with other children. Menarche took place when she was twelve and menses were always regular and not uncomfortable. She began school at the age of six and completed the third year of high school at seventeen or eighteen, leaving school when her father died. Although she had always done well in school she lost interest in her work and became quite depressed on her father's death. Thereafter she worked as a baby-sitter, waitress, domestic servant, and 5-and-10-cent-store clerk, changing jobs frequently. She was casually interested in several men and engaged to one for six years although the couple quarreled frequently. She had no sexual education at home and the paternal attitude toward sex was severely moralistic. In her adult years she had many somatic complaints.

*Personality.* The patient was described as being shy but tactless, fault-finding, and stubborn. She was sensitive to criticism of her figure. She had few interests although she enjoyed reading "pulp" magazines and listening to the radio.

*Hospital Course.* The patient's first hospitalization lasted only one month. She was discharged in July, 1943, as recovered, having had no specific treatment. In August, 1944, she was readmitted and was once more seclusive and hypochondriacal. Her return to Greystone was arranged after she had been admitted for an appendectomy at a local hospital but had become unmanageable and panicky. In Greystone she constantly sought medical examinations attributing her complaints to such things as a "nonfunctioning stomach valve" and "too much Lugol's solution." Insulin comas were instituted in November, 1944, but this treatment was discontinued when the patient became extremely fearful. In January, 1945, she was paroled but returned in October presenting the same picture as on previous admission. A course of forty-three insulin comas was started the same month. During treatment she made a general improvement although she began to express persecutory ideas for the first time. She was paroled in January, 1946, but at home she was markedly suspicious and expressed ideas of reference. This paranoid trend expanded until it was necessary (November, 1946) that she be returned to Greystone.

*Mental Status.* The patient was neatly dressed. She was generally cooperative but suspicious. Affect was displayed mainly in the form of hostility and she was not unusually productive of speech. The thoughts centered about physical complaints (such as pain in the leg, weakness, anemia, and nausea) and persecutory delusions. The latter involved ideas that she was being poisoned and that she was marked for rape. She was markedly hostile toward the physicians. Although the sensorium was clear and she was correctly oriented, insight was completely lacking.

*Operation.* On June 2, 1947, a partial removal of area 24 was carried out bilaterally.

*Follow-Up Notes.* The patient was examined on June 4, 1947. Her immediate post-operative course was stormy and marked by severe vomiting, including hematemesis. She was markedly retarded, confused, and semistuporous much of the time.

The patient was again interviewed on July 4, 1947. After a period of uninhibited aggressive behavior she had returned to a condition similar to that which was present before operation. Her delusional system remained unchanged and she continued to be critical, but somatic complaints were less prominent. Her affective responses were unchanged.

Further examinations were made on September 9, 1947, January 18, 1948, and May 7, 1948. No change from the condition of July 4 was noted during this period except that the delusional material was extracted with less difficulty than formerly. The patient continued to be suspicious, defensive, and sarcastic.

**Patient 44.** *Age:* 38. *Sex:* female. *Marital status:* married. *Occupation:* book-keeper. *Religion:* Catholic. *Informant:* husband. *Diagnosis:* schizophrenia, hebe-phrenic type.

*Presenting Picture.* The patient was admitted to a general hospital in September, 1942, and transferred to Greystone after two weeks during which she was agitated and having hallucinations.

*Present Illness.* After the extraction of all her teeth, six months before admission, the patient was fearful of dying. Subsequently she complained of headaches, was irritable during her menses, and was sexually more eager. Thereafter she became "confused," developed ideas of reference, and was admitted to a general hospital.

*Previous Personality Disorders.* No personality disorders had been manifest prior to the present illness.

*Family History.* The patient's father was a stockbroker who became mentally ill in 1911 and drowned in 1912. The patient's mother was sixty-six years of age at the time of the patient's admission. She had been in a mental hospital for more than twenty years, the diagnosis being "dementia praecox, paranoid type." An older brother and sister of the patient were in good health. The patient was always more fond of her sister than of her brother.

*Personal History.* This patient was born in New Jersey in February, 1909. It is known that she was enuretic until she was ten years old and that she had frequent nightmares after her father's death which occurred when the patient was three. For a few years the patient and her brother were placed in a foster home, and then were left to look after themselves while their mother worked. During the early years a maternal uncle made frequent sexual advances to the patient's mother and in later years to the patient although intercourse between him and the patient never actually occurred. The patient began school at seven, was bright, and skipped at least one grade. After grammar school she went to business school, worked as a bookkeeper for three years and, at the age of twenty, married. Her husband was nine months her junior and an insurance clerk. The marriage was happy although the patient was sexually timid. The first child, a girl, was a surprise to the patient and she tried unsuccessfully to abort the second. Thereafter she often refused sexual relations and her husband began to drink excessively although not enough to interfere with his job.

*Personality.* The description given was that of a quiet, rather shy woman who worried excessively about small things and who was interested chiefly in her home.

*Hospital Course.* On admission the patient was untidy, disoriented, and had hal-lucinations. At times she was assaultive. After two months insulin, electroshock, and metrazol treatments were given with improvement during treatment but immediate relapse when it was stopped. Shock therapy was resumed in February, 1943, and was followed by the disappearance of hallucinations and delusions. The patient was paroled but remained home only one week. Until she was transferred to the project she was untidy, seclusive, uncooperative, and assaultive at times. She was obviously responding to auditory hallucinations.

*Mental Status.* The patient was unkempt, restless, and preoccupied. Her mood appeared to be labile and superficial but no subjective description could be obtained. She was obviously responding to auditory hallucinations as indicated by her attitudinizing. Her stream of speech was mumbling. She was frequently facetious or irrelevant. For example, in response to the question, "How are you feeling?" she answered, "With hands. My friends asked me to come in and settle the dispute about the gorilla." She was oriented for person and place but not for situation or time.

*Operation.* On June 4, 1947, area 47 was removed bilaterally.

*Follow-Up Notes.* For one day after operation much of the psychotic material disappeared but the preoperation mental picture soon returned. On interview on July 4, 1947, this patient appeared to be the same as before operation.

Further interviews took place on September 9, and October 20, 1947. Throughout this period the patient continued to be impulsive, irritable, disoriented, silly, and to have hallucinations.

On October 28, 1947, a bilateral prefrontal lobotomy was performed.

On interviews of October 30, and November 3, 1947, it was noted that the patient continued to be silly, inappropriate, disoriented, and to have hallucinations. Perseveration was also noted on the interview of October 30.

On January 18, March 14, and May 7, 1948, the symptoms continued as before but the patient was responding almost constantly to hallucinations and it was almost impossible to make contact with her.

**Patient 47.** *Age:* 31. *Sex:* female. *Marital status:* single. *Occupation:* dye worker. *Religion:* Protestant. *Informants:* mother, friend. *Diagnosis:* schizophrenia, hebephrenic type.

*Presenting Picture.* On admission to Greystone in January, 1942, the patient was described as excited, destructive, and disoriented.

*Present Illness.* One day in January, 1942, the patient began to complain of fatigue and appeared to have lost interest in her boy friends. The next day she acted as though dazed, made unintelligible conversation, and was at times noisy and denudative. Her unpredictable behavior continued and she was admitted to an observation ward within a week after the initial onset of symptoms.

*Previous Personality Disorders.* There were no personality disorders prior to the present illness.

*Family History.* The patient's father was an Italian-born Presbyterian minister who died in 1915 (at the age of thirty-six) of pneumonia. He was supposedly unusually intelligent and sociable, although quick-tempered. The patient's mother was nine years younger than her husband. After the father's death her mother married an Italian jeweler who was described in opposite terms by the two informants. The patient was an only child by the first marriage, but there were two half-brothers by the second marriage. The younger had a stormy adolescence but was doing well when the patient was admitted. There was a history of alcoholism in one maternal uncle and of severe mental illness in another. A paternal aunt was also mentally ill.

*Personal History.* The patient was born in New Jersey in December, 1915. Birth was difficult but development was not unusual. She started school at five and almost completed high school, leaving in her fourth year to take a business course. She soon gave this up in order to work with the co-informant. The patient was interested in boys at fourteen and there was much family strife about this since her stepfather opposed this interest. One informant stated that the patient's stepfather had sexual relations with her during this period but this was not confirmed. The patient wanted to marry at sixteen, but this was opposed by her mother. For five years before admission she worked in dye factories with the co-informant who was married and had several children. She had regular sexual intercourse with him during this period and it was said that her sexual responses were normal. She tried many times to induce him to divorce his wife but he was unwilling to take this step.

*Personality.* Both informants agreed that the patient was stubborn and sensitive to criticism although they disagreed on other personality traits.

*Hospital Course.* On admission the patient was noisy, overactive, and disoriented. She complained that people were watching her and that she had been discriminated against on the job. In May, insulin, electric shock, and metrazol treatments were started. There was great improvement during the treatments but immediate relapse when treatments were stopped. For four and a half years the patient remained essentially the same, her behavior being marked by excitement and assaultiveness.

*Mental Status.* The patient was neatly dressed and well groomed. When seated she looked from side to side and over her shoulder and periodically broke out in spontaneous, rapid, illogical talk which was delivered in the manner of a soap-box orator. She was neither depressed nor elated. The thought content was inappropriate to the questions asked and was apparently dissociated from the environment. Her talk ran along these lines: "Anyone looked on Mrs. Murphy's—once close on human, there is never any other statement—public or private, Roosevelt the service is necessary." There was frequent mention of registration, doctors, presidents, women's suffrage, and words like "toxic," "lay," "rectum," and "teeth" occurred frequently. Orientation, information, and insight could not be tested.

*Operation.* On May 28, 1947, area 44 was removed bilaterally.

*Follow-Up Notes.* On May 29, 1947, one day after operation, the patient was not alert but she spoke with no speech defect.

Interviews were made on the following dates: June 2, 4, 25; September 9, 1947; January 1, and May 7, 1948. Throughout the one-year postoperative period this patient showed no clinical improvement. She continued to have hallucinations and to be manneristic. Her word salad continued as it had before operation and her affective responses remained unchanged.

## IMPROVEMENT GRAPHS

Any criteria of improvement have many shortcomings. In evaluating improvement, we found the only objective criterion was a comparison of the patient's preoperative with his postoperative social status. The principal shortcoming of this scheme is that individual differences between patients are not shown. For example, the recovered schizophrenic still has basic schizoid traits, even though he may be working, and these are not present in the patient who has recovered from an affective psychosis. Likewise, patients with residual organic changes may be able to work. These individual variations are more apparent in the case abstracts and will also be discussed in more detail in the material to follow.

**Scale of Improvement.** The following scale for measuring improvement was devised:

Patients on most disturbed ward—5
Patients on moderately disturbed ward—4
Patients still institutionalized but on ground parole—3
Patients at home under supervision—2
Patients at home and working or capable of working—1.

The improvement rating was the difference between the postoperative and the preoperative score. All of these stages are not of equal importance. For example, if a patient moved from a greatly disturbed to a less disturbed ward he was given the same score as the patient who moved from ground parole to home, even though his improvement was less significant. To more evenly balance this scale, the following weighted score was devised:

One additional bonus point was given for each of the following:
1. A change from the most disturbed ward to ground parole
2. A move from any place in the hospital to home
3. The ability to work at reduced capacity
4. The ability to work at former capacity.

On the original score, therefore, it was possible for a patient to gain a maximum of four points by moving from the most disturbed ward to a job at his former capacity. With the additional four bonus points, the maximal improvement became eight.

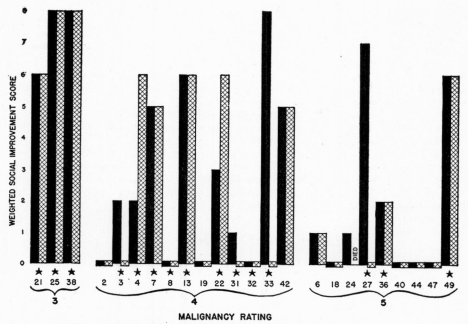

Fig. 103.   Figure correlating clinical improvement seven and one-half months and one year after operation with the estimated malignancy of the psychosis.

**Correlation of Diagnosis and Clinical Improvement with Area Removed.** The clinician is aware that the diagnostic category into which the patient falls is of considerable significance in judging a patient's chance of improving. The patient with an agitated depression on a disturbed ward has a much better prognosis than an equally disturbed deteriorated schizophrenic. In figure 103 the improvement according to the weighted scale is shown on each patient. In addition, patients are grouped according to the malignancy of their psychosis. Patients with a purely affective psychosis were graded as 3. Those with schizophrenic features plus considerable affect and with little evidence of deterioration were graded as 4, and those with schizophrenia with deterioration were graded as 5. The stars on this graph indicate the patients who had the region of areas 9, 10, and 46 included in the operative removal. The reason for singling out this region becomes clear in table 78.

In table 78 the patients have been arranged according to degree of clinical improvement and the area or areas removed are indicated opposite the case number. This table is based on the condition of the patient seven and one-half months after operation. At one year following operation, 3 of the patients were not as well as at seven and one-half months and 2 others had shown

TABLE 78. CORRELATION OF THE DEGREE OF CLINICAL IMPROVEMENT WITH AREA REMOVED

| Degree of improvement (weighted social score) at 7½ months | Case No. | Areas involved† | | | | | | | | | | | Weighted social rating at one year‡ |
|---|---|---|---|---|---|---|---|---|---|---|---|---|---|
| | | 6 | 8 | 9 | 10 | 11 | 24 | 32 | 44 | 45 | 46 | 47 | |
| 8 | 25 | | x | x | a | | | | | | x | | 8 |
| | 33 | | | | a | | | | a | x | a | | 0− |
| | 38 | b | b | b | | | | | | | | | 8 |
| 7 | 27 | a | a | a | a | | | | | | | | 0− |
| 6 | 49 | | | | x | a | | | | | a | | 6 |
| | 13 | | | a | a | | | | | x | x | | 6 |
| | 21 | | | | x | | | | | | | | 6 |
| 5 | 7 | | x | a | a | | | | | | | | 5 |
| | 42 | | | | | x | | | | | | | 5 |
| 3 | 22 | | | x | x | | | | | | x | | 6+ |
| 2 | 3 | a | | a | | | | | | | | | 0− |
| | 4 | | | | a | | | | | | x | | 6+ |
| | 36 | | | | x | x | | | | x | x | x | 2 |
| 1 | 6 | a | a | | | | | | | | | | 1 |
| | 24 | a | | | | | | | | | | | died |
| | 31 | | | | x | | | | | | | | 0− |
| 0 | 2 | a | x | | | | | | | | | | 0 |
| | 8 | a | a | a | a | | | | | | | | 0 |
| | 18 | | | | | x | | | | | | | 0 |
| | 19 | | | | | | | | | x | | | 0 |
| | 32 | | a | x | a | | | | | | | | 0 |
| | 40 | | | | | | x | | | | | | 0 |
| | 44 | | | | a | | | | | | | x | 0 |
| | 47 | | | | | | | | x | | | | 0 |

* In comparing this table with tables 41 and 59 see page 78.
† x, Indicates complete removal; a, indicates partial removal; b, indicates venous ligation.
‡ Plus sign following the social rating at one year indicates that the patient improved over his or her seven-month rating; minus sign indicates the patient became worse.

continued improvement. The improvement rating at one year after operation is shown in the last column; those who continued to improve are indicated with a plus sign (+) and those who became worse are indicated with a minus sign (−).

Using the weighted scale, a score of 3 or more is considered an indication of significant benefit and comparing those patients with a 3 to 8 weighted score with those patients whose score was 2 or less, we find that areas 9, 10, and 46 are the only ones which appear more often in the benefited group than they appear in the relatively unbenefited group. Area 9 appears six times in the benefited group, as against four times in the unbenefited. Similarly, the figures for area 10 are five times as against two and the figures for area 46 are four as against three. In contrast, all other areas, except 11, are represented only in the unimproved group or are represented in equal numbers in the two groups. It thus appears that the general region which produced significant clinical improvement is that which includes areas 9, 10, and 46. Since many of the patients had several areas removed in combination, it has not been possible to make finer distinctions. We cannot say from the figures alone whether area 9 is more important than area 10 or whether area 46 is less important than the other two, although several considerations make it appear that this may actually be the case. Area 11 is the only other area which produced significant improvement (in 1 patient) and this deserves further investigation even though 2 other patients showed no improvement when the same area was removed.

Table 79 shows the correlation between diagnosis and clinical improvement and the relationship to area removed.

Several points stand out. Most important is the superiority of the operation implicating the region of areas 9, 10, and 46, which improved 9 patients three points or more at seven and one-half months and 8 patients at one year, and failed to produce improvement of at least three points in only 6 patients at seven and one-half months and 7 patients at one year following operation. This is contrasted to improvement in only 1 patient (and this seems to have been spontaneous) and failure in 8 following removal of other areas.

The figure of 4 patients improved without operation is no longer valid. One of these 4 patients, a paranoid, received shock treatment when he became very disturbed. His improvement from this was only temporary and his psychotic symptoms returned at about seven months following operation. Another improved after developing lobar pneumonia but only slightly, although he was able to leave the hospital. Actually, only 3 patients have maintained spontaneous improvement and only one is gainfully employed. This makes the over-all ratio of patients able to leave the hospital between the operatee and control group 9:3.

Seven months following operation, 11 operatees were at home and 10 (or 42 percent) were working at old capacity and could be considered much improved. At one year following operation, 9 were at home, 8 working at old capacity. This figure is as high as those generally reported for lobotomy. When it is considered that many of the twenty-four operations, that is, those which did not implicate areas 9, 10, and 46, were ineffective, this figure becomes even more impressive.

Seventeen of the 24 patients operated upon were schizophrenics. Seven, or 41 percent, are now working at old capacity. At one year following operation this dropped to five, or 30 percent. All who were working had the regions of 9, 10, and 46 included in the operation. Only 3 schizophrenics in whom areas 9, 10, and 46 were included were not working at seven and one-half months and at one year, 5 patients who had this operation were unable to work. This series is too small to make much of this impressive 50 percent improvement in schizophrenics. In contrast, however, an over-all review of results with lobotomy in schizophrenics between 1936 and 1942, by Walker, showed that 18 percent made social recoveries. A recent report by Freeman

TABLE 79. CORRELATION OF IMPROVEMENT[a] WITH DIAGNOSIS

| | Total number in diagnostic category | | Improved 3 points or more following area 9, 10, 46 removal | | Improved 3 points or more after removal of other areas | | Improved 3 points or more without operation | | Improved less than 3 points following area 9, 10, 46 removal | | Improved less than 3 points after removal of other areas | | Improved less than 3 points without operation | |
|---|---|---|---|---|---|---|---|---|---|---|---|---|---|---|
| | 7½ mos. postop. | 1 yr. postop. | 7½ mos. postop. | 1 yr. postop. | 7½ mos. postop. | 1 yr. postop. | 7½ mos. postop. | 1 yr. postop. | 7½ mos. postop. | 1 yr. postop. | 7½ mos. postop. | 1 yr. postop. | 7½ mos. postop. | 1 yr. postop. |
| Schizophrenia, all types | 39 | 38 | 6 | 5 | 0 | 0 | 3 | 2 | 3 | 4 | 8 | 7 | 19 | 20 |
| Schizophrenia, paranoid type | 14 | 14 | 4 | 5 | 0 | 0 | 2 | 1 | 3 | 2 | 1 | 1 | 4 | 5 |
| Schizophrenia, catatonic type | 4 | 3 | 1 | 0 | 0 | 0 | 0 | 0 | 0 | 1 | 1 | 0[c] | 2 | 2 |
| Schizophrenia, hebephrenic type | 20 | 20 | 1 | 0 | 0 | 0 | 1 | 1 | 0 | 1 | 5 | 5 | 13[b] | 13 |
| Schizophrenia, other types | 1 | 1 | 0 | 0 | 0 | 0 | 0 | 0 | 0 | 0 | 1 | 1 | 0 | 0 |
| Manic-depressive psychosis | 5 | 5 | 2 | 2 | 1 | 1 | 1 | 1 | 1 | 1 | 0 | 0 | 0 | 0 |
| Involutional psychosis | 3 | 3 | 1[b] | 1 | 0 | 0 | 0 | 0 | 2 | 2 | 0 | 0 | 0 | 0 |
| Psychopathic personality (schizoid) | 1 | 1 | 0 | 0 | 0 | 0 | 0 | 0 | 0 | 0 | 0 | 0 | 1 | 1 |
| Total | 48 | 47 | 9 | 8 | 1 | 1 | 4 | 3 | 6 | 7 | 8 | 7 | 20 | 21 |

[a] Improvement measured by weighted social score.
[b] Organic brain disease coexisting in one patient.
[c] One patient dead at one year (patient 24).

and Watts indicated that about one third of their lobotomized schizophrenics have made social recoveries.

SUMMARY

1. All but 1 patient who showed marked clinical improvement had regions of areas 9, 10, and 46 removed at operation.

2. Over-all statistical results in this small series compare favorably with other types of surgery in the treatment of the psychoses.

CORRELATION OF FACTORS IN THE PATIENTS' BACKGROUNDS WITH IMPROVEMENT

In the following graphs and tables, various factors in the patients' background and in the operation itself have been arranged to indicate their relationship, if any, to the clinical course after operation. Correlating data for area removed, diagnosis, and malignancy rating have already been considered and will not be taken up here.

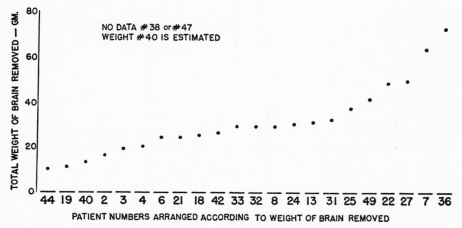

FIG. 104. Distribution of patients according to weight of cortex removed at operation.

In figure 104 the weight of brain removed has been plotted on the ordinate and the case numbers of the operatees arranged on the abscissa from left to right in increasing order of weight of brain removed. A reverse S curve results, showing that the usual amount of tissue removed was 20 to 40 gm. and that 5 patients had a smaller amount removed and 5 other patients had larger amounts ablated. If any direct relationship exists between weight of brain removed and clinical results, then a similar curve should appear when the values of the weighted social improvement score are substituted for the weight of brain removed. This has been done in figure 105 and it is apparent that no simple or direct relationship exists between the amount of cortex removed and the clinical change seen following operation.

In the following series of tables, a consistent arrangement has been used in which total figures are given first, followed by the data on significantly improved patients and then by the data on unimproved patients. Figures are given at seven and one-half months and one year after operation. All the tables suffer from the weakness which accompanies any comparison of a small group of patients, but some trends do appear which may serve to direct the attention of investigators in other projects of this type. In a larger series such tables should be drawn up separately for the various diagnostic categories, but this was not possible with such a small group and the data have (reluctantly) been treated *en masse*. The discussion centers around those patients who had areas 9, 10, or 46 removed since the remaining patients were generally an inert group as far as clinical improvement was concerned.

Table 80 indicates that the sex of the patient was not a determining factor in the response to operation. Thirty males and 18 females were studied in the series and, allowing for differences in the operative procedure which was performed, comparison does not indicate that the sex of the patient played a role in the therapeutic response to operation.

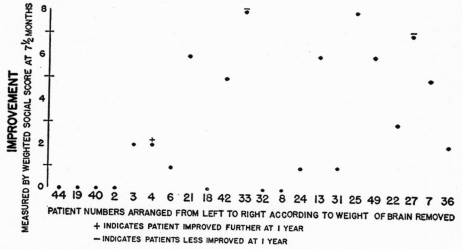

FIG. 105.  Comparison of patients, indicating the lack of correlation between weight of brain removed and degree of clinical improvement.

Tables 81, 82, and 83 present the data on age at the time of operation, age at onset of illness, and duration of the illness up to the time of operation. The figures suggest that those patients in the older age group and those who had their illnesses more than ten years did less well than the younger patients and those having a shorter period of illness, but no definite conclusions can be drawn from this small number of patients.

The type of illness is presented in table 84 where the patients are classified as having insidious, acute, or probably acute onsets. The figures do not indicate any noticeable trend nor do they appear to relate to the factor of precipitating stress. Data for the latter are given in table 85.

In table 86 the data on previous spontaneous remissions are presented. For this table a spontaneous remission was arbitrarily defined as a home visit of six months or longer which was not induced by shock treatment. There is nothing in the figures which would suggest that the therapeutic effects of topectomy are related to the patient's previous history of remissions. On the contrary, 6 of 9 patients who had had no spontaneous remissions were much benefited at seven and one-half months (5 out of 9 at the end of one year). It is interesting to note in this connection that the only patient showing a great

TABLE 80. CORRELATION OF IMPROVEMENT[a] WITH SEX

| | Total number in sex grouping | | Improved 3 points or more following area 9, 10, 46 removal | | Improved 3 points or more after removal of other areas | | Improved 3 points or more without operation | | Improved less than 3 points following area 9, 10, 46 removal | | Improved less than 3 points after removal of other areas | | Improved less than 3 points without operation | |
|---|---|---|---|---|---|---|---|---|---|---|---|---|---|---|
| | 7½ mos. postop. | 1 yr. postop. | 7½ mos. postop. | 1 yr. postop. | 7½ mos. postop. | 1 yr. postop. | 7½ mos. postop. | 1 yr. postop. | 7½ mos. postop. | 1 yr. postop. | 7½ mos. postop. | 1 yr. postop. | 7½ mos. postop. | 1 yr. postop. |
| Male............ | 30 | 29 | 6 | 6 | 0 | 0 | 2 | 1 | 3 | 3 | 5 | 4[b] | 14 | 15 |
| Female.......... | 18 | 18 | 3 | 2 | 1 | 1 | 2 | 2 | 3 | 4 | 3 | 3 | 6 | 6 |
| Total........... | 48 | 47 | 9 | 8 | 1 | 1 | 4 | 3 | 6 | 7 | 8 | 7 | 20 | 21 |

[a] Improvement measured by weighted social score.
[b] One male patient dead at one year (patient 24).

TABLE 81. CORRELATION OF IMPROVEMENT[a] WITH AGE AT OPERATION

| | Total number in group | | Improved 3 points or more following area 9, 10, 46 removal | | Improved 3 points or more after removal of other areas | | Improved 3 points or more without operation | | Improved less than 3 points following area 9, 10, 46 removal | | Improved less than 3 points after removal of other areas | | Improved less than 3 points without operation | |
|---|---|---|---|---|---|---|---|---|---|---|---|---|---|---|
| | 7½ mos. postop. | 1 yr. postop. | 7½ mos. postop. | 1 yr. postop. | 7½ mos. postop. | 1 yr. postop. | 7½ mos. postop. | 1 yr. postop. | 7½ mos. postop. | 1 yr. postop. | 7½ mos. postop. | 1 yr. postop. | 7½ mos. postop. | 1 yr. postop. |
| 20–29 years......... | 8 | 8 | 1 | 0 | 0 | 0 | 0 | 0 | 1 | 2 | 1 | 1 | 5 | 5 |
| 30–39 years......... | 12 | 12 | 3 | 2 | 0 | 0 | 1 | 1 | 0 | 1 | 4 | 4 | 4 | 4 |
| 40–49 years......... | 15 | 14 | 3 | 3 | 1 | 1 | 2 | 1 | 1 | 1 | 2 | 1[b] | 6 | 7 |
| 50–61 years......... | 13 | 13 | 2 | 3 | 0 | 0 | 1 | 1 | 4 | 3 | 1 | 1 | 5 | 5 |
| Total.............. | 48 | 47 | 9 | 8 | 1 | 1 | 4 | 3 | 6 | 7 | 8 | 7 | 20 | 21 |

a Improvement measured by weighted social score.
b One patient dead at one year (patient 24).

398    PROBLEMS OF THE HUMAN FRONTAL LOBE

TABLE 82.  CORRELATION OF IMPROVEMENT[a] WITH DURATION OF ILLNESS

| | Total number in group | | Improved 3 points or more following area 9, 10, 46 removal | | Improved 3 points or more after removal of other areas | | Improved 3 points or more without operation | | Improved less than 3 points following area 9, 10, 46 removal | | Improved less than 3 points after removal of other areas | | Improved less than 3 points without operation | |
|---|---|---|---|---|---|---|---|---|---|---|---|---|---|---|
| | 7½ mos. postop. | 1 yr. postop. | 7½ mos. postop. | 1 yr. postop. | 7½ mos. postop. | 1 yr. postop. | 7½ mos. postop. | 1 yr. postop. | 7½ mos. postop. | 1 yr. postop. | 7½ mos. postop. | 1 yr. postop. | 7½ mos. postop. | 1 yr. postop. |
| 5 years or less[b] | 13 | 13 | 5 | 4 | 0 | 0 | 1 | 1 | 1 | 2 | 2 | 2 | 4 | 4 |
| 6 to 10 years[b] | 11 | 11 | 0 | 0 | 0 | 0 | 0 | 0 | 1 | 1 | 2 | 2 | 8 | 8 |
| More than 10 years[b] | 20 | 19 | 4 | 4 | 1 | 1 | 2 | 1 | 4 | 4 | 3 | 2[d] | 6 | 7 |
| Total | 44[c] | 43 | 9 | 8 | 1 | 1 | 3 | 2 | 6 | 7 | 7 | 6 | 18 | 19 |

a Improvement measured by weighted social score.
b Calculated from onset of symptoms, not first hospitalization.
c Patients 5, 15, 37, and 40 omitted because data are incomplete.
d One patient dead at one year (patient 24).

TABLE 83. CORRELATION OF IMPROVEMENT[a] WITH AGE AT ONSET OF ILLNESS

| | Total number in group | | Improved 3 points or more following area 9, 10, 46 removal | | Improved 3 points or more after removal of other areas | | Improved 3 points or more without operation | | Improved less than 3 points following area 9, 10, 46 removal | | Improved less than 3 points after removal of other areas | | Improved less than 3 points without operation | |
|---|---|---|---|---|---|---|---|---|---|---|---|---|---|---|
| | 7½ mos. postop. | 1 yr. postop. | 7½ mos. postop. | 1 yr. postop. | 7½ mos. postop. | 1 yr. postop. | 7½ mos. postop. | 1 yr. postop. | 7½ mos. postop. | 1 yr. postop. | 7½ mos. postop. | 1 yr. postop. | 7½ mos. postop. | 1 yr. postop. |
| Below 20 years..... | 7 | 7 | 2 | 2 | 1 | 1 | 0 | 0 | 0 | 0 | 0 | 0 | 4 | 4 |
| 20–29 years........ | 16 | 15 | 3 | 1 | 0 | 0 | 2 | 1 | 2 | 4 | 4 | 3[c] | 5 | 6 |
| 30–39 years........ | 13 | 13 | 2 | 2 | 0 | 0 | 1 | 1 | 1 | 1 | 3 | 3 | 6 | 6 |
| 40–56 years........ | 8 | 8 | 2 | 3 | 0 | 0 | 0 | 0 | 2 | 1 | 0 | 0 | 4 | 4 |
| Total............. | 44[b] | 43 | 9 | 8 | 1 | 1 | 3 | 2 | 5 | 6 | 7 | 6 | 19 | 20 |

[a] Improvement measured by weighted social score.
[b] Patients 5, 15, 37, 40 are omitted because data are incomplete.
[c] One patient dead at one year (patient 24).

TABLE 84.  CORRELATION OF IMPROVEMENT[a] WITH TYPE OF ONSET

| | Total number in group | | Improved 3 points or more following area 9, 10, 46 removal | | Improved 3 points or more after removal of other areas | | Improved 3 points or more without operation | | Improved less than 3 points following area 9, 10, 46 removal | | Improved less than 3 points after removal of other areas | | Improved less than 3 points without operation | |
|---|---|---|---|---|---|---|---|---|---|---|---|---|---|---|
| | 7½ mos. postop. | 1 yr. postop. | 7½ mos. postop. | 1 yr. postop. | 7½ mos. postop. | 1 yr. postop. | 7½ mos. postop. | 1 yr. postop. | 7½ mos. postop. | 1 yr. postop. | 7½ mos. postop. | 1 yr. postop. | 7½ mos. postop. | 1 yr. postop. |
| Onset, insidious.... | 25 | 25 | 5 | 5 | 1 | 1 | 1 | 1 | 5 | 5 | 5 | 5 | 8 | 8 |
| Onset, acute........ | 18 | 17 | 4 | 3 | 0 | 0 | 2 | 2 | 1 | 2 | 3 | 2[c] | 8 | 8 |
| Onset, probably acute............ | 4 | 4 | 0 | 0 | 0 | 0 | 1 | 0 | 0 | 0 | 0 | 0 | 3 | 4 |
| Total............. | 47[b] | 46 | 9 | 8 | 1 | 1 | 4 | 3 | 6 | 7 | 8 | 7 | 19 | 20 |

[a] Improvement measured by weighted social score.
[b] No data available on type of onset for patient 30.
[c] One patient dead at one year (patient 24).

TABLE 85. CORRELATION OF IMPROVEMENT[a] WITH FACTOR OF PRECIPITATING STRESS

| | Total number in group | | Improved 3 points or more following area 9, 10, 46 removal | | Improved 3 points or more after removal of other areas | | Improved 3 points or more without operation | | Improved less than 3 points following area 9, 10, 46 removal | | Improved less than 3 points after removal of other areas | | Improved less than 3 points without operation | |
|---|---|---|---|---|---|---|---|---|---|---|---|---|---|---|
| | 7½ mos. postop. | 1 yr. postop. | 7½ mos. postop. | 1 yr. postop. | 7½ mos. postop. | 1 yr. postop. | 7½ mos. postop. | 1 yr. postop. | 7½ mos. postop. | 1 yr. postop. | 7½ mos. postop. | 1 yr. postop. | 7½ mos. postop. | 1 yr. postop. |
| Well established precipitating stress[b] | 9 | 8 | 1 | 1 | 0 | 0 | 2 | 2 | 3 | 3 | 1 | 0[d] | 2 | 2 |
| Questionable precipitating stress[c] | 8 | 8 | 1 | 1 | 0 | 0 | 0 | 0 | 1 | 1 | 1 | 1 | 5 | 5 |
| No history of precipitating stress | 31 | 31 | 7 | 6 | 1 | 1 | 2 | 1 | 2 | 3 | 6 | 6 | 13 | 14 |
| Total............. | 48 | 47 | 9 | 8 | 1 | 1 | 4 | 3 | 6 | 7 | 8 | 7 | 20 | 21 |

[a] Improvement measured by weighted social score.
[b] Including financial loss, death of close relatives, divorce proceedings by mate, rejection by fiance, childbirth, combat Army service.
[c] Including "overwork," unemployment, fear of political persecution, extraction of teeth, induction into Army.
[d] One patient dead at one year (patient 24).

TABLE 86. CORRELATION OF IMPROVEMENT[a] WITH HISTORY OF PREVIOUS SPONTANEOUS REMISSIONS

| | Total number in group | | Improved 3 points or more following area 9, 10, 46 removal | | Improved 3 points or more after removal of other areas | | Improved 3 points or more without operation | | Improved less than 3 points following area 9, 10, 46 removal | | Improved less than 3 points after removal of other areas | | Improved less than 3 points without operation | |
|---|---|---|---|---|---|---|---|---|---|---|---|---|---|---|
| | 7½ mos. postop. | 1 yr. postop. | 7½ mos. postop. | 1 yr. postop. | 7½ mos. postop. | 1 yr. postop. | 7½ mos. postop. | 1 yr. postop. | 7½ mos. postop. | 1 yr. postop. | 7½ mos. postop. | 1 yr. postop. | 7½ mos. postop. | 1 yr. postop. |
| No spontaneous remissions[b] | 26 | 26 | 6 | 5 | 0 | 0 | 2 | 2 | 3 | 4 | 4 | 4 | 11 | 11 |
| One spontaneous remission[b] | 11 | 10 | 0 | 1 | 0 | 0 | 2 | 1 | 2 | 1 | 3 | 2[c] | 4 | 5 |
| Two or more spontaneous remissions[b] | 11 | 11 | 3 | 2 | 1 | 1 | 0 | 0 | 1 | 2 | 1 | 1 | 5 | 5 |
| Total | 48 | 47 | 9 | 8 | 1 | 1 | 4 | 3 | 6 | 7 | 8 | 7 | 20 | 21 |

[a] Improvement measured by weighted social score.
[b] Spontaneous remission indicates home six months or longer without preceding shock treatment.
[c] One patient dead at one year (patient 24).

TABLE 87. CORRELATION OF IMPROVEMENT* WITH PREVIOUS RESPONSE TO SHOCK THERAPIES

| | Total number in group | | Improved 3 points or more following area 9, 10, 46 removal | | Improved 3 points or more after removal of other areas | | Improved 3 points or more without operation | | Improved less than 3 points following area 9, 10, 46 removal | | Improved less than 3 points after removal of other areas | | Improved less than 3 points without operation | |
|---|---|---|---|---|---|---|---|---|---|---|---|---|---|---|
| | 7½ mos. postop. | 1 yr. postop. | 7½ mos. postop. | 1 yr. postop. | 7½ mos. postop. | 1 yr. postop. | 7½ mos. postop. | 1 yr. postop. | 7½ mos. postop. | 1 yr. postop. | 7½ mos. postop. | 1 yr. postop. | 7½ mos. postop. | 1 yr. postop. |
| Able to return to home for at least 6 months.......... | 10 | 10 | 4 | 3 | 0 | 0 | 1 | 1 | 0 | 1 | 0 | 0 | 5 | 5 |
| Able to return to home up to 3 months: general quieting effect..... | 9 | 9 | 1 | 1 | 0 | 0 | 2 | 1 | 1 | 1 | 0 | 0 | 5 | 6 |
| No change or immediate relapse when treatment discontinued.......... | 14 | 13 | 1 | 1 | 0 | 0 | 0 | 0 | 3 | 3 | 7 | 6[b] | 3 | 3 |
| Total............ | 33 | 32 | 6 | 5 | 0 | 0 | 3 | 2 | 4 | 5 | 7 | 6 | 13 | 14 |

* Improvement measured by weighted social score.
b One patient dead at one year (patient 24).
NOTE: Thirty-seven patients had shock treatments. Patients 1, 22, 31, 32 not included here for lack of data. A patient is included in benefited group if he responded on one occasion to treatment, regardless of subsequent failures and regardless of type of treatment used (insulin, metrazol, electric shock).

therapeutic response following operation on an area other than 9-10-46 was a woman who had had four remissions (patient 42).

In table 87 the 37 patients who had various forms of shock therapy before this study are compared in respect to their improvement. A patient was considered as having benefited from shock treatment if he or she responded on one occasion, regardless of subsequent failure to respond and regardless of the type of shock treatment used (insulin, metrazol, or electroconvulsive). The figures suggest that those patients who responded best to shock treatment also responded best to removal of areas 9-10-46, and that those in whom shock treatment was ineffective did least well with operation. Thus all 4 of the patients who were capable of a six-month home visit after shock treatment were also much improved seven and one-half months after operation. Only 1 of 4 patients showing no response to shock made a similar improvement after operation. If such a trend is maintained when larger numbers of patients have been studied, the temporary response to shock treatment may serve as a general prognostic guide to the more permanent improvement which may be expected after surgery.

## SUMMARY

The statistics which can be derived from this study are drastically limited by the small numbers involved and must be considered only suggestive and exploratory.

1. No evidence was found which would relate the weight of brain removed, the sex of the patient, or the previous history of remissions to the therapeutic effects of area 9-10-46 removals. Similarly, the therapeutic response could not be correlated with the type of onset of illness or the factors of precipitating stress.

2. Clinical improvement occurred more often among the younger patients and among the patients whose illnesses were of shorter duration.

3. A favorable response to shock therapy earlier in the illness was a common finding among those patients who responded well to operation.

### REVIEW OF BEHAVIOR CHARTS

#### EXPLANATION OF CHARTS

Behavior charts of the Payne Whitney or Phipps Clinic type were kept for all patients on the project. The charts used were those currently in use at the Payne Whitney Psychiatric Clinic of The New York Hospital in which various observable aspects of behavior are listed down one side of a sheet, the remainder of the space being occupied by a grid in the spaces of which the ward nurse checks daily those items of psychopathologic behavior which she notes in each patient. Space is also provided for recording sleep, weight, and menstruation. These charts were initiated by the nurses five to seven weeks before the scheduled period of operation and were maintained as long as the patient was on the special ward. They were terminated with the patient's discharge from the hospital or transfer to another ward. Most of the charts were carried to the nineteenth week after operation but some were maintained a few weeks beyond or short of that figure. (Entries on one chart, patient 3, were not made after the eleventh week, and therefore this patient was omitted from this analysis.) Daily entries were made on all cases.

To condense these daily records for presentation they were converted to weekly records and a vertical line was drawn indicating operation, to separate graphically preoperative from postoperative behavior (see figs. 107-112). In addition, the unwieldy list of forty-eight items of psychopathologic data was compressed down to fifteen categories. A serious attempt was made to combine

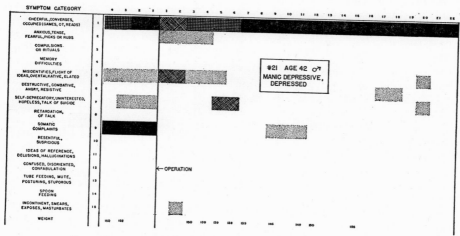

FIG. 106. Payne Whitney weekly behavior chart for patient 21.

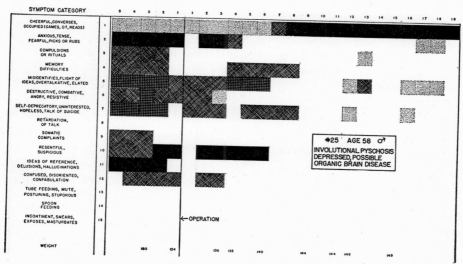

FIG. 107. Payne Whitney weekly behavior chart for patient 25.

in each symptom category various behavior trends which are psychiatrically related to one another. Thus many evidences of depression were included in category number 7, of elation in category number 5, of catatonia in category number 13, and so on. These categories were then arranged from top to bottom in a generally increasing order of severity, beginning with criteria of normal behavior (category number 1) and continuing through "neurotic" change (numbers 2, 3) into affective disturbances (numbers 5 through 9) and finally into "projective," disorganized, and regressive behavior (numbers 10 to 15). In some cases symptoms which did not relate well with others were allowed to stand alone (spoon-feeding, number 14; and memory difficulties, number 4), constituting a category in themselves. (See figs. 106-112.)

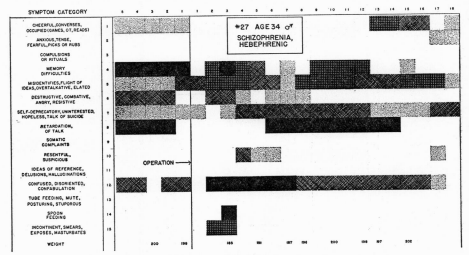

FIG. 108.   Payne Whitney weekly behavior chart for patient 27.

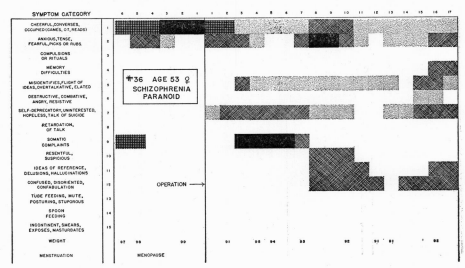

FIG. 109.   Payne Whitney weekly behavior chart for patient 36.

Some attempt was made to represent the intensity of abnormal behavior quantitatively although it must be emphasized that the results represent only a very gross approximation. The charts are shaded with three intensities of gray indicating mild to moderate abnormalities, and black to indicate severe behavior disturbances. No category was checked for the week unless at least two daily entries were recorded in that seven-day period.

These charts are of value in that they direct the nurse—a trained observer—
to the observation of specific behavior problems and permit her to record
behavior on a day-to-day basis with a minimum of writing. The short-comings
of such a system lie in the problems of changing personnel and in the interpretations given by various nurses to the behavior which they see. It may not

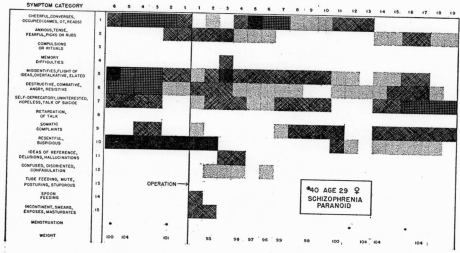

FIG. 110.  Payne Whitney weekly behavior chart for patient 40.

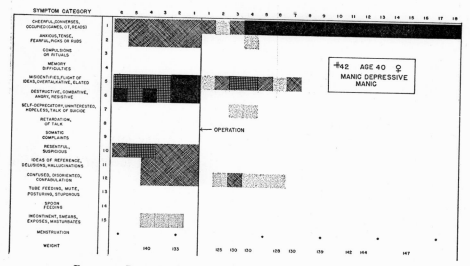

FIG. 111.  Payne Whitney weekly behavior chart for patient 42.

be easy, for example, to distinguish the depressed patient from the patient
who is preoccupied or to distinguish the overactivity of a manic from that
of a schizophrenic excitement. Delusions not freely expressed by the patient
are often unknown to the nurse and very often such symptoms were not recorded on the Payne Whitney charts even though the psychiatrist was aware
of their existence. All the nurses had been recently trained in psychiatric ob-

servation but no special instruction was given before the project began, a deficiency which should be remedied in future studies. The interpretation of these charts is also complicated by condensing the various types of behavior into a smaller number of categories, but none of these objections appears crucial.

Menses (in the women patients) and weight are included on the charts, but sleep is not, since it was found that nearly all patients slept well both before and after operation, often with a brief period (one-to-four days) of hypersomnolence immediately after operation. Perhaps, if closer observation of the patients had been possible during sleep, some deviations in the sleep rhythm might have appeared but no such data are available.

Figures 106-112 are the Payne Whitney weekly behavior charts of patients 21, 25, 27, 36, 40, 42, and 49. Table 88 gives a condensation of the behavior changes derived from all the Payne Whitney charts.

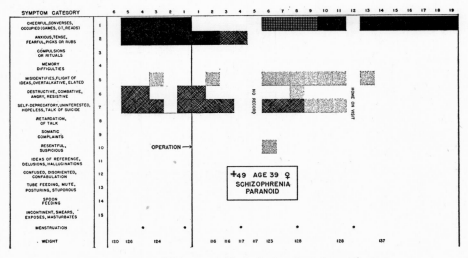

FIG. 112. Payne Whitney weekly behavior chart for patient 49.

### EFFECTS OF TOPECTOMY AS INDICATED BY CHARTS

Only the patients operated upon will be considered in what follows, since the control group maintained its preoperative behavior with very few exceptions. (Patient 9 developed an acute episode of confusion, resistance, and flight of ideas for which electroshock treatment was necessary. Following this treatment, his behavior improved markedly. Throughout his hospital stay, patient 15 displayed little psychopathologic behavior which could be recorded, and following an intercurrent illness with pneumonia he was paroled. Patient 34 was another whose record showed little throughout the observation period, and she, too, was paroled. Finally, the record of patient 39 indicates spontaneous recovery from marked symptoms of overactivity, suspiciousness, and anxiety with eventual parole.)

The following discussion centers about the categories of symptoms covered by the Payne Whitney charts and no attempt is made here to account for psychiatric or psychologic findings which may have been detected by other observers using other methods.

Many new symptoms appeared transiently following operation, nine of fourteen categories being represented in this temporary increase in symptomatology (categories numbers 2, 4, 5, 7, 10, 12, 13, 14, 15). These new symptoms were of varying degrees of severity and were characterized by a course which may be broken down as follows: (1) The greatest incidence occurred between the third and fifth postoperative weeks. (2) Beginning usually in the sixth to tenth postoperative weeks the number of patients exhibiting such symptoms began to decrease. (3) In no symptom category was the inci-

TABLE 88. CONDENSED TABLE OF BEHAVIOR CHANGES DERIVED FROM PAYNE WHITNEY CHARTS

| SYMPTOM CATEGORY | 2 ANXIOUS, TENSE, FEARFUL, PICKS OR RUBS | | 3 COMPULSIONS OR RITUALS | | 4 MEMORY DIFFICULTIES | | 5 MISIDENTIFIES, FLIGHT OF IDEAS, OVERTALKATIVE, ELATED | | 6 DESTRUCTIVE, COMBATIVE, ANGRY, RESISTIVE | | 7 SELF-DEPRECATORY, UNINTERESTED, HOPELESS, TALK OF SUICIDE | | 8 RETARDATION, OF TALK | | 9 SOMATIC COMPLAINTS | | 10 RESENTFUL, SUSPICIOUS | | 11 IDEAS OF REFERENCE, DELUSIONS, HALLUCINATIONS | | 12 CONFUSED, DISORIENTED, CONFABULATION | | 13 TUBE FEEDING, MUTE, POSTURING, STUPOROUS | | 14 SPOON FEEDING | | 15 INCONTINENT, SMEARS, EXPOSES, MASTURBATES | |
|---|---|---|---|---|---|---|---|---|---|---|---|---|---|---|---|---|---|---|---|---|---|---|---|---|---|---|---|---|---|
| | PRE OP. | POST OP. | PRE OP. | POST OP. | PRE OP. | POST OP. | PRE OP. | POST OP. | PRE OP. | POST OP. | PRE OP. | POST OP. | PRE OP. | POST OP. | PRE OP. | POST OP. | PRE OP. | POST OP. | PRE OP. | POST OP. | PRE OP. | POST OP. | PRE OP. | POST OP. | PRE OP. | POST OP. | PRE OP. | POST OP. |
| TOTAL NUMBER | 15 | 18 | 2 | 1 | 6 | 10 | 19 | 23 | 13 | 13 | 16 | 23 | 4 | 4 | 6 | 4 | 10 | 14 | 6 | 4 | 11 | 15 | 2 | 3 | 1 | 4 | 4 | 8 |
| POST-OPERATIVE DURATION — WEEKS 1 | | 9 | | 0 | | 2 | | 18 | | 6 | | 8 | | 1 | | 1 | | 3 | | 0 | | 5 | | 2 | | 2 | | 6 |
| 2 | | 11 | | 0 | | 4 | | 21 | | 7 | | 10 | | 2 | | 0 | | 5 | | 0 | | 9 | | 2 | | 0 | | 6 |
| 3-5 | | 16 | | 0 | | 9 | | 21 | | 7 | | 19 | | 3 | | 1 | | 8 | | 2 | | 12 | | 2 | | 2 | | 6 |
| 6-10 | | 6 | | 0 | | 4 | | 17 | | 6 | | 18 | | 2 | | 4 | | 8 | | 2 | | 7 | | 1 | | 2 | | 2 |
| 11-15 | | 5 | | 1 | | 3 | | 9 | | 5 | | 13 | | 3 | | 2 | | 2 | | 3 | | 4 | | 1 | | 0 | | 1 |
| 16- | | 6 | | 0 | | 2 | | 9 | | 5 | | 10 | | | | | | 3 | | 1 | | 6 | | 1 | | | | 0 |

TOTAL NUMBER OF OPERATED PATIENTS IN WHOM SYMPTOMS OCCURRED BEFORE AND AFTER OPERATION WITH BREAKDOWN OF POST-OPERATIVE DURATION BY WEEKS

| | PRE OP. | POST OP. | PRE OP. | POST OP. | PRE OP. | POST OP. | PRE OP. | POST OP. | PRE OP. | POST OP. | PRE OP. | POST OP. | PRE OP. | POST OP. | PRE OP. | POST OP. | PRE OP. | POST OP. | PRE OP. | POST OP. | PRE OP. | POST OP. | PRE OP. | POST OP. | PRE OP. | POST OP. | PRE OP. | POST OP. |
|---|---|---|---|---|---|---|---|---|---|---|---|---|---|---|---|---|---|---|---|---|---|---|---|---|---|---|---|---|
| | 15 | 7 | 2 | 0 | 6 | 4 | 19 | 11 | 13 | 8 | 16 | 13 | 4 | 2 | 6 | 1 | 10 | 4 | 6 | 2 | 11 | 6 | 2 | 1 | 1 | 1 | 4 | 0 |

TOTAL NUMBER OF OPERATED PATIENTS IN WHOM SYMPTOMS OCCURRED BEFORE OPERATION (PRE-OP.) AND IN THE 15th TO 19th WEEKS AFTER OPERATION (POST-OP.)

| | 9 | 6 | 2 | 0 | 3 | 2 | 12 | 8 | 8 | 5 | 11 | 8 | 2 | 0 | 5 | 0 | 6 | 3 | 4 | 1 | 4 | 4 | 1 | 0 | 0 | 0 | 0 | 0 |
|---|---|---|---|---|---|---|---|---|---|---|---|---|---|---|---|---|---|---|---|---|---|---|---|---|---|---|---|---|

TOTAL NUMBER OF PATIENTS WITH PARTIAL OR COMPLETE REMOVALS OF AREAS 9,10 OR 46 IN WHOM SYMPTOMS OCCURRED BEFORE OPERATION (PRE-OP) & IN THE 15th TO 19th WEEKS AFTER OPERATION (POST-OP.)

| | 6 | 1 | 0 | 0 | 3 | 2 | 7 | 3 | 5 | 3 | 5 | 5 | 2 | 2 | 1 | 1 | 4 | 1 | 2 | 1 | 7 | 2 | 1 | 1 | 1 | 1 | 4 | 0 |
|---|---|---|---|---|---|---|---|---|---|---|---|---|---|---|---|---|---|---|---|---|---|---|---|---|---|---|---|---|

TOTAL NUMBER OF PATIENTS WITH OPERATIONS NOT INVOLVING AREAS 9,10 OR 46 IN WHOM SYMPTOMS OCCURRED BEFORE OPERATION (PRE-OP) & IN THE 15th TO 19th WEEK AFTER OPERATION (POST-OP.)

dence greater at the end of the postoperative observation period (fifteenth to nineteenth weeks) than it was before operation. Thus operation did not usually produce lasting symptomatology as measured by the behavior charts, although a brief increase in recorded behavior was the rule in most categories.

The three patients whose records did indicate new and lasting changes after operation deserve special attention. Patient 36 (fig. 109) had a large mass of cortex removed (areas 10, 11, 45, 46, 47) and thereafter she is recorded as being confused, misidentifying, and showing much in the way of paranoid and depressive behavior. It is interesting that some of these qualities were present and known to the psychiatrists before operation but that they were not appreciated by the nurses until operation had accentuated them. Patient 6 was charted as being retarded after operation and patient 44 was charted as having memory difficulties and ideas of reference after operation. These characteristics of behavior were also known to the psychiatrists preoperatively and they can only be considered as accentuated after operation rather than actually produced by operation.

Operation reduced the incidence of many types of disturbed behavior. One exception to this statement is category number 14, spoon-feeding, where only one catatonic patient was represented—without improvement. The change in the patients began usually in the sixth to tenth weeks after operation and continued to the end of the observation period.

Operations other than area 9-10-46 removals produced a reduction in the incidence of symptoms although there was no change from the preoperative situation in five categories (nos. 7, 8, 9, 12, 13). There appears to be a difference in favor of removing frontal areas other than 9-10-46 in reducing the expression of anxiety and tension (category no. 2). This finding has little meaning when considered alone, however, and the entire question of emotional response is one which is better evaluated in terms of the whole personality before and after operation. Four patients whose behavior was markedly disturbed (category no. 15) were relieved by similar area removals but direct comparison with areas 9-10-46 is not possible, since none of the latter group showed such markedly regressive behavior before operation.

Area 9-10-46 removals were effective in relieving completely 5 patients with functional somatic complaints (category no. 9), 2 patients showing retardation of talk (category no. 8), and 2 who demonstrated compulsive or ritualistic behavior (category no. 3). Unfortunately, none of the patients operated on in other areas had compulsive behavior before operation, so again direct comparison is not possible. Area 9-10-46 operations were of no benefit in eliminating symptoms of confusion, disorientation, and confabulation (category no. 12) (compare with category no. 5). The remaining symptom categories showed no difference in their response to area 9-10-46 removals as compared with other areas of cortical removal. It should be noted that many patients were relieved of depressive symptoms (category no. 7), "elation" (category no. 5), suspiciousness (category no. 10), hallucinations and delusions (category no. 11), and destructive or combative behavior (category no. 6). The response of such symptoms was not apparently influenced by the site of operation.

Other possible variables such as sex, age, diagnosis, duration, and type of onset of illness and clinical improvement could not be related to the type of response to operation although much time-consuming effort was spent in investigating such factors.

**Summary of Effects of Topectomy.**

1. Regardless of area removed, a transient increase in abnormal behavior took place, reaching its height three to five weeks after operation and decreasing thereafter.

2. Ablation of frontal cortex did not produce prolonged abnormal behavior as measured by behavior charts except in 3 patients.

3. Regardless of areas removed and despite temporary exacerbation, operation produced a decrease in the incidence of many symptoms.

4. The removal of areas 9, 10, and 46 appeared to be of special value in relieving retardation of talk and somatic complaints. Compulsive and ritualistic behavior may also have responded specifically to these operations.

The removal of other areas appeared to be more effective in reducing the incidence of disturbed behavior and the expression of anxiety and tension although anxiety was also relieved by 9, 10, and 46 operations.

The authors feel that such indications of personality alterations following operation are only suggestive of the use to which behavior charts might be put in future studies. More accurate nursing observation on a larger series of patients is needed before the findings can be considered significant. This is especially true of the observations on emotional reactivity which appear to be crucial to the therapeutic effects of this operation and must be considered in a broad setting of personality structure in order to be meaningful.

5. Age, sex, diagnosis, length of illness, or type of onset could not be related with the response to operation.

CHARTS ON LOBOTOMY SUBJECTS

Payne Whitney charts were kept for the 8 patients who were operated on by the conventional lobotomy technique. Unfortunately these records were not maintained for the same length of time as were the Payne Whitney charts of the original topectomy patients. Because of administrative problems the longest behavior chart of a lobotomy patient extends to the tenth postoperative week and the usual observation time after operation was only six or seven weeks. The records on patients 2 and 11 extend only one week after operation and cannot be interpreted.

Patient 5 was the only one whose record indicated improvement during the six weeks he was followed after operation. He continued to be retarded but the chart indicated less confused thinking and the appearance of more general interest in his environment following operation than prior to it. Patient 23 showed less pressure of speech and ideas for the first two weeks after operation and less expression of delusions and hallucinations during that time. All of these symptoms returned, however, and continued until the end of the ten-week recording period. Patient 28 was hypersomnolent and showed marked feeding difficulties in the first ten days after operation. These signs were relieved and he returned to his preoperative type of behavior, according to the charts which were kept for six weeks after operation on this patient. One patient, 46, showed some increase in symptomatology during the first seven postoperative weeks when she was destructive at times and paid less attention to her environment at other times. Patient 20 showed no change in the first seven weeks after lobotomy. Patient 44 was a woman who had previously had a partial removal of area 10 without improvement. In the first six weeks after lobotomy the Payne Whitney charts indicated that this procedure, too, had been of no benefit to this patient.

EFFECT OF FRONTAL LOBE SURGERY ON PSYCHOTIC BEHAVIOR

Alterations of behavior in man as a result of frontal lobe damage have been described in the literature for over a century. Since 1825 it has been shown that patients with frontal lobe damage became carefree and showed lack of concern for their environment. The word *Witzelsucht* was coined by Jastrowitz to refer to clownish behavior and Moniz developed the lobotomy procedure in 1935. In 1936 the technique was refined by Freeman and Watts and since then a number of otherwise incurable patients have been restored to society.

The most frequently voiced objections to this procedure are: (1) that often, owing to lack of social inhibitions in the patient following operation, the behavior following treatment is almost as bad as that due to the preceding illness and (2) that, since so many pathways are cut, it is difficult to explain physiologically the changes that the patients undergo.

Until recently, very little work has been done to determine behavior changes resulting from removal of cortical tissue in man. Ody, in 1936, performed unilateral resection of cortical tissue in a schizophrenic. He reported good results. This apparently was not pursued by Ody and in the hands of others the operation proved ineffective. Freeman and Watts ('42) report: "No patient with bilateral lobectomy has yet been able to work for a living."

Theories of frontal lobe function have been formulated on the basis of extensive studies of patients with existing organic disease in the frontal lobes. This data can hardly be considered relevant, however, since in all these studies parts of the brain other than the frontal lobe were involved, either by pressure or distortion secondary to the actual lesion. This includes the cases of Ackerly ('35), Brickner ('36), Nichols and Hunt ('40), and Mixter, Tillotson, and Wies ('41). An exception is the patient of Hebb and Penfield (Hebb, '45) operated on for epilepsy resulting from an injury and subsequent scarring of the frontal poles, with bilateral removal of frontal cortex. This patient made a good social and economic adjustment over a six-year follow-up period. Hebb noted that the patient's behavior did not conform to that which would have been expected if any of the existing theories were correct.

Since the inception of lobotomy, many observations of changes in behavior have been reported following the operation. This procedure, however, is very inexact and the resulting damage widespread, as we were able to show during our studies. Additional theories have, nevertheless, been postulated on the basis of these observations. Study of our patients did not support any existing theory of frontal lobe function.

The first four topectomies were performed at the Neurological Institute, the first in October, 1946. The region selected for removal was the junction of areas 9 and 10, and this was chosen on the basis of primate experiments. Richter and Hines ('38) and later Mettler ('44) reported specific changes in behavior following removal of area 9 that did not occur with bilateral removal of other single areas of prefrontal cortex. Animals so operated upon did not show the great defect in behavior that would have been anticipated from the clinical reports.

The results of our first 4 cases were encouraging. Overt psychotic symptoms disappeared in the first 2 patients and, despite the chronicity of their illness (hospitalization periods were twenty-eight years and seven years, respectively), they were able after a few months to function at pre-illness capacity. The third patient, a deteriorated schizophrenic, institutionalized six years but with a history of disordered behavior from early childhood, did not improve. The fourth patient was also a deteriorated schizophrenic with inappropriate affect. Incontinence and paroxysms of violence created a problem in management. Following operation the violence and incontinence subsided but the basic schizophrenic picture was unchanged. The subject was able to adjust outside the institution with supervision. His brother states, "He gets along OK but figuratively speaking we 'have him on a leash.'" The gross deterioration in social behavior so frequently seen following lobotomy was not present in any of the cases.

It appeared, therefore, that the improvement might be related to removal of only a fraction of frontal cortex and that this might have advantages over undercutting all the frontal association area, as in lobotomy.

THERAPEUTIC RESULTS

Because of chronicity of the patients' illness and the preponderance of schizophrenics the cases reported here had a poor prognosis with any type of treatment.

**Control Group.** In consideration of the possibility that some of the patients might have improved from the increased attention they received during this project, 24 patients in addition to those subjected to operation were included in the study. The same work-up was carried out on all patients and those to be operated upon were not selected until two or three days before operation. Methods for determining which patients would be in the operatee group and which in the control group are discussed on pages 21-22. Patients from the control group were anesthetized during the operative period and blood was taken from them to be used for transfusions. All of them felt they too had a special treatment. Postoperative or postanesthesia studies were also the same in the two groups. Three of the 24 control patients are now out of the institution. Abstracts of patients of this group are to be found on pages 315-319. One of the 3 (patient 34) is making an excellent social adjustment. She had been placed in the control group because: (1) marked spontaneous improvement was evident at the onset of the project and (2) x-ray studies revealed a duodenal ulcer. The second patient (39) whose acute elation partially subsided during the preoperative work-up period remains hypomanic but capable of making a marginal social adjustment and the third (patient 15) resides in a veterans' camp gaining his subsistence by doing odd jobs; he is still incapable of finding gainful employment.

**Operatee Group.** In 13 patients of the 24 in the operatee group psychiatric examination revealed definite interruption of psychotic behavior. Two additional operatees showed social improvement but it is questionable how much their improvement can be attributed to operation.

Improvement was temporary in some. Seven months after operation 11 of the operatees were at home and working. Ten were gainfully employed of whom only one was working below his pre-illness capacity. This subject was sixty-one years of age and the company for which he worked before becoming ill, eight years prior to operation, had reorganized so that there no longer was a place for him. Other companies were reluctant to hire him in an important position because of his advanced age. The eleventh patient returned to housekeeping.

One year after operation 2 of the 11 patients in this group had a return of their psychotic symptoms and a third had returned to the institution for other reasons. All but one of the patients in the group of 13 in whom operation altered psychotic behavior had areas 9 and/or 10 removed completely or in part either alone or in combination with other areas, the most frequent additional area being the relatively small area 46 which is in propinquity to 9 and similar to 9 in cytoarchitecture. One of the 11 patients now working ostensibly had area 46 alone removed. Histologic study showed that in addition, a small amount of area 10 was also removed. Although schizophrenic, the subject's preoperative social adaptation was marginal. Operation produced definite but not as startling effects as that following removal of areas 9 and 10. Further explanation of the two patients who questionably improved from operation is necessary. Both patients (42, see pp. 373-374 and 38, see pp. 371-373) were manic depressives with histories of spontaneous remissions. In patient 42, elation was subsiding before operation. Area 11 was removed bilaterally. During the one-year follow-up period the patient became depressed but improved following a spontaneous grand mal convulsion. Patient 38 was also elated prior to operation which consisted of ligating the veins draining the cortex of the frontal association area. After operation the elation subsided somewhat so that the patient could be paroled. During the one-year follow-up period she remained somewhat euphoric, overly talkative and scattered, but was able to hold her job.

### NATURE OF THE CHANGE IN BEHAVIOR RESULTING FROM SURGERY

When clinically observable change in behavior resulted from operation it was essentially of the same nature, regardless of parts of frontal cortex removed. No patients were made worse and most of the areas removed produced very slight or no improvement. The ideas of specific localization for different personality patterns in the frontal lobes, including Kleist's fanciful chart, can be discarded. Changes were consistently in the sphere of affective response. Emotion was not absent nor even noticeably blunted. Rage, fear, and joy were still felt; the change being that these reactions did not affect the patient so profoundly. Emotions were readily and more appropriately discharged. Repression of unpleasant emotions with resultant tension and subsequent regression into overt psychotic behavior no longer occurred. There was not an over-all dampening of emotional response. Patients reacted to real external dangers as they always had. The difference was a marked lessening of the painful affect that accompanied memories. When questioned as to the effect of operation, patients, regardless of the type of psychopathologic illness, gave similar answers, such as: "The tensions don't pile up," "I don't feel like I'm now carrying a tremendous load any longer," "I'm not full of fear like I used to be."

Several patients did not have areas 9 or 10 included in the removal. Previously it was mentioned that all who benefited had all or part of cortical areas 9 and/or 10 removed. Several confusing points remain unanswered. Why did some improve only temporarily? Why weren't all patients who benefited discharged from the hospital? Did only patients with areas 9 and/or 10 removed benefit by operation? We shall now attempt to clarify these points.

### REVIEW OF RESULTS IN PATIENTS HAVING CORTEX FROM AREAS OTHER THAN 9 AND/OR 10 REMOVED

Area 6 alone was removed in 2 patients. Following operation, one of these patients became slightly more tractable for a period of a few weeks, then regressed to his preoperative behavior level; the other was unchanged.

Area 8 alone was removed in one patient. He became slightly more tractable and cooperative after operation, but the psychosis remained unchanged.

Removal of area 45 alone produced no change. One patient had area 44 (Broca's area) alone removed. Her word salad, delusions, and hallucinations were unaffected.

As we have previously mentioned, one patient was paroled to return to her duties as a housewife, following area 11 removal. No immediate change followed her operation and it seems likely this was a spontaneous remission. Another patient had area 11 alone removed. For a few weeks this patient became slightly more tractable than he was prior to operation, although delusions and hallucinations remained unchanged and he regressed shortly to his preoperative state.

Case 40, in which the cingulate gyrus was removed, takes on a great significance in view of the attention that has been directed toward this area by other investigators. Papez ('37) theorized that this area was the cortical representation of a pathway for emotions. In their writings, Freeman and Watts ('41) have reasoned that the stupor often seen immediately following lobotomy is due to cutting the pathways connecting with this area. Recently Ward has singled out this area for further study. He attempted to cut specific pathways connecting with this area. Our patient was one who seemed to have a very favorable prognosis utilizing criteria of lobotomy. She was an early paranoid schizophrenic, who had been ill less than a year, with considerable affective component to her illness. Although considerable physical discomfort, manifested by vomiting, occurred during the first few postoperative days, stupor did not result and there was no clinical improvement. Six months following operation further emotional deterioration was evident; delusions were more fixed and there was less emotional response. One year after operation she was openly suspicious.

### REVIEW OF RESULTS IN PATIENTS STILL INSTITUTIONALIZED FOLLOWING REMOVAL OF AREAS 9 AND/OR 10

It was emphasized that the patients who definitely benefited sufficiently from operation to leave the institution had areas 9 and/or 10 removed wholly or in part. This would suggest that the specific desirable effect follows removal of this region. Of the 14 patients who had these areas implicated in the removal, however, 5 were not able to live outside the institution following operation. A review of these 5 cases is revealing. In contrast to the minimal change or no change that followed removal of other areas, these patients obtained the desired effect and remain hospitalized despite this. In 3 patients, overt symptoms of the psychosis disappeared but because of impulsiveness, tactlessness, and irresponsibility these patients remain hospitalized; however, they are on less disturbed wards. All 3 had a large amount of cortex removed in addition to areas 9 and/or 10 and we feel that this accounts for the appearance of the deleterious symptoms. The fourth patient in this group of five was in an elated state when operated upon. The fifth improved considerably and was paroled. We believe that her return to the institution was necessitated by lack of proper support in the home.

A more detailed description of these patients follows:

Patient 8, a paranoid schizophrenic, was very self-centered and preoccupied with his hypochondriasis. He was preoccupied with thoughts of homosexuality and delusions that various bodily organs were disintegrating. Considerable affect accompanied these symptoms. He was irritable but well contained. At operation the entire middle frontal gyrus was removed bilaterally, including large parts of areas 9 and 10. Postoperative behavior contrasted sharply. Somatic complaints and his self-centered attitude immediately disappeared. He became impulsive; there were great variations in mood.

Although generally carefree, garrulous, and outgoing, sudden explosive periods would occur in which he became obstreperous and assaultive. On a few occasions he cut his fist by thrusting it through a window. This and the assaultiveness occurred only in the immediate postoperative period. Remorse did not follow. Marked deterioration in social behavior occurred. He insulted patients and attendants, hoarded prized foods, and demanded special privileges. He was less conscientious in his work. Six months following operation his sister, a nun, visited him. Before operation he had displayed a great respect for her. Now he swore and was so insulting that she found it necessary to shorten her visit. Another relative could not understand his lack of remorse and refusal to apologize. One year after operation his behavior was essentially the same. Of special interest, however, was his changed behavior in the sexual sphere. Before operation he occasionally indulged in overt homosexual behavior. During the one-year postoperative period he felt no homosexual impulses and stated that an interest in women had developed. Occasionally he masturbated with some heterosexual fantasies.

This patient shows not only the changes in the affective responses, but also exhibits gross deterioration in social behavior. We attribute his lack of concern, absence of tact, and lack of conscientiousness to removal of too much of the frontal lobe. This type of behavior resembles that which we have seen in some of our lobotomy patients and is similar to that reported by others to sometimes follow lobotomy.

Patient 22 displayed paranoid trends throughout his adult life but actual breakdown did not occur until the fifth decade of life. Prior to operation he was negativistic, obstreperous, often disturbed and assaultive, with a well-developed paranoid delusional system. Areas 9, 10, and 46 were removed. Almost immediately following operation he became pleasant, cooperative, tractable, and paranoid ideation disappeared. Ground parole was granted and in this controlled setting his behavior was satisfactory except for some evidence of irresponsibility. Three months after operation he was paroled to his home. Although the overt psychotic symptoms were not in evidence, his judgment was quite defective and he lacked his former sense of responsibility. Emotional reactions toward his wife were somewhat unrestrained. Because of lack of education and understanding, and remembering irascible trends that accompanied his previous breakdowns, the patient's wife called the police and he was returned to the hospital. On the ward he remained cooperative without the preoperative impulsiveness, but evidenced, at six months after operation, obvious impairment of judgment and some confusion. Speech was rambling, at times irrelevant, and often centered about remote happenings. This defective judgment had lessened considerably by one year after operation. He was then better oriented on current events, rambled less, and was considered quite responsible by his ward physician. He had ground parole and was free to visit the neighboring village frequently. The ward psychiatrist considered him fit for discharge and felt that the chief impediment to his making a satisfactory social adjustment was his wife's unstable condition. Persistent defective judgment was, however, apparent in this patient's reluctance to live elsewhere than with his wife. Here again the specific alteration of affect occurred and overt psychotic symptoms disappeared, but owing to the removal of too much frontal cortex, deterioration in judgment with irresponsible behavior resulted, making his early return to society impractical. (Note: Just before this was submitted for publication this patient was paroled.)

Patient 36 first displayed evidence of "beginning paranoid development with hypochondriasis" at the age of twenty-one years. Gross deterioration with development of ideas of reference, persecutory delusions, and auditory hallucinations occurred four years prior to this study, necessitating institutionalization, at the age of forty-eight. Before operation the subject, a woman, displayed the fully developed paranoid picture minus grandiosity but with moderate tension and agitation. Agitation was so great during the first two years of hospitalization that ambulatory shock was necessary. The affect, however, spontaneously flattened to a considerable degree during the year preceding operation. Areas 10, 11, 45, 46, and 47 were removed. The principal change following operation was the disappearance of remaining agitation and tension. The patient's paranoid development was not markedly changed. Adaptation at home following parole was inadequate, primarily because of indolence and irresponsibility and also because the patient continued to express the persecutory delusions. One year after operation her delusions were unchanged. Behavior on the ward, however, was markedly improved. The ward physician described her as a model patient. When interviewed, she told in detail of the horrible things that people were doing to her but throughout remained in complete equilibrium.

Here, too, the alteration of affective response was achieved and it is necessary to consider two factors in analyzing this patient's failure to adjust adequately. As in the two preceding cases, extensive amounts of cortex were removed, probably accounting for the indolence and tactlessness. Secondly, the regressive reparative processes of the psychosis had gone far, so that affect was largely divorced from ideation. We believe this accounts for persistence of the paranoid picture despite lessened emotion.

Patient 32 was a manic depressive operated upon at the height of a period of elation. Although areas 8 and 9 were removed, behavior was unchanged and remained the same one year after operation. Several investigators have also reported poor results in elation with lobotomy. One can only speculate why this procedure fails in the treatment of elated states. The most logical explanation, based on clinical observation, is that tension and painful affect of depression are removed through the reparative manic reaction. The operation which acts in the same direction cannot be expected to help. It will be interesting to see, with the passage of time, if the operation eliminates future depressions and thereby the need for repair through elation. Further experience with manics will be necessary to clarify these points.

Patient 31 developed persecutory ideas accompanied by considerable agitation during the fifth decade of life. Following removal of area 9 the agitation lessened markedly and almost immediately. Paranoid ideation, divorced from affect, subsided considerably but more slowly and was still slightly evident at the time of this patient's discharge. One day following release she was returned by a drunken husband who found her too much trouble—an impediment to his new and freer life. We believe her chances for further improvement were impaired by lack of support at home. Seven months after operation she continued to be improved, and was granted ground parole privileges. Soon after, however, she began to slip, the old agitation returned with increasing paranoid ideation, and one year after operation she was much as she had been at the onset of the project. This patient must, therefore, be considered in the group that only temporarily improved.

## TEMPORARY IMPROVEMENT VERSUS LASTING IMPROVEMENT—RELATIONSHIP TO CORTICAL AREAS REMOVED

Three patients in the group who made definite improvement and were paroled following operation later had a recurrence of their psychotic symptoms, which necessitated re-hospitalization: one eight months after operation (patient 3), another eleven months after operation (patient 27), and the third twelve months after operation (patient 33).

Patient 31, referred to in the preceding paragraph, showed definite improvement for eight months following operation (although she remained institutionalized for sociological reasons) then relapsed to her former psychotic state.

Patient 3, a sixty-one-year-old male, ill for eight years, the diagnosis being "involutional psychosis mixed" with symptoms of depression and persecutory ideas, had hallucinations in the auditory sphere. Several years before operation, he improved for a few weeks with electroshock but was able to remain outside the hospital for only one day. Symptoms immediately disappeared after operation and for a short time he was quite euphoric. When paroled three months after operation he adjusted well but shortly afterward mild depressive symptoms returned. The company for which he formerly worked had reorganized and could not rehire him. He worked at menial tasks but gradually lost interest and self-confidence. Depression increased and eight months after operation re-hospitalization became necessary. One year after operation he was retarded and depressed. The persecutory ideas had not returned, and he stated the voices had no meaning to him although he occasionally heard them. In referring to the immediate postoperative period he said, "I was on top of the world but it didn't last." This marked improvement lasted only two weeks. The intention at operation was to remove area 9. Studies showed, however, that the removal was caudal to the intended site and included the caudal part of areas 9, 8, and even part of area 6.

Patient 27 was a hebephrenic schizophrenic who improved sufficiently to return to work at old capacity despite untoward features which will be described later (p. 419). His adjustment was satisfactory until eleven months after operation when he suddenly became confused, delusional, exhibited blockage of speech, and again began having hallucinations.

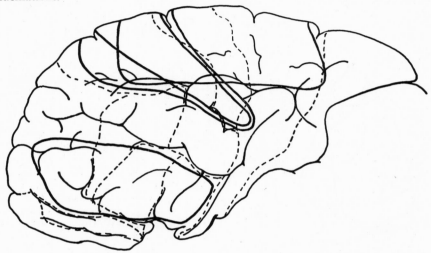

FIG. 113. Region removed in patients who showed temporary improvement (patients 3, 27, 31, and 33). The removals depicted here are not exact, but are based on x-ray studies, photographs, and cytoarchitectural reports. (Dotted lines indicate Brodmann's areas; solid lines the regions removed.)

Patient 33 was in catatonic stupor prior to operation, was negativistic, sat on the floor in knee-chest position, and was mute except for screaming when an attempt was made to gain her cooperation for testing. Following removal of the inferior frontal gyrus she gradually improved so that at three months after operation she was able to begin work. Gainful employment continued until ten months after operation when she was laid off. Gradually she became more preoccupied and retarded and finally, one year after operation, took to bed with recurrence of stupor. Removal included part of area 10 which probably interfered temporarily with circulation to other parts of areas 9 and 10.

The sites removed in each of these patients who temporarily improved are sketched on a Brodmann's map, figure 113, and in figure 114 sites removed in the patients who had lasting recovery are sketched.

All patients in whom improvement was related to operation had at least part of area 9 or 10 removed. Those who remained well had the junction of areas 9 and 10 included in the removal; whereas, temporarily improved patients had only partial removal of other regions in area 9 or 10.

### REVIEW OF PATIENTS SHOWING DETERIORATION IN SOCIAL BEHAVIOR

In the group of 5 patients who were unable to leave the institution for any prolonged period, 3 were described as unable to leave because they were too deteriorated in the social-ethical sphere. Several patients temporarily made adjustments outside the institution despite these symptoms.

One patient (27) worked for several months. The family said he did not care about his dress and was often disheveled. He was inane and forgot his manners when alone with his family, but pulled himself together fairly well at work. He was not concerned if he arrived late for work and sometimes took one and one-half or two hours for lunch. He did his work satisfactorily, but was not at all conscientious. Despite this his carefree attitude made him an excellent salesman and until overt psychotic symptoms returned he earned more money than at any period of his life. At operation the entire superior frontal gyrus was removed bilaterally.

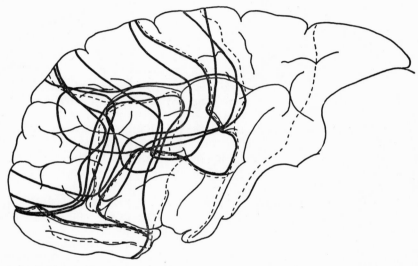

FIG. 114. Region removed in patients who showed lasting improvement. The removals depicted here are not exact, but are based on x-ray studies, photographs, and cytoarchitectural reports. (Dotted lines indicate Brodmann areas; solid lines the regions removed.)

Patient 7 was a paranoid schizophrenic with hypochondriasis and ideas of reference. These symptoms disappeared after areas 8, 9, and 10 were removed. Three months after operation he returned to his old job as a skilled machinist and performed well. His domestic life, however, was not tranquil and we received several letters from his wife accusing him of very pathologic behavior. Seven and one-half months after operation the wife was interviewed along with the patient. Her behavior was pathologic; she was suspicious, complained the room was wired for sound, was tense, cried readily and obviously was quite paranoid. The patient was advised to live elsewhere and did so for a short time. Two months later, however, he attempted a reconciliation with his wife and she had him arrested and returned to the institution. Further attempts were made to convince him that living with his wife was impossible. When we felt this was accomplished his wife visited him and the couple again decided to live together. The patient was jubilant, and it was impossible to deter him on this course of action. One year after operation he was again paroled, resumed living with his wife, and was re-employed as a skilled machinist. Our observations reveal no other defects in judgment. Socially the patient adjusts well, he is neat in dress and conscientious on the job.

In all of the 5 patients in whom social deterioration appeared with operation a large surface area of cortex was removed. It did not occur in any patient who had only one or two large areas or several small areas removed and is not a necessary accompaniment of clinical improvement. Also the degree of impairment varies considerably in different patients. No correlation can be made between area or region removed and this defect. No single area produced it and there was no consistent area involved in the various patients who showed it. There was one other patient who temporarily recovered (patient 33) (inferior frontal gyrus) who had large areas of cortex removed without resulting deterioration of social behavior. It is therefore difficult to say definitely how much cortex can be removed before this syndrome results. Individual thresholds vary, but when more than two of the larger areas are removed the social deterioration will appear in a large percentage of cases.

These complicating side effects frequently appear after lobotomy. Recovery was explained by some authors to be due to this attitude and it was interpreted as lessening of consciousness of self.

### EFFECT OF TOPECTOMY ON SPECIFIC CLINICAL SYNDROMES

Methods of describing improvement that are universally used in evaluating lobotomy results are of very limited usefulness in conveying what the operation actually does. Our improvement graphs (pp. 391-403) have this same shortcoming. To tell what percentage of schizophrenics recover, what percent improve, and so on, as compared to recovery and improvement in depressions, involutionals, obsessive compulsives, or other psychiatric manifestations, gives a spurious impression. The result of operation on a schizophrenic is entirely different from that on a patient having an affective psychosis, even though both subjects may be classified as recovered because they have returned to work. Impressions of members of the families as to degree of recovery likewise are valueless except in the broadest sense. Detailed studies on a large number of patients—and this requires living with the patient over a prolonged postoperative period—are necessary to determine what the operation has done. We have the humble beginnings of such a study.

Patient 21, successfully operated upon for an affective psychosis of twenty-one years' duration, is employed as diener in the laboratory. During the twenty-one years of illness he had only a few short visits from the hospital. When operated upon he was retarded and depressed. Patient 49, successfully operated upon for schizophrenia of twenty-three years' duration, was employed as a maid in the home of one of us for four months and lived there. These 2 patients, who had the same area (10) removed, have been observed in their daily routine duties for several months. Both are considered by their respective families to be the same as they were before becoming ill, and both are working at their pre-illness capacity. By virtue of this they rate the best score on our improvement charts. Over-all behavior, however, differs considerably.

Patient 21, the diener, performs excellently in his job. He is conscientious, almost too much so, and very anxious to please. He keeps the operating room orderly and clean. When activities are scheduled in the laboratory, he anticipates what will be needed and is prepared. He readily learns routine procedures and executes them well. Each morning he reports to work early, does not prolong his lunch hour, and often works overtime without complaining. After observing that two of us used an old bucket as a receptacle in our office and frequently missed it with our cigarette butts, he retired to the shop and in remarkably short time returned with a waste basket that he had ingeniously constructed from plywood. It was well built and nicely stained. Recently he suffered from a mild dysuria. A medical workup revealed prostatitis for which he is now being treated. In speaking to associates in the laboratory and on one occasion to a visiting doctor, he attributed his past mental illness to this condition. However, when speaking to the psychiatrist whom he feels knows more about him he does not use this camouflage. He shows no hesitancy about discussing his illness. In so doing he gives a good description of depression and has considerable insight into contributing dynamic factors.

Patient 49, the maid, was also very conscientious. She arose on time each morning and prepared the breakfast. She, too, was very anxious to please and was very neat in personal appearance. In the house she was at all times friendly and pleasant. She smiled appropriately, appeared fond of the children, but was quite reserved. The neighbors did not suspect that she had been ill. They felt that she was just a shy person, rather ineffective, like so many people seen in everyday life.

There were, however, at the time she was first employed many abnormal behavior traits not seen in patient 21, which markedly reduced her efficiency. There was considerable autistic thinking when she was not active. She worked well and with remarkable energy if someone told her what to do in detail, but she seldom saw things to do on her own initiative. She was unable to see a job in its entirety. If asked to sweep the floors she began, but if she saw a small collection of debris her entire attention became centered on this and she sometimes neglected to sweep the entire floor. In making cereal in the mornings she found it difficult to use proper proportions of cereal and water. Frequently the cereal was lumpy or too runny. In cleaning the bathroom, she often failed to notice obvious spots in need of cleaning.

It was necessary to make repeated suggestions before she responded. For example, it was her custom to put garbage in the waste basket instead of the proper receptacle. Only after being told several times did she change in this habit. She was unusually forgetful, especially if told more than one thing at a time. She remembered one thing and forgot the others. This seemed to be attributable to preoccupation and not to a fundamental defect of memory.

After a few weeks these symptoms lessened and eventually largely disappeared. The girl was more at ease, exhibited more interest, and functioned quite efficiently in the house. She was a satisfactory cook and baked excellent cakes and pies.

No defect in planning was apparent. She looked forward to her day off and planned activities well. These included shopping trips and excursions to the movies. Seldom, however, did she do these things alone. Days off were spent with her sister toward whom she had a strong dependence.

She has an excellent grasp of current events. One of us had a lengthy discussion with her when the Communists moved into Czechoslovakia. She showed appropriate concern, and discussed at some length the horrible possibilities of a future atomic war. She talked of the futility of war, noted that no one profited by it, and that it merely made for new and different conflicts.

She socialized very little and was abnormally shy. She made no effort to make friends in the community and immediately disappeared when neighbors arrived. She stated that this was because she was embarrassed over having spent so much time in a mental institution. (It must be remembered that she has been hospitalized almost continuously throughout her adult life.)

She slept well and admitted dreaming but did not care to discuss the dreams. This patient showed many limitations, especially in the sphere of community activity, but continued to improve until one year after operation when several events occurred which precipitated a partial temporary setback. Because of illness in the family her work was increased. She performed very well and showed more initiative than at any previous period. A few days later one of the children of the household fell and sustained a moderately severe concussion. The patient was quite perturbed over this, frequently peered into the child's room, and asked many questions about the severity of the injury. About the same time her sister began spending week ends at her cottage in the country. The patient spoke at considerable length of this, implying that she was being left out, giving the impression that she was abused. She did not speak to the psychiatrist of feeling badly and outwardly she appeared well when departing for her day off in the last week in May. Later her sister called saying the patient was not well, that she complained of insomnia and fatigue, and expressed fears that her illness was returning. When assured she need not return to work unless she felt able, she began to sleep better. The one-year follow-up study was conducted the next week and at that time the patient appeared worn, had a distraught look, and was quite irritable and depressed. Her sister said that the thought of reporting back to the hospital had caused apprehension as it had on such occasions previously. During the interview the patient stated that she felt the work had been too hard, and that she had developed considerable fear that one of the children might be injured. Two weeks later when seen by the social service worker she was much improved, was again quite relaxed, was sleeping well, and was talking of taking a new job with shorter hours, nearer home, so that she could be close to her sister and spend week ends with her at their summer home. A short time later she acquired another job as a domestic and is reportedly performing well on the job. From the mental content it seems apparent that the precipitating factor in her relapse was the fear of injury to the children. This had reactivated the nucleus of her conflict (fear of mutilation to herself) which had originally been prominent in the paranoid development.

Close observation over a considerable period of time revealed that painful affect had been markedly lessened by operation. Now the old conflict had been strongly reactivated by a realistic incident. Could the reduction of affect prevent regression into a psychotic state? The subsequent improvement indicated that the effect of operation was sufficient to accomplish this. Unfortunately psychotherapy could never be given. It seems plausible to assume that considerable insight could have been given if psychotherapy had been available. A more detailed account of the degree and manner in which patients integrated the psychotic symptoms during the postoperative period is given in succeeding material (p. 426).

Operation had a similar effect on both patients. Patient 21 said it lifted a weight from him and relieved the depression. Patient 49 said, "I don't develop the extreme tension any longer."

It would have been difficult to determine if the abnormal behavior seen in patient 49 was due to operation or to her schizoid makeup if we had not also studied patient 21 with the same operation for a different psychosis. In view of the contrast in behavior between the 2 patients it seems likely the abnormalities were due to basic personality difficulties rather than the operation. Patient 49 could hardly be expected immediately to assume an independent way of life since she had never done so before in her life.

The pre-psychotic personality of the patient with an affective psychosis is usually quite well integrated. The real manic-depressive patient tends toward extraversion whereas those with involutional psychosis are apt to be meticulous, approaching the compulsive. Following operation this type of behavior is again seen. The patient with schizophrenia is, however, quite different. Pre-psychotic history indicates a loosely organized person never able to feel or act as the normal individual. The degree of disintegration, of course, varies in different schizophrenics and is seldom as marked as in patient 49. Operation, by removing the intense emotion, makes subsequent inferior reparative behavior unnecessary but does nothing toward restoring the pre-psychotic lack of organization.

Observing these patients as they improve following removal of the intense emotional reaction sheds added light on the dynamic processes of the psychosis and indicates why the operation is successful in some clinical types and not in others. It is quite apparent why operation is successful in the affective states where patients clearly describe inwardly directed emotions. Why it works in many schizophrenics and not in others needs further elaboration. The paranoid type will be used for illustration as it is the best understood of the schizophrenic categories.

Psychoanalytic observations indicate that the basis of the paranoid development is the intense castration anxiety, from which evolves the impending fear of bodily harm and the hypochondriasis. In the male, apprehension of losing the penis develops into fears of behaving as a female in the sexual role from which originates the fear of anal rape. Parental threats to the effect that he will be a social outcast for his misdemeanors underlie the ideas of reference and persecutory delusions of the paranoid. The final stage of grandiosity is one of marked spontaneous repair which neutralizes the emotion and produces complete equilibrium. The auditory hallucinations are thought to be repetitions of the parental threats. When this development takes place in a schizoid person, disintegration into a full-blown schizophrenic reaction results. Since the driving force is the intense fear reaction to parental threats, the operation which alters the affective response should relieve this symptom. Excerpts from a few cases will be given to illustrate.

Patient 7 exhibited all stages of the paranoid development except grandiosity. Hypochondriasis was foremost and was accompanied by ideas of reference and persecution. Evidence of vaginalization of the anus was obvious when this patient referred to an enema as a douche and declared his guilt over taking it. Removal of the fears made the subsequent paranoid developments unnecessary and led to disappearance of the presenting symptoms.

Patient 49 suffered hypochondriasis, expressed delusions that she had been used sexually, and was very irritated by accusing voices. After operation, which she said removed the strong tension, she was quite at a loss to explain her delusions and said the voices were those of an authority accusing her of nasty things.

Patient 27, a hebephrenic who had hallucinations before operation, had a history of impotency before the onset of his psychosis. When seen eight months following operation, overt psychotic symptoms were no longer present and because they produced less pain, he was able to verbalize conflicts previously hidden by the schizophrenic process. His conversation centered largely around his sex life. He boasted of his prowess and spoke of his desire for sexual activity. The following impotency dream was related: "I dream of riding through woods and seeing deer. I aim at them with my gun and then I decide, to heck with them, they are just animals, and I walk off without firing and I then feel they don't have any sense—they don't know I'm after them at all. Why not give them a sporting chance, why pull the trigger at all? They keep on feeding without knowing that the hunter was near." (As mentioned previously psychotic symptoms recurred in this patient eleven months after operation.)

These cases serve to illustrate the point long known from psychiatric observation, that a schizophrenic illness is an inferior attempt on the part of the patient to adapt to the intense and disturbing emotions. Following the operation which lessened the intensity of the emotions the inferior regressive attempt at adaptation was no longer necessary.

As the disease process continues in the schizophrenic patient and more regressive repair takes place, the ideation becomes more divorced from affect until a state of relative equilibrium with inner harmony is achieved. For example, the paranoid, through grandiosity, may counteract all of his stress and achieve this equilibrium. Logically, an operation which specifically removes the disturbing affect could not help this condition.

In our group of 48 patients we had one grandiose paranoid. Although he served as a control for the topectomy group, he was later subjected to lobotomy, following which all preoperative symptoms remained, plus irresponsibility and tactlessness. Most workers agree that the most important change following frontal lobe surgery is the alteration of the affective response. Some, however, have postulated that symptoms disappear because of lessening of consciousness of self and lack of foresight. Freeman and Watts ('47a) say a paranoid loses *his* delusions and *his* hallucinations because he is less concerned with himself. If such were the case, then the grandiose paranoid who is just as self-centered if not more so than the disturbed persecuted paranoid should also lose his symptoms following operation. That such a patient does not improve appears to be related to the absence of a strong affective component. The only patients in our group who had lessening of consciousness of self after operation were those in the group who had large amounts of cortex removed. This group was also less conscious of many other things.

At the seven months' follow-up study we carefully questioned members of the patients' families in an attempt to detect if there were defects in the patients' ability to orient to the future. No positive evidence was forthcoming. All patients were declared able to plan as well as ever. Unfortunately, there were no talented artists in this group, so we are as yet unable to determine from this study if topectomy impairs creative ability.

We cannot agree with those who postulate that the tension is lessened after the operation because of lack of concern for the future. In the group who improved there was less concern not only for the future but also for the past and present.

### REASONS FOR IMPROVEMENT

Evidence thus far accumulated indicates that clinical improvement results from removal of a specific region of cortex involving areas 9 and/or 10. Both these areas, however, are granular cortex and are quite large. When other single areas of granular cortex were removed improvement did not result, but they are all smaller and, in order to get a combination as large as areas 9 or 10, it was often necessary to infringe on these areas. On the basis of the one-year follow-up which revealed that those patients who did not have the junction of 9-10 included in the removal improved only temporarily, it seems likely that improvement is not quantitative, but rather due to removal of a specific site. Patients 33 and 27, for example, who had large surface areas which could have only partially removed the important site and also temporarily impaired the function of the specific site by vascular or other changes, did not remain well.

### EFFECTS OF LOBOTOMY

In September, 8 patients underwent lobotomy in accordance with the Freeman-Watts technique. Two patients who originally had topectomy without improvement were included; they also failed to improve after lobotomy. Three of the remaining 6 showed improvement. This was maintained over the eight-month follow-up period in 2. The third patient (5), a catatonic in stupor, became slightly more active following operation so that parole to his home was possible. At no time was he able to work, and seven months after operation retardation with stupor returned necessitating return to the hospital. Patient 11 showed the greatest improvement of the lobotomy group. He was a paranoid schizophrenic with persecutory delusions, auditory hallucinations, and ideas of influence to which he reacted with considerable affect. Following parole he obtained a job beneath his former capacity and has held it successfully for several months. Patient 20, a stuporous catatonic, became slightly more active following lobotomy, was paroled to his home and has been able to help to a limited extent on his father's farm.

In both patients who maintained improvement in behavior there was no disappearance of the psychotic symptoms. When seen eight months after operation patient 11 was euphoric and carefree. He laughed, was inane, and regularly punctuated his statements with profanity. The principal change over his preoperative condition was his complete lack of concern for both his psychotic symptoms and everyday happenings. When questioned about the voices he replied, "Hell yes, they're still there but they don't bother me. Sure there's a plot against me but whoever's behind it ain't worth bothering about." When questioned about the world situation and the atomic bomb he laughed heartily and said, "Hell, if it's coming it's coming; no sense worrying about it." When reminded he had a son of military age he replied without changing this inane grin, "If he has to go he has to go." There was no insight and judgment was lacking, but intellect and memory in gross testing were unimpaired. There was no separation of the psychotic material from reality, no realization that his delusions were symptoms of an illness.

The other improved lobotomy patient was much the same in that there was no integration. He continued to hear voices as he had before operation and showed no realization that he had been ill and that the delusions and hallucinations had been symptoms of an illness.

Despite persistence of the psychotic symptoms, these two patients were socially improved and it was because they showed little concern either about their own thoughts or the present environment.

In the topectomy group there were patients who presented a clinical picture similar to the improved lobotomized patients. Some who had 9 and/or 10 area operations also improved and returned to jobs of their old capacity.

Of the remaining 3 lobotomy patients, one was catatonic, one was a grandiose paranoid without disturbing affect, one was a deteriorated hebephrenic. These did not improve.

Although 3 of the lobotomy patients are now devoid of overt psychotic behavior by virtue of the same alteration of affective response described for topectomy they are, nevertheless, considerably different from the patients benefiting from topectomy in that they all show the tactless, carefree, irresponsible behavior with lack of initiative and absence of remorse that was characteristic of the topectomy patients who had too large an area of cortex removed.

It becomes apparent from this comparative study that these changes in behavior are essentially the same when cortex is removed as when it is undercut. In both procedures the corticifugal and corticipetal fibers are interrupted. In the cortical operation, long and short cortical association fibers are also interrupted and this does not happen in lobotomy. The corticifugal and corticipetal fiber tracts are, therefore, much more important in determining the behavior than are the cortical association fibers.

### POSTOPERATIVE BEHAVIOR OF THE PATIENTS

All operations produced an immediate effect in all patients. Symptoms varied considerably and consisted primarily of confusion, diminished awareness, and distractibility. The intensity of these symptoms varied in different patients and could not be correlated with the type of operation. Generally it was less marked on the first postoperative day than during the succeeding two weeks. After that it began to diminish so that usually by six weeks following operation it had largely disappeared. Because this reaction was universal and unrelated to type of operation we feel that it is the result of trauma to the brain. The appearance of these symptoms did not necessarily alter the basic psychotic picture, but often did make the patients more difficult to manage (see figs. 106-112).

In addition to these nonspecific changes, the patients who had 9 and/or 10 area operations and the lobotomy patients had an almost immediate diminution in painful affect; fears, tension, anger, and similar reactions largely disappeared. This did not occur in the patients having other areas removed.

The course after the immediate nonspecific operative effects had subsided varied considerably in different patients. Those with areas other than 9 and/or 10 removed did not change and will be excluded from the subsequent discussion. In reviewing behavior during the one-year follow-up period in the patients with 9 and/or 10 removals and the lobotomy patients (eight months), several factors stand out.

First is the problem of altered affect. All patients with these areas implicated in the removal had lessening of painful affect. In some this effect was greater than in others. It was also noted than in some patients this alteration was much greater during the first few weeks. These variations, we feel, are due to the physiologic changes that follow operation. We discussed the anatomic correlation with duration of improvement earlier in this discussion. It was stated that although removal of any part of areas 9-10 produced some lessening of affect, it was not marked unless a specific site at the junction of areas 9 and 10 was included in the removal. It seems plausible to explain the immediate marked alteration which subsided in a few weeks on the basis of temporary damage (interference with circulation and edema) beyond the site of actual removal. It also seems plausible that those patients in whom only slight but persistent lessening of painful affect was achieved had only part of the specific area removed. When this happened it gave less protection against recurrence of the psychosis.

The second factor that varied considerably in this group was the manner and degree to which the subjects managed to integrate during the follow-up period. Some of the patients developed complete understanding of the nature of their previous psychotic symptoms, realized that they had been delusional and that the voices they heard were imaginary. The lobotomy patients represented the opposite extreme where psychotic behavior remained unchanged but was ignored, there being absolutely no integration. Between these extremes, many patients had varying degrees of integration. The process of integration, when it occurred, was not immediate and usually was accompanied by considerable stress. As the patients became aware of the old behavior patterns and conflicts there was sometimes considerable stress associated with separating them from reality. There was a partial re-living of the old psychotic period. Usually for a period of one to three weeks there were times when fleeting patterns of the old psychotic behavior would appear. When patients who subsequently went on to recovery were questioned, during these episodes, they would state that they could recognize the old patterns as unrealistic. Once integration had taken place, the psychotic period was referred to as something past. The subjects were able to realize it as a past illness. The lessened emotional reaction to the conflict was always apparent in the patients who successfully reintegrated. As an example, if insomnia had accompanied the psychosis, these patients would manage to sleep soundly during the period of reintegration.

Patient 13 (pp. 355-357) was one of the patients who was able only partially to integrate the past psychotic symptoms. He developed the realization that his auditory hallucinations and intense depression were symptoms of an illness, but several things were never completely understood. He insisted that he had been doped and also some of his persecutory ideas persisted. He showed little concern over these symptoms, however, and said he did not discuss them because people would not understand. Patient 49 had more completely integrated in that she recognized the true nature of all her psychotic symptoms and referred to them as a past illness.

The third factor that must be considered in reviewing the postoperative behavior of the patients is the fact that they have returned to society and are subject to realistic vicissitudes which might conceivably reactivate the original conflicts. Patient 49, the maid, had a partial relapse when one of her employer's children was injured. From observing her it was apparent that this incident had activated her basic fears of mutilation which had led to the paranoid development.

With these factors in mind we shall discuss the problem of temporary versus lasting improvement. A partial parallel can be drawn to infectious disease where the final outcome is determined by two things: the virulence of the organism and the resistance of the host. The lessening of painful affect following operation can be likened to giving some immunity. If the basic disease process is too malignant, it cannot be controlled despite this change. In some of the cases this effect was minimal, so that when reintegration occurred or when patients experienced disturbing events in everyday life, the psychosis recurred.

Patient 27 was able to make a social adjustment following operation despite the fact that basic conflicts (intense mutilation fear) remained apparent in his productions and dreams until he arranged to have a date and became sexually aroused. Regression into psychosis then returned despite the alteration of affective response (the degree of alteration was not marked in this case).

Patient 33 who also had obtained only partial protection as a result of operation suffered a recurrence of her psychosis when confronted with increasing frustration over speech difficulty which led to loss of her job.

On the other hand, patient 49, cited above, who had a greater effect from operation was able to reintegrate following a painful realistic event which had activated her basic conflict.

Patient 4 (pp. 349-351) illustrates a subject who achieved only minimal alteration of affect as a result of operation. Nevertheless, because this individual's illness was of a milder degree, the minimal effect of operation has enabled him to return to society.

## ROLE OF TOPECTOMY IN PSYCHIATRIC TREATMENT

From this survey one is able to judge where topectomy should fit into the psychiatrist's therapeutic armamentarium. Its specific effect is to alter the affective response so that tensions do not accumulate, thereby making regressive-reparative behavior unnecessary. A thorough psychiatric evaluation, keeping this point foremost, is the only method of selecting patients for operation. Haphazard recommendations will result in an increased percentage of failures and will include patients who could have been helped by more conservative measures. This must be guarded against.

The conventional diagnostic categories cannot be the only criteria in determining whether or not a patient is a suitable candidate for operation. Patients with agitated depressions and the agitated involutional paranoid, because of the intense affective component to their illness and its appropriateness to ideation, have a very favorable prognosis.

The manic depressive in the depressed state, suffering from inwardly directed emotion responds well, but when the compensatory manic period intervenes to spontaneously interrupt his suffering, the operation is of no avail. Further study of the effect of operation in manics is necessary.

A most thorough preoperative psychiatric study is imperative in order to determine whether or not schizophrenics will benefit by operation. Consideration of clinical subcategories is of little help. Only schizophrenics in whom there is affect appropriate to ideation have a reasonable chance for improvement. Clinicians are well aware that this is more apt to prevail in the earlier stage of the disease. Other more conservative types of therapy are sometimes sufficient to arrest the schizophrenic development, but the psychiatrist should always be alert for signs of beginning deterioration so that operation can be undertaken before it is too late.

On the basis of this study we are in no position to discuss its effects on psychopaths. There is, of course, considerable tension in these patients and all other treatments are notable failures. The tension, however, bears a different relationship to the underlying conflict than it does in the neuroses and psychoses. Clinicians are aware that pressure developing from fear of detection and competition frequently precipitates overt psychopathic behavior in these individuals. Investigation of the effects of operation should be undertaken with great caution. Our evaluation of the efficacy of this treatment in this disease must await further experience.

We touch on the problem of psychoneurosis with great trepidation. Our clinical studies and the psychologic tests undertaken thus far indicate that relatively little is sacrificed by the patient as a result of a small specific area removal. Regardless of this, we must consider first and foremost that brain tissue is being removed and it can never be replaced. This procedure cannot become a substitute for adequate and skillful psychotherapy. No psychoneurotic patient was included in this series, but it is readily apparent from the description of the effects of operation (and the authors can add that a few neurotics with intractable tension which could not be resolved by the most skillful psychotherapy have been included in another series) that relief can be obtained. Until considerably more time has elapsed to provide much more extensive evaluation of this procedure, one should be hesitant to recommend operation for any but the most severe neurotics, and then only if intensive and skillful psychotherapy has proved valueless.

Some are certain to note that the psychologic tests in this series indicate less impairment of function following topectomy than appears following the shock therapies. Despite this, we do not feel that surgery can replace shock. We are not aware of the exact nature of the change produced by shock, but certainly brain tissue is not removed as it is with operation. In certain schizophrenics who are in danger of rapid deterioration, the operation is immediately indicated and should replace shock which is known to be ineffective.

Patients of other types who do not respond to shock should not be given one series of treatments after another of a so-called ambulatory type merely to make them more tractable. This frequently leads to extensive damage and masks signs of underlying deterioration. The illness in many of these patients can be markedly shortened by operation.

## SUMMARY

1. Beneficial effects resulting from frontal lobe surgery were due to alteration of the affective responses.

2. This effect appeared only if areas 9 and/or 10 were encroached upon at operation.

3. When the rostral part of area 9 and caudal part of area 10 were not included in the removal the full effect of operation was not obtained. The effects of infringement on other parts of 9-10 were, nevertheless, often adequate to produce improvement in milder cases. Patients who were very ill and also patients who encountered traumatic events in everyday life which reactivated or intensified basic conflicts sometimes became so disturbed that, despite the protection provided by operation, they again regressed into a psychotic state.

4. A large percentage of patients in whom more than two large areas or several small cortical areas were removed showed signs of deterioration in social behavior. This also occurred in our lobotomy patients when large amounts of cortex were undercut.

5. Patients whose overt psychotic symptoms disappeared following operation showed essentially the same basic personality traits that were present before the illness began. This occurred only if complete reintegration took place. Reintegration began anytime between three weeks and four months after operation. During this period psychotherapy should be very helpful.

6. In chronic psychotics, affect was divorced from ideation to varying degrees. This seldom occurred in patients other than schizophrenics and manics. As this dissociation increases, the prognosis with operation becomes less favorable.

*Chapter 26*

# Neurology

J. LAWRENCE POOL, ROBERT G. HEATH, FRED A. METTLER,
AND H. HARVEY GASS

---

W ITH the exception of patient 24 (who displayed a condition resembling parkinsonism) none of the patients in the series exhibited any very marked preoperative evidence of neurological disorder. Minor disorders in patients (other than 24) subsequently operated were: moist, clammy extremities (27, 40), tic (7), resistance to passive movement (6, 18, 27, 38, 47), and inequality of tendon reflexes (6, 19, 22, 32, 49).

## SENSORY SYSTEMS

Olfaction, gustation, and thermal sensibility were especially examined in only 1 or 2 patients and then only by crude tests. No gross changes were observed in these modalities but it cannot be denied that subtle changes may easily have gone unnoticed. Vision, audition, and vestibular function were the subjects of especial examination and are considered elsewhere. We shall concern ourselves here with pain and with deep sensation and light touch.

### PAIN

It is, of course, well-known that the reaction of lobotomized patients to painful states is altered but the precise nature of this alteration is still undefined. Thus, although patients commonly bear intractable pain more easily after lobotomy than before, it is generally believed that certain types of pain, notably phantom-limb pain, is relatively more refractory than other types. Another peculiarity of the behavior of lobotomized patients to pain is the fact that their initial reaction to even slightly painful stimuli is enhanced even though a chronic painful state may be better borne. With the exception of one or two laboratories, really valid physiologic studies of the sense of pain have not been carried out after lobotomy and the present observations are based upon the crude and imprecise methods of ordinary bedside examination. More precise methods were impractical in the great majority of patients in the series.

Three patients (10, 13, 24) showed some general insensitivity to pain prior to operation. Of these three, patients 13 and 24 were operated upon. After the visit to surgery sensitivity to pain returned to normal limits in patient 13 but not in patient 24. It is believed that this improvement was merely a reflection of general psychiatric improvement. Only 1 patient (6) showed any reduction in sensitivity to pain after operation and this was of but two days' duration, immediately after operation, and localized to one upper extremity which was temporarily paralytic following removal of part of area 6. Acuity to pain returned before the extremity had recovered full motor power.

That many of the patients over-reacted to but slightly painful stimuli following operation was frequently remarked by the physicians and technicians engaged in venipunctures and finger-pricking. These patients also over-reacted to other noxious but not necessarily painful stimuli and restraint was more frequently required in the immediate postoperative period than before, in the case of many patients. Unfortunately no records were kept of which patients fell into this group. Not all did.

DEEP SENSATION

Observations relating to deep sensation fell into two categories: (1) observations of the appreciation of the passive movement of joints and vibratory sense and (2) ability to perceive pressure touch as disclosed by two-point sensitivity and the motor indication of local sign.

**Passive Movement of the Joints and Vibratory Sense.** The psychiatric condition of many of the patients was too profound to recommend testing by more than crude methods (goniometric records were not made nor was the frequency of the vibrating stimulus altered) which failed to disclose any evidence that any of the operative procedures (with the exception of the temporary change in patient 6 already noted) exerted an influence upon these tests other than may have resulted from general psychiatric improvement.

**Two-Point Sensibility and Local Sign.** Curiously enough, more reliable data were secured in respect to these functions than the two former and rather accurate recording of these functions was possible in 18 of the 24 patients subsequently operated upon. Of these 18, 14 showed a prompt postoperative drop in threshold for two-point sensitivity. Five of these 14 showed an additional later drop and 4 a subsequent rise but not to their preoperative levels. It is significant that these changes were quite unrelated with psychiatric improvement or with area or amount of cortex removed. One of these 18 patients showed no change and 3 displayed a rise in threshold for two-point sensibility.

Local sign, insofar as this is tested by a blindfolded patient's ability to touch with his finger a spot previously touched by the examiner, was apparently uninfluenced (patient 6 again excepted) by any of the operative procedures.

LIGHT TOUCH

Physiologically satisfactory testing of light touch was not attempted. The method of testing which was used was to touch the blindfolded patient on various parts of his body (no attention being paid to whether this was glabrous or hirsute) with a wisp of cotton, and asking him to touch the stimulated spot with his finger. By this crude method, no alteration (patient 6 excepted) in the sense of light touch could be detected following any of the operations.

## Motor Systems

### MOVEMENTS OF THE EYES

Only one of the patients (33) exhibited permanent abnormality in eye movements, but inability to use the eyes to follow moving objects and freely to direct central vision about the visual field was common. Convergence was more frequently impaired than lateral movement and the former function was evidently more easily affected by a frontal lesion than was the latter. Disability of lateral movement of the eyes was bilateral in some cases and predominantly unilateral or purely unilateral in others reflecting, no doubt, in the latter cases inequality in the cortical excisions. In patients with bilateral paresis of lateral gaze the eyes were directed somewhat internal from the straight forward position, producing a peculiar staring gaze with a suggestion of strabismus.

Disorders in extraocular movements did not invariably follow excision of area 8 or of the upper parts of 9 and 10 and the evidence indicates that injury restricted to the superior frontal gyrus does not impair extraocular movements. Impairment in movements of the eyes in patients with injury in the inferior frontal gyrus and caudal half of middle frontal was very common.

### SPEECH AND DEGLUTITION

Speech could not be induced in patient 6 (areas 6 and 8) for nine days after operation; in patient 24 (area 6) for twenty-three days; and in patient 33 (inferior frontal gyrus) for approximately three weeks.

It is of interest that all three of these patients had cortical lesions extending into or close to the foot of the precentral gyrus on both sides. Yet, patient 47 (area 44 removal) showed no apparent changes in her speech after operation (see p. 452).

Of special interest is patient 33, a twenty-six-year-old catatonic schizophrenic, who was mute before operation. Following bilateral excision of the inferior frontal gyri she remained mute for the first three weeks after surgery, and made little effort to feed or help herself, while saliva flowed constantly and profusely from her mouth, soaking the pillow. Approximately three weeks after operation drooling became progressively less pronounced as the patient became more cooperative, able to eat and drink, and finally to speak. At first she spoke only in monosyllabic fashion. Five weeks after operation she was able to speak only in unintelligible phrases, and three weeks later, though seldom volunteering conversation, she began to speak rationally in connected sentences. This condition has persisted during the twelve-month follow-up period to date, with no evidence of aphasia or anarthria, but with definite dysarthria and dysphagia.

The cortical excision included area 44, the bulk of area 45, and parts of areas 46 and 10. As the result of circulatory interference it is quite possible that the function of at least part of the second frontal convolution (middle frontal gyrus) was also jeopardized. While care was taken not to interfere with the integrity of circulation of the gyri breves of the island of Reil, the foot of the central gyrus or the superior temporal convolution may have been affected by the operation in either patient 33 or 47. In patient 47, area 44 was excised.

While there was no evidence of true aphasia in patient 33, the examination was marked by failure to volunteer conversation, some difficulty in enunciating with clarity, especially consonants, and a tendency for mucus and saliva to collect in the mouth. In addition, there seemed to be impairment of volitional as contrasted with emotional facial movements; there was difficulty in moving the tongue; and finally, an extremely hypoactive gag reflex despite preservation of pharyngeal, palatal, and buccal sensation, and taste on all parts of the tongue. The patient's chief neurological deficit therefore appeared to consist of dysarthria and dysphagia, of cerebral rather than of bulbar or peripheral origin. In this connection, the otolaryngologist, Dr. Edmund Fowler, Jr. stated: "I believe that this woman's voice difficulty is cortical rather than motor in origin."

The failure to volunteer speech seemed, in part at least, due to embarrassment occasioned by the patient's difficulty in articulation. It is, however, equally, if not more probable that this fault represents a fragment of motor aphasia and might therefore be termed motor, verbal, or expressive dysarthria.

The marked hypoactivity of the gag or pharyngeal reflex remains unexplained, as it was not possible to test it prior to operation. One might speculate that cortical components of the gag reflex may have been interrupted bilaterally by the cortical removals, which in this case were so close to the cortical motor representation of the facial, lingual, pharyngeal, and laryngeal muscles. The difficulty in volitional movements of the tongue and facial musculature is in keeping with this possibility. It is possible therefore the hypoactive gag reflex may be the result of the bilateral supranuclear surgical lesion which interrupted cortical components of the gag reflex just as loss of the abdominal reflexes may follow certain supranuclear lesions.

Turning now to the chief interest in this case, it is apparent that Broca's area, or at least its major part, had been bilaterally removed without resulting in the full-blown aphasia of motor, verbal, or expressive type, that is, inability to articulate (Weisenburg, and McBride, '35) which is commonly said to follow its destruction.

There appears to be a certain lack of unanimity not only regarding the exact limits of Broca's area but also as to the effect consequent to its destruction. Grinker ('34), for example, refers to a type of anarthria manifested by a profound defect in word formation, with preserved comprehension of word meaning, which may lead to a monosyllabic, telegraphic form of speech known as verbal, motor, or expressive aphasia, following a lesion of Broca's area in the left cerebral hemisphere of right-handed individuals. However, in many of the illustrative cases cited by Grinker ('34), Weisenburg and McBride ('35), and Moutier ('08), it is clear that the extent of the lesions far exceeded that of Broca's area. Moreover, Marie ('06) and also Moutier ('08) in extensive and careful analyses showed plainly that complete destruction of Broca's area frequently occurred without aphasia of any type; and conversely, that motor aphasia (anarthric) occurred in many cases with gross and microscopic preservation of all of Broca's area bilaterally. On the basis of his study, Moutier felt that anarthric aphasia must be attributed rather to lesions of the lenticular zone ("zone lenticulaire"). Jackson inclined to a similar view: "Whilst I believe the hinder part of the left third frontal convolution is the part most often damaged, I do not localize speech in any such small part of the brain . . . the nearer the disease is to the corpus striatum, the more likely is the defect of articulation to be the striking thing, and the farther off, the more likely is it to be one of mistakes of words." (Jackson, '32.) Recently J. P. Robb described a right-handed patient who exhibited a complete recovery of speech after removal of Broca's area on the left side, and suggested that speech function might have been taken over by the opposite Broca's area. Similar cases have been described by F. Cramer (personal communication), and J. E. Scarff (personal communication). J. M. Nielsen has referred to the possibility of *bilateral* cortical representation of speech mechanisms.

Our 2 cases (33, 47) of bilateral removal of Broca's area militate against the views (a) that destruction of the left Broca's area in right-handed individuals necessarily results in anarthria or motor aphasia; and (b) that the opposite

Broca's area takes over speech function. These 2 cases therefore lend support to the contention of Marie ('06), Moutier ('08), and Jackson ('32) that the function of motor speech is presided over by a part of the brain other than Broca's area (perhaps the insula or adjacent parts of the brain). The implications of this finding are, of course, of particular importance both to the neurologist and the neurosurgeon.

In patient 47, Brodmann's area 44 was excised. Following operation the patient spoke well without logorrhea for several days and then relapsed into garrulous, rambling word-salad speech that did not differ from that of her preoperative state as far as could be determined. Owing to her psychotic condition, it was impossible to carry out any accurate tests of speech mechanisms, but certainly no gross evidence of anarthria, dysphagia, or motor aphasia could ever be demonstrated.

It is suggested that the impairment of volitional control of the facial, pharyngeal, and lingual musculature in patient 33 is probably not due to removal of areas 44 or 45 since no such disability followed removal of area 44 in patient 47, nor of area 45 in patient 19 and 36. It seems more likely that the observed dysarthria and impairment of volitional (but not of emotional) movements of the face in patient 33 may have been secondary to operative manipulation of area 6 or 4, or possibly to some interference with the circulation of the insula.

### OTHER PARETIC PHENOMENA

Patient 6 exhibited postoperative temporary flaccid paralysis of the right upper extremity (thirteen days) and a right facial paresis (nine days).

Patient 27 had a brief postoperative paresis of the brachial movements of the left upper extremity without impairment of the movements of the antebrachial or manual muscles. Area 6 was involved in both of these cases. The masticatory disabilities in patient 33 have been referred to in the preceding section. In addition to patients 6 and 33, patient 40 showed some facial weakness which was still detectable, though in minimal degree, a year later (this patient had exhibited some facial asymmetry prior to operation).

In the lobotomy series, 3 patients (28, 44, 46) showed difficulty in chewing and swallowing for seven days after operation and patient 5 for thirty-six days. The latter patient displayed a flaccid paresis of the right arm for three days and patient 23 had a left facial weakness for seven days after operation.

### EXTRAPYRAMIDAL PHENOMENA

**Cerebellar Signs.** Ataxia and other so-called "cerebellar" signs are frequently encountered in cases of frontal lobe tumors but it is by no means clear that these should be attributed to dysfunction of the frontal lobe itself. In none of the operatees did ataxia, dysmetria, or past-pointing emerge.

**Abnormal Movements and Tonic Postures.** Patient 7 showed a facial tic before operation. Temporarily absent after operation this gradually returned but, a year later, its intensity and frequency were still reduced. Patient 24 displayed a wide and rapidly shifting variety of tonic postures, tremors, and akinesia prior to operation. In fully developed form this patient's picture was one of semiflexed catatonic rigidity. In remissions he walked about slowly in a slightly flexed, hypokinetic manner, his eyes staring, a slow smile slowly appearing and disappearing on his frozen face; he spoke in monosyllables only, and only when addressed. In passing from a remission to full rigidity, a process generally taking about a week, he became stiffer, unable to move about, and displayed almost continuous rapid tremors in the lower extremities. These tremors resulted in heel-tapping movements which were usually but not invariably bilaterally synchronous. Asynchronicity with identical frequency, bilaterally different frequency, and unilateral tremor were all observed. The patient was subjected to bilateral area 6 operation during a remission and promptly relapsed into catatonic rigidity. After passing of this rigidity the patient's tremor was exactly the same as before operation.

Deviation of the head as well as eyes to the right side, together with a definite but indeterminate influence upon movements of the upper extremity, was observed as a temporary phenomenon in patient 33.

### RIGIDITY, SPASTICITY, REFLEX CHANGES

**Rigidity.** Rigidity or evidence of abnormal innervation of muscles in what should be conditions of rest was observed as a preoperative phenomenon in patient 24. It was not encountered as a novel postoperative result of any of the topectomies of the original series. Bilateral removal of most of area 6 in patient 24 did not abolish or reduce the rigidity. Indeed, the condition was more prominent following than before operation, presumably owing to a worsening of the patient's general catatonic state rather than as a specific result of the operation.

**Spasticity and Reflex Changes.** Spasticity or increased susceptibility to proprioceptive stimulation, as measured by resistance to passive movement and a lowering of threshold and increase in speed and force of myotatic reflexes, was generally unchanged or reduced as a result of operations on granular cortex. The latter result is not interpreted as a specific phenomenon but only as a result of lessening of general tension owing to bed rest, some slight muscular weakness, and perhaps reduction in psychic tension in the immediate postoperative period. Removal of none of the areas under study invariably produced any definite enhancement in spasticity or myotatic reflex responses. Neither can the appearance of any abnormal reflexes or signs, such as the Babinski, Hoffmann, or forced-grasping, be attributed to the removal of any of the parts of cortex ablated in the present study. Faint evidences of such phenomena or dubious congeners of them were encountered on one day and not the next, in a very few of the patients. It was impossible to correlate the appearance of these obscure, fleeting signs with any of the variables of the study.

### AUTONOMIC FUNCTION

**Urinary Incontinence.** Twelve patients had incontinence of urine after topectomy, 5 patients only once, 7 more than once (eight to seventeen days). One patient experienced urinary *retention* (four days). Eleven patients never had incontinence. Thus, of the 23 patients having had bilateral cortical excision, 8 suffered significant vesical dysfunction. Six of the 8 patients having had bilateral prefrontal lobotomy suffered urinary incontinence lasting eighteen to thirty-six days. Not only was the percentage of cases higher in this group, but the duration of incontinence was longer and 3 of the lobotomy subjects were also incontinent of feces for about eighteen days. Every patient with area 6 removal had incontinence. All of these observations strongly suggest that urinary incontinence is more apt to be associated with removal of area 6, than with ablations of any other frontal area. The only patient having a lesion *confined* to areas 8 and 9 (patient 32) suffered urinary *retention* (four days). This suggests the possibility of an inhibitory-activatory system at the cortical level, for voluntary vesical control.

**Gastrointestinal Function.**    Postoperative vomiting occurred in 5 cases (25, 27, 32, 33, 40). The common factor in cases 25, 27, and 32 was bilateral excision of areas 8 and 9. In case 33 it may be that removal of area 44 accounted not only for the vomiting, but also increased salivation. Patient 47 (area 44 removal) suffered bloody diarrhea for eleven days after operation. (The only other patient having diarrhea, on one day only, was patient 42, one of the 3 having removal of area 11, which it is believed, represents a cortical end-station for vagal afferents.)

Vomiting, both fecal and nonfecal, occurred in patient 40 along with fecal incontinence and gross transitory changes of the peripheral circulation, following subtotal removal of area 24 bilaterally (cingular gyri). While these autonomic changes may well be due to removal of area 24, two other factors must be considered: (1) the presence of blood in the cerebrospinal fluid; (2) the fact that the circulation of areas 6, 8, 9, may have been affected as the result of retraction of the right frontal lobe or vasospasm of the blood supply to these areas owing to operative manipulation along the course of both anterior cerebral arteries. In the experience of one of us (JLP) the latter usually does not lead to such changes. Moreover in 1 lobotomy patient (5) having blood in the cerebrospinal fluid neither fecal nor nonfecal vomiting occurred. It therefore seems reasonable to suggest that the marked autonomic disturbances in patient 40 may be attributed to removal of area 24.

**Somatomotor Activity.**    Reliable records on the amount of activity in which the patients engaged is not available. It was not until late in the study that we were able to obtain pedometers (the instrument is still impossible to purchase commercially) and basal metabolic studies were not conducted. There is a distinct impression that the most notable degree of overactivity occurred in those individuals from whom the largest number of areas (and largest amount of cortex) was removed. In peculiar contrast to this we know that the measurements we do have on the lobotomy cases demonstrated a definite reduction in the amount of activity. Additional and more precise data is needed to resolve this important question.

### ABSTRACTS OF NEUROLOGICAL EXAMINATIONS

**Patient 2.**    *Preoperative.*    This patient was generally quiet and subdued. The patellar reflex and plantar responses were within normal limits. The eye movements were normal. Two-point discrimination: palmar, 6 mm.; digital, 2 mm.

*Postoperative.*    For four or five days immediately after operation this patient was unusually quiet and subdued, but was able to respond quite rationally to simple questions. Thereafter he became gradually more alert and well adjusted. His myotatic reflexes developed a progressively lower threshold and greater force and briskness. There were no periods of restlessness; eye movements were unaffected. He had incontinence of urine on the third postoperative day. Two-point discrimination rose, in the week after operation, to 9 and 4 mm. and then fell in the following month to 4 and 2 mm. respectively for the palms and fingers. Shortly before reoperation on October 29 it had climbed to 10 and 4 mm. respectively.

*Reoperation, Lobotomy (10/29/47).* On the day after lobotomy the patient was stuporous. His eyes were not turned to the left or to the right. His right hand tended to close on objects put into it but this "grasp" was not well sustained. There was no clonus. Stroking of the plantae resulted in up-going toes and down-going halluces. The following day general plantar flexion was encountered and the day after, general dorsiflexion. The patient was very apathetic and tended to fall asleep easily during the first two weeks after operation. By November 12, 1947, he had developed a tremendous appetite. On January 17, 1948, the patient's color was considerably better than on previous examinations. He was physically more active and was generally in movement around the hall. His gaze tended to shift about abnormally but on the whole he gave no notable evidence of abnormality. The threshold of the right patellar reflex was lower than that of the left but he had no motor disability with the exception of a very slight fine tremor of the right hand, when this was held in full extension with the fingers spread. Two-point sensibility was 4 and 1 mm. respectively for the palms and fingers.

**Patient 3.** *Preoperative.* This patient was unusually quiet, cooperative, subdued, and unresponsive. Patellar reflexes had a very low threshold, no spread, force slight, pendular character, and was slight in amplitude. Responses to plantar stimuli showed almost no movement of the toes. Two-point sensibility was 11 and 2 mm. for the palms and fingers.

*Postoperative.* The patient was very restless during the first three postoperative days; he was talkative, somewhat facetious, and disoriented with regard to space. By the eighteenth day he had become almost as subdued as preoperatively. The only reflex changes consisted in a persisting high instead of low threshold, with a direct instead of pendular quality and some irregularity in the plantar response (no Babinski sign). For six days the eye movements were sluggish and there was a tendency for the bulbi to remain slightly converged. These changes gradually disappeared during the ensuing three days, and eye movements thereafter remained normal. There was urinary incontinence once, on the fourth day. Three weeks after operation two-point sensibility had dropped to 6 mm. in the palm, staying at 2 mm. in the fingers. After operation this patient protested abnormally about slightly noxious stimuli. He subsequently volunteered the information that he was more active than before. He was a chess player and his postoperative playing was about the same as his preoperative. He had previously worked in the record room and his work after operation was as efficient as before though he was said to be more cheerful and to smile, an accomplishment which he had not achieved previously.

**Patient 4.** *Preoperative.* This patient was an agitated, complaining individual. The patellar reflex threshold was high, there was no spread, the force was variable, the character irregular and brisk, the amplitude often increased, the uniformity variable, and relaxation incomplete. The plantar response was normal. Two-point sensibility was 10 and 2 mm.

*Postoperative.* This patient showed no evidence of restlessness or agitation after operation. He never had incontinence. Following operation he was more relaxed and his patellar reflexes became more regular. Plantar stimulation during the first seventeen days resulted in plantar flexion on the right and dorsiflexion of the left toes and hallux. Shortly thereafter the plantar response became flexor on the left also, and remained so. Postoperatively the eyes tended to a position of partial convergence. This disappeared in two weeks after operation. For forty-six days the left pupil was 2 mm. larger than the right. Two-point sensibility rose to 13 mm. on the palm (five days after operation) and then (three weeks postpostoperatively) dropped to 6 mm,

**Patient 5.** *Preoperative.* This was a quiet, subdued, staring patient with an expressionless face. He showed no neurological abnormalities except that both plantar responses were irregularly dorsiflexor and were accompanied by contraction of the adductors of the thigh.

*Postoperative (Lobotomy on 10/30/47).* The day following lobotomy the patient was absolutely unresponsive. He was re-explored on the second day and rallied but then had a unilateral convulsion. His next week was a stormy, febrile one. On November 8 he had rallied to the point where he lay quietly in bed playing with a hair. His finger and eye movements were good though he looked to the left more frequently than to the right. Possibly there was a right grasp response. Stroking the right sole sent all digits into dorsiflexion. Pressure on the right tibia resulted in dorsiflexion of the hallux alone. (These phenomena disappeared before November 13.) On the right, the threshold of the patellar response was lower than on the left. Two-point sensibility could not be measured.

**Patient 6.** *Preoperative.* This patient was very deteriorated and silly, rather quiet, sometimes surly, and given to periodic outbursts of aggressive excitement. The patellar reflex threshold was low on the right, high on the left, being brisker, more forceful and of greater amplitude on the right, with no spread on either side. The other tendon reflexes were difficult to elicit. There were almost no plantar responses on the right; flexor on the left. There seemed to be some increased resistance to passive movements of the joints of both upper extremities. Two-point sensibility was 10 and 2 mm. respectively for the palms and fingers. The left pupil was slightly larger than the right.

*Postoperative.* During the first two postoperative days this patient was extremely lethargic, unresponsive to commands, and apparently unable or unwilling to speak, although he occasionally sat up in bed. He then seemed to be elated for a few days, but on the tenth day became violently destructive. The destructive attitude gradually subsided during the following week. Nine days after operation he began to speak, and tended for the next few days to reiterate resounding though irrelevant words and phrases (he had shown this tendency before operation). Thereafter his speech became progressively more rational, with no aphasia or dysarthria.

Immediately upon the conclusion of the operation all four extremities were moved voluntarily, but the right arm, including the fingers, was moved only feebly. The other three extremities never exhibited any appreciable weakness.

On the first postoperative day a left facial paresis of cortical type was noted. Resistance to passive movements became much as it was before operation. At no time could any "spasticity" be elicited.

No reflexes could be elicited in the right arm on the second day after operation. By the sixth day reflexes had returned in the right brachial musculature (excepting in the triceps) but were still absent in the antebrachial musculature. Some degree of flexor power had returned in the right hand and the patient could move the humeroscapular joint but not the humero-ulnar joint. On the eleventh day the fingers were still kept in semiflexion and the left upper extremity was preferred though the patient was right-handed. By the twenty-fourth day no evidence of paresis could be detected.

No pathologic toe-signs could be elicited by any of the customary tests; plantar stimulation resulted in plantar flexion of all toes bilaterally. There was no Hoffmann sign. It was thought by one observer (JLP), on the eleventh postoperative day and only on that day, that a slow forced-grasp was elicited several times on light tactile stimulation of the left palm but not the *right*, with the patient supine in bed. Proprioceptive (stretch) stimuli did not yield a forced grasp at that or at any other time.

For the first two days the patient looked only toward the right, the eyes being directed forward when at rest. The chin was turned over the right shoulder. The eyes seemed on slightly different planes. On the sixth day there was slight internal deviation of each eyeball. On the eleventh day the eyes tended to stare straight ahead.

By the twentieth day eye movements had become normal. (The left pupil remained slightly larger than the right, as it was before operation.)

Apparently there was no perception of pain (pin-prick) in the paralyzed right arm during the first two postoperative days, for the patient showed no signs of discomfort when it was tested, although when tested anywhere else there was always an obvious response. By the twenty-fourth postoperative day, two-point sensibility could easily be tested on both sides and had dropped to 5 mm. for the palms, staying at 2 mm. for the fingers.

Urinary incontinence occurred through the twelfth postoperative day.

Three months after operation there was still some tendency to prefer the use of the left hand, though the right upper extremity was also well employed. There was also a tendency to look toward the right more frequently than to the left. Two-point sensibility was 6 mm. in the palms. Stimulation of the right sole provoked no response or only slight plantar flexion. The patellar reflexes had a high threshold, low amplitude, poor force, and matured slowly.

Four months after operation the left arm was loosely held in walking and failed to show associated movements. Locomotion was peculiarly loose at all joints and performed with a strange up-and-down movement of the body in which the weight was brought down on the right leg, the right foot being squarely brought in contact with the floor. Passive movement of the upper limbs revealed rapid, regular, fine cogwheeling resistance, especially to extension. A similar phenomenon was occasionally encountered in the right lower extremity. The biceps reflex was more marked on the left than right.

*Reoperation—Unilateral Ablation of Remainder of Right Area 6 (10/27/47)* (see fig. 62). Following operation the head and eyes were directed toward the right and this situation continued for somewhat over four days. The eyes were not moved to the left of the midline in this period but occasionally the head was. Occasionally, when the patient wished to look to that side, the head was rotated. The pupils were equal. There was a left facial paresis and a flaccid paralysis of the left upper extremity. No reflexes and no grasp response could be elicited on the upper extremity of the left side. The left lower extremity was not paretic. The left abdominal reflexes were poor but present. They were active on the right. Both plantar responses were flexor, the right somewhat irregularly so. The left hand sweated more than the right and this extremity was apparently insensitive to pin-prick. On November 6, 1947, this patient had a generalized convulsion.

By November 8 the patient was up and about, moving with the same sort of gait as before operation, the left arm dangling and not being used for any kind of activity. There was still a trace of left facial paresis and the gaze was directed predominantly toward the right.

The right arm exhibited the same sort of resistance to passive movement previously mentioned. The left displayed no resistance. The left biceps reflex had a greater amplitude (+3) than the right (+2), its force was greater and it matured faster. There was no grasp reflex on either side. The left patellar reflex had a lower threshold, greater force and amplitude, and was brisker than the right. Sweating of the hands was equal.

On December 1, the left arm still exhibited a flaccid paralysis and was not involved in any voluntary or associated movements or postures.

Passive movement of the left fingers and wrist disclosed no resistance and there was no clonus. Passive flexion of the elbow elicited no resistance but, upon passive extension, some resistance could be felt in the second half of the movement. Slight resistance to passive movement of the shoulder could also be detected.

When the arm was passively placed in abduction or protraction it could be held for a short time but slowly descended under the influence of gravity. Passively superimposed positions of the wrist or fingers could not be maintained.

There was definite overactivity of the left biceps reflex and Hoffmann's sign was present on the left. No difference in two-point sensitivity could be detected between the upper extremities.

On January 17, 1948, the same general postural stance was used in walking. The right foot turned out somewhat more than the left and there was diminished swing of the left arm. Progression was good and strong. The right biceps measured 26 cm. and the left 25. The right forearm measured 24.2 cm. and the left 23.2. The left gastrocnemius was 33.2 cm. and the right 32.5. The left arm was held somewhat loosely to the side of the body. There was no evidence of contractures at any of the joints. The left arm was somewhat straighter than the right and the fingers of the left hand were more open. Both arms were well extended in front of the body. The left wrist dropped slightly and there was slight supination of the forearm, with the first finger definitely higher than the little finger. During elevation of the arm there were slow, clonic contractions of the flexors of the fingers, more marked in the little finger and occurring at the rate of about three to two per second. Such clonic contractions could also be seen when the arm was hanging loosely at the side, at which time they were particularly active in the little finger, spreading occasionally to the other fingers and thumb, the first finger and thumb being rarely involved in this movement. The arms were well extended to the side, though the left perhaps a little less fully than the right. The left arm was also somewhat supinated and the wrist slightly dropped. When the arms were extended to the sides of the body, supination and pronation of the left arm was less pronounced than on the right. In flexion of the forearms, from this position, the left brachium was dropped somewhat from the horizontal line and approached the side of the body. Reaching above the head was well performed but the left arm did not rise as far as the right and the fingers were not so fully extended. Supination was performed much better than pronation when the antebrachium was resting. Clonic contractions of the flexors of the fingers and the thumb appeared intermittently and involved all digits and the wrist. There were occasional clonic contractions of the deltoid at the same frequency. The left shoulder was lower than the right. Movements of apposition of the fingers and thumb could be performed with both hands but were less complete in the left hand. Given an object, the thumb was not well extended but kept along the side of the hand. The fingers were neither well flexed nor extended and there was a tendency to move the hand without flexing the wrist but by elevating and shifting the shoulder as a whole. With the hands flat on the knees the thumbs could be extended away from the knee and both were well flexed. Extension of the left thumb was less pronounced than the right. The fingers could not be extended from the knee nor could the wrist be elevated without shifting the forearm as a whole. Movements involving the flexor carpi radialis and flexor carpi ulnaris were not performed. The clonic contractions seen in the hand were apparently movements of the intrinsic muscles of the palms and did not extend to the muscles of the forearms. The focal point was the little finger and the focal movement was flexion of this. There was no resistance to passive movement in an initial movement. With repeated movement the patient developed some cogwheeling in the antebrachium of both arms, more particularly the left. There was no resistance to flexion of the arm nor, as indicated above, to initial extension of it. The patellar reflexes showed slight inequality the threshold of the *right* being lower than that of the left. The response on the right was brisker and the amplitude greater. The right reflex matured more rapidly and was more forceful. The pupils were equal and extraocular movements were well performed in all directions. Facial movements were equal and well performed.

The plantar responses were flexor on both sides. Percussion of the tibia and Achilles tendon and forceful stroking of the tibia produced plantar flexion of the toes and hallux.

With the patient in the dorsal decubitus there was no resistance to passive flexion of the forearm. Passive extension elicited a certain amount of resistance which was entirely of a cogwheel nature. There was also cogwheel resistance to passive pronation and supination, to abduction but not to adduction. There was no resistance to protraction. There was no resistance to the fingers in any direction nor to movements in any direction of the wrist. There was no forced grasp in any phase. Examination was frequently interrupted by clonic contractions of the small finger and the other fingers.

Vibratory sense was equal on both sides. There did not appear to be any difference in the ability to appreciate passive movements of the digits of the left hand. Light touch was easily appreciated. Two-point sensibility was 4 mm. for the palms and 1 mm. for the fingers. This man's postoperative paralysis had almost entirely cleared. The only evidence of resistance to passive movement which was seen was of an interrupted type which was clearly clonic. *There was no sustained resistance to passive movement.* An entirely unexpected feature of his condition was the spontaneous clonic movements he displayed, chiefly in his hand and little finger.

Cursory re-examination in May, 1948, still showed an inability to approximate the left thumb and forefinger and difficulty in holding objects in that hand.

**Patient 7.** *Preoperative.* This patient was quiet and cooperative. The patellar reflex threshold was very low, the spread slight, the force marked, the character brisk, amplitude high. Plantar stimulation resulted in a struggle reaction. Occasional tic-like twitching affected the left facial and platysma muscles. The swing of the right arm was less than that of the left. Two-point sensibility was 5 mm. and 2 mm.

*Postoperative.* The patient was moderately restless and irritable the postoperative first day, but gradually improved until by the ninth day he was quiet and cooperative.

There were no appreciable postoperative changes in the reflex status, but on testing passive movements there seemed to be fine tremulous interruptions on flexion or extension bilaterally. Eye movements were normal in all respects. Two-point discrimination was unchanged during the first four months after operation but by the eighth month it had dropped to 4 and 1 mm. in the palm and fingers respectively. There was no incontinence. The left facial tic was replaced by a slight facial twitch of lesser frequency than the original movement.

**Patient 8.** *Preoperative.* This patient was usually active about the ward, and sporadically helpful, but often became suddenly violently aggressive.

Patellar reflexes were irregular, threshold low, spread slight, force often increased, character brisk, amplitude often extreme, uniformity variable. Plantar stimulation evoked a struggle reaction. Two-point sensibility was 6 and 2 mm.

*Postoperative.* The patient was extremely restless and boisterous during the first thirteen postoperative days, then cooperative and cheerful. He was relaxed and the patellar reflex threshold was higher than before operation, the character of the reflexes was sluggish, and the right was slightly more active than left; otherwise there were no significant changes. Dorsiflexion of all toes and hallux of both feet were instantly evoked by plantar stimulation. For six days the eyes were usually directed forward and somewhat inward. There was incontinence on the third and fifth postoperative days. Vibratory sense was impaired in the right upper arm five days after operation. Six days postoperatively two-point sensibility in the right palm and fingers was 40 mm. (but by the seventeenth day this had dropped to 6 mm. for both palms and 2 mm. for right as well as left fingers). On the seventh day a grand-mal seizure occurred. During an insulin tolerance test, forty-four days after operation, the patient went into coma though he said he could hear during this. There were no further convulsions until three months after operation. Thereafter grand-mal seizures occurred about every two weeks, though postoperative months six and seven were free from these.

Three months after operation two-point sensibility stood at 5 and 2 mm.

**Patient 11.** This patient was a euphoric, active man without abnormal neurological findings. He was subjected to lobotomy which did not produce any abnormal neurological reactions.

*Patient 13. Preoperative.* This patient was mild and apprehensive. The patellar reflexes had a variable threshold, with occasional spread, moderate force, low amplitude, and were irregular in character and uniformity. Plantar stimulation evoked a struggle reaction which involved dorsiflexion of the left hallux.

*Postoperative.* The patient was restless for the first two days, then very inactive for several days. With increased relaxation, patellar reflexes showed very high threshold; there was no spread, poor force, irregularity in character and uniformity, and low amplitude. Plantar responses: flexor. There was marked forward fixation of gaze with internal deviation of both eyes which were directed on different horizontal planes for at least two days and forward fixation for a longer period. By the nineteenth day this had disappeared but side-to-side movements were still irregular.

*Patient 18. Preoperative.* The patient was a detached, ethereal individual smiling to himself and given to elaborate circumlocution and circumstantiality. No tendon reflexes were obtainable except the biceps. There was flexor response on plantar stimulation. On testing passive resistance, slight extra contractions of arm movements were noted. Two-point sensibility was 4 and 1.5 mm.

*Postoperative.* The patient was very quiet and subdued following operation. He was cooperative from the first postoperative day onwards, but extremely restless on the third postoperative day. He was hungry, but not excessively so on the first day. He slept poorly requiring sedation the first eight days; then he slept eight to ten hours at night. Three months after operation he was more active than before operation. There was no change in reflex status. The eye movements at times showed questionable "cogwheel" type of irregularity for eighteen days. Two-point sensibility was 8 and 2 mm. (eighteen days after operation); thereafter 4 mm. palmar. There was no incontinence.

*Patient 19. Preoperative.* This patient was frequently overactive, usually very voluble. The reflex status was within normal limits throughout except that the left biceps reflex was slightly more active than the right. Plantar response: flexor. Two-point sensibility was 7 and 4 mm.

*Postoperative.* The patient was quiet and cheerful immediately after recovery from anesthesia; the context of speech was wild and confused for eight days. He was very depressed on the thirteenth day. His appetite was good. The reflex status reflected postoperative muscular relaxation. There was slight tremor of outstretched hands for fifteen days. There was slight irregularity of eye movements for fifteen days, with fine nystagmus, the rapid component being toward the right. A defect in ocular convergence was observed forty days after operation. Two-point sensibility was 9 and 3 mm. on the fifteenth day, later dropping to 4 mm. palmar. There was no incontinence.

*Patient 20. Preoperative.* This was an uncommunicative powerful individual who was extraordinarily inactive. No information could be coaxed from him about any of the phases of the examination requiring his comment. There was notable, irregular resistance to passive extension of the upper extremities and some degree of stiffness in all muscles. The myotatic reflexes were all difficult to elicit. A barely perceptible patellar reflex could be evoked on the right. Plantar stimulation resulted in generalized struggling with dorsiflexion and fanning of all toes and dorsiflexion of both halluces.

*Postoperative (Lobotomy on 10/31/47).* Following operation the patient was stuporous for several days and his neurological status was similar to that before operation except that the toes and halluces turned down in response to plantar stimulation. Stroking the periosteum of the left tibia resulted in dorsiflexion of the toes and hallux. Similar stimulation on the right produced flexion.

By the end of the week the patient was more active. A convulsion occurred on November 8, 1947. Two and a half months later the patient responded to questions and was reasonably active. Two-point sensibility was now measurable and unequal on the two sides, right palm 5 and left 2 mm., right fingers 1 mm. and left somewhat less.

**Patient 21.** *Preoperative.* The patient was quiet, depressed, and relatively inactive. The patellar reflex threshold was very low, the spread slight, the force considerable, very brisk, of moderate amplitude, the right slightly greater than left, many local contractions. There was flexor response to plantar stimulation. Two-point sensibility was 9 and 2 mm.

*Postoperative.* The patient spent the first nine days after operation sleeping most of the time. He ate well. There was no change in reflex status. His gaze was internally convergent for eighteen days, with occasional jerking on conjugate movement. There was incontinence of urine on the third day and on the sixth through the thirteenth days. Nine days after operation two-point sensibility was as before operation but three months later had dropped to 5 and 2 mm. respectively in palms and fingers. The patient went through several phases of depression in these three months each of which became shorter than the one preceding. Activity gradually increased to a condition of continued spryness.

**Patient 22.** *Preoperative.* This patient was confused, inactive, and aggressive when disturbed. When his confidence was obtained he tried to cooperate but had difficulty in keeping his mind on what he was asked. Reflexes were difficult to test. At times myotatic reflexes seemed more active on the right. Plantar stimulation evoked nothing or a struggle reaction. Two-point and other sensory modalities could not be properly tested.

*Postoperative.* This man was more restless than patient 4, less than 3 and 8. He had incontinence. He had only one aggressive episode and was fairly talkative. He was cheerful and cooperative, and ate well. Reflexes were within normal limits after operation. On the third day a convergence defect of eye movements was noted. Two-point sensibility was 10 and 2 mm. twenty days after operation, and 4 mm. two and one-half months later. As this man's negativism and aggressiveness faded it became apparent that beneath this he was confused as to time and sequence. His thoughts were jumbled and he was very circumstantial and rambling. He was reputed to have had a convulsion several months after operation.

**Patient 23.** *Preoperative.* This patient was a thoroughly disoriented individual with marked delusions and hallucinations. Reflexes were lively, the patellar reflex threshold was low, elicitable from a wide zone, strong and rapid with wide amplitude and uniform in repetition and from side to side. Two-point sensibility was 6 and 3 mm. on the left, less on the right.

*Postoperative (Lobotomy on 10/29/47).* There were irregular flexor movements upon plantar stimulation. This result was regularly seen for three days after operation. Two and a half months after operation this patient was much the same as before operation.

**Patient 24.** *Preoperative.* This patient, a catatonic schizophrenic, exhibited coarse generalized tremors of about two-to-three per second frequency during catatonic episodes. These tremulous movements were most marked in the lower extremities, and might involve either side alone or both sides together. There was resistance to both passive flexion and extension of all extremities. On the left side this was of cogwheel character. On the right, cogwheeling was not notable. There was bilateral finger and ankle clonus. Atrophy of muscles of hands and lower forearm was manifest. The toes and hallux were kept in dorsiflexion. The facies were masked. The tendon reflexes of the right extremities were more active than those on the left. No pathologic reflexes could be elicited.

The patient, when he could be induced to walk, had a shuffling type of gait, stooped posture, and no associated movements of the arms, which were carried in partial flexion.

Both patellar reflexes were brisk in character. The right showed marked force and amplitude, no spread, and a very low threshold. The left did not seem abnormal as to force or amplitude; its threshold was high and there was no spread. Local taps produced local and partial contractions in various muscles. Plantar stimulation resulted in prompt plantar flexion of all digits bilaterally.

The eyes were fixed in a forward, staring position. When not in catatonic rigidity, pin-prick was apparently felt all over. Two-point sensibility was 9 mm. for the right palm and absent from the left palm. There was no ability to distinguish two points on any fingers. Other sensory modalities were difficult to evaluate.

The neurological picture closely resembled that of parkinsonism.

#### TABLE 89. REFLEXES, PATIENT 24, THIRD POSTOPERATIVE DAY

| | Right | Left | | Right | Left |
|---|---|---|---|---|---|
| Pectoral | 3+ | 3+ | Hamstrings | 4 | 4 |
| Biceps | 3+ | 3+ | Achilles | 5 | 5 |
| Triceps | 3+ | 3+ | U. lat. abdom. | 1+ | 1 |
| Radial | 3+ | 3+ | Cremasteric | 3 | 3 |
| Ulnar | 3 | 3 | Plantar flexion | 2 | 0 |
| Suprapatellar | 3 | 3 | Babinski | 0 | + |
| Patellar | 3+ | 3+ | Hoffmann | + | + |

*Postoperative* (see figs. 63-66, and tables 89 and 90). For the first two postoperative days this patient was very quiet and listless, but thereafter he became quite restless. On the third postoperative day, he lay with his head flat on the pillow (in previous rigid states it was clear of this by several inches). The head was not moved and the mandible was fixed against the maxilla. The eyes were open without evidence of convergent abnormality. The pupils were equal and reacted well to light. When the eyes were closed they drifted back and forth in a horizontal movement requiring two seconds to complete the cycle. This kept up indefinitely (and was previously observed in the patient after shock therapy). If the patient was aroused, and with eyes open, conjugate movements could be obtained to the fullest extent. The upper extremities were extended, adducted, retracted, and internally rotated. The fingers were flexed with the thumb protruding between the second and third finger (this posture was observed before operation). The lower extremities were internally rotated and extended. There was bilateral ankle but no patellar clonus. When the legs were lifted by the heel a suggestion of rotatory clonus at the hip occurred.

Occasional undirected movement was observed in all extremities, the right greater than the left in the arms, equal in the legs. Movements were slow and strong, such as: flexion of the knees almost to the chest, then extension, then a long rest. During movements quite bizarre positions often resulted, e.g. crossing of legs. Occasionally there was coarse shaking movement of various extremities—flexion, extension and abduction, and adduction. There were generalized writhing movements; chief of which was the tendency to pull the knees to the chest followed by rigid extension.

Very slight resistance to passive extension of the left lower leg was noted while the right was quite flaccid. There was marked bilateral equal resistance to extension of the elbows; flexion was not resisted. There were free movements at the wrists. No grasp reflex was elicited. Pin-prick produced a slow withdrawal of the extremity being tested.

On the fifth postoperative day, the patient's condition had slightly improved. He now fixed his gaze on the examiner and the oscillating movements of the eyes had ceased. Conjugate movement was poor. The left eye was about thirty degrees to the left, while the right looked straight ahead. This angle of difference changed from time to time. Reflexes were the same and the abnormal involuntary movements continued.

On the sixth day, resistance to passive flexion of the upper extremities seemed greater and equal on both sides. The left Babinski sign was no longer elicitable but ankle clonus persisted and was more marked on the left than on the right. Gaze to the right was more frequently observed than to the left.

TABLE 90. REFLEXES OF PATIENT 24 JUST PRIOR TO REOPERATION

|  | Right | Left |
|---|---|---|
| Pectoral, biceps, radial, triceps.... | 3 | 3 |
| Upper abdominal............... | Not elicited | Not elicited |
| Lower abdominal............... | 1 | Not elicited |
| Cremasteric.................... | 2 | 1 |
| Hamstrings, ankle.............. | 3 | 3 |
| Clonus........................ | At the wrist there was cogwheeling which resembled clonus bilaterally but was not real clonus | |
| Patellar....................... | No clonus | No clonus |
| Ankle......................... | Two reduplications | Two reduplications |
| Hoffmann..................... | Not tested | Not tested |
| Babinski...................... | Plantar response | Plantar response |
| Chaddock, Oppenheim, Rossolimo | 0 | 0 |
| Patellar: | | |
|    Threshold.................. | Medium | Medium |
|    Reflexogenous zone.......... | Lower ⅓ of thigh | Lower ⅓ of thigh |
|    Spread.................... | To adductors | To adductors |
|    Force..................... | Medium | Medium |
|    Character................. | Brisk | Brisk |
|    Amplitude................. | Very short | Very short |
|    Nature.................... | Restricted by rigidity | Restricted by rigidity |
|    Irregularity in sides.......... | None | None |
|    Uniformity in succession....... | Constant | Constant |
|    Special features.............. | Normal amplitude of reflex seems checked by rigidity | Normal amplitude of reflex seems checked by rigidity |

On the eighth day the patient lay on his back, his eyes staring straight ahead, his pupils equal. No speech was elicited even with urging. He could move all four extremities, but when the right arm was placed in vertical position from the bed, it remained where placed. The left arm, however, fell slowly (in straight position) to the bed. At times the arms, both together or one independently, would stiffen straight out and turn inward as though a decerebrate posture were forming. The legs tended to maintain an antigravity position: when so placed by the examiner they fell slowly, though faster than the left arm. No forced grasp could be elicited with either tactile or stretch stimuli. The reflex status was the same as on the sixth day.

On the tenth day the patient was in definite catatonic rigidity. The left eye was not directed to the left of the midline. The right moved satisfactorily. There was marked ankle clonus on the left but not on the right. The plantar response was flexor. On the right but not the left the patellar reflex spread to the adductors. The upper extremities occasionally exhibited slow movements together. Usually they were internally rotated and flexed. There was marked resistance to passive extension of the forearms to an angle of 90 degrees, beyond which they could not be extended. The most notable resistance was in the biceps, internal rotators, adductors, and retractors. A dose of 0.25 gm. of amytal temporarily abolished all resistance. There was little change in the following week.

On the seventeenth postoperative day the patient was quiet in bed but moved all four extremities at times slowly and deliberately. He stared straight ahead most of the time, but occasionally his eyes wandered from side to side. The right arm was completely flaccid and limp while the left was quite resistant. The legs were not resistant. The patient turned in bed on request. He had incontinence of urine. There was no speech. The left fingers were clenched most of the time. At times both leg and arm showed coarse rhythmical tremors. No Hoffmann's sign was elicited on the left but there was positive reaction on the right with secondary clonus on the right of the hand and forearm. There was questionable forced grasp on the left only. Transitory (three-to-four times) bilateral ankle clonus was present on the left; clonus was sustained on the right. The Babinski sign was positive on the left with no fanning (plantar flexion of toes: up-going of hallux). No Babinski sign was elicited on the right. Reflexes of the right arm and leg were more active than those of the left. Abdominal reflexes: 1−, equal: cremasters 2−, equal. (The patient had no incontinence after this day.)

By the twenty-eighth day the patient was able to move about and obey instructions but he still could not speak. An adduction-abduction tremor had appeared which was sometimes replaced by a flexor-extensor tremor at one or both hips. The pupils reacted well to light but eye movements were still abnormal. The right bulbus did not move laterally very well and a little nystagmus was present on lateral gaze. A cinematographic record was made on the following day.

On the thirty-third day the patient was more alert. He was able to chew and swallow fairly well when fed and urged. Masked facies persisted. Voluntary movements of the extremities were slow.

The patellar reflex threshold was very low bilaterally, with high amplitude, no spread, and marked force. Plantar stimulation resulted in plantar flexion of each hallux and the toes of the right foot, but dorsiflexion of the left toes. There was marked resistance to the extremes of both passive flexion and extension, very marked on the left and characterized by some interruptions, suggestive of cogwheeling.

During the next week no definite abnormalities in movements of the eyes could be observed nor could any evidence of a group reflex be detected.

Three months after operation the patient was in about the same state as before operation. He sat about smiling in a frozen manner or walked as before. He was unable to speak and showed a tremor of the right leg of about two-to-three per second. Plantar stimulation produced general flexion on the right but of only the toes on the left. The left hallux remained stationary or might flex slightly once or twice during the stimulus. When supine in bed, the position was sufficiently flexor to keep the head 12 inches above the pillow. If the head was pushed down it slowly rose again. The digits of all extremities were adducted and flexed but not the knees or elbows. Passive movement to extend digits met with alternating resistance in all but the right toes. The threshold of all deep reflexes was very, very low, their amplitude and speed great and the action of the antagonists very marked. Antigravity postures of the arms were maintained for four minutes and then began to subside. By the following week the patient was able to talk and two-point sensibility could be tested. He was unable to distinguish two points as distinct, even at great distances.

During the next month the patient's condition changed very little. His catatonic rigidity waxed and waned and his tremor subsided and reappeared. Just before reoperation he was about as he had been before his first operation. At times, especially at the beginning of the examination, if left standing alone, he tended to show retropulsion, but only for a few steps, unless an effort was made to catch him, in which case it became more marked. With repeated trials he could be pushed backwards to either side or forward without pulsion, and except for restricted range of movements his response was normal. When pushed hard enough he could be made to run, and then his body resisted the pushing hand at his back. Straight-line walking could not be tested.

*Postoperative.* Second Operation on 10/28/47 (see figs. 63-66). On the day after operation the patient was again mute. The left but not right extremities were spontaneously moved. There was definite resistance to passive movement of the left arm but less than before operation. The right resisted passive extension of elbow and extension of fingers in all ranges. The left plantar response was flexor. On the right, adduction of the thigh only was produced. Stroking the right tibia caused dorsiflexion of the toes. A right Achilles jerk was present but not a left. There was no ankle clonus. On the afternoon of this day the patient suddenly went into coma and was placed in an oxygen tent (apparently he developed his cerebral thrombus at this time, see figs. 63-66).

On the second postoperative day the right arm showed notable resistance to passive protraction and abduction and to flexion of both the elbow and wrist. Movements in the opposite direction were not resisted and the left arm opposed passive movement only slightly with but a trace of irregular cogwheeling during flexion. There was no grasp reflex on either side.

Both legs equally resisted passive extension of the knee; there was no clonus in the lower extremity. A complex mass movement (not a Babinski reflex) appeared upon right plantar stroking. This consisted in simultaneous contraction of internal rotators of the thigh, adductors, quadriceps femoris, and anterior tibial muscles together with dorsiflexion of the hallux. The eyes were well moved in all directions.

On the third postoperative day there was now a definite sustained posture of the right arm. This consisted of pronation of the forearm, marked flexion and adduction of the wrist, and inward rotation of the scapula. Attempts to flex or extend the elbow were strongly opposed. There was resistance to extension but not flexion of the leg. Plantar stimulation produced the same result as previously.

On the fourth postoperative day, the position of the right upper extremity was now clearly an established one. Passive extension of the elbow met sudden resistance when the antebrachium was brought to slightly over 90 degrees and dorsiflexion of the wrist met sudden resistance when this was in line with the antebrachium. The fingers exhibited general resistance without sudden change at any place. The arm was not moved in response to painful stimuli. There was no resistance of any sort in the left arm. No grasp response was present.

The legs were as previously noted and there was no evident impairment in the movement of the eyes.

The patient's motor state continued in much the same manner (except that dorsiflexion of the hallux began to disappear from the mass response by November 6, 1947) until the patient's sudden demise on November 19, 1947, twenty-two days after operation. He ran a low-grade fever, which showed a tendency to spike, throughout his postoperative period. During the period November 4 to 7 his temperature ranged about 102° F. and then slowly descended to 100°. He was allowed up in a chair November 16. Autopsy showed that death was due to aspiration pneumonia.

**Patient 25.** *Preoperative.* This patient was an agitated individual in almost constant activity. There were no abnormal neurological findings. Two-point sensibility was 8 and 2 mm.

*Postoperative.* The patient was rather quiet and subdued for the first two days following operation. Then he became extremely irritable, depressed, and uncooperative for about thirty days. Several times during the first fourteen days restraint was necessary for several hours at a time. His stock phrases did not begin to abate until after about thirty days. He frequently cried out demanding a drink of water which he would sip and then demanded another and so on. He had no incontinence but vomited the first day.

There was slight depression in force and amplitude of tendon reflexes for eight days, with a higher threshold on the left. A slight convergence defect of eye movements was noted thirty-eight days after operation. There was gradual abatement of somatic overactivity. Two-point sensibility became only slightly more acute.

**Patient 27.** *Preoperative.* This patient was a surly, uncommunicative, relatively inactive individual. The reflex status was within normal limits, except that the right plantar response was practically nil; the left was flexor. Resistance to passive movements was slightly irregular. Two-point sensibility could not be properly tested.

*Postoperative.* The patient was restless and disoriented, and occasionally bawled loud, brief, senseless phrases for the first thirty days following operation. The reflexes were difficult to elicit. Both plantar responses were slightly flexor. For six days, the lateral eye movements were slightly impaired; the right eye did not move to the right of the midline until the twenty-fifth day; thereafter the eye movements were normal. There was incontinency of urine through the sixteenth and of feces on the twelfth and the sixteenth day. The patient vomited on the first day, after eating. He did not begin to speak until the seventh day.

In the second month he began to wander around, examining objects, and was more amiable. By the eight month after operation it was obvious that this patient had been altered from a taciturn, sullen individual to a garrulous person who smiled and occasionally tried to make a joke. He had some difficulty in keeping his thoughts in order and occasionally in finding the word he wanted. The difficulty he had with words was very slight and not like an aphasia but rather suggested that he rambled on in a garrulous manner and that occasionally his thoughts only caught up with his words some time after he had uttered them.

**Patient 28.** *Preoperative.* This patient was a slow, slovenly, stuttering, confused man who made futile efforts to cooperate. There was some resistance to passive movements of all extremities. On plantar stimulation there was plantar flexion with a tendency for a mass response to appear. Two-point sensibility was 10 and 5 mm.

*Postoperative, Lobotomy (11/1/47).* (Cortical electrical stimulation at the time of operation disclosed a very high threshold.) There was defective internal deviation of the left eye during convergence. Incontinence was present. The patient was slow in chewing and swallowing. Two-point sensibility was 6 and 2 mm.

**Patient 31.** *Preoperative.* The patient was a depressed, inactive woman with many varied complaints. Her reflex activity varied with apprehension. Plantar responses: flexor on right, irregular on left. Two-point sensibility was 10 and 3 mm.

*Postoperative.* This patient spoke as soon as operation was concluded. She was somewhat confused for ten days. Her tendon reflexes were difficult to elicit. Right hallux: plantar flexion; left, dorsiflexion; other toes of each foot gave flexor responses for the first month; thereafter the plantar responses were normal bilaterally. The eye movements were normal. There was incontinence of urine through the eighth day and of the feces on the first two days. There were no notable eye signs. Two-point sensibility was 7 and 2 mm.

On the fourth postoperative day the patient suffered a temporary state of apparent surgical shock with blood pressure reading 76/64. At no time following operation was the patient unusually restless or apathetic.

**Patient 32.** *Preoperative.* This patient was a restless, voluble, petulant woman, oscillating between euphoria and temper outbursts.

Her patellar reflex threshold was higher on the right than on the left; force and amplitude were poor bilaterally, with no spread. The plantar response showed poor reaction or struggle reaction. Two-point sensibility was 10 and 4 mm. on the right and 8 and 2 on the left.

*Postoperative.* The patient was able to smile and to speak immediately after operation. She was rather quiet but cheerful for the first two days. Thereafter she became increasingly active (more so than in the preoperative state), voluble, and restless and apparently there was a shortening of hours of sleep. She commented on the fact that she had a greater awareness of environment and various forms of sensory experience, including physical and psychic sex stimuli and appetite for food. Her patellar reflexes showed a low threshold (equal), no spread, poor force, brisk character, and high amplitude. Plantar responses; stroking of one sole produced bilateral dorsiflexion of all digits on both feet on the first postoperative day; thereafter, there was dorsiflexion of the right digits, but not the left, through the fourteenth day; thereafter reaction was normal. Two-point sensibility dropped to 5 and 2 mm. bilaterally, then rose to 8.5 mm. four months after operation. There was urinary retention on the third and fourth days. The patient vomited on the first and third day.

Seven months after operation this patient was still overactive. At this time she volunteered the following: "I'll tell you one thing you have done, you fixed it so I can't cry any more. I can't even start to cry."

**Patient 33.** *Preoperative.* This patient was a violent, resistive woman who haunted the corridor in an effort to escape. She was said to have spoken in monosyllables in the early part of project. The examiner did not hear the patient speak. She could not be examined.

*Postoperative.* The first day she moved all four extremities with great strength. She was usually quiet and asleep but periodically she thrashed about, moaning a little, and making sucking movements with her mouth. She persistently lay on her abdomen, face downward. There was profuse salivation. Slight left facial weakness was noted. The left eye deviated laterally, the right was in the midline. On the second day the patient retched frequently, and vomited bile-stained liquid three or four times. Nausea and retching were also noted on the eighth day. For eight days the patient was unreactive except for bulbar and reflex movements. Her eyes were divergent and were directed toward the right. She turned her head toward the right. These movements disappeared after twenty days. It was difficult to elicit any tendon reflexes during the first twenty-one days. On the eighth day there was dorsiflexion of the right and plantar flexion of left digits on plantar stimulation. By the twenty-first day a flexor response was elicited bilaterally. Two-point sensibility was impossible to determine before six weeks after operation; then it was found to be 5 mm. and, five months later, 9 mm.

The patient began to speak in thick monosyllables four weeks after operation. The speech slowly improved thereafter but up to twelve months it was still dysarthric. Tongue and lip movements were deficient. The patient was unable to swallow unless the food was in the back of her throat; she pushed it there herself with her finger as part of her method of eating.

Urinary incontinence occurred nearly every day for fourteen days. Profuse drooling continued indefinitely. There was little or no reaction to stimulations of inside of the mouth, fauces, and pharynx.

Six months after operation the furrowing of the tongue was limited to the anterior third. Its corpus could be moved to either side but protrusion was absent. When an attempt was made to protrude the tongue the corpus was elevated but no forward movement occurred. The soft palate was well elevated and the constrictors of the pharynx moved but not as much as they should. There was no upward movement of the hyoid in the attempt to swallow. The pharynx appeared to be completely insensitive to stimulation and none of the usual intrapharyngeal reflexes could be evoked. The larynx was not visualized but sounds of a hoarse nature were produced.

Nine months after operation there was no evidence of ataxia, incoordination, nor weakness of the extremities. The sense of smell was intact bilaterally. There was no gross impairment of vision. The pupils were equal and normally reactive; they were 3 mm. in diameter. Ocular movements were normal. There was difficulty in opening the mouth fully, but this may have been owing in part at least to the fact that the operative procedure involved incision through both temporal muscles. There was no facial asymmetry, and smiling was naturally and fully carried out, but there was difficulty in showing the teeth on volitional effort. The voluntary facial movements were limited in contrast with involuntary facial movements. Uvula was in the midline and moved symmetrically with phonation but a gag reflex was elicited only upon strong stimulation of the posterior pharyngeal wall on both sides, but never to its fullest extent. Salivation was normal in amount with a tendency for thick saliva to collect in the mouth owing to difficulty in swallowing. The patient could swallow food or liquids with ease. The function of the vocal cords was reported as normal by Dr. Edmund Fowler, Jr. There was no weakness of the muscles supplied by the spinal accessory nerve on either side. The tongue showed no fibrillation nor atrophy, but was moved and protruded with obvious difficulty though in the midline. Sensation for light touch, pin-prick, and pressure was intact over the entire face, nostrils, buccal mucosa, tongue, and pharynx; corneal reflexes were preserved and brisk.

The patient spoke rationally and answered questions accurately and promptly in connected sentences with correct usage of nouns, verbs, and articles. However, she did not volunteer any conversation and her articulation was not clear, there being a tendency to slur words, particularly initial consonants of long words. Speech was not "nasal" nor was there a "bulbar" quality.

During the course of several interviews there was no evidence of aphasia. Rather, the patient's mode of speaking showed a severe degree of dysarthria in which the mandibles and lips were energetically moved but the tongue was not moved at all. On reading or speaking the first few words were intelligible but after that one could not tell what she was saying unless she spoke slowly and took time to wipe away the saliva which collected. The patient always understood everything that was said, and could correctly interpret written as well as spoken requests, whether simple or somewhat complicated. Repeated examinations showed no difficulty in naming test objects or describing their use. She wrote and spelled correctly within the limits of her education. Her penmanship was unusually neat, her spelling was accurate, and the context of written words faultless. She could read newspaper paragraphs without error, recount later what she had read, and comment quite intelligently upon their context. Simple mathematical problems were solved accurately in her head without undue delay. See chapter 25 for further course of this case.

**Patient 36.** *Preoperative.* The patient was a depressed, inactive woman. There were no abnormal neurological findings. Two-point sensibility was 7 and 2 mm.

*Postoperative.* The patient was alternately listless and moderately restless for three days following operation. There was no appreciable change in reflexes. There was internal strabismus of the right eye for five days; the left pupil was 2 mm. larger than the right for twenty days. Two-point sensibility was 5 and 2 mm. Urinary incontinence was noted on the first day; constipation for four days. The patient tended to remain in bed but claimed she did not sleep much.

**Patient 38.** *Preoperative.* This patient was a very active, voluble woman. Her patellar reflexes had a very low threshold, considerable spread, force and amplitude; there was struggle reaction on plantar stimulation. There was fine tremulous resistance on passive movements of extremities. Two-point sensibility was 8 and 2 mm.

*Postoperative.* The patient was somewhat restless for the first few days following operation. There were no abnormal eye signs until the fourth day when some convergence appeared which was gone on the following day.

For two months the patellar reflexes had a high threshold, no spread, poor force and amplitude, and were characterized by a narrow reflexogenous zone. There was a struggle reaction on plantar stimulation. There was no resistance to passive movements. There was no change in two-point sensibility at first; three months later it was down to 5 mm. palmar; six months after operation it was again 8 and 2 mm. There was no incontinence. Two convulsions occurred in the first three postoperative weeks.

**Patient 40.** *Preoperative.* This patient was a suspicious, quiet woman with many somatic complaints. Her palms and soles were dripping, cool, and pale. Two-point sensibility was 8 and 2 mm. She was unable to report accurately on vibratory perception or topographic recognition. Tendon reflexes showed a very low threshold throughout. Plantar response: flexor bilaterally.

*Postoperative.* Following operation there was fecal and bilious vomiting. When the patient was touched she began to retch. She said she was not dizzy but was very nauseated. Vomiting continued two days more. On the third day (only) she complained that food tasted "poisoned" and milk tasted "like ammonia"; yet the sense of smell and taste were apparently intact bilaterally. She had a stiff neck for ten days; blood-tinged cerebrospinal fluid was obtained on lumbar puncture. Her hands and feet were warm, dry, and of excellent color for the first twenty days after operation, then they reverted to their cool and clammy state noted before operation.

There was incontinence of urine through the fifteenth day and of feces on the first postoperative day.

On the third day there was a very low tendon reflex threshold with increased force and amplitude, but no inequality. On plantar stimulation there was bilateral withdrawal, fanning, and dorsiflexion of all digits. Left facial weakness (slight) was apparent for a year (facial asymmetry existed before operation). There was temporary paresis of the left upper extremity on the seventh postoperative day. No abnormal eye movements were observed at any time. Two-point sensibility was 6 and 2 mm.; six months after operation the palmar was over 10 mm., the digital continued at 2 mm. This patient is believed to have had at least three convulsions several months after operation.

**Patient 42.** *Preoperative.* This patient was a woman of variable attitude. Patellar reflexes showed a high threshold, no spread, poor force, weak character, and small amplitude; plantar response: up-going of toes in struggle reaction, the hallux gave no response. Slight resistance of the left extremities was noted on passive movements. Two-point sensibility was unsatisfactory.

*Postoperative.* For twenty-two days following operation the patient slept a great deal; she also ate a great deal and her weight climbed. On the ninth day the tendon reflexes were within normal limits, on the twelfth the amplitude of the left patellar was greater than that of the right and there was spread from this. All digits dorsiflexed on plantar stimulation. No further changes in reflex patterns ensued during the twelve-month follow-up period and there was no postoperative resistance to passive movement.

For nine days the patient gazed towards the right more than toward the left. On the twelfth day a slight jerking quality of eye movements was noted; thereafter no abnormalities were observed. Olfactory acuity was normal. Taste was objectively normal although on the seventh day subjective distortion was reported. Two-point sensibility on the ninth day was 7 and 3 mm.; two months later it was 5 mm. palmar. There was no incontinence of urine or feces.

**Patient 44.** *Preoperative.* This patient was a grossly disoriented woman who babbled to herself and gestured to the walls. Reliable neurological examination was not possible. She squinted and shielded her eyes with her hands. There were no evident gross neurological disabilities.

*Postoperative.* Following operation the patellar reflex threshold was low; the force and amplitude were increased. The reflexogenous zone was increased. Responses occurred to all strengths of stimulation. Plantar responses: halluces dorsiflexed, probably as part of a struggle response. Resistance to passive movement was slightly increased for seventeen days. There were no abnormal eye movements. Sensory condition could not be examined. There was incontinence of urine once on the day of operation only.

*Reoperation, Lobotomy (10/28/47).* No abnormal neurological signs were noted after this operation. There was no essential change in the patient's condition.

**Patient 46.** *Preoperative.* This patient was a fatuous incoherent woman who assumed theatrical attitudes of prayer and meditation. Although inaccessible to many phases of the examination, she showed no evident neurological disorder.

*Postoperative (Lobotomy on 10/30/47).* This patient became belligerent and obscene after operation. Satisfactory examination was not possible. There were no obvious neurological disabilities other than incontinence. There were no eye signs. Plantar stimulation produced struggling. Masturbation, not noticed preoperatively, was now overt. Except for a brief period of improvement in the second month after operation the patient's condition continued essentially unchanged to the present time.

**Patient 47.** *Preoperative.* This patient displayed bizarre posturing and confused "word-salad" speech; she was hyperactive. Tendon reflexes were essentially within normal limits. There was slight resistance to passive movements in the lower extremities. She was unable to respond to sensory tests.

*Postoperative.* For about five days following operation the patient's speech was greatly improved with little or no babbling. She answered questions directly and accurately. When asked, while reading a book on twenty-third day, who wrote it, she turned to the front and read the authoress' name correctly. When asked if the authoress had written other books, she turned to the back in search of a list of these which she read off correctly. When asked to spell she did this in absolutely disorganized fashion. Her letters were a marvel of misspelling. Attempts to obtain samples of her pre-illness spelling and of her school work disclosed no definite evidence of such disorder but no information could be obtained about any written productions following the onset of her illness.

Patellar reflexes had an elevated threshold, no spread, and were brisk. Positive Hoffmann's sign was elicited on the left; the plantar responses were normal. There was no unusual resistance to passive movements. There was little if any abnormality in eye movements. The sensory examination was unsatisfactory. Within three months the patient was speaking as before operation, i.e. word-salad effect. There was no dysarthria and no dysphagia.

Diarrhea was present on the first through the eleventh postoperative day, with gross blood in the stools on the first day. (No parasites were detected in stools.)

**Patient 49.** *Preoperative.* This patient was a depressed, quiet woman. There was a high reflex threshold, somewhat more so on the right; there was no spread, poor force, and low amplitude. Plantar response: plantar flexion of all digits on the right and the toes on the left; no response of the left hallux. Two-point sensibility was 7 and 3 mm.

*Postoperative.* The patient was cooperative but depressed directly after operation and thereafter. There was no change in tendon reflexes. On plantar stimulation, there was dorsiflexion of all digits on the right (plantar flexion on left) for four days. There was internal deviation of the eyes for four days. Two-point sensibility was 5 and 2 mm.

*Chapter 27*

# Pathology

ABNER WOLF AND DAVID COWEN

A NUMBER of investigators have studied biopsy specimens of cerebral tissue obtained from psychotic patients at operation. Elvidge and Reed ('36) examined small cylinders of cerebral cortex and white matter, 4.5 cm. in length and 3 to 4 mm. in diameter, removed by means of gentle suction through a cannula inserted into the brain. Kirschbaum and Heilbrunn ('44) excised pea-sized specimens of frontal cortex bilaterally for histologic study prior to lobotomy in schizophrenic subjects. Hydén and Hartelius ('48) made observations on small pieces of frontal cortex removed from psychotic individuals in the course of lobotomy. It would seem that such fresh specimens of cerebral tissue removed from the living patient and fixed immediately would be superior to postmortem material in a search for specific lesions in psychoses. In fact, it was with this thought in mind that the present study was initiated.

## MATERIAL AND METHODS

Fifty blocks of cerebral tissue obtained at operation from a series of 28 patients were examined. These patients included cases of schizophrenia (of which 9 were diagnosed as hebephrenic, 2 as catatonic, 9 as paranoid, and 1 as schizophrenia with affective and psychopathic features). Three were designated as instances of manic-depressive psychosis (2 in the manic and 1 in the depressed phase), and 3 were diagnosed as examples of involutional psychosis (in 1 of whom there was a suspicion of organic brain disease).

Since the project as a whole was not oriented toward the obtaining of ideal specimens for a histologic search for specific changes of etiologic significance, patients were not selected as to optimum age, short duration of illness, or freedom from previous treatment. Of the 20 patients from whom cerebral specimens were taken, 5 were in their twenties, 10 in their thirties, 7 in their forties, 5 in their fifties, and 1 over sixty. Twenty-two were therefore under fifty and 15 under forty years of age. Sixteen of the patients were first admitted six to nine years before biopsy and the remaining 6 were first seen thirteen to twenty-one years before they were operated upon. All but 4 of the patients received insulin, metrazol, and electroshock therapy, only 5 having been treated with metrazol. The great majority had both insulin and electroshocks. The greatest number of insulin treatments in a single individual were 114, and the greatest number of electroshocks, forty-eight. All patients received sodium pentothal-nitrous oxide anesthesia. The anesthesia was kept light, but averaged five and a half hours in duration, and was sometimes considerably longer.

A variety of fixatives were prepared in advance of operation, and were available in the operating room for prompt use after excision of the specimens. The time elapsing between removal of the blocks of tissue and immersion in the appropriate fixative varied from two to fifteen minutes and usually ranged from five to ten minutes. The interval was used for weighing, drawing, and subdivision of the specimen. In nearly every instance the tissue was partitioned and subdivided among the following fixatives: 10 percent formalin (one to five weeks), formalin ammonium bromide (one day to thirty-one days), cold absolute acetone (twenty-four hours), and formol-alcohol (2 days). Pieces were frozen with carbon dioxide ice and preserved in the cold. The formalin, acetone, and formol-alcohol fixed blocks were embedded in paraffin and frozen sections were made of the formalin ammonium bromide and some of the formalin material. Staining methods for demonstrating all of the neuroectodermal and mesodermal structures were applied to sections of appropriate thickness. These included the Nissl, Mahon, Bodian, hematoxylin-eosin, Laidlaw, Perl's iron, and scarlet red stains, and Cajal's gold chloride sublimate, and Hortega's silver carbonate impregnations. In addition, the Gomori ('39, '41a, 41b) technique for the histochemical demonstration of acid and alkaline phosphatases was applied to the acetone-fixed paraffin-embedded material. Microincineration was carried out on the formol-alcohol material for estimation of the mineral content of the tissue. The Ziehl-Neelsen stain was applied for the demonstration of "ceroid" pigment.

## RESULTS

**Patient 2.** Male, 46 yrs. Diagnosis: schizophrenia: hebephrenic. Duration: 9 yrs. Shock treatment: none. Operation: topectomy: area 8, part of 6 bilaterally and right 9.

Histologic findings: Left: (Time between removal and fixation: 6 minutes; weight: 5.8 gm.) Mild diffuse loss (?) of ganglion cells. Many remaining nerve cells disoriented, distorted, shrunken, deeply staining. Some pallid with coarsely vacuolated cytoplasm. Oligodendroglia and microglia normal. Mild increase of astrocytes in cortex with conversion to fibrillary form. Small to moderate amounts of ceroid pigment in small numbers of nerve cells. No abnormal iron deposition. Axons and myelin sheaths: normal. Alkaline and acid phosphatase normal in amount and distribution. Leptomeninges, vascular pattern, and blood vessel walls: normal.

Right: (Time between removal and fixation 7 minutes; weight 7.1 gm.) Cortical architecture and nerve cell numbers normal. Nerve cell structure normal except for rare shrunken, distorted, deeply stained forms near cut surfaces. Moderate number of nerve cells half filled with scarlet-red-staining material. Oligodendroglia in subcortical white matter: rare examples swollen. Microglia and astrocytes: normal. Other findings as on left.

**Patient 3.** Male, 61 yrs. Diagnosis: involutional psychosis: mixed. Duration: 7 yrs. Treatment: shock: insulin: 14; metrazol: 19. Medical history: typhoid fever at 22 yrs. Operation: topectomy: parts of areas 9, 6, and 4 on left and of 9 and 6 on right.

Histologic findings: Left: (Weight 6.3 gm.: mostly white matter.) Available cortex uncapped to fourth layer or lower: most nerve cells deeply stained and distorted. Moderate amount scarlet-red-stained material in scattered nerve cells and in walls of few cortical blood vessels. Ceroid pigment: small amounts in scattered nerve cells. No abnormal iron deposition. Myelin sheaths: normal. Alkaline and acid phosphatase: normal in amount and distribution. Leptomeninges, vascular pattern, and blood vessel walls: normal.

Right: (Weight: 6.4 gm.) Cortical architecture and nerve cell numbers: normal. Scattered, shrunken, darkly staining nerve cells. Moderate amounts of scarlet-red-stained material in scattered nerve cells and walls of occasional cortical blood vessels. Ceroid pigment: small to moderate amounts in one-fifth to one-half of nerve cells, in occasional oligodendroglia and some mural cells of capillaries. Other findings similar to those on right, except for lack of success in demonstration of alkaline phosphatase.

Patient 4. Male, 55 yrs. Diagnosis: schizophrenia: paranoid. Duration: 13 yrs. Treatment: electroshock: 23. Medical history: alcoholism. Operation: topectomy: area 46 and parts of 9 and 45 on left; area 46 and part of 10 on right.

Histologic findings: Left: (Time between removal and fixation: 10 minutes; weight: 5.8 gm.) Cortical architecture and nerve cell numbers: normal. Scattered, distorted, darkly staining nerve cells especially near surfaces. Small to moderate amounts of scarlet-red-staining material in moderate numbers of nerve cells. No abnormal deposition of iron pigment. Axons and myelin sheaths: normal. No success in impregnation of oligodendroglia and microglia. Astrocytes normal. Alkaline and acid phosphatase normal in amount and distribution. Leptomeninges, vascular pattern, and blood vessels walls: normal.

Right: (Weight: 4.8 gm.) Scattered focal nerve cell losses (?) in cortex. Scattered, deeply staining, deformed nerve cells. Ceroid pigment: small to moderate amounts in occasional nerve cells and in occasional mural cells of capillaries. Microglia: normal. Other findings as on left.

Patient 5. Male, 35 yrs. Diagnosis: schizophrenia: hebephrenic. Duration: 2 yrs. Treatment: shock: insulin: 62; electroshock: 21. Operation: lobotomy: later: cortical biopsy: right frontal; white matter disrupted by hemorrhage.

Histologic findings: Cortical architecture and nerve cell numbers: normal. Great many dark, distorted, shrunken nerve cells. No scarlet-red-stainable material. Ceroid pigment: small to moderate amounts in roughly one third of nerve cells. Axons and myelin sheaths: normal. Impregnation of oligodendroglia and microglia: unsuccessful. Astrocytes: normal. Glycogen: none. Leptomeninges and blood vessel walls: normal.

Patient 6. Male, 32 yrs. Diagnosis: schizophrenia: hebephrenic. Duration: 7 yrs. Treatment: shock: insulin: 114; metrazol: 14; electroshock: 26. Operation: topectomy: parts of areas 6 and 8 bilaterally.

Histologic findings: Left: (Time between removal and fixation: 6 minutes; weight: 9.6 gm.) Diffuse moderate loss (?) of nerve cells. Scattered dark, distorted nerve cells and focal collections of blanched neurones. Small amounts of scarlet-red-staining material in scattered nerve cells and occasional mural capillary and pericapillary cells. Ceroid pigment: small to moderate amounts in occasional nerve cells. No abnormal iron deposition. Axons and myelin sheaths: normal. Oligodendroglia, astrocytes, and microglia: normal. Alkaline and acid phosphatase: normal in amount and distribution. Leptomeninges, vascular pattern, and blood vessel walls: normal.

Right: (Time between removal and fixation: 9 minutes; weight: 16.3 gm.) Cortical architecture and nerve cell numbers: normal. Rare dark, distorted, shrunken nerve cells. Other findings as on left.

Patient 7. Male, 40 yrs. Diagnosis: schizophrenia: paranoid. Duration: 5 yrs. Treatment: shock: insulin: 35; electroshock: 43. Operation: topectomy: area 8 and parts of 9, 10, and (?) 46, bilaterally.

Histologic findings: Left: (Time between removal and fixation: 5 minutes; weight: 25 gm.) Cortical architecture and nerve cell numbers: normal. Nerve cell structure: normal except for few shrunken, distorted, dark forms. Moderate amount of scarlet-red-stained material in scattered nerve cells and walls of occasional cortical blood vessels. Ceroid pigment: small amounts in rare nerve cells. No abnormal iron deposition. Axons and myelin sheaths: normal. Oligodendroglia: moderate numbers of swollen forms in subcortical white matter. Astrocytes and microglia: normal. Alkaline phosphatase: normal in amount and distribution. Acid phosphatase demonstration: unsuccessful. Leptomeninges, vascular pattern and blood vessel walls: normal.

Right: (Weight: 20 gm.) Cortical architecture and nerve cell numbers: normal. Widespread shrinkage, but only moderate hyperchromatism of nerve cells. Small to moderate amounts of scarlet-red-staining material in moderate numbers of nerve cells. Ceroid pigment: small amount of pigment in rare nerve cells. No abnormal iron deposition. Oligodendroglia: frequent swollen forms in subcortical white matter. Other findings as on left.

Patient 8.    Male, 29 yrs. Diagnosis: schizophrenia: paranoid. Duration: 5 yrs. Treatment: shock: insulin: 56; electroshock: 16. Medical history: head injury in childhood. Operation: topectomy: areas 9 and 10 on left and 6 and 8 on right.

Histologic findings: Left (Weight: 7.8 gm.) Cortical architecture and nerve cell numbers: normal. Nerve cell structure normal except for distorted, dark, shrunken forms near surfaces. Moderate amount of scarlet-red-stainable material in occasional nerve cells. Ceroid pigment: small amount in rare nerve cells. No abnormal iron deposition. Axons and myelin sheaths: normal. Impregnation of oligodendroglia unsuccessful. Astrocytes and microglia: normal. Alkaline phosphatase: normal in amount and distribution. Acid phosphatase demonstration: unsuccessful. Leptomeninges, vascular pattern, and blood vessel walls: normal.

Right: (Weight: 8.7 gm.) Histologic findings: like those on left.

Patient 11.    Male, 44 yrs. Diagnosis: schizophrenia: paranoid. Duration: 4 yrs. Treatment: shock: insulin: 51; electroshock: 48. Medical history: suicide attempt by gas, 40 yrs. of age; rheumatic fever, 39 yrs. of age; gastric ulcer (?), 38 to 39 yrs. of age. Operation: lobotomy and later, cortical biopsy.

Histologic findings: Right frontal lobe: Cortical architecture and nerve cell numbers: normal. Great many dark, shrunken, distorted nerve cells near torn, cut, and other surfaces. Small amounts of scarlet-red-stainable material in rare nerve cells, in walls of capillaries and pericapillary cells, and rarely in phagocytes in perivascular spaces in white matter. Ceroid pigment: small amount in scattered nerve cells. No abnormal iron deposition. Some swollen oligodendroglia in white matter. Microglia: normal. Focal astrocytosis in white matter. Axons and myelin sheaths: normal. Alkaline and acid phosphatase normal in amount and distribution. Leptomeninges, vascular pattern, and blood vessel walls: normal.

Patient 13.    Male, 43 yrs. Diagnosis: schizophrenia: paranoid. Duration: 3 yrs. Treatment: shock: insulin: 56; electroshock: 36. Operation: topectomy: areas 9, 46 and 45 on left and 9, 10, 45, and 46 on right.

Histologic findings: Left: (Time between removal and fixation: 12 minutes; weight: 13.5 gm.) Cortical architecture and nerve cell numbers: normal. Nerve cell structure normal except for some shrunken, distorted forms. Moderate to considerable amounts of scarlet-red-stainable material in many nerve cells. Ceroid pigment: small amount of pigment in rare nerve cells, oligodendroglia, and capillary walls. No abnormal iron deposition. Small number of swollen oligodendroglia in subcortical white matter. Microglia and astrocytes: normal. Myelin sheaths: normal. No adequate axonal stains. Alkaline phosphatase: normal in amount and distribution. Acid phosphatase demonstration: unsuccessful. Leptomeninges, vascular pattern, and blood vessel walls: normal.

Right: (Time between removal and fixation: 12 minutes; weight: 14 gm.) Similar to left with the following exceptions. The fat stain and oligodendroglia impregnation were inadequate.

Patient 18.    Male, 39 yrs. Diagnosis: schizophrenia: hebephrenic. Duration: 4 yrs. Treatment: shock: insulin: 35; electroshock: 12. Medical history: struck by lightning at 18 yrs., unconscious 1½ hrs., ill 7 weeks. Operation: topectomy: area 11, bilaterally.

Histologic findings: Left: (Weight 4.2 gm.) Cortical architecture and nerve cell numbers: normal. Nerve cell structure normal except for scattered, shrunken, deeply staining, distorted forms. Occasional nerve cells contained considerable amounts of scarlet-red-stainable material and moderate amounts were encountered in the walls of occasional cortical blood vessels. Ceroid pigment: small amounts in rare nerve cells. No abnormal iron deposition. Occasional oligodendroglia in subcortical white matter swollen. Microglia and astrocytes: normal. Myelin sheaths: normal. Axons: no adequate preparations. Alkaline and acid phosphatase demonstration: unsuccessful. Leptomeninges and blood vessel walls: normal.

Right: (Time between removal and fixation: 7 minutes; weight: 4.3 gm.) Histologic findings like those on left with following exceptions: moderate to considerable amount of scarlet-red-stainable material in moderate numbers of nerve cells; numerous swollen oligodendroglia in lower layers of cortex and adjacent subcortical white matter.

**Patient 19.** Male, 50 yrs. Diagnosis: schizophrenia with affective and psychopathic features. Duration: 7 yrs. Treatment: shock: insulin: 17. Operation: topectomy: area 45 with encroachment on 46 bilaterally.

Histologic findings: Left: (Time between removal and fixation: 10 minutes; weight: 1.8 gm.) Cortical architecture and number of nerve cells: normal. Nerve cell structure normal except for deeply staining, shrunken, distorted elements near surfaces. Rare nerve cells contained small amounts of scarlet-red-stainable material. Ceroid pigment: small amounts in roughly half of nerve cells. No abnormal iron deposition. Occasional swollen oligodendroglia in subcortical white matter. Microglia and astrocytes: normal. Axons and myelin sheaths: normal. Alkaline and acid phosphatase: normal in amount and distribution. Leptomeninges, vascular pattern, and blood vessels: normal.

Right: (Time between removal and fixation: 6 minutes; weight: 1.8 gm.) Histologic findings like those on the left with following exceptions: piece used for Nissl stains much smaller; many more shrunken, distorted, deeply staining forms; no swollen oligodendroglia.

**Patient 20.** Male, 28 yrs. Diagnosis: schizophrenia: hebephrenic. Duration: 5 yrs. Treatment: shock: insulin: 54; electroshock: 32. Operation: Lobotomy with subsequent cortical biopsy.

Histologic findings: Cortical architecture and nerve cell numbers: normal. Nerve cell structure normal except for shrunken, distorted, dark forms where cortex was uncapped and undermined. No fat stain or metallic impregnations. Ceroid pigment: small amounts in scattered nerve cells. No alkaline or acid phosphatase studies. Axons and myelin sheaths: normal.

**Patient 21.** Male, 42 yrs. Diagnosis: manic-depressive psychosis: depressed. Duration: 21 yrs. Treatment: no shock treatment. Operation: topectomy: area 10 on left; area 10 and some of areas 45 and 46 on right.

Histologic findings: Left: (Time between removal and fixation: 7 minutes; weight: 8.2 gm.) Cortical architecture and number of nerve cells: normal. Fresh hemorrhages due to operative trauma. Some shrunken, distorted nerve cells, only occasionally deeply staining. Some nerve cells pale and coarsely vacuolated. Small to moderate amounts of scarlet-red-stainable material in few nerve cells. Ceroid pigment: small amounts in occasional nerve cells. No abnormal iron deposition. Some swollen oligodendroglia in subcortical white matter. Microglia and astrocytes: normal. Axons and myelin sheaths: normal. Alkaline and acid phosphatase: normal in amount and distribution. Leptomeninges, vascular pattern, and blood vessel walls: normal.

Right: (Time between removal and fixation: 15 minutes; weight: 5.2 gm.) Histologic findings similar to left with following exceptions: small piece, fresh hemorrhages; scattered, shrunken, dark nerve cells, sinuous apical dendrites. Nearest hemorrhages: nerve cells swollen, pale, rarefied cytoplasm. Where best preserved: cortex normal.

**Patient 22.** Male, 50 yrs. Diagnosis: schizophrenia: paranoid. Duration: 3 yrs. Treatment: shock: insulin: 11. Medical history: lead poisoning at 14 yrs. Head injury at 18 yrs., resulting in headaches for 2 weeks. Operation: topectomy: areas 9, 10, and 46, bilaterally.

Histologic findings: Left: (Time between removal and fixation: 15 minutes; weight: 23.1 gm.) Cortical architecture and number of nerve cells: normal. Nerve cell structure normal except for rare shrunken, deeply staining elements. Ceroid pigment: small to moderate amount of pigment in scattered nerve cells and occasional normal and swollen oligodendroglia. No abnormal iron deposition. Oligodendroglia and microglia: impregnation unsuccessful. Astrocytes: normal. Axons and myelin sheaths: normal. Alkaline phosphatase: normal in amount and distribution. Acid phosphatase demonstration inadequate. Leptomeninges, vascular pattern, and blood vessel walls: normal.

Right: (Time between removal and fixation: 9 minutes; weight: 19.5 gm.) Histologic findings similar to left with following exceptions: many more shrunken, dark, distorted nerve cells chiefly related to numerous petechiae; moderate amounts of scarlet-red-stainable material in small numbers of nerve cells; microglia stained and normal.

**Patient 23.** Male, 39 yrs. Diagnosis: schizophrenia: paranoid. Duration: 5 yrs. Treatment: shock: insulin: 28. Medical history: diphtheria at 7 yrs. with paralysis of legs. Operation: Lobotomy with subsequent cortical biopsy, right frontal lobe.

Histologic findings: Cortical architecture and number of nerve cells: normal. Nerve cell structure normal except for moderate number of dark, shrunken, distorted forms. No scarlet-red or acid-fast stains. Metallic impregnations inadequate. No abnormal iron deposition. Alkaline and acid phosphatase: normal in amount and distribution. Leptomeninges, vascular pattern, and blood vessel walls: normal.

**Patient 24.** Male, 41 yrs. Diagnosis: schizophrenia: catatonic. Duration: 14 years. Treatment: shock: metrazol: 28; electroshock: 7. Medical history: intrinsic atrophy of small muscles of hands. Operation: topectomy: area 6, bilaterally.

Histologic findings: Left: (Time between removal and fixation: 8 minutes; weight: 7.6 gm.) Cortical architecture and number of nerve cells: normal. Nerve cell structure normal except for occasional distortion, shrinkage, and deep staining of nerve cells. Small to moderate amounts of scarlet-red-stainable material in some nerve cells and in walls of occasional, smaller, cortical blood vessels. Ceroid pigment: small amounts in rare nerve cells. No abnormal iron deposition. Some swollen oligodendroglia in subcortical white matter. Microglia and astrocytes: normal. Axons and myelin sheaths: normal. Alkaline and acid phosphatase: normal in amount and distribution. Leptomeninges, vascular pattern, and blood vessel walls: normal.

Right: (Time between removal and fixation: 8 minutes; weight: 10.9 gm.) Histologic findings similar to left with following exceptions: rare focal loss (?) of nerve cells in third cortical layer; moderate amount of scarlet-red-stainable material in many nerve cells. Many swollen oligodendroglia in lower layers of cortex and subcortical white matter.

**Patient 25.** Male, 57 yrs. Diagnosis: involutional psychosis: depressed. Suspected of organic brain disease. Duration: 2 yrs. Treatment: electroshock: 21. Medical history: head injury in childhood. Operation: topectomy: areas 8, 9, and 46 on left and 8, 9, 46, and part of 10 on right.

Histologic findings: Left: (Time between removal and fixation: 10 minutes; weight: 11.3 gm.) Described as firm and rubbery at operation. Cortical architecture and nerve cell numbers: normal. Nerve cell structure normal except for moderate number of shrunken, distorted, dark elements and coarsely vacuolated, pallid nerve cells in sixth layer in some areas. Small amount of scarlet-red-stainable material in rare nerve cell and in wall of occasional cortical capillary. Ceroid pigment: small amounts in scattered nerve cells and oligodendroglia. No abnormal iron deposition. Rare partially swollen oligodendroglia in subcortical white matter. Microglia and astrocytes: normal. Axons and myelin sheaths: normal. Alkaline phosphatase normal in amount and distribution. Demonstration of acid phosphatase unsuccessful. Leptomeninges, vascular pattern, and walls of blood vessels: normal.

Right: (Time between removal and fixation: 9 minutes; weight: 14.1 gm.) Findings similar to those on left.

**Patient 27.** Male, 33 yrs. Diagnosis: schizophrenia: hebephrenic. Duration: 8 years. Treatment: shock: insulin: 53; electroshock: 13. Operation: topectomy: areas 10 and 6 bilaterally.

Histologic description: Left: (Time between removal and fixation: 10 minutes; weight: 16.9 gm.) Cortical architecture and nerve cell numbers: normal. Nerve cell structure normal except for occasional, distorted, darkly staining elements. Moderate amounts of scarlet-red-stainable material in many nerve cells and walls of some small cortical blood vessels. Ceroid pigment: small amount of pigment in rare nerve cells. No abnormal iron deposition. Swollen oligodendroglia in moderate numbers in subcortical white matter. Microglia and astrocytes: normal. Axons and myelin sheaths: normal. Alkaline and acid phosphatase: normal in amount and distribution. Leptomeninges, vascular pattern, and blood vessel walls: normal.

Right: (Weight: 17.8 gm.) Histologic findings similar to those on right except for no swelling of oligodendroglia.

**Patient 28.** Male, 27 yrs. Diagnosis: schizophrenia: hebephrenic. Duration: 3 yrs. Treatment: shock: insulin: 30; electroshock: 21. Medical history: struck head while diving at 13 yrs. Operation: lobotomy with subsequent cortical biopsy. Right frontal lobe.

Histologic findings: Cortical architecture and number of nerve cells: normal. Nerve cell structure normal except for many dark, shrunken, distorted forms. Small amounts of scarlet-red-stainable material in rare nerve cells and moderate amounts in occasional cortical capillaries. Few oligodendroglia in subcortical white matter in various stages of swelling. Microglia and astrocytes: normal. Alkaline and acid phosphatase: normal in amount and distribution. No glycogen. Leptomeninges, vascular pattern, and blood vessel walls: normal.

**Patient 31.** Female, 51 yrs. Diagnosis: involutional psychosis: paranoid type. Duration: 6 yrs. Treatment: shock: insulin: 28; electroshock: 15. Operation: topectomy: area 9, bilaterally.

Histologic findings: Left: (Time between removal and fixation: 2 minutes; weight: 13 gm.) Focal nerve cell losses (?) in third cortical layer. Some distorted, shrunken, darkly staining nerve cells. Group of pallid, distorted, vacuolated nerve cells beneath leptomeningeal hemorrhage. Small amounts of scarlet-red-stainable material in rare nerve cells and moderate amounts in some cortical capillaries. Ceroid pigment: small amounts in occasional nerve cells. No abnormal iron deposition. Myelin sheaths: normal. Axonal stains inadequate. Oligodendroglia, astrocytes, and microglia: normal. Alkaline and acid phosphatase: normal in amount and distribution. Leptomeninges, vascular pattern, and blood vessel walls: normal.

Right: (Time between removal and fixation: 10 minutes; weight: 10.7 gm.) Similar to left with following exceptions: no pale vacuolated nerve cells; small to moderate amounts of scarlet-red-stainable material in many nerve cells. Axons demonstrated as normal. Occasional swollen oligodendroglia in subcortical white matter.

**Patient 32.** Female, 41 yrs. Diagnosis: manic-depressive psychosis: manic phase. Duration: 13 years. Treatment: shock: metrazol: 22. Operation: topectomy: area 9 on left and area 9 and parts of 8 and 10 on right.

Histologic findings: Left: (Time between removal and fixation: 4 minutes; weight: 12.5 gm.) Cortical architecture and nerve cell numbers: normal. Nerve cell structure normal except for some shrunken, deeply stained elements with sinuous apical dendrites. Ceroid pigment: small amounts in occasional nerve cells. No abnormal iron deposition. Myelin sheaths normal. Axonal stains inadequate. Scattered oligodendroglia in subcortical white matter swelling or swollen. Microglia: normal. Astrocytes: focal astrocytosis in zonal layer. Alkaline and acid phosphatase: normal in amount and distribution. Leptomeninges, vascular pattern, and blood vessel walls: normal.

Right: (Time between removal and fixation: 4 minutes; weight: 17 gm.) Similar to left with following exceptions and additions. Nerve cell structure entirely normal. Small amounts of scarlet-red-stainable material in nerve cells, walls of cortical capillaries, and in phagocytes in perivascular spaces in subcortical white matter. Some oligodendroglia in subcortical white matter and sixth cortical layer in various stages of swelling. No astrocytosis. Microglia normal. Axons demonstrated as normal.

Patient 33. Female, 27 yrs. Diagnosis: schizophrenia: catatonic. Duration: 3 yrs. Treatment: shock: insulin: 42; electroshocks: 34. Operation: topectomy: area 10 and part of 44 on left and area 10 and part of 45 on right.

Histologic findings: Left: (Time between removal and fixation: 8 minutes; weight: 12.9 gm.) Cortical architecture and nerve cell numbers: normal. Nerve cell structure: normal. Ceroid pigment: small amounts in rare nerve cells. Axons and myelin sheaths normal. Some swollen oligodendroglia in superficial subcortical white matter. Microglia and astrocytes: normal. Demonstration of alkaline phosphatase unsuccessful. Acid phosphatase normal in amount and distribution. Leptomeninges and blood vessel walls: normal.

Right: (Time between removal and fixation: 10 minutes; weight: 7 gm.) Similar to left with following exceptions: Hemorrhages into cortex, architecture distorted; moderate numbers of distorted, deeply stained nerve cells. No scarlet red-stainable material in nerve cells; moderate amounts in walls of occasional cortical capillaries and in phagocytes in perivascular spaces of larger blood vessels in subcortical white matter. Alkaline phosphatase demonstrated: normal in amount and distribution.

Patient 36. Female, 53 yrs. Diagnosis: schizophrenia: paranoid. Duration: 2 yrs. Treatment: electroshock: 22. Operation: topectomy: areas 10, 11, 45, 46, and 47, bilaterally.

Histologic findings: Left: (Time between removal and fixation: 7 minutes; weight: 23.8 gm.) Cortical architecture and nerve cell numbers normal. Nerve cell structure normal except for shrinkage, distortion, and deep staining of elements, especially near surfaces and hemorrhages. Small amounts of scarlet-red-stainable material in walls of cortical capillaries. Ceroid pigment: small amounts in occasional nerve cells and oligodendroglia. No abnormal iron deposition. Axons and myelin sheaths: normal. Many swollen oligodendroglia in subcortical white matter. Microglia and astrocytes: normal. Alkaline and acid phosphatase: normal in amount and distribution. Leptomeninges, vascular pattern, and blood vessel walls: normal.

Right: (Time between removal and fixation: 5 minutes; weight: 29 gm.) Similar to left with following exception: small to moderate amounts of scarlet-red-stainable material in many nerve cells.

Patient 40. Female, 29 yrs. Diagnosis: schizophrenia: paranoid. Duration: 4 yrs. Treatment: shock: insulin: 41; electroshock: 1. Operation: topectomy: partial removal of area 24, bilaterally.

Histologic findings: Left: (Time between removal and fixation: 7 minutes.) Cortical architecture and nerve cell numbers: normal. Nerve cell structure normal except for very frequent distorted, deeply stained forms (small specimen). Small to moderate amounts of scarlet-red-stainable material in occasional nerve cells. Ceroid pigment and axonal demonstration inadequate. Myelin sheaths: normal. Occasional swollen oligodendroglia in subcortical white matter. Astrocytes and microglia normal. Demonstration of acid phosphatase unsuccessful. Alkaline phosphatase normal in amount and distribution. Leptomeninges, vascular pattern, and blood vessel walls: normal.

Right: Only acid phosphatase studied: normal in amount and distribution.

**Patient 42.** Female, 40 yrs. Diagnosis: manic-depressive psychosis: manic phase. Duration: 19 yrs. No shock treatment. Operation: topectomy: subtotal removal of area 11, bilaterally.

Histologic findings: Left: (Time between removal and fixation: 3 and 10 minutes; weight: 2.9 and 2 gm.) Cortical architecture and nerve cell numbers: normal. Nerve cell structure normal except for scattered, shrunken, distorted, dark elements. Small amounts of scarlet-red-stainable material in occasional nerve cells and in the walls of moderate numbers of cortical capillaries. Ceroid pigment: small amounts in scattered nerve cells. Axons and myelin sheaths normal. Oligodendroglia, astrocytes, and microglia: normal. Alkaline phosphatase normal in amount and distribution. Demonstration of acid phosphatase unsuccessful. Leptomeninges, vascular pattern, and walls of blood vessels: normal.

Right: (Time between removal and fixation: 5 minutes; weights: 2 and 5 gm.) Similar to left with following exceptions: no scarlet-red-stainable material in nerve cells. Impregnation of oligodendroglia unsuccessful.

**Patient 44.** Female, 38 yrs. Diagnosis: schizophrenia: hebephrenic. Duration: 5 yrs. Treatment: shock: insulin: 37; electroshock: 34. Operation: topectomy: removal of area 47 bilaterally and subtotal removal of area 10.

Histologic findings: Right: (Time between removal and fixation: 3 minutes; weight: 2.5 gm.) Cortical architecture and nerve cell numbers: normal. Nerve cell structure normal except for some shrunken, distorted, deeply staining forms. No fat stain. Ceroid pigment: small amount in rare nerve cells. Axons and myelin sheaths: normal. Oligodendroglia, astrocytes, and microglia: normal. Alkaline and acid phosphatase normal in amount and distribution. Leptomeninges, vascular pattern, and blood vessel walls: normal.

Left: (Time between removal and fixation: 3 minutes; weight 2 gm.) Similar to right with following exception: moderate amount of scarlet-red-stainable material in occasional nerve cell.

**Patient 47.** Female, 31 yrs. Diagnosis: schizophrenia: hebephrenic. Duration: 5 yrs. Treatment: shock: insulin: 41; electroshock: 20; metrazol: 12. Operation: topectomy: area 44, bilaterally.

Histologic findings: Right: (Time between removal and fixation: 5 minutes; weight 3.0 gm.) Cortical architecture and nerve cell numbers: normal. Nerve cell structure normal except for many shrunken, distorted, dark elements. No fat stain available, nor any demonstration of ceroid pigment. No abnormal iron deposition. Axons and myelin sheaths: normal. Occasional oligodendroglia swollen in subcortical white matter. Microglia normal. Some conversion of protoplasmic astrocytes into fibrillary form in cortex. Alkaline and acid phosphatase normal in amount and distribution. Leptomeninges, vascular pattern, and blood vessel walls: normal.

Left: (Time between removal and fixation: 5 minutes; weight: 3.6 gm.) Findings similar to those on right except for small focal nerve cell losses (?) in third cortical layer.

**Patient 49.** Female, 39 yrs. Diagnosis: schizophrenia: paranoid. Duration: 18 yrs. No shock treatment. Operation: topectomy: area 10 and portions of 11 and 46 on left and area 10 and a portion of 11 on right.

Histologic findings: Left: Cortical architecture and nerve cell density: normal. Nerve cell structure normal except for occasional shrunken dark forms. Small to moderate amounts of scarlet-red-stainable material in moderate numbers of nerve cells. Ceroid pigment: small amounts in rare nerve cells. No abnormal iron deposition.

Axons and myelin sheaths: normal. No adequate impregnation of oligodendroglia. Microglia and astrocytes: normal. No successful demonstration of alkaline and acid phosphatase activity. Leptomeninges and blood vessel walls: normal.

Right: Findings similar to those on left with following exceptions: few swollen oligodendroglia in subcortical white matter; no fat stain; alkaline phosphatase normal in amount and distribution. Vascular pattern: normal.

## SUMMARY OF HISTOLOGIC FINDINGS

**Cortical Architecture.** The cortical architecture was normal in each instance except insofar as distortion of the tissue had resulted from operative tears and hemorrhages and immediate postoperative manipulation in the unfixed state. In such instances, disorientation of layers and of individual nerve cells occurred. The nerve cell stratification was normal. There was no clear-cut loss of nerve cells observed in any of the Nissl material of the cortex. In six instances doubtful focal (fig. 115) or diffuse (fig. 116 left) diminution of neural elements, usually in the third layer and in some in the fifth and sixth layers as well, was recorded in specimens from the cortex of one cerebral hemisphere while a roughly symmetrical specimen from the opposite hemisphere appeared relatively normal in this respect. This difference on the two sides raises a question as to the validity of the impression of nerve cells diminution on the one side. Five of these cases were diagnosed as schizophrenia, 3 of which were classified as hebephrenic, 1 as catatonic, 1 as paranoid, and the sixth was an instance of involutional psychosis, paranoid type.

**Nerve Cell Structure.** The vast majority of the nerve cells in the specimens examined appeared normal in size, shape, content of Nissl substance, and nuclear appearance as seen in the Nissl stain. The neurofibrils did not stain consistently but where visualized were normal in caliber and number. In each of the specimens examined (from the 28 subjects), darkly staining, distorted, shrunken nerve cells (figs. 116, 117) were encountered in the cortex and this was bilateral in all cases except 2. These shrunken cells were narrowed, showed agglomeration of their Nissl substance, were frequently misshapen, and occasionally had sinuous apical dendrites. Their deeper color made them stand out sharply from the surrounding nerve cells. In the specimens from 11 patients these cells were frequent; in 5 of these 11 only one cortical specimen was available; in another 5 the specimen from the opposite symmetrical cortical area showed only rare or scattered cells of this type; in the remaining patient the symmetrical specimen contained numerous shrunken, deeply staining cells. Ten of the patients from whom these specimens were taken were suffering from schizophrenia and 1 had an involutional psychosis. Of those with schizophrenia, 5 had the paranoid type, 4 the hebephrenic, and 1 had schizophrenia with affective and psychopathic features. In specimens from 5 patients, pallid, sometimes coarsely vacuolated nerve cells were encountered but were relatively infrequent. These 5 patients included 2 with the hebephrenic type of schizophrenia, 2 with involutional psychosis, and 1 with manic-depressive psychosis in the depressed phase.

Fatty material, seen in the scarlet red stain (fig. 118), was encountered in nerve cells of 23 of the patients. In the 5 others no fat stains were available in 3 and no fat was present in nerve cells in the remaining 2. In 16, it was present in small amounts in scattered neurones, in 6 in small to moderate amounts in moderate numbers of nerve cells, and in 1 in considerable amounts

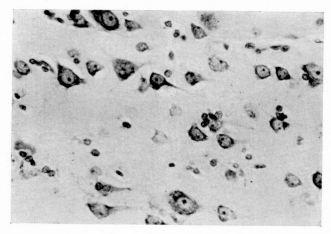

FIG. 115. Focal diminution (?) in nerve cells in cerebral cortex of schizophrenic paranoid patient. (Patient 4. Nissl stain. X250.)

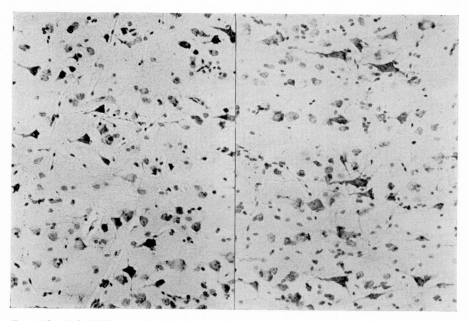

FIG. 116. Left. Diffuse reduction in number of nerve cells in cerebral cortex of patient with hebephrenic schizophrenia. Note hyperchromatism and distortion of some nerve cells and pallor of others. (Patient 6. Nissl stain. X125.)

Right. Distortion, shrinkage, and hyperchromatism of nerve cells in cerebral cortex of patient with hebephrenic schizophrenia. Note sinuous apical dentrites. (Patient 6. Nissl stain. X125.)

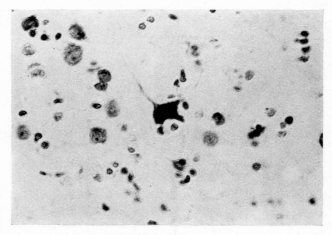

FIG. 117.  Shrunken, distorted, hyperchromatic nerve cell in cortex of schizophrenic hebephrenic individual. (Patient 5. Nissl stain. X250.)

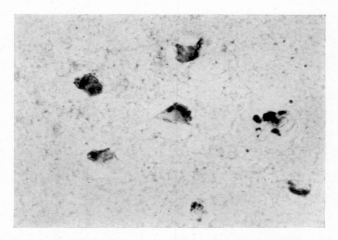

FIG. 118.  Scarlet-red-stainable lipid in nerve cells and in pericapillary space in cortex of
patient with catatonic schizophrenia. (Patient 24. Nissl stain. X250.)

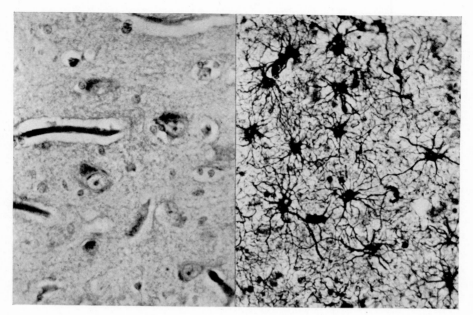

Fig. 119.   Acid-fast (ceroid) pigment seen in nerve cells of the cerebral cortex in a patient with hebephrenic schizophrenia. (Patient 2. Ziehl-Neelsen stain. X250.)

Right. Focal area of astrocytosis in subcortical white matter in a patient with paranoid schizophrenia. (Patient 11. Cajal gold-chloride sublimate stain. X250.)

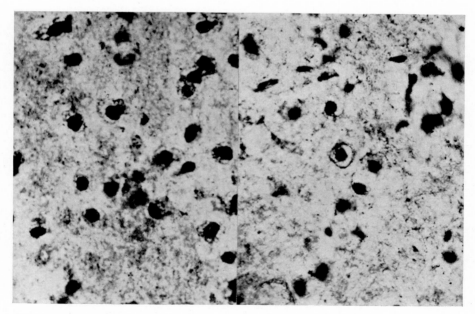

Fig. 120.   Left. Partial and complete swelling of the oligodendroglia in the subcortical white matter of a catatonic schizophrenic individual. (Patient 33. Hortega's silver carbonate stain. X450.)

Right. Swelling of oligodendroglia in subcortical white matter of a patient with manic depressive psychosis in the manic phase. (Patient 32. Hortega's silver carbonate stain. X450.)

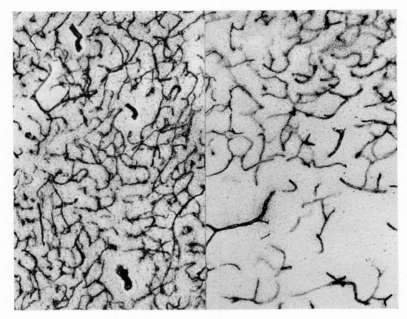

Fig. 121. Left. Normal distribution of alkaline phosphatase and normal vascular pattern in the cerebral cortex of a patient with catatonic schizophrenia. (Patient 33. Gomori's method. X50.)

Right. Normal alkaline phosphatase distribution in cerebral cortex and subcortical white matter in a patient with catatonic schizophrenia. (Patient 33. Gomori's method. X50.)

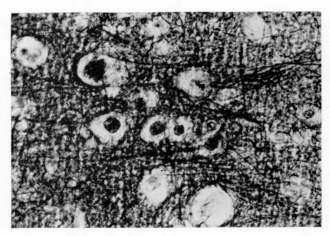

Fig. 122. Normal distribution of acid phosphatase in the cerebral cortex of a patient with catatonic schizophrenia. Phosphatase most concentrated in nuclei and nerve fibers. (Patient 24. Gomori's method. X250.)

in many nerve cells. The individual with the most lipid was forty-three years old and had schizophrenia of the paranoid type. The 6 with the moderate amounts of lipid ranged from thirty-three to fifty-five years of age; they were all schizophrenics—2 had the hebephrenic type, 3 the paranoid, and 1 the catatonic. The patients having little lipid ranged from twenty-seven to sixty-one years of age; 5 of these had schizophrenia, 2 manic-depressive psychosis, (1 in the depressed and 1 in the manic phase), and 1 had an involutional psychosis.

Since some of the lipid referred to above was judged to be lipochrome, it seemed necessary to determine whether a portion of it was acid-fast. This feature of lipochrome relates it to so-called "ceroid" pigment. The term "ceroid" was first applied by Lillie and his associates ('42) to a coarsely globular, yellow, waxlike pigment found in the cirrhotic livers of rats on low-protein, low-fat diets. This pigment is characterized, in addition to its acid-fastness when stained by the Ziehl-Neelsen method, by its insolubility in lipoid solvents, its affinity for fat stains and for basic aniline dyes, and its fluorescence. By analogy with the acid-fast material of the tubercle bacillus, it seems probable that this quality of acid-fastness is due to the presence in the compound of unsaturated fatty acids of high molecular weight. Such acid-fast pigment (fig. 119 left) was present in every specimen examined. In specimens from 4 patients this pigment was more abundant than in those from any of the others, being present in small to moderate amounts in many of the nerve cells. Of these 4 patients, 2 had schizophrenia (1 had the hebephrenic type and the other the affective with psychopathic features), 1 had a manic-depressive psychosis in the depressed state, and the fourth an involutional psychosis with paranoid trends. These 4 varied from thirty-five to fifty-one years of age. The remainder of the patients had only small to moderate amounts of acid-fast pigment in rare or scattered nerve cells. Similar pigment was encountered occasionally in the cytoplasm of oligodendroglia and in the walls of cortical blood vessels.

**Axons and Myelin Sheaths.** These were normal both in number and structure in gray and white matter.

**Glia.** *Astrocytes.* The protoplasmic and fibrillary astrocytes were normal in nearly all the specimens examined. In two instances, metallic impregnations were not obtained. In 3 patients there was a mild astrocytosis. In 1 of these, a forty-six-year-old man who had schizophrenia of the hebephrenic type and who had had no shock therapy, there was a mild generalized conversion of protoplasmic astrocytes into the fibrillary form in the cortex. The other 2 had focal astrocytosis; in 1 it was localized in the white matter (fig. 119 right) (this patient was a man of forty-four with schizophrenia of paranoid type who had had fifty-one insulin and forty-eight electroshock treatments) and in the other in the zonal layer of the cortex (this patient was a woman of forty-one with manic-depressive psychosis in the manic phase who had had twenty-two metrazol shocks).

*Oligodendroglia.* Swelling of the oligodendroglia as demonstrated in Hortegas' silver carbonate stain was a very frequent finding (fig. 120). In six instances adequate stains could not be obtained. In the remainder of the cases there was a varying degree of impregnation but, since many sections were prepared from each block, the total picture, as derived from the series of sections in each instance, gave a usable index of the state of the oligodendroglia. In the specimens from 9 patients there was swelling of small numbers of these cells in the subcortical white matter, and at times in the lower layers of the cortex, while in those from 11 this change occurred in moderate numbers of oligodendroglia in the same areas. Of the 9 patients showing mild changes, 6 had schizophrenia (2 hebephrenic, 2 paranoid, 1 catatonic, and 1 affective and psychopathic features), 1 had a manic-depressive psychosis in the manic stage, and 2 had involutional psychosis. Of the 11 patients who exhibited moderate swelling of the oligodendroglia, 9 were schizophrenics (4 hebephrenic, 4 paranoid, and 1 catatonic) and 2 had manic-depressive psychosis (1 in the depressed phase and the other in the manic phase). In 2 patients the oligodendroglia appeared entirely normal. One of these patients had an involutional psychosis and the other schizophrenia of the hebephrenic type. Observations of the oligodendroglia in the Nissl stain revealed swelling of these cells, often of considerable degree, in most instances. This was seen not only in the white matter but in most of the cortex. It is doubtful whether this appearance of "swelling" in the Nissl stain, as in other common laboratory stains, is significant, since it is so regularly encountered even in the freshest postmortem material.

*Microglia.* In three instances, impregnation by Hortega's silver carbonate method was unsuccessful. In the other 25, a sufficient number of adequate specimens was obtained to indicate that no abnormal changes had occurred in the microglia. This impression of a normal number of microglia, of unaltered structure, was sustained by observations in the Nissl and other stains, where it was found that the number of microglial nuclei, and their size, were within normal limits.

**Phosphatase.** *Alkaline Phosphatase.* Phosphatases demonstrable at a $pH$ of 9.2 using sodium beta-glycerol phosphate as a substrate, according to the method of Gomeri ('39, '41) were present (fig. 121) in all 20 cases in which appropriate material was examined. It was found in the endothelial lining of the leptomeningeal and parenchymal blood vessels, the pia and arachnoid, particularly in arachnoid cells, and to a much lesser degree diffusely in the cortex and white matter, being more abundant in the former. The distribution, and relative quantity of alkaline phosphatase appeared to be similar in each instance to those observed in the brains of nonpsychotic individuals obtained at autopsy. Specimens from patients with all the types of schizophrenia, of manic-depressive psychosis, and involutional psychosis included in this study, showed the same normal picture.

*Acid Phosphatase.* Material obtained from 20 of the patients was examined histochemically for acid phosphatases by Gomeri's ('41b) method as modified by Kabat and his co-workers (Wolf, Kabat, and Newman, '43). Enzyme demonstrable at a $pH$ of 4.7, using sodium beta-glycerol phosphate as a substrate, was found to be present in all structures of the cortex (fig. 122) and white matter, being particularly rich in nuclei and axons. The distribution and relative concentration of acid phosphatase was similar to those in cerebral tissue of nonpsychotic persons. The 20 psychotic patients whose specimens showed a normal content of acid phosphatase in the cerebral cortex and white matter included those having all types of schizophrenia, manic-depressive psychosis, and involutional psychosis included in this investigation.

**Leptomeninges and Blood Vessels.** The histological structure of the pia and arachnoid membrane, and of the leptomeningeal and parenchymal blood vessels, was essentially normal except for the effects of operative trauma and the presence of fatty material, referred to below. The vascular architecture of the cortex and subcortical white matter (fig. 121) could be observed in the alkaline phosphatase preparations and appeared to be of normal type in all the cases examined by this method. In 19 cases there were small to moderate amounts of scarlet-red-staining lipid in the walls of occasional capillaries and less often larger vessels in the cortex. In 3 instances such lipid was seen in small amounts in phagocytes in perivascular spaces in the subcortical white matter.

**Microincineration.** The results of these studies will be reported later.

## DISCUSSION

**Autopsy Findings in the Psychoses.** Alzheimer ('13) described focal losses of nerve cells in the upper layers of the cerebral cortex in patients with schizophrenia. Similar observations were made by Sioli ('09) and later confirmed by Zingerle ('10), Wada ('10), Zimmermann ('15), the Vogts ('22), Naito ('24), Fünfgeld ('27), Boumann ('28), Josephy ('30), Hechst ('33), Meyer ('34), Watanabe ('34), Miskolczy ('33; '37), and others. Josephy ('30) recorded the greatest changes in the frontal lobes, with less frequent involvement of the temporal and parietal lobes and the fewest changes in the occipital region. The cortical layers affected in the order of their frequency were the third, fifth, fourth, and second. Boumann ('28) insisted that all layers could be implicated and believed that this occurred in the following order of frequency: third, second, fifth, sixth, and fourth. Hechst ('33) agreed with Boumann that all layers were involved but in a differing order: third, fifth, second, sixth, and fourth. Fünfgeld ('27) found that there was no constancy of localization of the process in any cortical areas. For instance, areas 38, 46, 8, and 11 were severely changed in one case and showed little, if any, alteration in another. On the other hand, area 17 was always free of lesions, and areas 4 and 7 almost always clear. These findings were later confirmed by Josephy ('30). Naito ('24), however, found lesions of moderate intensity in area 4 in all cases. He agreed that there was a greater tendency to changes in the frontal lobes. Hechst ('33) subsequently described the most intense changes in the prefrontal area, supramarginal and angular gyri, regio parietalis basalis and superior temporal gyrus, while least involved were the area striata, pre- and postcentral convolutions, and the gyri of Heschl. The changes were not always symmetrically distributed in the two hemispheres.

All of the investigators referred to above, who described nerve cell losses in the cerebral cortex, in instances of schizophrenia, also recorded abnormal changes in cortical neurones. These were described by Alzheimer ('13) and confirmed by the others, including Josephy ('30), who summarized them as being of two main types: cell sclerosis and fatty degeneration. Josephy pointed out that clusters of normal cells mingled with the abnormal and that the large-celled layers were affected more than the small-celled. Fünfgeld ('27) and later Hechst ('33) described a rarefaction of the nerve cell cytoplasm and hyperchromatism of the nucleus which might end in cell shadows or sclerosis. Josephy ('30) confirmed this finding but denied it any specificity.

Naito ('24), Marburg ('24), and Fünfgeld ('27) described a diminution in, and pallor of, the tangential myelin sheaths in the upper layers of the cortex. Ferraro ('34, '43) has reported 3 cases diagnosed clinically as dementia praecox in which autopsy revealed diffuse demyelination of the cerebral white matter, the process being marked in the frontal lobes. Marcus ('36) reported focal areas of demyelination throughout the brain, found primarily in the basal ganglia and in the cortex and white matter of the frontal and temporal lobes in instances of schizophrenia.

Glial changes have been recorded as absent or mild. In postmortem material, limited focal areas of astrocytic proliferation most often seen at the junction of cortex and white matter have been reported by Alzheimer ('10), Walter ('19), Josephy ('30), and others and these were present only in some cases. Cardona ('34) noted a moderate degree of swelling of the oligodendroglia in the frontal lobes in autopsy material of schizophrenic patients. In cases of involutional melancholia there was a slight degree of such swelling in the cortex and more in the nuclei of the thalamus. Roberti ('31b) described microglial activation in a single instance of schizophrenia and felt that this was parallel to the nerve cell changes. Josephy and others have referred to the finding of "glial rosettes," presumably a focal proliferation of microglia or oligodendroglia.

The leptomeninges and blood vessels have generally been described as normal. Phagocytes containing fat or yellow pigment have been seen in the perivascular spaces of the cortex and white matter in some instances.

The pathologic changes of manic-depressive psychosis are virtually unknown. Such postmortem studies as those of Marchand ('28) and Meyer ('35), describing changes in the leptomeninges and cerebral vessels, and in Meyer's material, describing degeneration and disappearance of cortical nerve cells chiefly in the frontal and temporal lobes, are still unsubstantiated. The pathologic picture of involutional psychosis is equally poorly documented.

Another group of workers, studying postmortem material from psychotic individuals, doubted the significance of the reported positive findings in these conditions. Spielmeyer ('31) summarized the histopathologic findings in schizophrenia and concluded that the pathologic anatomy of the disease had not yet been determined. He pointed out several sources of error in his material as well as in that of other investigators. Changes in the central nervous system, occurring in the course of an acute terminal illness or chronic disease involving other organs, might mask, or be mistaken for, specific lesions of the psychosis. Findings repeatedly described in instances of schizophrenia, such as areas in the cortex free of nerve cells, and fatty deposits in cortical elements, have been seen consistently in supposedly normal individuals. The fresh areas of degeneration occasionally encountered in catatonic attacks of schizophrenia have the earmarks of vascular lesions and would seem to be an acute complication of schizophrenia rather than part of its specific pathologic picture. They are seen in a great variety of other conditions in which circulatory abnormalities occur. Dunlap ('24; '28), a few years earlier, stressed the errors introduced by fixation and technical defects, and those which arose from erroneous conceptions of what was normal.

Dunlap attempted to minimize the sources of error by studying material only from young patients whose course was uncomplicated and of reasonably short duration and controlling these with tissues from the best available normal subjects of the same age range. It was clear that under these circumstances, the schizophrenics and the normal controls were often mutually indistinguishable. During the next decade, Peters and Roeder-Kutsch were able to confirm Dunlap's findings of changes in normal individuals identical with those in schizophrenics. Each of these workers examined the brains of nonpsychotic individuals as controls. Spielmeyer ('31) and Peters ('37) used the freshly fixed brains of newly executed individuals, while Dunlap ('28) and Roeder-Kutsch

('39) used medical and surgical patients who died suddenly, or following a very short illness. In these patients, nerve cell losses in the cerebral cortex, and changes in cortical nerve cells identical with those described as cell sclerosis, fatty degeneration of nerve cells, and shadow cells were encountered. These findings are exactly similar to those described in schizophrenics, and indeed Dunlap who mixed unidentified sections of normal individuals with those from schizophrenics was unable to distinguish between them. Spielmeyer and Peters made direct comparisons between these two types of material and found no differences. Even those who have contended that nerve cell losses in the cortex and degenerative changes in the remaining nerve cells particularly in the frontal lobes constitute the pathologic picture of schizophrenia and cause its symptoms, have admitted that such changes were absent in some clear-cut instances of this condition. Josephy ('30), for instance, pointed out that in a long-standing case of his own, and in another described by Rosenthal ('14, cited by Josephy '30), no abnormalities were encountered in the brain in spite of the chronicity of the condition.

**Cerebral Biopsies in Psychotic Individuals.** Foerster ('12) introduced the procedure of brain biopsy by means of cerebral puncture in the diagnosis of disease of the brain. In this early work he did not examine material from any individuals with so-called functional psychoses. It remained for Elvidge and Reed ('36) to apply this technique to the study of specimens from 13 patients with schizophrenia, 5 with manic-depressive psychoses, and a patient with "encephalitis." In each, they encountered generalized or patchy swelling of the oligodendroglia in which some elements showed nuclear pyknosis. This oligodendroglial swelling was limited to the cerebral white matter and was greatest at a depth of 1 cm. or more below the cortex. Specimens were taken from the occipitoparietal regions of the cerebral hemispheres. There was often an accompanying mild hypertrophy of the astrocytes. Nerve cells were described as normal except for pyknotic elements in some cases which were considered to be artefacts. There were no differences between the schizophrenic and manic-depressive patients. In a series of 16 control patients, chiefly epileptics, similar changes were encountered in a small group. These were described as epileptics who showed mental symptoms between seizures and others who had convulsive seizures during the operation.

Kirschbaum and Heilbrunn ('44) excised pea-sized specimens of frontal cerebral cortex prior to lobotomy in 11 individuals with schizophrenia. In all but 1 patient pathologic alterations in the nerve cells, glial cells and blood vessels were found. Nerve cell losses in the cortex were present in 1 patient and doubtful in another. Ganglion cell changes were encountered in all but 1 patient and these consisted of fatty degeneration, swelling and vacuolization, cell shrinkage and pyknosis, and cell shadows. Satellitosis and neuronophagia were present but were not prominent. In most instances there was insufficient white matter to permit study of the oligodendroglia in that tissue, but in specimens from 2 patients Hortega stains revealed "vacuolation" of these cells. In one instance mild swelling of the cortical oligodendroglia was noted. Fat was found in glial cells and in the walls of blood vessels and phagocytes in perivascular spaces in many cases. The authors raised the question as to whether the fat in the ganglion and glial cells, and in the blood vessels, might be due to ether anesthesia. The brains of 2 young nonschizophrenic individuals who had died during abdominal operations were used as controls and showed no such changes postmortem. The protoplasmic astrocytes were hypertrophied in all cases and multiplied in some. The fibrillary astrocytes had frequently proliferated but not as often as the protoplasmic. The authors ascribed much of this to the insulin and metrazol shock treatments.

The studies of Hydén and Hartelius ('48) were confined to a histochemical examination of the cortical nerve cells in biopsy specimens obtained during the course of lobotomy. They report that the polynucleotides and protein substances in certain ganglion cells of the cerebral cortex in persons suffering from psychoses, chiefly schizophrenia, are considerably decreased in amount as compared with that in corresponding cells from psychically healthy persons. No attempt was made to do any more extensive histologic studies which might be compared with those in the present study.

In the present material, the problem of nerve cell losses was a difficult one. Unless such losses are gross, subjective impressions of a diminution of neurones may be quite misleading. Until cell counts are available in a large series of normal subjects and can be compared with many similar counts in psychotic individuals, statements of mild focal or diffuse nerve cell losses must be viewed with suspicion. Hechst ('33) reported reduced counts in 3 cases (as compared with the values of von Economo). Both normal and pathologic data on this score, however, are quite insufficient. On the other hand, Dunlap found that nerve cell counts in the cortices of normal and schizophrenic individuals were practically identical. The majority of cortical specimens examined in this study showed no nerve cell losses. In 6 subjects, 5 of whom had schizophrenia and 1 an involutional psychosis, appearances such as others have described as focal and diffuse cell losses, were encountered. They were observed in the third cortical layer and less often in the fifth and sixth layers. The ages of the patients in this group ranged from thirty-one to fifty-five years; the duration of the illness in the schizophrenics from five to fourteen years, and six years in the patient with involutional psychosis. All of these patients, except a schizophrenic who had received no treatment, were exposed to shock therapy. Each had been given numerous electroshocks, the fewest being seven and the greatest twenty-six. In addition 3 were exposed to insulin shock, 1 having twenty-eight, another forty-one, and the third, 114 such treatments. Two of these were further treated with metrazol, 1 twelve times and the other fourteen times. Another patient who had had electroshocks without insulin had twenty-eight metrazol convulsions. One schizophrenic, who received twenty-three electroshocks, also had a history of alcoholism. The remaining twenty-two patients who showed no apparent nerve cell losses in their cortical specimens, varied in age from twenty-nine to sixty-one years of whom 5 were over fifty years of age. The duration of illness varied from two to twenty-one years, and was five years or less in 15. They had received from one to forty-eight electroshocks, eleven to sixty-two insulin shocks, and nineteen to twenty-two metrazol treatments. Three of the 22 received no treatment of this type. Four of the 22 patients had had head injuries in the past, 1 had attempted suicide by gas, 1 had suffered from lead poisoning, and 1 had been struck by lightning.

In assessing the significance of the apparent nerve cell losses in the 6 patients referred to above, it was noted that the specimen removed from a symmetrical portion of the cortex of the opposite cerebral hemisphere in 5 did not show any diminution in neurones. In the sixth instance, cortex from only one cerebral hemisphere was available. If the cell losses were real, one might expect them to be bilateral although this might not necessarily be so. The fact that individuals of equivalent ages, having psychoses of the same sort for equal or longer periods, who had received comparably frequent shock therapy, and who had been exposed to a series of possible brain-damaging incidents, were free of nerve cell losses, would seem to cast considerable doubt upon the etiologic significance of the apparent cell losses in the 5 schizophrenics and 1 patient with involutional psychosis. The work of Dunlap ('24; '28), Spielmeyer ('30), Peters ('37), and Roeder-Kutsch ('39) would appear to indicate that such apparent diminution of nerve cells is of doubtful significance and the present material tends to support this view.

Abnormal changes in nerve cells were in the main infrequent and of two chief types. The most frequent abnormality was shrinkage, deep staining, and distortion of neurones. It was striking that this was seen most often near the surfaces of a specimen, both superficial and deep, and near tears, cuts, and other injuries to the parenchyma. It was most frequent in small blocks of tissue with their relatively greater surfaces. It would appear that this type of nerve cell change is an artefact since it seems to be related to adventitious factors such as nearness of neurons to surfaces of the tissue, trauma to the tissue, and size of the tissue block. Its frequency in a biopsy from one cerebral hemisphere and rarity in an equivalent specimen from the opposite hemisphere in some cases of this series, tend to cast further doubt upon any possible relationship between this change and the condition from which the patient was suffering. The fact that it was encountered to some degree in specimens from every patient further weakens the probability that it has etiologic significance for any of the diagnostic categories. This type of cell shrinkage and hyperchromatism has been noted repeatedly in surgical biopsy specimens of cerebral tissue from nonpsychotic individuals, examined in this laboratory, which proved to be free of tumor or other lesions. Its frequency seemed to be inversely proportional to the size of the specimen and directly to the degree of trauma it had sustained.

Another common but less frequent change in the nerve cells in these cases was the accumulation of scarlet-red-stainable lipid material in them. This was encountered in 23 patients, most of whom were schizophrenics. Since most of the patients studied were schizophrenics this is not especially significant. No comparable lipid material was found in 2 of the patients with this psychosis. In this laboratory, scarlet-red-stainable lipid has been encountered in the nerve cells of the cerebral cortex in variable amounts from early middle age on, and often earlier, in nonpsychotics. This was within the range encountered in the present series of psychotic individuals. It is therefore difficult to accept this fatty change as a special characteristic of schizophrenia and the other psychoses under consideration. This lipid accumulation and the deep staining and shrinkage of nerve cells referred to above, have been the two most commonly emphasized neuronal changes in the literature on the pathologic anatomy of schizophrenia. One can only emphasize, with Spielmeyer ('31), Dunlap ('24; '28), Peters ('37), and Roeder-Kutsch ('39), that such deviations from the normal can be encountered in nonpsychotic control individuals and thus are probably of no etiologic significance. Further the nerve cell shrinkage may well be an artefact as suggested above.

One must also consider the possibility that any or all of the neuronal changes in these cases may have been the result of the shock therapy to which most of the patients were exposed. Kobler ('38), Leppien and Peters ('37), Cammermeyer ('38), Ferraro and Jervis ('39), and many others have described nerve cell losses in the cerebral cortex and degenerative changes in the remaining cells in schizophrenics following insulin therapy. Petersen ('39), and Weil and Liebert ('40) described abnormal changes of varying degree in the cerebral cortex of psychotics who had received metrazol shock treatments. Mild changes in the cerebral cortex of psychotics receiving electroshock therapy have been noted by Ebaugh, Barnacle, and Neubuerger ('43). It must be noted that 4 of the twenty-eight patients in the present series received no shock therapy, 2 of these having schizophrenia and 2 manic depressive psychosis, and that these showed cortical changes of the same type seen in the treated patients.

Acid-fast pigment was present in the nerve cells of every patient. Its distribution and quantity were quite similar to those in nonpsychotic individuals.

The findings of Naito ('24), Marburg ('24), and Fünfgeld ('27) of a diminution in, and pallor of, the tangential myelin sheaths in the upper layers of the cortex in cases of schizophrenia, could not be confirmed in the present material. The myelin sheaths, as well as the axons, were intact and appeared to be normal in number.

The oligodendroglia showed some degree of swelling in the subcortical white matter and less often in the lower layers of the cortex in 20 of the 22 instances in which impregnation was successful. The specimens included those from schizophrenics and from patients with manic-depressive and involutional psychoses. These findings conform to those of Elvidge and Reed ('36) with the following exceptions. The oligodendroglial swelling in the present series of cases was much less intense, the lower layers of the cortex were sometimes involved, and specimens from 2 patients with involutional psychosis showed the same feature. Elvidge and Reed believe this to be a definite part of the pathologic picture of schizophrenia and manic-depressive psychosis. They suggest that the same process which produces the oligodendroglial change may adversely affect conduction in the axons of the cerebral white matter and thus interfere with the passage of associative impulses from one portion of the brain to another, disrupting thought processes. In view of the ease with which oligodendroglia swell postmortem, and the possibility that a similar process might be active during fixation itself, the pathologic significance of this phenomenon might be questioned. Elvidge and Reed, however, point out that rapidly fixed material from normal animals, and a series of human control biopsies, revealed no comparable oligodendroglial swelling. Penfield and Cone ('26) examined six neurosurgical biopsy specimens from nonpsychotic patients and found the oligodendroglia normal in four and swollen in two. The four normal specimens were from tumor suspects and a patient with a glioma of the brain; one of the two specimens showing swollen oligodendroglia was from a patient having a cerebral embolus and the other from an epileptic. On the other hand, Andrew and Ashworth ('45) contend that there is an "adendroglial" type of oligodendroglia which can be found in promptly fixed animal and human brain, in which the swollen state is a normal phase and does not indicate the presence of a pathologic process. Ferraro and Jervis ('39) have described swelling of the oligodendroglia following insulin therapy in the schizophrenic. That swollen forms of oligodendroglia occur in the brains of psychotics seems clear. It is not at all certain, however, that this swelling is the result of the etiologic mechanism at work in these psychoses, or is indicative of the site of activity of such factors in the brain.

Roberti ('31b) reported microglial activation in a patient with schizophrenia. Josephy ('30) and others have spoken of glial rosettes presumably referring to foci of microglial or oligodendroglial proliferation. The present material yields no evidence of reaction on the part of the microglia. Weil and Liebert ('40) have described hypertrophy and hyperplasia of these cells following metrazol convulsions in psychotics. Ferraro and Jervis ('39) have seen microglial activation following insulin therapy for schizophrenia.

Limited astrocytosis has been described in postmortem material of schizophrenia, and this only in some cases. The biopsies of Elvidge and Reed ('36) frequently revealed a mild astrocytosis accompanying the oligodendroglial swelling in both schizophrenics and manic-depressive individuals. Kirschbaum and Heilbrunn ('44) reported hypertrophy of protoplasmic astrocytes in all their patients with schizophrenia and multiplication of these cells in some. There was a lesser reaction of the fibrillary astrocytes. The authors attributed the severer grades of astrocytosis to shock therapy. Weil and Liebert ('40), studying patients with schizophrenia, manic depressive psychosis, and involutional psychosis treated with metrazol, found a considerable astrocytosis. In experimental hyperinsulinism, as in the work of Weil, Liebert, and Heilbrunn ('38), astrocytosis is rarely encountered, and it has been as inconspicuous among the findings following insulin shock in man (Ferraro and Jervis, '39; Cammermeyer, '40). Ebaugh and his co-workers ('43) have described a slight localized astrocytosis following electroshock in psychotics. Only 3 cases, of the 26 in the present series in which astrocytes were impregnated, showed a mild degree of astrocytosis in the cortex or subcortical white matter. One of the patients had received no shock therapy and, of the other 2, one had had fifty-one insulin and forty-eight electroshock treatments, and the other twenty-two metrazol shocks. Four other patients who had received from twelve to twenty-eight metrazol treatments, in addition to other forms of shock therapy, showed no astrocytosis. In the remaining patients who had received insulin or electroshocks, but no metrazol, astrocytosis was also absent. Weil and Liebert ('40) found that astrocytosis was more vigorous in patients with an illness of short duration than in those with long-standing psychosis treated with metrazol. The 5 patients treated with metrazol in the present series had been ill from five to fourteen years. In summary, no significant astrocytosis was encountered in our biopsy material.

The histochemical demonstration of phosphatases in the cerebral specimens in this series yielded uniformly normal results. In the alkaline phosphatase preparations the vascular pattern of the cortex and subcortical white matter was found to be normal.

## COMMENT AND CONCLUSIONS

In the present material it was remarkable that so few histologic abnormalities were encountered in spite of the chronicity of many of the cases and the vigorous shock treatment which most of the patients received.

Nerve cell losses were observed in the third cortical layer in a few cases and less often in the fifth and sixth layers. These appeared to bear no apparent relationship to the type of case, duration of illness, treatment, or area of brain examined. At times, they were present in a specimen removed from one side of the cerebrum and absent in that removed from the other side. In the majority of instances where this could be truly estimated in the absence of distortion, the cortical architecture and nerve cell density appeared to be within normal limits. Scattered nerve cells or clusters of such elements showed the picture of cell sclerosis and variable numbers contained fatty material and appeared vacuolated in Nissl stains. It did not seem that the fat content of these nerve cells was beyond what is encountered in nonpsychotic patients, and the shrunken, deeply staining nerve cells were often so distributed as to seem to be the result of artefact. Such artefacts have been stressed by Spielmeyer ('31), Dunlap ('24; '28), and others as a great source of error in postmortem material of schizophrenia. Unfortunately, it is obvious that such artefacts are added to, rather than subtracted from, in biopsy material. Aside from the effects of the nitrous oxide anesthesia, cautery, silver clips, and saline wash which were used as sparingly as was possible, the effects of physical manipulation and drying during subdivision of the specimen for special fixation must be taken into account. In addition, the fixation of small biopsy specimens of brain tissue has in our experience led to numerous artefacts in nerve cells near surfaces and such appeared to be the case in the present circumstances.

Furthermore, we must be clear in our minds as to the limited possibilities for discovering significant etiologic alterations in the brain when examining only small fragments of it, and without examining other organs and tissues. Is the brain the site of primary lesions in these conditions, or is it the instrument through which metabolic, internal secretory, or other disturbances initiated elsewhere are recorded? If lesions primary in the brain produce the manifestations of the disease, are these symptoms the results of changes in one or another area of the frontal cortex, a combination of such areas, such areas in association with others such as the hypothalamus, or a reflection by, without organic change in, the frontal cortex, of a process proceeding elsewhere in the brain? It is clear that many of these questions are crucial, and cannot be answered by the present material.

Last, but not least, for obvious reasons, no true control material removed in the same fashion from nonpsychotic individuals, was available for study.

It would appear from these studies that application of the usual neurohistologic techniques to biopsy specimens from the brains of psychotics, does not reveal any constant or specific pathologic changes. The addition of some histochemical methods such as the demonstration of alkaline and acid phosphatase, and of ceroid pigment, brought to light no deviations from control material.

If histopathology is to contribute to the solution of the etiologic factors of the psychoses in question, it must do so by the application of additional histochemical and other techniques.

SECTION V

# Summary

# Introduction

At the present point in the presentation it was originally hoped that a correlative interpretative chapter might have been presented but this proved to be unobtainable—at least within the time limits of reasonable publication. Even if it had been possible to arrange the schedules of all the responsible investigators so that they would have been able to sit down together, in a reflective mood after having assimilated all the available data, it is still doubtful whether it would have been possible to follow through, step by step, in an orderly manner and in a reasonable length of time, the collective cogitations necessary to arrive at a consensus. Moreover, certain honest differences of opinion were apparent which, it soon became obvious, can only be resolved by additional investigative work. In such situations, where the weight of evidence is not great enough to compel an inevitable decision, it has been our experience that any tentative opinion, however attractive, is likely to fall short of the mark. We come therefore to this point in the presentation without complete agreement as to just why it has been possible to return a palpable number of apparently incurable psychotic patients to society. The reflective reader will have no reason to regret this state of affairs for it puts him on a par with the present writers. The data have been presented and his general conclusions, if he keeps these data firmly in mind, are probably as valid as any we might evolve. There are at least two other good reasons why we should refrain from an ambitious effort to construct a grand hypothesis from the data before us. If we were to do so it is possible that new psychosurgical therapeutic procedures and further research might be adversely affected. Moreover, we ourselves are too well aware of the limitations of our data to feel that we have built the most solid foundation we can by the methods of investigation we have evolved. Had we no opportunity to gather more data, theoretical generalizations might be pardonable but this is not the case so we need be in no hurry to raise another, and probably temporary, theoretical elaboration on the medical horizon. Even though we have not attained the ultimate in the understanding of the mysteries of being we have no reason to feel that we have wasted our time and energy. It is just possible that entirely too much esoteric doctrine has been attached to the frontal lobe. We are inclined to content ourselves with the belief that we have been able to dispel a certain number of misconceptions and that future work, freed of some of these incubi, will be able to move forward more rapidly and certainly.

At the present place, as a concession to the urgent, but not always laudable, demands for interpretation of data we shall, in view of what has been said above, limit ourselves to an attempt to answer but two questions: (1) What bearing do the present data have upon current ideas relating to the frontal lobe, apart from psychoses? (The present commentator and Professor Landis will attempt to deal with the question.) (2) What bearing do present data have upon current ideas of psychoses? (This question has been assigned to

Dr. Heath.) In order to make clear that these opinions are purely personal and are not necessarily concurred in by any person other than the author each of these sections is separately distinguished.

The spheres of information relating to the "normal" upon which the present data have a direct bearing are neuroanatomy (chapter 5), neurophysiology (chapters 6-12, 26), and psychology (chapters 13-24). In spite of the fact that the information applicable to all of these spheres is to some extent influenced by the subjects' residence in an institution for the mentally ill, such residence, insofar as application of these data to the "normal" individual is concerned, is of less importance in the case of information gained by objective means than it is in the case of data which must be obtained from the patients' own reports. Obviously a change in gastrointestinal motility following ablation of the cortex is of greater significance for the normal than is a change in auditory acuity, which may be merely a reflection of the patient's ability to report upon his subjective state and may not represent any real change in the acuity of the auditory system at all.

*Chapter 28*

# Anatomy and Physiology

FRED A. METTLER

All students of the cytoarchitecture of the frontal cortex are agreed that this consists of two major territorial categories, agranular and granular divisions, and that the former (precentral and cingular regions) is mesocortical on the cingular gyrus and parolfactory area and specifically isocortical over the paracentral lobule and precentral region. All students also agree that the granular cortex is not entirely homogeneous and that there is a region of transition between the lateral agranular and granular regions. The more common maps of the frontal region shown in figures 54-59 indicate wherein various authorities differ regarding their manner of subdividing the granular region.

As a purely anatomic study, the present work might perhaps have been better done on "normal" material. Still, if the psychotic state results in changes in the cytoarchitectural pattern such changes were not sufficiently marked in the present cases to render the locus of origin of samples unrecognizable.

Indeed one lesson to be learned from the present investigation is that so little "normal" material, free from postmortem change, has been available that our criteria of what is normal require serious reinvestigation. Perhaps the major anatomic contribution of the present work is the conclusion that any of the existing cytoarchitectural plans of the frontal cortex are sufficiently accurate to be used in accordance with the criteria of the plan in question, and that mutual conversion between plans is possible. This is not to say that the most detailed plans are easily followed, that the broader plans are completely satisfying, nor that more desirable plans cannot and will not be developed. It is, however, concluded that one can work in a practical manner with the schemata which are available, and that there is no real cause to reject completely one scheme and to cleave in an uncompromising manner to another now in existence. An uncritical acceptance of any existing plan for the human cortex could easily usher in an era of confusion such as occurred in the experimental physiologic field as a result of referring to printed maps and neglecting actual histologic specimens.

## PHYSIOLOGY
### SUPPOSED FUNCTIONS OF THE REGIONS STUDIED

The parts of the brain which were under present study have been reported to have the following normal functions as determined by the following techniques.

**Experimental Bilateral Simultaneous Ablation (Chiefly Simian Data).** *Of Both Frontal Lobes.* Over-all activity is reduced. The following capacities are abolished: true locomotion, climbing, self-feeding, reactions of placing and contact. The following functions are impaired: speed of complex movement, range of movement (including that of the eyes), chewing, swallowing, peripheral vasoconstriction. Tonic and vestibular reflexes become marked; plantar responses abolished; the proprioceptive reflexes show a decreased reflexogenous zone, a tendency to spread, the threshold is elevated, the force increased, maturation rapid, quality stiff. The limbs assume mid-postural positions (fingers and toes flexed and adducted, the wrist is partially pronated and it and the ankle are flexed, the upper limb is partially pronated and the lower internally rotated and adducted, the elbow is flexed to mid-posture, the knees partially extended). Passive movement, tending to displace these postures, is strongly resisted and clasp-knife reflexes are present. A forced grasp is present if the most caudal part of area 4 is intact. The pupils are somewhat dilated and the gastrointestinal system shows increased muscular activity.

*Of Both Granular Areas.* Over-all activity is increased. This is a true over-reactivity to stimulation in contrast to essential intrinsic overactivity. Cursive hyperkinesia appears, particularly in response to visual stimulation. Excessive vocalization occurs. No specific somatomotor function is abolished or notably impaired (a temporary reduction in the freedom of movements of the eyes may be seen). The width of the palpebral fissure is increased. The plantar response becomes extensor (both of toes and hallux). The proprioceptive reflexes show some restriction of reflexogenous zone and occasional spread; the amplitude is increased; quality is loose. Voracity appears.

*Of Both Granular Areas Rostral to Area 9.* Although a variety of defects have been reported following such procedures, none of those so far published and of which we are aware have been encountered in the laboratories of the Department of Neurology of the College of Physicians and Surgeons of Columbia University.

*Of Both Areas 9.* The principal result is mild spontaneous overactivity (rather than over-reactivity) which is depressed by external stimulation.

*Of Both Areas 8.* No notable effect.

*Of Both Areas 6.* Stolidity, repetition of stereotyped movements, manual apraxia. Plantar response: flexion of hallux, extension of toes. Proprioceptive reflexes: reduction of threshold, quality loose. Occurrence of a phase I grasp reflex.

**Experimental Stimulation (Simian and Human).** These data may be most briefly presented in tabular form (table 91).

**Observational Methods Applied to Neurological Clinical and Psychiatric Clinical Material.** Simple examination of clinical material has suggested that the frontal lobe may have a number of physiologic functions in addition to those noted above.

*Autonomic and Metabolic Functions.* Over and above the autonomic functions mentioned above, a wide range of autonomic alterations and profound changes in metabolism have been reported (the recent literature has repeatedly been reviewed and Bechterew ['08-'11] has summarized most of the data of the four decades preceding his publication) to occur in organisms with lesions of the frontal lobe. The great difficulty in evaluating these data derives from the difficulty in being certain that such changes are really due

TABLE 91. RESULTS OF ELECTRICAL STIMULATION OF THE FRONTAL LOBE

| Area | Activatory | | Inhibitory | |
|---|---|---|---|---|
| | Somatic | Autonomic | Somatic | Autonomic |
| 12 F, L | Inactive | Inactive | Inactive | Inactive |
| 11 F, L | Inactive | Inactive | Inactive | Respiratory arrest |
| 10 F, L | Inactive | ? | Inactive | ? |
| 9 F | Rostrally, inactive Caudally, conj. eye deviation and ear movements | ? | Inactive | ? |
| 9 L | Postural adjustments Acts | ? | Generalized and marked | ? |
| 8 F | Conj. eye deviation and ear movements | Pupillary dilatation | Inactive | ? |
| 8 L | Same and flexor adjustments | | Generalized | ? |
| 6 F | Conj. eye deviation and head and eye movements | | Inactive | ? |
| 6 L | Rostrally, flexor or extensor adjustments Caudally, simple movements | Spinal sympathetic and parasympathetic effects | Of flexion | ? |
| 4 (Rostral) F | Conj. eye and head movements | | Inactive | ? |
| 4 (Rostral) L | Extensor adjustments and simple movements | | Of extension | ? |
| 4 (Caudal) F | Simple, localized movements* | | Of activity other than that stimulated | ? |
| 4 (Caudal) L | Phasic patterns | | | |

\* Individual muscle contractions can be elicited from the cortex, though, of course, late ontogenetic movements are abolished by bilateral cortical ablation.
F = Full surgical anesthesia.
L = Light anesthesia.
? = no data available.

to dysfunction of the frontal lobe itself. Since extensive lesion of the frontal lobe is not invariably accompanied by them, such negative evidence would seem to indicate that they are due to involvement of other structures.

*Enhancement of Appetite.* Bulimia came to be regarded as a symptom of frontal lobe disease as a result of its frequent association with Pick's disease in which the brunt of the pathologic change may fall, but not necessarily so, upon the frontal lobe.

*Enhancement of Sex Drive.* This has been mentioned by Freeman and Watts ('42) as an occasional but not invariable consequence of lobotomy. This has not been reported to extend to homosexual activities.

*Ataxia and Other Cerebellar and Vestibular Signs.* Ataxia has figured prominently in the symptomatology of the frontal lobe since the days of

Bruns (1892). Thus Williamson (1896) encountered it in 14 of his 50 cases. Bruns (1898) thought it occurred in 50 percent of frontal lobe tumors and was generally absent when the tumor lay in the motor region. Here again, such phenomena are not usually encountered unless the lesions are large and usually neoplastic.

*Aphasia and Agraphia.* Reference has already been made (p. 62) to Broca and Maubrac's (1896) attribution of *aphémie* or motor aphasia to dysfunction of the pars opercularis of the inferior frontal gyrus. The present data indicate clearly that this region may be bilaterally decorticated without invariably producing such a phenomenon. This should not be interpreted to mean that deeper lesions, or lesions which reach farther caudally, may not produce such a phenomenon or that there may not be individual variation in this respect. Rather, one simply cannot assume that damage of the cortex of the pars opercularis on either or both sides will produce it.

It is possible that the suitability of patient 47 as a crucial test of Broca's hypothesis may be questioned on the basis of the pre-existing logorrhoea. "As is well known, persons suddenly attacked with word-deafness exhibit in addition to paraphasia, a special symptom, logorrhoea." (Mettler, Lee H., '04.) Logorrhoea in itself, however, does not conversely argue for the invariable pre-existence of word-deafness. Attention is further directed to the spelling difficulty noted in this patient. No such phenomenon was encountered in patient 33 so one would have to conclude that this was part of the original psychotic disorder and not a result of the operation.

A word of caution appears to be due at this place to avoid confusion. That motor deficits, like those in other parts of the body, can and do occur in the muscles of the glossopalatal and manual apparatus after destruction of the corresponding cortical motor sites, is perfectly clear in the present series. It is possible that, in the presence of an established preconception, hasty or cursory examinations might leave the examiner with the erroneous impression that such patients suffered from aphasia or agraphia but it is difficult to see how such a fundamental error could be made.

Agraphia has been attributed to damage of the caudal part of the middle frontal gyrus. The original report on this phenomenon was probably that by Sciamanna ('01) who encountered the condition in a patient with a solitary tubercle in that location. No such phenomenon was encountered in the pertinent present cases (temporary apraxia was, however, seen when the part of area 6 immediately in front of the hand area was excised).

*Convulsions.* Myoclonic epilepsy has long been known to be a frequent sequel of brain injury, especially injury of the frontal lobe but no one would now regard this (or convulsions, in a more general sense) either as an invariable consequence of frontal damage or as particularly restricted to such a circumstance.

*Ill-Defined "Higher" Functions.* The attribution of *changes in personality* to frontal lobe damage is not so old as might be supposed. Although some psychic disorders were attributed to cerebral dysfunction even in the early post-Galenic period (Mettler, C.C. '47) it was not until the second half of the nineteenth century that any evidence was brought forward to suggest that the frontal lobe is specifically concerned with psychic processes. There is nothing in Greisinger's (1867) book to this effect and the suggestion that Harlow's (1848) patient, Phineas Gage, of the so-called "crow-bar case," owed his personality changes (the phrase that he was "no longer Gage" appears in the record, Harlow, 1869, p. 14) to frontal lobe damage was an afterthought on the part of Ferrier. (For Harlow and most of his contemporaries the most significant feature of the case was the survival of the patient, and others, overzealous to defeat the phrenologists, were almost willing to argue that the brain was practically useless in order to achieve their purpose. It is interesting to observe, in passing, that one of the first cases in which a personality change was observed to follow a brain injury was a psychotic case in which the psychosis disappeared after attempted suicide by shooting through the head [Nobele, 1835].)

Welt's (1888) case of Franz Binz of Zürich was probably the first verified example of serious alterations of character and moral behavior due to a frontal lesion, the extent of which was established at autopsy. Franz Binz, like Phineas Gage, changed from a peaceful, gay, polite and cleanly person to a violently quarrelsome sloven. Goltz, Hitzig, and Ferrier had previously described similar changes. Ferrier (1890) believed that removal of cortex rostral to the electrically excitable area produced "a form of mental degradation which appears to me to depend on the loss of the faculty of attention, and my hypothesis is that the power of attention is intimately related to the volitional movements of the head and eyes." Ferrier attributed the opinion that intellectual degradation may follow lesion of the rostral part of the brain to a number of previous authors, including Brissaud. Welt had been unable to demonstrate any true degradation of intellectual capacity in the case of Binz. Hitzig (1883) also thought that intelligence is impaired by injury of the frontal lobe in the dog, a belief controverted by Loeb ('02), and Bruns could find no evidence of impairment of intellect in one extensive tumor case of his own.

An unpleasant, nasty character was one of the triad of symptoms of release which Goltz felt succeeded frontal lobe changes. (The full triad was [1] general excitement [the capstone of the theory that injury of the cortex brought about a phenomenon of "release" was laid by Charcot, 1876-1880], [2] lack of self-control, [3] violence of spinal and bulbar activity.)

*Clownish behavior* (*Witzelsucht, mania bel esprit, lazzi, moria*) as a symptom of rostral frontal lobe damage appeared in Jastrowitz's articles of 1888 (Jastrowitz, 1888; see also Leyden and Jastrowitz, 1888; and Bruns, 1892) and formed a part of Bruns' (1897) table of frontal lobe symptomatology. Jastrowitz referred to the condition as moria.

*Difficulties in the associational process* entered the symptomatology of the frontal lobe through the work of Flechsig who argued that two (originally he said three) "association" centers existed in the brain (a large parieto-occipito-temporal and a smaller frontal one) which gave rise to no projections but only associational fibers, for the purpose of inter-relating afferent impulses. Flechsig felt that the frontal association field was primarily concerned with the association of impulses of bodily sense, as contrasted with vision and audition as special senses (he thought of the frontal lobe as containing sensory as well as motor capacities, as indeed its caudal part does), and that injury of it produced defects in personality and self-awareness. Association fibers from it were supposed to deal especially with memory images (Flechsig, 1896). Flechsig's theory was not widely accepted (Oppenheim, '00) but the theory that psychiatric disorders depend upon an essential difficulty in the associational process long endured in the literature. Thus Bolton ('11) divided psychotic processes into two categories: (1) those in which there is defective control of the processes of lower association and (2) those in which there is independent activity of the "centers of lower association." He placed apathetic, hebephrenic, and manic syndromes in the first category and illusory and hallucinatory states in the second.

*Loss of initiative or apathy* as symptoms of frontal lobe disease appeared in Bruns' tabulation and *loss of complex emotional behavior* probably should also be included here together with *defective recognition, due to a degradation in perceptual ability.* In contrast to simple apathy, *ambulatory hyperkinesia* was attributed by Baraduc (1876) as, much earlier, by Magendie, to frontal lobe lesion—specifically by Baraduc, to atrophy of the left inferior frontal convolution.

*Persistence of fear and the occurrence of panic reactions* have been described as signs of frontal damage, and apparently, in cases of thrombosis of the arteries supplying the frontal region, may be so severe as to amount to *delirium tremens.* Perhaps these phenomena are to be related with Goltz's listing of release phenomena, though this is far from clear.

*Memory defects for the past without impairment of the ability to learn and lack of planning for the future (deterioration of insight)* are also listed as results of frontal lobe damage.

It may be justifiably said that these so-called "higher" functions discussed in the foregoing paragraphs are so ill-defined as to be scarcely worth scientific consideration. This depends upon one's point of view. One common criticism of the scientific method as applied to the present sphere is that it has not yielded quantitative support of phenomena which anyone, using merely observation, can easily perceive. Since scientific tests answer only the questions they have been designed to ask, it is, of course, possible that the proper tests have not been devised. On the other hand, it is perfectly possible that these "higher" functions are not functions of the frontal lobe at all or, at best, require damage of very large parts of the frontal lobe in such a way as to compound simple functional deficits into complex patterns of deficit.

The premier question which must receive an affirmative answer in order to conclude that the "higher" functions under discussion are frontal lobe functions, is, "Do such deficits invariably appear if the frontal lobe is quite dysfunctional?" Under such scrutiny the allocation of most of the preceding phenomena (slovenliness is an exception) fails to be substantiated. We must therefore conclude either that special circumstances, beyond the factor of frontal lobe damage, must be present for their appearance or that they are not true functions. One might conclude that some portion of the frontal lobe must be functional for a particular phenomenon to appear (as, for example, the motor region for aggressive behavior) or that an additional process must develop (such as scar tissue, before myoclonic epilepsy will result).

In order to examine these possibilities one must inquire very closely into the correlation between impairments of the above type and the location and extent of the concurrent pathologic change. Other than the present study only two groups of data are available to help us to inquire into this matter— correlation with pathologic findings and the effects of lobotomy.

**Physiologic Correlations Available from Pathologic Findings.** There is little data obtained from pathologic findings to suggest that changes can be found in specific parts of the brain in patients with impairment in higher functions. An effort in the direction of determining which portons of the brain are responsible for psychiatric abnormalities and psychophysiologic functions had been made, in a rather crude way, by Meynert, and this method was applied by Tigges (1889), and other students of Meynert. Somewhat later, Bolton ('11) substituted a combined method, involving not merely the weighing of gross material but also the measurement of microscopic sections taken from various portions of the brain of psychotics. According to Bolton, the processes giving rise to psychotic alterations are either failure of development (subinvolution), or the destruction of parts of the brain already developed (dissolution). According to Bolton, the average weight of the brains of psychotic patients, when these brains showed no gross pathologic changes, is less than the average weight of the brain of psychotic patients who do exhibit gross pathologic processes. He explained this apparent paradox by pointing out that psychotic processes could not be expected to be found in individuals with normal brains unless rather marked pathologic change had occurred, whereas in the case of those individuals who were psychotic, without obvious disease, the brain, though of normal appearance, was distinctly smaller in size. Bolton believed that in dementia, the greatest amount of pathologic change was to be found in the prefrontal region. The next most markedly affected region was the first temporal gyrus and insula and next the superior and inferior parietal lobules. Bolton attempted to discover changes in specific cellular layers of the cortex, and believed that such differences to be seen in the depths of the layers of the prefrontal regions in amentia and dementia are not specific but part of a generalized process which tended to destroy first the layers which were latest evolved. His terminology is somewhat different from that of Brodmann, but, converted into Brodmann's nomenclature, the polymorphic layer is evolved first, and is best preserved in psychotic processes. He considered it an emissive rather than receptive layer, and thought it dealt with instinctive functions. Brodmann's third layer, Bolton felt, was most seriously affected in dementia. In amentia, different layers suffer in different degrees, but since the inner layers evolved first, they are more perfectly developed, and the process is to be regarded as one of subinvolution. Changes in the internal granular layer are considered nonspecific and in proportion to the severity of the process. The layer was regarded as a receptive one. According to Bolton, the prefrontal region, which for him consisted largely of Brodmann's area 10 and the adjacent parts of 9, 11, and 47, is the last region to be evolved and the first region to undergo dissolution in mental decadence (dementia). In amentia, or subinvolution, the degree of evolution of the prefrontal region is incomplete by virtue of the fact that it was considered to be the last of the cerebral regions to be evolved. Such subsequent positive evidence as exists has tended to confirm the belief that the frontal pyramidal layer is most frequently affected, but no evidence has been forthcoming as to which parts of granular area of the frontal lobe are concerned with what functions and as pointed out in chapter 27, only a small part of the available evidence is of a positive nature.

**Functional Deficits Due to Deprivation of the Granular Cortex (Lobectomy and Lobotomy).** It is not surprising that patients have been reported to have shown, after lobectomy or lobotomy, evidence of more or less involvement of the physiologic activities already noted. What would be surprising (if one were not aware that the situation has existed for over sixty years) is the fact that the results of cerebral operations, presumably rendering dysfunctional the same parts of the frontal lobe, are so variable, running, as it were, the gamut from a complete catalogue of disabilities to near normalcy. Since the data in the literature have been gathered from wholly inequivalent surgical material it is, of course, obvious that one cannot lump all the data together and strike an arbitrary average. Less obvious but very real complications in the literature are due to the facts that the time elapsing between operations and study are extremely variable and that by the use of different methodologies of study, various inquiries have been oriented in very different directions. On the whole, the most rewarding studies have been those which have been conducted by skilled observers applying adequate methods in both the initial postoperative period and also for at least the ensuing year, and which have disclosed the fewest defects. One such is a study by Hebb ('45) who, in discussing the frequently quoted paper of Jacobsen ('36) observes that although some of the results were generalized "beyond the actual laboratory conditions in which they were obtained," concludes that lower animals may be more seriously incapacitated by frontal lobe damage than man. This is an interesting conclusion for it is just the reverse of that commonly encountered—notably that lower animals show much less by way of defect than does man. Another explanation might be drawn if one considers that not all of the wide assortment of physiologic defects which have been reported in experimental communications have withstood the test of repeated investigation.

In sharp contrast to the report of Hebb is the very common opinion that disconnection of the greater part of the granular cortex produces notable and serious deterioration. When, however, the nature of this supposed deterioration is fairly stated it is found to be difficult to evaluate. A good résumé has just been made by Solomon ('48) who lists the defects as slight impairment in the ability to generalize, as measured by Goldstein-Scheerer but not Shipley-Hartford Retreat examinations, a tendency to perseverate (as measured in the Rorschach test), "euphoria, apathy, lack of interest, procrastination, facetiousness, profanity, temper outbursts and distractability." Also impaired are "judgement, planning for the future, discrimination, laudable ambition, fine sentiment and creative imagination." Electroencephalographic changes occur in most patients but tend to subside within three months. With the exception of the last-named finding it is apparent that disabilities of the type named are exceedingly difficult to detect in psychotic patients and, indeed, are exactly the kind of disability which sends an individual to a mental hospital and from which he might be least expected to recover. In any event they fall almost entirely in the psychologic rather than physiologic sphere. The defects (other than flicker-fusion) defined by Halstead ('47) similarly belong in that category.

### RELATION OF PRESENT DATA TO PHYSIOLOGY OF FRONTAL LOBE

In some respects the literature is clear enough—the results which follow deprivation of certain general territories of frontal cortex are entirely different. One class of results may be expected if all frontal cortex is dysfunctional, another if area 4 is spared, and still another if areas 4 and 6 are spared and only the granular regions rendered dysfunctional. Beyond this point agreement is poor but one is immediately struck by the fact that data gathered by different observers, using the same technique or type of material, lead to reasonably reconcilable opinions, while data gathered by diverse methods often cannot be correlated at all. Thus, it should be apparent that there is no necessary correlation between information obtained by stimulating and ablational techniques. Quite apart from the possibility of false results due to current spread and also apart from the fact that all stimulating procedures are highly artificial, it must be recognized that, after ablation, homeostasis tends to obliterate a functional hiatus. Only rarely can one observe a physiologic deficit directly; more usually what one sees is the organism's compensatory behavior in the presence of such a deficit. If the deficit is slight and easily compensable no change may be detectable at all; biologic organisms are not such shoddy structures that they are easily set awry by the insults which the circumstances of living, as well as experimenters, constantly offer them. Such considerations force us to recognize that data obtained by stimulation are frequently falsely positive and that the appearance of intactness in organisms with actual organic damage is often deceptively negative. This is one important reason why scientific agreement in the field under consideration is less than perfect though it should be apparent that much of the disagreement is excessively naïve and certainly some of it is unnecessary.

Even when we deal with one technique—such as the ablational—the circumstances of particular cases must be kept in mind. Observations made in the acute stages of an ablational study cannot be forced into a Procrustean bed with those made during the chronic phase of another ablational study. The number of immediate physiologic sequelae of bilateral removal of individual Brodmann areas, or the combinations of these ablated in the present studies, are not inconsiderable. Under such circumstances there might be a tendency to disregard troublesome, early, fleeting phenomena as inconsequential simply because they are difficult to explain. To shirk the task of analyzing these changes by attributing them all to some hypothetical general cause—such as edema—is merely self-narcotization and actually may ignore one of the most promising opportunities which may present itself. It is perfectly possible, and indeed laboratory work indicates the probability, that more defects are lost as a result of rapid compensation than appear as a result of early nonspecific causes. That nonspecific effects do exist none will deny but the absence of evident dysfunction in a chronic organic discontinuity does not indicate that such dysfunction never resulted from the organic discontinuity. In order to know the whole story both the chronic and acute physiologic phenomena must be described. Since the former are more easily disposed of, we may begin with them.

**Permanent Physiologic Effects of Bilateral Ablation of Parts of the Frontal Cortex.** The present data demonstrate fairly conclusively that removal of none of the Brodmann areas by themselves, or in the combinations in which they were ablated in this study, produces (with certain possible exceptions) any notable permanent physiologic effects if one spares area 4 and the most caudal part of 6. The most notable exception is the possibility of convulsions.

*Convulsions.* We agree that convulsions may follow ablation of frontal cortex. They do not invariably follow the ablation of any specific area. Although a definite convulsive pattern was established in only one case (8), and this happened to be a case of a removal (middle frontal gyrus) which extended close to the motor region, the series is too small to lay down the rule that scar tissue near the motor area is more dangerous in this respect than that elsewhere in the frontal lobe. Solitary or occasional convulsions succeeded removal of various parts of the medial, orbital, and lateral surfaces of the hemisphere and at considerable distance from the motor region.

*Electroencephalographic Changes.* Our data do not support the belief that a cortical ablation necessarily sets up an "irritative focus," as it were, and that this produces reverberating effects, and thus continuing physiologic activity, which produces a more or less enduring shift in homeostasis and thereby improvement in the psychiatric state. As in the case of other physiologic indicators, there was more abnormality in the electroencephalograms of the acute than chronic postoperative phase. Thus, of the 13 patients exhibiting abnormal records in the first postoperative month, 9 continued to show abnormalities in the third month though usually of decreased severity. Of the ten originally abnormal records which showed localizing signs, six continued to show these. Removal of no specific area invariably resulted in electroencephalographic abnormalities lasting three months but such durable abnormalities might be seen following removal of any area. Neither was there any correlation between the amount of cortex removed and the durability of abnormal findings. Finally there was no correlation between abnormality in the electroencephalogram and any other physiologic function (except convulsions) or psychiatric state or improvement. Although all patients who developed convulsions had electroencephalograms which were abnormal postoperatively, not all continued to have such abnormal records. From the point of view of the cause of the electroencephalographic abnormality itself our data support the belief that this is caused by alterations at the edge of the cortical discontinuity. Whether this should be correlated with the rather specific cytoarchitectural change we have found to develop at such sites should be easy enough for future workers to determine.

Other possible exceptions to the general rule that no permanent effects followed the removals indicated were the following: increased appetite, increased sex drive, increased over-all activity, decreased sensitivity to pain, increased distractibility, and, what may be the same thing, greater sensitivity or responsiveness to external stimulation resulting in a phenomenon of externalization.

In the evaluation of all of these possible phenomena we are confronted by two considerable difficulties. With one exception, none can be said to have been measured proximally by reliable objective techniques and the interpretation of all changes, if such changes really exist, is seriously complicated by the existence of a psychosis. Let us, nevertheless, thread our way through the pertinent considerations and see where we emerge.

*Increased Appetite as Measured by Weight Increase.* Our data do not support the belief that removal of a particular Brodmann frontal area invariably produces bulimia or that this is an invariable result of lobotomy. It is important to observe that a *preoperative* trend toward increase in weight was apparent, dating from the time the patients were brought under study and that this trend continued in the control group following their visit to surgery. Nevertheless, the operatees as a whole showed a relatively greater increase in weight than did the controls. "Neither the type of operation nor the patient's response to it could be correlated with changes in weight" (p. 102). In the experience of Sharp and Baganz ('40) mere increase in the caloric value of the diet received by institutionalized psychotic patients does not increase their weight and it is therefore difficult to explain the upward trend displayed by our unoperated cases on the basis of increased food intake alone. A correlation of weight with changes in general activity will be needed in the future.

*Increased Sex Drive.* Our data do not support the belief that lobotomy invariably produces a sexually more active individual. Neither is there evidence that removal of one or another of the Brodmann frontal areas has such a specific effect. Evidently the personality of the individual is an important variable in such a result and this must be further defined in order to detect which cerebral mechanisms are of importance. Although some of the patients showed a recrudescence or enhancement of sex drive in the preoperative period upon being first brought under study, ablation of none of the regions removed here, invariably produced any evidence of such a phenomenon nor of any change in fundamental sex patterns, according to observations made by Dr. Pomeroy, using the study method now so familiar as the result of his collaboration with Dr. Kinsey. Individuals showing possible enhancement of sexual interest were patients 32 (area 9 and parts of 8 and 10) and 44 (lobotomy).

*Increased Over-all Activity.*   It is interesting to observe that apathy is frequently reported after lobotomy, that our lobotomy patients showed a decrease in activity, and that a similar result is achieved in the laboratory when the line of frontal removal is carried too far caudally. In order for "a marked increase in general bodily activity" to occur "both agranular frontal areas must be intact" (Mettler, '44, p. 131). On the other hand, restricted cortical ablations did not invariably produce apathy. Indeed, in some cases activity was notably increased. Since measurable data are unavailable it is impossible to correlate such increase with the circumstances of operation but none of the patients with notable involvement of the agranular area showed any evidence of increased activity. Before it is possible to conclude that agranular ablations should be carried out on patients with overactivity and granular on patients with decreased activity, precise measured data are required. Moreover, it will always be necessary to take into consideration the dynamics of the fundamental psychotic state, for some definitely agitated individuals who were subjected to granular ablations lost their overactivity with a lessening of their agitation.

*Decreased Sensitivity to Pain.*   There is no evidence from our studies that the threshold for pain was increased. Indeed there is a suggestion that it, as well as sensitivity to other forms of noxious stimuli, was decreased. This need not necessarily indicate that results such as those reported by Le Beau and Gaetano de Barros ('48) are incorrect but merely that the toleration of pain may be independent of its threshold level. More data are required.

*Increased Distractibility.*   The behavior of some of the operatees during various postoperative tests suggested that their performance was interfered with in a certain specific manner. Required responses of a repetitive nature were unusually prompt and accurate for an initial brief period, but then would cease and some prodding was necessary in order to get the subjects to proceed. Such a phenomenon was observed in various sensory tests—notably the determination of two-point sensibility. The impression arose that the phenomenon might have been due to increased distractibility or to "blocking." Some attempt to arrive at an estimate of such causes was made in the psychologic battery but definite correlations have not emerged. It is possible that all the information available in these directions has not yet been obtained.

*Greater Sensibility to External Stimuli.*   It is only in the fields of two-point sensibility, audition, vestibular function, and vision that measurable data on the thresholds of sensation are available. In the case of audition the rises in auditory acuity are probably to be correlated with improvement in the psychiatric condition of the patient. In vision the levels of the sensitivity of the tests are not low enough to give useful information about small variations in threshold of acuity. In vestibular function, reflex motor responses were used as the indicator of sensitivity. There is some evidence that the duration of this motor response was temporarily decreased by cortical ablation but information as to the minimal amount of stimulation necessary to produce a response and of the time interval between the application of a stimulus and the appearance of a response is still lacking. In the field of two-point sensibility, acuity was generally increased and this increase often tended to outlast the three-month postoperative period. There is no evident correlation between this phenomenon and the nature of the operation or the patient's response to this and it is possible that the apparent improvement merely represents a learning effect. In order to exclude this, repeated preoperative testing will be necessary in the future. Against this was the information volunteered by patient 32 that she felt "more sensitive to a variety of sensory stimuli" and the observation that with additional testing almost as many patients (4) showed a rise as showed a further decrease (5) in their threshold.

*Paralytic Phenomena.*  Permanent paralytic phenomena did not succeed removal of any of the areas ablated except in the following circumstances: dysarthria and dysphagia followed bilateral ablation of the inferior frontal gyri with possible injury to the foot of the precentral gyri and/or cortex of the lateral cerebral fossa.

Unilateral reoperation in two patients (6, 24), in whom an area 6 ablation was carried caudally to encroach upon the front of the electrically excitable area, produced, in patient 6, a temporary contralateral *flaccid* paralysis which ultimately resolved itself into paresis (except for the muscles of the hand). With the disappearance of the flaccidity, resistance to passive movement became somewhat more pronounced than before operation. In the second patient (24), who showed evidence of pre-existing organic damage, a postoperative thrombosis compromised the greater part of the blood supply of the precentral gyrus. This patient developed an upper extremity such as is commonly seen in an extreme hemiplegic picture, with total paralysis and fixation of posture, passing into contracture. It is worth emphasizing that electrical stimulation, at the time of reoperation, had disclosed much of the precentral gyrus to have been inexcitable at that time even though this was not suspected by observing the patient's movements before operation.

Our data do not support the assumption that removal of area 24 produces any notable evidence of somatomotor "release," such as might be expected from the effects reported to follow stimulation of that area.

*"Higher" Functions.*  Definition of the extent and precise nature of defects in so-called "higher functions"—notably personality changes, clownish behavior, difficulties in the associational process, loss of initiative (apart from decrease in somatomotor activity), persistence of fear, memory defects (deterioration of insight)—were originally attributed to the frontal lobe on the basis of simple observation or pure theoretical speculation, not as a result of the consideration of data obtained by specialized tests, as the dates of the articles already cited above indicate. If the discovery of such defects is really based on observation and if they really follow frontal lobe damage they might well have been expected to become glaringly apparent in the present studies. That they did not invariably appear in such obvious form (and whether they did in less obvious form is the problem of the psychologist and psychiatrist) under a given set of circumstances can have only two explanations. Either attribution of them to frontal lobe damage is false or they involve a combination of factors not present under the circumstances of this investigation. Such combinations might require the removal of a minimal amount of tissue, or the addition of a

minimal number of "specific" areas, or the combination of an extraneural factor (such as a particular basic personality set), in addition to the factors of removal here present. There is some evidence in favor of each of these hypotheses. We know (Mettler and Mettler, '42) that whereas frontal decortication makes but little difference in the "personality" of an experimental animal the addition of significant striatal to frontal cortical damage produces a profound alteration of what might be called psychic state. Further, it is well known that lesions which do not exceed the factor of physiologic safety of a neural system do not produce notable physiologic deficits (Mettler, Finch, Girden, and Culler, '34) and that the addition of deficit of one specific system to that of another may produce an entirely new kind of deficit (Carrea and Mettler, '47). Finally, there is an abundance of evidence to indicate that physiologic deficits produce different personality effects in individuals whose basic personality is essentially different. What weight should be attached to these various explanations will require more work to determine.

**Transitory Physiologic Effects of Bilateral Ablation of Parts of the Frontal Cortex.** It is obvious that audition, vestibular, and painful sensation need not be reconsidered here, having just been discussed in the preceding sections. No adequate data are available for olfaction, gustation, or thermal sensation and we are therefore unaware of any transitory as well as permanent effect upon these.

*Touch and Deep Sensation.* Alterations in two-point sensibility were noticed in the preceding section. Impairment in tactile or deep sensibility was encountered only in such instances in which paralytic phenomena appeared but not always so long as they endured, nor in every paralytic case. In the original topectomy series such alterations were of a temporary nature and only occurred after ablation of cortex situated far caudally, notably area 6.

*Vision.* There was no evidence of any visual-field defects in any of the cases studied. It is possible that previous investigators who have reported such impairment may have been confused by the transient impairment in movements of the eyes which is commonly encountered after frontal ablations.

Temporary impairment in cortical flicker fusion occurred in a number of individuals and in some lasted as long as three months. There was no correlation between this phenomenon and the area nor amount of brain tissue excised. Correlation was probably impeded by the fact that only individuals with initially high critical flicker fusion showed such loss. We agree with Halstead that such a defect may be seen in frontal lobe injury but not that it invariably occurs. No correlation between visual acuity (variation in stimulus strength) and flicker (variation in stimulus frequency) was made.

A temporary loss in autokinetic movements was observed in a number of patients. Since autokinesis is not clearly related to extraocular movement this phenomenon cannot be simply attributed to impairment in movements of the eyes. Further study and correlation with studies of the latter function are indicated.

*Blood Substances.* There is no evidence that ablation of any of the cortical areas, removed in the present studies, exerts any influence upon circulating electrolytes or upon the leucocytic system. It is possible that the red cell system (erythrocytes, hemoglobin, and reticulocytes) may be affected but more data must be accumulated to exclude absolutely, unspecific operative effects. In general more notable erythrocyte drops occurred following dorsocaudally situated ablations, and reticulocyte rises after removals of area 10, 45, 44, and the ventral part of 6. If removal of the areas ablated in these studies exerts any influence upon fasting, blood reducing substances the influence would appear to be nonspecific for areas and in the direction of a temporarily increased (for about two weeks) level of such substances. Data from glucose tolerance tests suggests that ablation of granular but not agranular cortex tends to impair the patient's ability to tolerate sugar for about a month after operation. Removal of the orbital surface does not invariably produce such a result. There is some evidence that ablation of the frontal cortex may produce a temporary increase in the blood sugar response to epinephrine but that this falls below preoperative values within three months.

*Gastrointestinal Function.*  Ablation or disconnection of granular frontal cortex may be followed by an increase in gastric and intestinal motility. No definite correlation with subregions within the granular region has been developed. It is possible that removal of area 6 may ultimately be shown to result in slowing of gastrointestinal motility.

Results on gastric acidity following localized ablation are unclear.

Remarkable diarrhea occurred in one case following removal of area 44.

*Blood Pressure.*  Although there is a tendency for blood pressure to fall following topectomy the responsible factors in such a circumstance have yet to be elucidated.

*Vascular and Sudomotor Control.*  No definite measurable data are available to indicate that any of the areas ablated exerted any influence upon these functions. Suggestive temporary changes occurred in two patients in one of whom area 6 had been involved. The other suffered an ablation of cingular cortex with entry into the ventricular system. Other area 6 cases failed to show such an effect and it evidently only follows dysfunction of the caudal part of area 6 (vasodilatation). There was but one area 24 case.

*Urinary Bladder.*  Every patient with involvement of area 6 had temporary incontinence of urine though urinary incontinence was not limited to this category of cases.

*Vomiting.*  Vomiting occurred in a number of cases. It was not clearly correlated with the nature of the operative removal but was very prominent in the single case in which area 24 was involved (and the ventricular system opened).

*Movements of the Eyes.*  Movements of the eyes were temporarily impaired in a considerable number of patients. Movements of convergence were more frequently impaired than were conjugate movements to the side. These effects did not invariably follow removal of area 8 nor the upper parts of 9 and 10, and the evidence indicates that more ventrally situated cortex is primarily concerned with extraocular movements in the human being. When the ablation was reasonably symmetrical the usual gaze was one of forward staring with the eyes directed somewhat internal to straight forward. Occasionally, the vertical level of the gaze of the two eyes was different. If the lesion was predominently unilateral, gaze was directed toward the side of greater injury.

*Aphasia and Agraphia* (see p. 432).  It may be repeated here that motor aphasia did not follow removal of any of the areas of cortex studied. Motor disability (dysarthria) followed bilateral ablation of the inferior frontal gyri with possible interference with the foot of the precentral gyri or cortex of the lateral cerebral fossa.

*Dysphagia.*  Dysphagia occurred under the circumstances just cited. This patient also exhibited a hypoactive gag reflex.

*Somatomotor Paralysis.* Somatomotor paralysis other than that noted above, occurred as a temporary phenomenon in only two patients in both of whom the ablation involved area 6. Since other area 6 operations were not followed by paralysis, and longer enduring and permanent paralysis occurred only in patients in whom the pathologic damage is known to have extended farther caudally, it may safely be assumed that paralysis is not a necessary sequel to removal of most of area 6. We agree that manual apraxia, as a temporary phenomenon, succeeds removal of that part of area 6 immediately rostral to the excitable hand area.

*Abnormal Reflexes.* In none of the patients was removal of any area consistently followed by the appearance of even a temporary abnormal reflex, including the Babinski or any of the various aspects of the grasp phenomenon. In general, there was a postoperative relaxation of muscular tension during the examination and this was reflected in some looseness of the myotatic reflexes which were sometimes difficult to elicit (difficulty in obtaining myotatic reflexes in some cases of frontal lesion has long been known; Williamson [1896] found the patellar reflex absent in 20 percent of his series of cases). The evidence indicates that relatively large amounts of frontal cortex (including all of the rostral part of area 6) can be bilaterally removed without producing a grasp reflex in the human being. If damage of that area does invariably produce it, the responsible region must be very close to area 4 or on the medial hemispheric surface. The phenomenon, closest to the Babinski, which invariably resulted from operation, was a complex mass response seen in the two patients in whom the rostral part of the Betz cell area was removed. Such a mass response bears a close resemblance to the classical Babinski but does not have its precise specific limitations.

*Cerebellar Signs.* No ataxia nor other cerebellar signs were encoutered.

# Chapter 29

# Psychology

## CARNEY LANDIS

---

THE enormous literature relevant to the psychologic functions somehow associated with the human (or animal) frontal lobes was competently summarized by Freeman and Watts ('42). The critical survey by Hebb ('45) adequately pointed out the scientific weakness of many current observations, hypotheses, and conclusions. Various chapters in the present volume have considered critically certain formulations which were related to the Columbia-Greystone findings. It remains to consider the wider psychologic implications of the entire study.

### CRITIQUE OF METHOD

Two questions must be borne in mind in trying to evaluate the outcome of the panel of psychologic experiments and tests used in this study: (1) Were the procedures used those which might give some indication of the changes which did occur? (2) Were the procedures sensitive enough to give evidence of changes which may have occurred?

When the psychologic side of this investigation was formulated more than 100 test and experimental approaches, drawn from many sources were considered. We wanted a test battery which would touch upon as wide a range of psychologic functions as possible as well as a group of tests which would give objective evidence of the changes in psychologic function following frontal lobe injury or ablation as reported by previous investigators. Limitation in time as well as overlapping in the nature of the procedures involved caused us to limit the test battery to thirty-five procedures. These were, as previous chapters indicate, most diverse. They touched upon practically every phase of mental life. We know of no other group of patients who have ever been given such a systematic and diverse group of tests. We believe that if any *generality* in function was altered by topectomy these tests should have given evidence of it. If the function or functions altered were limited and highly specific then our tests might have missed the changes. There is no evidence from the general observations or clinical reports that any such specific alterations did occur.

Were the measures which we used too rough or insensitive to give evidence of changes which might have occurred? The sensitivity of a psychologic test depends on the nature and fractionation of the scoring based on the tests. None of the psychologic procedures was scored in one way only. Certain of our tests had standard or established ways of scoring, e.g. the Wechsler-

Bellevue, but even these established scores were set aside during the course of the study and other scoring methods tried in an attempt to obtain results indicative of change. The final scoring used with practically every one of our nonstandardized procedures was that which seemed to indicate the greatest dispersion of measures and hence greatest possibility of change. We gave these procedures as much sensitivity as possible.

### TEMPORARY NATURE OF PSYCHOLOGIC CHANGES

The time at which a patient is examined with reference to the occurrence of a pathologic process is of great importance in the testing of psychologic (and physiologic) function. Discrepancies in this respect have, in all probability, caused part of the conflicting evidence present in the literature.

No permanent psychologic defect, detectable by the testing methods used, was discovered. The loss in mental age score on the Porteus Maze Test, the decrease in ability to perform verbal shifts on the Capps Test, the loss of the ability to shift the basis of sorting on the Weigl Test, and the decrease in CFF acuity were alterations shown by the tests three weeks after operation which usually disappeared four months postoperatively. In similar fashion the Per-cent of Loss shown by the method of marked deviation (chapter 24) was greatest (17 percent) three weeks after operation and decreased to 14 percent four months after operation. That changes hitherto thought to be more or less permanent proved to be temporary depended on the fact that the tests were repeated several times during the postoperative year.

The decrease in CFF means that there must be a greater time interval between flashes of light before there is a functional restoration of some mechanism which when tripped off sets up the visual process. If before operation this mechanism was so efficient that it was restored twenty-four times a second then flicker would be perceived at 24 or any rate less than 24. If the maximum rate of restoration was twenty-five times a second then flashes at 25.5 or 26 would overlap the restoration process and the result would be fusion which is perceived as a continuous light. If the operation reduced the speed of restoration of the mechanism so that it was restored only twenty times a second then the CFF would be reduced. This was what we found. In patients who had a slow restoration mechanism to start with— one which restored itself only eighteen times a second—little change might be produced and in such instances we did not find a change.

These temporary changes must for the present be regarded as isolated and very specific phenomena. For every test which showed a change (except CFF) there was one or more very similar psychologic test or experiment carried through with the same patients without any consistent or regular change in performance following operation. For example there is no obvious explanation of the change in the Capps without a similar or equivalent change in the Analogy or Essential Differences Test since *a priori* it seems to involve the same sort of mental processes.

These losses in efficiency shown by the Porteus, Capps, and Weigl were similar only in that they were decreases in efficiency of psychologic function. When tested three weeks after operation the patients were unable to perform as adequately as before operation or four months after operation. The loss seemed similar to that shown in fatigue states and the restoration similar to that occurring after rest.

### RELATION OF PSYCHOLOGIC CHANGE TO AREA OF ABLATION

There was some evidence that excision of certain portions of the frontal cortex tended to be associated with certain kinds of psychologic alterations. In chapter 24 it was shown that the largest Percent of Change was associated with excision of area 6 and that the percentage decreased in a regular fashion as one moved rostrally to area 11. The same gradient of change was shown for the Sorting Test results (chapter 16) and for the changes on the Word Association Test (chapter 17).

Unfortunately we do not have very complete psychologic test results from patients from whom area 6 was removed nor were the results from patients with area 8 excised as complete as one might desire. From the fragmentary results which we do have there is the clear indication that ablation of areas 6, 8, and 9 results in more temporary changes than does the removal of any other areas. Area 8 (and possibly part of area 9) ablation results in a transient interference with nonverbal performance efficiency (chapter 14). The changes are not pronounced nor, more significantly still, were they shown in every area 8-9 case.

The changes following excision of 9-10-46 (reduction in Anxiety and Complaint scores) are nonspecific to the ablation, particularly when one recalls that patient 38, who showed these reductions, had no tissue removed but only a venous tie of the veins draining the 9-10-46 region was performed. The reduction in Anxiety and Complaint scores was nonspecific and more quantitative than qualitative in nature.

Ablation of areas 11, 44, and 47 resulted in no regular psychologic change that we could determine.

Areas 45-46 seemed to give a somewhat different pattern of changes than did 8-9 or 9-10-46. The clearest changes (which were usually temporary) in the ability to shift on the Capps Test or Weigl Test were shown when area 45 or 46 was involved. The loss in PI-1 Grouping score (chapter 16) when area 9 was excised did not occur if both 9 and 46 were removed.

### RELATION OF PERSONALITY CHANGES TO OPERATION

The psychiatric descriptions and diagnoses, the Rorschach characterizations, and the personality sketches given in connection with Word Association Test or the Anxiety and Complaint Inventories are in essence portraits of these patients viewed from differing angles. There is no clear-cut evidence of a consistent or uniform personality change which resulted from any particular variety of topectomy in which the operation could clearly be said to be solely responsible for the change. The amelioration from psychosis and social improvement which occurred in many of the operatees is easiest understood as an indirect effect of the operation. If any operation specifically changed behavior some clear-cut regular phenomena should have been evoked. If any variety of operation had specifically resulted in the alleviation of some physical or mental disease or in the change of a particular personality structure then greater regularity of results should have been achieved.

It is an old clinical observation that any of a wide variety of physical injuries may be followed by a temporary amelioration of psychotic symptoms. Mentally disturbed patients are frequently relatively lucid during convalescence from an appendectomy, while recovering from a broken leg, or following an acute bout with an infectious disease. It is conceivable that the mental amelioration following topectomy might be basically the same sort of thing. But why does an appendectomy patient show a relapse when healing is complete while certain topectomy patients were still lucid at the end of a year?

The decrease scores on the Complaint and Anxiety Inventories are closely associated with the fact of related amelioration from psychoses and subsequent social recovery, but are they directly dependent on the operation? Several considerations argue against it. The decreased scores were nonspecific and quantitative rather than qualitative. The Anxiety scores showed a gradual decrease during the entire postoperative year. The Complaint score was decreased when the patients were tested three weeks after operation and it held constant at subsequent retest periods. The course of the Complaint and Anxiety changes might be compared to the alleviation of some specific source of acute, continuous physical pain by chordotomy. The specific pain disappears with the operation; associated physical and mental complaints would sharply decline when the primary pain disappeared while the anxieties and worries would decline as rehabilitation proceeded in a satisfactory fashion.

There is nothing which we know from any experimental or clinical evidence which indicates that the anxieties and complaints as indicated in our inventories had a specific biologic basis in the sense that flicker fusion is based on the efficiency of the retinal and cortical neural process or in the sense that the performance on the Porteus is based on definable psychomotor processes. No one has ever been able to define a biologic basis for anxiety—or for any other affective experience. All experimentation shows that there is a tendency for a wide variety of physiologic processes to be associated with affect (increased blood pressure with fright; regular respiration with contentment, and so on) but no specific one-to-one relationship between conscious experience of affect and physiologic process exists.

### REDUCTION IN "PSYCHIC PAIN" OF PSYCHOSIS

There is a theory which points out that the motor expressions of emotion are localized in the hypothalamus and that clinical evidence may be interpreted as indicating that hypothalamic lesions give rise to disturbances in conscious affective experience. Lashley ('38) made a critical evaluation of the evidence on which the theory rests and found it in part erroneous and in part unsatisfactory. We have no evidence which strengthens this theory and we see no point in using it as a basis of explanation.

An explanation which might be advanced is that there is functional physiologic imbalance somewhere in the body of the psychotic patient. This imbalance might be conceived as setting up reverberating sensory "pain" processes similar to those described by Livingstone ('43) for causalgia and intractable pain. Instances have been reported where causalgia and intractable pain has been relieved either by ablation of portions of the contralateral somesthetic cortex (Gutierrez-Mahoney, '44) or by prefrontal lobotomy (Scarff, '48). Since the somesthetic area is regarded as the principal terminus of the cutaneous sensory pathways, excision of the area might be expected to bring about a change in cutaneous sensibility. In patients from whom the contralateral somesthetic area has been removed in an effort to relieve intractable pain, relief is usually, though not invariably, the result. Furthermore, the removal of this area gives rise to an immediate disturbance in cutaneous sensibility from which after several days there is partial recovery. (There is no evidence that such an operation relieves the "psychic pain" of the psychotic patient.)

This hypothesis draws further support from the following evidence. There are centrifugal tracts connecting the medial thalamic nucleus with the prefrontal areas 9-10 (Le Gros Clark, '48). Scarff ('48) has shown that the interruption of these tracts either ipsilaterally, contralaterally, or bilaterally by lobotomy relieves intractable pain without producing disturbances in cutaneous sensibility. This leads to the notion that the decrease in anxiety following lobotomy (or topectomy) might be attributed to the removal of the terminus for some portion of the sensory impulses which serve as the physical basis for the conscious processes of "psychic pain" so prominent in psychosis. But if this is true then several other difficulties arise: (1) Direct stimulation of area 9-10 gives rise to no conscious experience while direct stimulation of the somesthetic area is reacted to as referred cutaneous sensation. (2) Ablation of the somesthetic cortex leads to a disturbance in cutaneous sensibility followed by partial recovery. Ablation of area 9-10 may lead to a remission from psychosis but there is no clear evidence of loss or decrease in the threshold for pain sensitivity. (3) There may be a reoccurrence of the psychotic state after remission which followed lobotomy (or topectomy). This would mean that other areas and other connecting pathways had taken over the mediation of the "psychic pain" of psychosis. (4) Removal of areas 9-10 by bilateral amputation of the frontal poles of the brain (Peyton et al., '48) is not regularly followed by a remission from psychosis (and psychic pain), and if remission does occur there are instances of relapse.

The hypothesis that the loss in press of anxiety (or affect) following ablation of areas 9-10 is specific to the areas, fails to meet the following points: (1) There is no hitherto known specific localization of affect. (2) Area 9-10 is silent from a sensory point of view and insofar as response to direct stimulation is concerned. (3) After ablation of area 9-10 these patients reported no alteration in emotional experience—fear, anger, pleasantness or unpleasantness—as ordinarily perceived. The report was that of diminution of anxiety as a derived or secondary experience. (4) This relief of anxiety was in certain cases temporary in that there was a relapse into the psychotic state not essentially different from that which they experienced originally.

No existing theory or hypothesis dealing with the psychologic significance of the human frontal lobes is tenable. There is no point in either propping up or demolishing established theories. They add only to the confusion of thought and had best be forgotten. With the body of evidence now available from this study there is no clear outline of a useful and unifying formulation which would readily replace the older theories. We believe that the way is clear for a comprehensive investigation which should lead to new knowledge which will be meaningful.

## Chapter 30

# Psychiatry

ROBERT G. HEATH

A STUDY such as the present one might be expected to shed some light on the psychotic process.

In this project patients were studied extensively and uniformly before and after operation from the standpoint of several different disciplines. They were divided into two groups, one acting as a control and the other subject to various types of frontal lobe surgery which was successful in removing psychotic behavior in many patients.

Various authors have noted many—although vague—biologic differences between the chronic psychotic and normal individuals. It is generally accepted that the chronic psychotic is not well integrated. Hoskins ('46) states: "The malintegration could conceivably exist at any level from the atomic to the social. Whether the psychosis is singularly or multiply caused and the nature and level of operation of the etiological factor or factors remain for research to determine. Until such knowledge comes to hand attempts at prevention of the disorder will be mere trial and error and treatment will be empirical shooting in the dark."

In reviewing and correlating our data we find nothing which promises to solve definitely this long-standing riddle. There are, however, some suggestive findings which will be described in the hope that they may prove worthwhile leads for future study.

### MEDICAL CONSIDERATIONS

The most consistent abnormal findings in the chronic schizophrenic are general lassitude, low blood pressure, mild anemia, and aberrations of sugar metabolism not accounted for by other reasons. Our patients generally presented these features.

On general physical examination the patients in the series presented a rather favorable picture to those of us who have been accustomed to considering institutional populations as rather neglected groups. It must be remembered that the present series was not medically screened prior to our study and that nearly all the cases came from "back" wards. Very little was turned up by our own medical studies which the hospital staff was not already aware of and this suggests that even under the understaffed conditions of heavy stress of the war and postwar period few medical conditions remain undetected long enough to become truly chronic without the knowledge of the staff. It is evidently the surgical emergency or acute medical condition which presents the greater problem in psychiatric institutional care.

Nutrition was surprisingly good. It is true that many of the patients gained weight in the preoperative period in the special ward of the project under conditions of unusual care, but on the whole the nutritional state of the patients was quite comparable with that seen in patients of comparable age in the out-patient departments serving the lower middle classes of metropolitan areas.

In the special medical studies which are included in the medical section, chapter 6, an important correlation worthy of further study is the finding that the most marked biologic changes occurred with ablation of granular cortex. It was removal of this same region of frontal cortex that produced definite clinical improvement.

The commonly reported aberration of sugar metabolism in the chronic psychotic is a supposed anti-insulin factor (Meduna *et al.*, '42; Romano and Coon, '42). Our studies on sugar metabolism were by no means complete. They consisted of evaluations of fasting sugars and of glucose tolerance curves before and at regular intervals after operation. For one to two months after granular cortex was ablated, the ability to tolerate sugar was impaired.

Similarly, it was ablation of granular cortex that produced the greatest (although not outstanding) alterations of gastric function as measured by the analysis of the stomach contents.

The preoperative blood pressure recording in our patients revealed that most were quite hypotensive, some were normotensive, and there was no hypertension. This finding is consistent with reports of others. Changes that did occur following surgery were of minor degree and temporary. These changes were toward further lowering of pressure and were usually associated with removal of granular cortex.

In the laboratory data there was a suggestive finding that supported the frequently reported finding of anemia in chronic psychotic patients. Blood studies indicated that a drop in hemoglobin may precipitate an acute disturbance in the psychotic individual.

### NEUROLOGICAL CONSIDERATIONS

The preoperative neurological findings were not outstanding. Perhaps the incidence of minor positive findings was slightly higher than it would be in the general populace but no major abnormal findings were present. Since many of the patients had previously had electroshock, it seems logical to consider that the findings might be residues of this treatment. Another valuable correlation from the neurological survey was that it became possible to gain a rough idea of the amount of cortex that could be removed before social deterioration appeared.

### CONTROLLING FACTORS

Two factors proved to be of considerable value in controlling this study. The first was the use of patients not subjected to operation to control the effect of total push. In this control group, 3 patients were able to be paroled even though they had no specific treatment. This seems quite important in view of the survey in chapter 2 where, on the basis of a statistical study of a large group of similar patients under ordinary hospital care, the expectation of discharge would have been practically nil. Only one of the 3 patients was making a completely satisfactory adjustment eight months after parole, but this nevertheless indicates that total push is an effective therapy which must be considered.

The second valuable control was the finding that the only patients in whom we felt improvement was definitely related to operation (patients 3, 4, 7, 8, 13, 21, 22, 25, 27, 31, 33, 36, 49) had areas 9 and 10 implicated in the removal. In the 9 patients who did not have parts or all of these areas included at operation, psychotic behavior was not altered. (The absence of a one-to-one correlation between alteration of psychotic behavior and the social ratings recorded in the improvement graphs is explained in the section on improvement ratings.)

### COMPARISON OF THE EFFECTS OF LOBOTOMY WITH THOSE FOLLOWING ABLATION OF FRONTAL CORTEX

Throughout the psychiatric section, when it was appropriate, comparisons were made between various features of topectomy and lobotomy. The number of cases in our lobotomy series is small, so references were made to the writings of others more experienced with the lobotomy procedure. A recent and very inclusive summary of the effects of lobotomy has been prepared by Solomon ('48) and it therefore seems pertinent that we should devote a few pages to comparing topectomy with lobotomy in regard to the specific points made by him.

**Possibility of Improvement.** *Lobotomy.* According to Solomon, although the percentage of improved patients cannot be accurately determined because of inequivalence in the data, a "fair estimate would be in the neighborhood of ten percent. It may be further judged that another 15 or 20 percent of operated patients are able to live a relatively happy life and be in part self-sustaining. Probably 80 percent of the patients subjected to this type of surgery become more contented individuals and have a more satisfactory existence than before operation."

*Topectomy.* The present series of topectomy patients is so small and contains so many variables that it would be a mistake to develop statistics relating to improvement. Significant, however, is the finding that many patients with poor prognostic expectations did improve. The assumption that this improvement was related to removal of areas 9-10 seems fairly logical since all patients who we felt definitely improved through operation had these areas implicated in the removal (patients 3, 4, 7, 8, 13, 21, 22, 25, 27, 31, 32, 33, 36, 38, 49). Fifteen patients had such operations and only 9 had other areas removed (patients 2, 6, 18, 19, 24, 40, 42, 44, 47), so the series was somewhat weighted* toward 9-10 operations. Nine patients without improvement following other operations is not quite an adequate number to rule out the purely somatic factor of craniotomy being responsible for improvement. More removals of areas other than 9-10 will be necessary before this point is definitely clarified. Results in the control series rule out the possibility of a wide range of nonspecific factors such as total push being responsible for the improvement.

To summarize the comparison of results in the two procedures, it can be

---

* The reason for the larger number of cases in the 9-10 group will be apparent on consulting chapter 1. In addition to a numerical weighting a prognostic weighting must be considered. Prognosis was more favorable in the 9-10 group, 80 percent being given a good prognosis prior to operation compared to 33 percent with good prognostic rating for the non-9-10 group.

said that the results which have followed ablations of smaller parts of cortex than are disconnected with lobotomy appear to yield results at least equally as good without producing the unwanted results of the latter operation.

**Mechanism of Improvement.** *Lobotomy.* It has been postulated that the improvement in the psychiatric condition of patients subjected to lobotomy is due to interruption of thalamocortical connections linking affective with intellectual mechanisms. The original essential link in this process of reasoning was the medial nucleus, as explained on page 425 where the conflict between the explanation and observable evidence has been pointed out.

Hebb also raised the question as to why relapses could occur after these fibers had been severed, since there can be no regeneration. We feel that this cannot be argued solely in terms of physiology and have attempted to explain it on the basis of our psychiatric observations (see chapter 25, p. 427). Also in this study our physiologic evidence does not support the explanation which Hebb offered to account for this temporary improvement.

Hebb has postulated that the improvement in lobotomy may be due to a reversible effect. He has in mind here a physiologic disturbance produced by the operation. "Electrical evidence and the clinical course . . . show clearly that surgical procedures are followed by a local cerebral disturbance. . . . If lobotomy tends to leave extensive scar formation and vascular damage, the physiologic disturbance could become chronic. . . ."

*Topectomy.* In the present work there is no evidence which can be used to prove Hebb's explanation. If it is correct, one would expect the largest ablations to produce the greatest disturbance and there should be a correlation between the amount of tissue removed and improvement. This is not the case. One would also expect a correlation to exist between abnormality in the electroencephalogram and improvement. There is none. One would also expect to find a correlation between disturbances, howsoever transient, in basic physiologic functions and improvement. If there is one, we have not found it.

In the psychiatric section we have discussed the mechanisms of improvement. Since others have given reasons for improvement that differ from ours, we shall discuss them briefly. From our observations, the factor producing improvement was the lessening of painful affect associated with mental conflict. Many others feel that this is the fundamental factor but some have explained improvement as being due to such things as "becoming externalized." It is then stated that patients become more interested in things outside themselves and forget their inner conflicts. Such is not the case. During the early postoperative period patients are attracted to many things in their environment but this is accompanied by general lessening of awareness: they are distractible and cannot center their attention on anything for reasonable periods and therefore go from one thing to another. The fallacy of explaining improvement on the basis of lessening of consciousness of self has been fully explained on page 424.

**Mortality.** In the case of lobotomy, "The mortality rate in the operation varies considerably . . . but may be estimated as in the neighborhood of three to four percent." (In the original series of topectomy cases there were no deaths. The demise of patient 24 occurred after a unilateral cortical operation performed long after the original procedure.)

**Convulsive Seizures.** According to Solomon, "Convulsive seizures occur in from four to ten percent of patients" who have had lobotomy. "Usually only a few attacks are suffered, but occasionally a patient will have repeated attacks." The same situation seems to obtain after localized ablations of frontal cortex. It is clear that statistics will differ on this point unless the occurrence of a single convulsion is regarded as placing the patient in the convulsive group. In the topectomy cases, 1 patient developed a definite convulsive pattern and 4 (including the patient just mentioned) have had more than one seizure. In all of these 4 patients the electroencephalogram was abnormal immediately after operation or became so before convulsions occurred. Not all individuals with abnormal electroencephalograms developed convulsions.

It was noted in the section in which psychiatry was correlated with neurological findings that no convulsions occurred in patients who had area removals confined to the site which produced best psychiatric results (anterior 9 and posterior 10). This suggests that in topectomy it may be possible to eliminate or markedly reduce the incidence of convulsions.

**Clinical Evaluation of the Psychiatric Condition.** According to Solomon, lobotomy may result in "A carefree attitude, with euphoria, [which] may be excessive for the best of personal relations. Apathy, lack of interest, procrastination, facetiousness, profanity, a temper outburst, and distractibility are among other undesirable conditions which have been encountered. There is a distinct tendency for these unfavorable reactions to improve during the course of months following the operation. The greatest concern is in relation to the loss of some of the important characteristics of personality integration such as judgment, planning for the future . . . ," (Hebb ['45] has previously pointed out that this last "deficit," which was extended by Freeman and Watts to a general explanation, is only part of a general process which includes lack of concern for the past.) . . . "Discrimination, laudable ambition, fine sentiments, and creative imagination."

On the positive side, Solomon indicates that after lobotomy:

"(1) Tension, apprehension, fear, concern, worry, and agitation are greatly reduced or abolished.

"(2) Excitement, aggressive and assaultive behavior, emotional outbursts and rage-like exhibitions, although not infrequently intensified shortly after operation, tended to diminish within a few weeks or months.

"(3) Paranoid ideas tend to lessen to the vanishing point, or, if continued in an attenuated form, cease to lead to overt expressions.

"(4) Obsessive thinking becomes less distracting, compulsive actions no longer occur, and ritualistic behavior ceases.

"(5) Long-standing hallucinations may lessen, or lead to a lessened response; only rarely do they disappear entirely.

"(6) Anergic states are occasionally transformed into states of greater activity but frequently are unchanged or activity may even be reduced."

The results of our study, although too small to be conclusive, indicate that with topectomy it is possible to achieve the positive effects and eliminate many of the negative ones.

**Indications for Operation.** According to Solomon, lobotomy may be used in the manic depressive psychoses and in involutional melancholia when such cases have reached a state of chronicity and recovery has not taken place after the benefit of the best environmental conditions, psychotherapy, and convulsive shock therapy. In obsessive compulsive neuroses, the operation may be used when the syndrome has existed for several years with an increasing intensity of symptoms progressing toward a state of incapacity, preferably in those cases which begin insidiously in puberty or early adolescence and progress inexorably to incapacity in the middle or late twenties or thirties. In the schizophrenic psychoses, lobotomy may be used if the patient has been ill for three years. Solomon feels that if the patient has been ill for ten years or longer, very little benefit can be expected to result from lobotomy. So far as subgroups are concerned, "Patients with a great deal of emotional turmoil, with catatonic-like behavior patterns and with circumscribed paranoid trends, appear to have a better prognosis if operated upon than the patients with little energy, little emotional turmoil, and with a hebephrenic syndrome." In the paranoid psychoses, "those patients whose paranoid systems are very well organized and who maintain good contact with reality tend to make a good readjustment after operation. On the other hand, individuals, sometimes considered to belong to this group, who are disorganized in their thinking processes and subject to vivid and continued auditory hallucinations, tend to have a less satisfactory outcome."

Solomon considers lobotomy of very little use in conditions of organic disease of the brain with the possible exception of the sequelae of chronic encephalitis. In psychopathic personality, lobotomy is advised against, on the basis of the possibility of rendering the individual less inhibited than previously and also because inadequate data are available. Lobotomy is advised for those individuals who are suicidal and for whom shock therapy is contraindicated. It is also indicated in patients having intractable pain which cannot be treated by less mutilating procedures.

On page 427 we discussed at some length the place for topectomy in the psychiatrist's therapeutic armamentarium. On most points our indications were similar to those advanced by Solomon. Patients with well-preserved affect, regardless of the diagnostic category into which they fall, respond best, whereas those who are more disorganized respond less well. We do not feel that duration of the illness is an important factor. In this series many successful results were obtained in patients who had been ill for periods much longer than ten years, some as long as twenty-five years. The important factor in their ultimate recovery seemed to be that affect was well preserved; the patients had not deteriorated. On the other hand, we do not feel that it is necessary for a patient to have been ill at least three years before surgery is undertaken. In some very malignant cases of schizophrenia there is danger of rapid deterioration and if more conservative treatments fail, surgery should be resorted to before it is too late.

This series is extremely small, especially when compared to the number of patients who have been lobotomized. It is, therefore, impossible at this date to draw accurate impressions. At a later date, after more patients have been topectomized, we will be in a better position to make comparisons with lobotomy and also will be able to better define indications for this procedure.

ACKERLY, S., 1935, Instinctive, emotional and mental changes following prefrontal lobe extirpation. *Am. J. Psychiat.* 92:717-729.

ALZHEIMER, A., 1897, Beiträge zur pathologischen Anatomie der Hirnrinde und zur anatomischen Grundlage einiger Psychosen. *Monatschr. f. Psychiat.* 2 : 90.

ALZHEIMER, A., 1910, Beiträge zur Kenntnis der pathologischen Neuroglia und ihre Beziehungen zu den Abbauvorgängen im Nervengewebe. *Nissl-Alzheimer Histologische Arb.*, 3 (Heft 3), 401-562.

ALZHEIMER, A., 1913, Beiträge zur pathologischen Anatomie der Dementia praecox. *Ztschr. f.d. ges. Neurol. u. Psychiat.* (Ref.) 7 : 621-622.

ANDREW, W., and ASHWORTH, C. T., 1945, The adendroglia. A new concept of the morphology and reactions of the smaller neuroglial cells. *J. Comp. Neurol.* 82 : 101-116.

ANDRUS, E. D., BRONK, D. W., GARDEN, G. A. JR., KEEFER, C. S., LOCKWOOD, J. S., WEARN, J. T., and WINTERNITZ, M. C., 1948, Advances in military medicine, 2 vols. Boston, Little Brown & Co.

BAILEY, P., and SWEET, W. H., 1940, Effects on respiration, blood pressure and gastric motility of stimulation of orbital surface of frontal lobe. *J. Neurophysiol.* 3 : 276-281.

BALLENGER, W. L., and BALLENGER, H. C., 1943, Diseases of the ear, nose, and throat, ed. 8. Philadelphia, Lea & Febiger.

BANG, I., 1913, Der Blutzucker. Weisbaden, J. F. Bergman.

BARADUC (no initial), 1876, Troubles cérébraux analogues à ceux de la paralysie générale. *Bull. Soc. anat.* pp. 277-279.

BARRIS, R. W., and INGRAM, W. R., 1936, The effect of experimental hypothalamic lesions upon blood sugar. *Am. J. Physiol.* 114 : 555-561.

BARTLEY, S. H., 1941, Vision. New York, Van Nostrand, pp. 117-119.

BECHTEREW, W. v., 1908-1911, Die Funktionen der Nervencentra. Trans. by Richard Weinberg, 3 vols. Fischer, Jena, (see vol. 3).

BECK, S. J., 1944, Rorschach's Test, vol. I. New York, Grune & Stratten.

BENTON, A. L., 1945, A visual retention test for clinical use. *Arch. Neurol. & Psychiat.* 54 : 212-216.

BERG, B. N., and ZUCKER, T. F., 1937, Blood sugar recovery from insulin hypoglycemia after section of the splanchnic nerves. *Am. J. Physiol.* 120 : 435.

BERGER, H., 1923, Klinische Beiträge zur Pathologie des Grosshirns. I. Mitt., Herderkrankungen der Präfrontal-region. *Arch. f. Psychiat.* 69 : 1-46.

BIANCHI, L., 1922, The mechanism of the brain and the function of the frontal lobes. Edinburgh, Livingston.

BODO, R. C., and BENAGLIA, A. E., 1938, Effect of sympathin on blood sugar. *Am. J. Physiol.* 121 : 728-737.

BOHM, R., and HOFFMAN, F. A., 1878, Beitrage zur Kenntnis der Kohlenhydratstoffwechsels. *Arch. f. exper. Path. u. Pharmakol.* 8 : 271.

BOLLES, M. M., 1937, The basis of pertinence. *Arch. Psychol.* 30 (no. 212) : 51 pp.

BOLLES, M. M., and GOLDSTEIN, K., 1938, A study of the impairment of "abstract behavior" in schizophrenic patients. *Psychiat. Quart.* 12 : 42-65.

BOLTON, J. S., 1911, A contribution to the localization of cerebral function based upon the clinico-pathological study of mental disease. *Brain* 33 : 26-148.

BOUMANN, K. H., 1928, Die pathologische Anatomie des Zentralnervensystems bei Schizophrenie. *Psychiat. en neurol. bl.* 32 : 517-539.

BRADLEY, C., 1937, Effect of encephalography on blood sugar level of children. *Am. J. M. Sc.* 193 : 259-264.

BRAZIER, M., and FINESINGER, J. E., 1945, Action of barbiturates on the cerebral cortex —electroencephalographic studies. *Arch. Neurol. & Psychiat.* 53 : 51-58.

BRICKNER, R. M., 1936, Intellectual functions of the frontal lobes: A study of a man after partial bilateral frontal lobectomy. New York, The Macmillan Company.

BRITTON, S. W., 1928, Neural and hormonal factors in bodily activity. The prepotency of medulliadrenal influence in emotional hyperglycemia. *Am. J. Physiol.* 86 : 340-352.

BROBECK, J. R., TEPPERMAN, J., and LONG, C. N. H., 1943, The effect of experimental obesity upon carbohydrate metabolism. Yale, *J. Biol. Med.* 15 : 893-904.

BROCA, A., and MAUBRAC, P., 1896. Traité de chirurgie cérébrale. Paris.

BROCA, P., 1861, Remarques sur le siége de la faculté du langage articulé, suivies, d'une observation d'aphémie (perte de la parole). *Bull. Soc. anat. de Paris.* Ser. 2, 36 : 330-357. Nouvelle observation d'aphémie produite par une lésion de la moitié postérieure les deuxième et troisème circonvolutions frontales. *ibid.* 398-407.

BRODMANN, K., 1908, Beiträge zur histologische Lokalization, IV, *J. f. Psychol. u. Neurol.* 10 : 231-246.

K. BRODMANN, 1925, Vergleichende Lokalisationslehre der Grosshirnrinde in ihren Prinzipien dargestellt auf Grund der Zellenbaues. Leipzig, Barth.

BROOKS, C. M., 1931, A delimitation of the central nervous mechanism involved in reflex hyperglycemia. *Am. J. Physiol.* 99 : 64-76.

BROUHA, L., CANNON, W. B., and DILL, D. B., 1939, Blood-sugar variations in normal and in sympathectomized dogs. *J. Physiol.* 95 : 431-438.

BRUNS, L., 1892, Ueber Störungen des Gleichgewichtes bei Stirnhirntumoren. *Deutsche med. Wchnschr.* 18 : 138-140.

BRUNS, L., 1897, Die Geschwülste des Nervensystems. Berlin.

BRUNS, L., 1898, Zwei Fälle von Hirntumor mit genauer Localdiagnose. *Neurol. Centralbl.* 17 : 770-788, 848-858.

BURCKHARDT, G., 1875, Die physiologische Diagnostik der Nervenkrankheiten. Leipzig.

BURCKHARDT, G., 1890-91, Ueber Rindenexcisionen. *Allg. Ztschr. f. Psychiat.* 47 : 463-548.

CAMMERMEYER, J., 1938, Uber Gehirnveränderungen, enstanden unter Sakelscher Insulin Therapie bei einem Schizophrenen. *Ztschr. f.d. ges. Neurol. u. Psychiat.* 163 : 617-633.

CAMMERMEYER, J., 1940, Recherches anatomo-pathologiques sur les lésions cérébrales dans la thérapeutique convulsivante de la démence précoce. *J. belge de neurol. et de psychiat.* 40 : 169-229.

CAMPBELL, A. W., 1905, Histological studies on the localization of cerebral function. Campbridge University Press.

CANNON, W. B., SHOHL, A. T., and WRIGHT, W. S., 1911, Emotional glycosuria. *Am. J. Physiol.* 29 : 280-287.

CAPPS, H. M., 1939, Vocabulary changes in mental deterioration. *Arch. Psychol.* 34 : 1-81.

CARDONA, F., 1934, Studio sul rigonfiamento acúto della oligodendroglia nella psichosi. *Rassegna di studi psichiat.* 23 : 271-281.

CARREA, R. M. E., and METTLER, FRED A., 1947, Physiologic consequences following extensive removals of the cerebellar cortex and deep cerebellar nuclei. *J. Comp. Neurol.* 87 : 169-288.

CASE, T. J., and BUCY, P. C., 1938, Localization of cerebral lesions of electroencephalography. *J. Neurophysiol.* 1 : 245-261.

CHAPMAN, W. P., ROSE, A. S., and SOLOMON, H. C., 1948, Measurements of heat stimulus producing motor withdrawal reaction in patients following frontal lobotomy. The frontal lobes. Res. Monogr., *A. Research Nerv. & Ment. Dis.* 27 : 754-768.

CHARCOT, J. M., 1876-1880, Leçons sur les localisations dans les maladies due cerveau et de la moelle épinière faites à la faculté de médecine de Paris, 1876-1880, 2 vol.

CLARK, E. P., and COLLIP, J. B., 1925, A study of the Tisdall method for the determination of blood serum calcium with a suggested modification. *J. Biol. Chem.* 63 : 461-464.

CLEVELAND, D., and DAVIS, L., 1936, Further studies on the effect of hypothalamic lesions upon carbohydrate metabolism. *Brain* 59 : 459.

COBB, S., 1944, Personality as affected by lesions of the brain. Chapter 18 in HUNT, J. M., Personality and the behavior disorders, Vol. 1. New York, Ronald, pp. 550-581.

COBB, W. A., 1944, The electroencephalographic localization of intra-cranial neoplasms. *J. Neurol., Neurosurg. & Psychiat.* 7 : 96-102.

COFFIN, JUDITH, 1946, The effect of electro-convulsive therapy on the learning and retention of meaningful and semi-meaningful material. Master's Essay, Columbia University.

COHN, R., 1945, Electroencephalographic study of prefrontal lobotomy—a study of focal brain injury. *Arch. Neurol. & Psychiat.* 53 : 283-287.

CONKEY, R. C., 1938-9, Psychological changes associated with head injuries. *Arch. Psychol.* 33 (no. 232) : 62 pp.

DANIEL, I., and MAXIM, M., 1929, Der Einfluss des Grosshirns auf den Zuckergehalt im Blute. *Klin. Wchnschr.* 8 : 1769-1770.

DAVIDSON, E. C., and ALLEN, C. I., 1925, The blood glucose curve in head injuries. *Bull. Johns Hopkins Hosp.* 37 : 217-230.

DAVIS, L., 1934, The relation of the hypophysis, hypothalamus, and the autonomic nervous system to carbohydrate metabolism. *Ann. Surg.* 100 : 654-666.

DAVIS, P. A., 1941, The technique and evaluation of the electroencephalogram. *J. Neurophysiol.* 4 : 92-114.

DONATH, J., 1925, The significance of the frontal brain with respect to the higher psychic functions. *J. Nerv. & Ment. Dis.* 61 : 113-141.

DONHOFFER, C., and MACLEOD, J. J. R., 1932, Studies in the nervous control of carbohydrate metabolism. III. The nature of the mechanism of the nerve control. *Proc. Roy. Soc., London,* 110B : 158-171.

DUNLAP, C. B., 1924, Dementia praecox. Some preliminary observations on brains from carefully selected cases, and a consideration of certain sources of error. *Am. J. Psychiat.* 3 : 403-421.

DUNLAP, C. B., 1928, The pathology of the brain in schizophrenia. A. Research in Nerv. & Ment. Dis., vol. 5 (Schizophrenia). New York, Paul B. Hoeber.

DUSSER DE BARENNE, J. G., and McCULLOCH, W. S., 1936, Some effects of laminar thermocoagulation upon the local action potentials of the cerebral cortex of the monkey. *Am. J. Physiol.* 114 : 692-694.

EBAUGH, F. G., BARNACLE, C. H., and NEUBUERGER, K. T., 1943, Fatalities following electric convulsive therapy. Report of two cases. *Arch. Neurol. & Psychiat.* 49 : 107-117.

ECONOMO, C. v., and KOSKINAS, G. N., 1925, Die Cytoarchitektonik der Hirnrinde des erwachsenen Menschen. Vienna and Berlin, J. Springer.

EISENSON, J., 1946, Examining for aphasia. New York, Psych. Corp.

ELVIDGE, A. R., and REED, G., 1936, Biopsy studies of cerebral pathologic changes in schizophrenia and manic depressive psychosis. *Arch. Neurol. & Psychiat.* 40 : 227-264.

FEINBLATT, H. M., 1923, Hyperglycemia based upon a study of 2000 blood chemical analyses. *J. Lab. & Clin. Med.* 8 : 500-505.

FERRARO, A., 1934, Histopathological findings in two cases clinically diagnosed dementia praecox. *Am. J. Psychiat.* 13 : 883-902.

FERRARO, A., 1943, Pathological changes in the brain of a case clinically diagnosed dementia praecox. *J. Neuropath & Exper. Neurol.,* 2 : 84-94.

FERRARO, A., and JERVIS, G. A., 1939, Brain pathology in four cases of schizophrenia treated with insulin. *Psychiat. Quart.* 13 : 207-228.

FERRIER, D., 1886, The functions of the brain. London, Smith, Elder & Co.

FERRIER, D., 1890, The Croonian lectures on cerebral localization. London, Smith, Elder & Company, p. 151.

FEUCHTWANGER, E., 1923, Die Funktionen des Stirnhirns ihre Pathologie und Psychologie. *Monogr. a.d. Ges. geb. d. Neurol. u. Psychiat.* 38 : 1-194.

FISHBEIN, M., 1941, Frontal lobotomy. *J.A.M.A.* 117 : 535-536.

FITZGERALD, G., CAWTHORNE, T. E., and HALLPIKE, C. S., 1942, Studies in human vestibular function. I. Observation on the directional preponderance of caloric
nystagmus resulting from cerebral lesions. *Brain* 65 : 115-137.

FLECHSIG, P., 1896, Die Lokalisation d. geistigen Vorgänge. Leipzig.

FLOURENS, M. J. P., 1842, Recherches experimentales sur les propiétés et les fonctions
du système nerveux. Paris, J. B. Bailliere.

FOERSTER, O., 1912, Die histologische Untersuchung der Hirnrinde intra vitam durch
Hirnpunktion bei diffusen Erkrankungen des Centralnervensystem. *Berl. klin.
Wchnschr.* 49 : 973-977.

FRANK, J., 1946, Clinical survey and results of 200 cases of prefrontal leucotomy.
*J. Ment. Sc.* 92 : 497-508.

FRANZ, S. I., 1907, On the functions of the cerebrum: the frontal lobes. *Arch. Psychol.*
1 (no. 2). New York, Science Press.

FREEMAN, H., and ELMADJIAN, F., 1947, The relationship between blood sugar and
lymphocyte levels in normal and psychotic subjects. *Psychosom. Med.* 9 : 226-232.

FREEMAN, W., 1937, New fields in psychiatry. *Clin. Med. & Surg.* 44 : 59.

FREEMAN, W., and WATTS, J. W., 1941, Frontal lobes and consciousness of self.
*Psychosom. Med.* 3 : 111-119.

FREEMAN, W., and WATTS, J. W., 1942, Psychosurgery. Springfield, Ill., Charles C.
Thomas.

FREEMAN, W., and WATTS, J. W., 1944, Physiological psychology. *Ann. Rev. Physiol.*
6 : 517-542.

FREEMAN, W., and WATTS, J. W., 1947, Retrograde degeneration of the thalamus following prefrontal lobotomy. *J. Comp. Neurol.* 86 : 65-93.

FREEMAN, W., and WATTS, J. W., 1947a, Psychosurgery during 1936-1946. *Arch.
Neurol. & Psychiat.* 58 : 417-425.

FRITSCH, G., and HITZIG, F., 1870, Ueber die elektrische Erregbarkeit des Grosshirns.
*Arch. f. Anat. u. Physiol.* 37 : 300-332.

FULTON, J. F., 1943, Physiology of the nervous system. Oxford University Press.

FÜNFGELD, E., 1927, Über die pathologische Anatomie der Schizophrenie und ihre
Bedevtung für die Abtrennung "atypischer" periodisch verlaufendes Psychosen.
*Monatschr. f. Psychiat.* 63 : 1-68.

GALTON, F., 1880, Psychometric experiments. Brain 2 : 149-162.

GARRETT, H. E., 1946, A developmental theory of intelligence. Am. Psychol. 1 : 372-378.

GELB, A., and GOLDSTEIN, K., 1925, Ueber Farbennamenamnesie nebst Bemerkungen
uber das Wesen der amnestischen Aphasie ueberhaupt und die Beziehung zwischen
Sprache und dem Verhalten zur Umwelt. *Psychol. Forsch.* 6 : 127-186.

GERMAN, W. J., and FOX, J. C., 1932, Observations following unilateral lobectomies.
*Proc. A. Research Nerv. & Ment. Dis.* 13 : 378-434.

GIBBS, F. A., and GIBBS, E. L., 1941, Atlas of electroencephalography. Cambridge,
Mass., Leu A. Cummings Co.

GILLETTE, A. L., 1936, Learning and retention: a comparison of three experimental
procedures. *Arch. Psychol.* 28 (no. 198): 56.

GLORIG, A., and FOWLER, E. P., JR., 1947, Tests for labyrinth function following strep-
tomycin therapy. *Ann. Otlol., Rhin. & Laryng.* 56 : 379-392.

GOLDSTEIN, K., 1923, Die Funktionen des Stirnhirnes und ihre Bedeutung für die
Diagnose der Stirnhirnerkrankungen. *Med. Klin.* 19 : 965-969.

GOLDSTEIN, K., 1936, The problem of the meaning of words based upon observations
of aphasic patients. *J. Psychol.* 2 : 301-316.

GOLDSTEIN, K., 1936a, The modifications of behavior consequent to cerebral lesions.
*Psychiatric Quart.* 10 : 586-610.

GOLDSTEIN, K., 1936b, The significance of the frontal lobes for mental performances.
*J. Neurol. & Psychopath.* 17 : 27-40.

GOLDSTEIN, K., 1939, The organism. New York, American Book Company.

GOLDSTEIN, K., 1939a, The significance of special mental tests for diagnosis and
prognosis in schizophrenia. *Am. J. Psychiat.* 96 : 575-587.

GOLDSTEIN, K., 1940, Significance of speech disturbances for normal psychology. *Tr. New York Acad. Sc.* 2 : 159-163.

GOLDSTEIN, K., 1944, Methodological approach to the study of schizophrenic thought disorder. In J. S. Kasanin (Ed.) Language and thought in schizophrenia. Berkeley, University of California Press.

GOLDSTEIN, K., 1944a, The mental changes due to frontal lobe damage. *J. Psychol.* 17 : 187-208.

GOLDSTEIN, K., and SCHEERER, M., 1941, Abstract and concrete behavior. An experimental study with special tests. *Psychol. Monogr.* 53 : 151.

GOLTZ, F., 1881, Ueber die Verrichtungen des Grosshirns. *Arch. f.d. ges. Physiol.* 26 : 1-49.

GOMORI, G., 1939, Microtechnical demonstration of phosphatase in tissue sections. *Proc. Soc. Exper. Biol. & Med.* 42 : 23-26.

GOMORI, G., 1941a, Distribution of phosphatase in normal organs and tissues. *J. Cell. & Comp. Physiol.* 17 : 71-83.

GOMORI, G., 1941b, Distribution of acid phosphatase in the tissues under normal and under pathologic conditions. *Arch. Path.* 32 : 189-199.

GREISINGER, W., 1867, Mental pathology and therapeutics, translation by Robertson, C. L., and Rutherford, J. London, The New Sydenham Society.

GRIFFITH, F. R., JR., LOCKWOOD, J. E., and EMERY, F. E., 1938, Adrenalin and blood lactic acid: effect of evisceration. *Am. J. Physiol.* 123 : 432-440.

GRINKER, R. R., 1934, Neurology. Springfield, Ill., Charles C. Thomas.

GUTIERREZ-MAHONEY, C. C., DE, 1944, The treatment of painful phantom limb by the removal of the post-central cortex. *J. Neurosurgery*, 1 : 156-162.

HALSTEAD, W. C., 1940, Preliminary analysis of grouping behavior in patients with cerebral injury by the method of equivalent and non-equivalent stimuli. *Am. J. Psychiat.* 96 : 1263-1294.

HALSTEAD, W. C., 1947, Brain and intelligence. University Chicago Press.

HANSEN, H. C., 1946, Effect of electric convulsive therapy on the recall and recognition of previously learned paired associates. Master's Essay, Columbia University.

HARLOW, J. M., 1848, Passage of an iron rod through the head. *Boston M. & S. J.* 39 : 389-393. See also BIGELOW, H. J., 1850, Dr. Harlow's case of recovery from the passage of an iron bar through the head, *Am. J. Med. Sc.*, N. S. 20 : 14-22; and also HARLOW, J. M., 1869, Recovery from the passage of an iron bar through the head. Boston, D. Clapp and Son., p. 20.

HARLOW, J. M., 1868, Recovery from the passage of an iron bar through the head. *Publ. Mass. Med. Soc.* 2 : 329-346.

HARRIS, A. J., 1946, Harris tests of lateral dominance. New York, Psych. Corp.

HEBB, D. O., 1939, Intelligence in man after large removals of cerebral tissue: report of four left frontal lobe cases. *J. Gen. Psychol.* 21 : 73-87.

HEBB, D. O., 1945, Man's frontal lobes: a critical review. *Arch. Neurol. & Psychiat.* 54 : 10-24.

HEBB, D. O., and PENFIELD, W., 1940, Human behavior after extensive bilateral removal from the frontal lobes. *Arch. Neurol. & Psychiat.* 44 : 421-438.

HECHST, B., 1933, Beiträge zur Histopathologie der Schizophrenie. *Monatsch. f. Psychiat. u. Neurol.* 87 : 32-47.

HECHT, S., 1934, A handbook of general experimental psychology. Worcester, Mass., Clark University Press.

HECHT, S., and SMITH, E. L., 1936, Intermittent stimulation by light. VI. Area and the relation between critical frequency and intensity. *J. Gen. Physiol.* 19 : 979-989.

HERRICK, C. J., 1926, Brains of rats and men. Chicago, Illinois, University of Chicago Press.

HESSER, F. H., LANGWORTHY, O. R., and KOLB, L. C., 1941, Experimental study of gastric acidity released from cortical control. *J. Neurophysiol.* 4 : 274-283.

HITZIG, E., 1883, Zur Physiologie des Grosshirns, Wandervers. d. Südwestd. Neurol. u. Irrenärzte in Baden, 17 Juni, 1883. In *Arch. f. Psychiat.* 15 : 270-275, 1884.

HOAGLAND, H., and KAUFMAN, C. I., 1946, Dominant brain wave frequencies as measures of physio-chemical processes in cerebral cortex. *Arch. Neurol. & Psychiat.* 56 : 207-215.

HOFSTATTER, L., SMOLIK, E. A., and BUSCH, A. B., 1945, Prefrontal lobotomy in treatment of chronic psychoses. *Arch. Neurol. & Psychiat.* 53 : 125-130.

HOSKINS, R. G., 1946, The biology of schizophrenia. New York, W. W. Norton and Co., Inc.

HUEBNER, DOROTHY M., 1938, A comparative study of verbal associations of normal adults and schizophrenic patients in repetitions of the Kent-Rosanoff association test. Unpublished Master's Essay, Johns Hopkins University.

HULL, C. L., and LUGOFF, L. S., 1921, Complex signs in diagnostic free association. *J. Exper. Psychol.* 4 : 111-136.

HUNT, THELMA, 1942, Personality profile studies. In W. Freeman and J. W. Watts, Psychosurgery. Springfield, Ill., Charles C. Thomas.

HURSH, J. B., 1945, Origin of spike and wave pattern of petit mal epilepsy—An electroencephalographic study. *Arch. Neurol. & Psychiat.* 53 : 269-282.

HUTTON, E. L., 1947, Personality changes after leucotomy. *J. Ment. Sc.,* 93 : 31-42.

HYDÉN, H., and HARTELIUS, H., 1948, Stimulation of the nucleoprotein-production in the nerve cells by malononitrile and its effect on psychic functions in mental disorders. *Acta psychiat. et neurol.,* suppl. XLVIII, p. 117.

INGRAM, W. R., and BARRIS, R. W., 1936, Evidence of altered carbohydrate metabolism in cats with hypothalamic lesions. *Am. J. Physiol.* 114 : 562-571.

JACKSON, J. H., 1932, Selected writings of. Edited by James Taylor. London, Hodder and Stoughton, vol. 2, pp. 3-237.

JACOB, CRISTOFORO, 1941, Cytology of the frontal cortex. Folia neurobiólogica, Argentina, B. Air., A. Lopez.

JACOBSEN, C. F., 1935, Functions of frontal association area in primates. *Arch. Neurol. & Psychiat.* 33 : 558-569.

JACOBSEN, C. F., 1936, Studies of cerebral function in primates. I. The function of the frontal association areas in monkeys. *Comp. Psychol. Monogr.* 13 : 1-60.

JACOBSEN, C. F., and NISSEN, H. W., 1937, Studies of cerebral function in primates. IV. The effects of frontal lobe lesions on the delayed alternation habit in monkeys. *J. Comp. Psychol.* 23 : 101-12.

JACOBSEN, C. F., WOLFE, J. B., and JACKSON, T. A., 1935, An experimental analysis of the functions of the frontal association areas in primates. *J. Nerv. & Ment. Dis.* 82 : 1-14.

JANIS, I., 1949, Psychological effects of electric convulsive treatments, II. *J. Nerv. & Ment. Dis.* In press.

JASPER, H. H., and HAWKE, W. A., 1938, Electroencephalography. IV. Localization of seizure waves in epilepsy. *Arch. Neurol. & Psychiat.* 39 : 885-901.

JASPER, H. H., KERSHMAN, J., and ELVIDGE, A., 1944, Electroencephalographic studies of injury to the head. *Arch. Neurol. & Psychiat.* 44 : 328-348.

JASTROWITZ, M., 1888, Beiträge zur Localisation im Grosshirn und über deren praktische Verwerthung. *Deutsche med. Wchnschr.* 14 : 81-83, 108-112, 125-128, 151-153, 172-175, 188-192, 209-211, see p. 111.

JEFFERSON, G., 1937, Removal of right or left frontal lobes in man. *Brit. M. J.* 2 : 199-206.

JOSEPHY, H., 1930, Dementia praecox (Schizophrenia). Handbuch der Geisteskrankheiten (O. Bumke), VII. Die Anatomie der Psychosen. Berlin, J. Springer.

JUNG, C. G., 1918, Studies in word association. London, William Heinemann.

KENNARD, M. A., 1939, Alterations in response to visual stimuli following lesions of frontal lobe in monkeys. *Arch. Neurol. & Psychiat.* 41 : 1153-1165.

KENNARD, M. A., 1943, Electroencephalogram of decorticate monkeys. *J. Neurophysiol.* 6 : 233-241.

KENNARD, M. A., and NIMS, L. F., 1942, Effect of electroencephalogram of lesions of cerebral cortex and basal ganglia in Macaca mulatta. *J. Neurophysiol.* 5 : 335-348.

KENT, G. H., and ROSANOFF, A. J., 1910, A study of association in insanity. *Am. J. Insan.* 67 : 37-96, 317-390.

KENT, G. H., and ROSANOFF, A. J., 1920, Free association test. In A. J. Rosanoff, Manual of psychiatry, 5th ed. New York, John Wiley.

KIRSCHBAUM, W. R., and HEILBRUNN, G., 1944, Biopsies of the brain of schizophrenic patients and experimental animals. *Arch. Neurol. & Psychiat.* 51 : 155-162.

KISKER, G. W., 1943, Remarks on the problem of psychosurgery. *Am. J. Psychiat.* 100 : 180-184.

KISKER, G. W., 1944, Abstract and categorical behavior following therapeutic brain surgery. *Psychosom. Med.* 6 : 146-150.

KISKER, G. W., 1945, The behavior sequelae of neurosurgical therapy: bilateral prefrontal lobotomy. *J. Gen. Psychol.* 33 : 171-192.

KLOPFER, D., and KELLEY, D. H., 1942, The Rorschach technique. Yonkers, World Book Co.

KNOX, G. W., 1945, The effect of practice, under the influence of various attitudes, on the CFF. *J. Gen. Psychol.* 33 : 121-129.

KOBLER, F., 1938, Histologischer Gehirnbefund nach Insulin Coma. *Arch. f. Psychiat.* 107 : 688-700.

KOHS, S. C., 1914, The association method in its relation to the complex and complex indicators. *Am. J. Psychol.* 25 : 544-594.

KRAMER, B., and GITTLEMAN, I., 1924-5, An iodometric method for the determination of sodium in small amounts of serum. *J. Biol. Chem.* 62 : 353-360.

KRAMER, B., and TISDALL, F. F., 1921, A clinical method for the quantitative determination of potassium in small amounts of serum. *J. Biol. Chem.* 46 : 339-349.

KREHT, H., 1936, Cytoarchitektonic und motorisches Sprachzentrum. *Ztschr. f. mikr.-anat. Forsch.* 39 : 351-54; and Zur Volumengrösse der architekonischen Felder 55-66 einiger menschlichen Gehirne in Vergleich zu der des Schimpansen und Orang-Utan. *ibid.* 409-14.

LASHLEY, K. S., 1929, Brain mechanisms and intelligence. Chicago, University of Chicago Press.

LASHLEY, K. S., 1938, The thalamus and emotion. *Psychol. Rev.* 45 : 42-61.

LASHLEY, K. S., and CLARK, G., 1946, Cytoarchitecture of cerebral cortex of Ateles; critical examination of architectonic studies. *J. Comp. Neurol.* 85 : 223-305.

LE BEAU, J., and GAETANO DE BARROS, MANOEL, 1948, Bilateral removal of some frontal areas (topectomy). Program, Int'nl. Conf. on Psychosurg., pp. unnumb.

LE GROS CLARK, W. E., 1948, The connexions of the frontal lobes of the brain. *Lancet* 254 : 353-356.

LEPPIEN, R., and PETERS, G., 1937, Todesfall infolge Insulinshockbehandlung bei einem Schizophrenen (klinische und pathologisch—anatomische Beschreibung) *Ztschr. f.d. ges Neurol. u. Psychiat.* 160 : 444-454.

LEWIS, J. T. and TURCATTI, E. S., 1935, abstr. le diabete pancréatique chez le chien prive du systeme nerveux sympathique. *Compt. rend. Soc. de biol.* 120 : 274-276.

LEWY, ALFRED, 1947, The symptomatology of vertigo. *Ann. Otol. Rhin. & Laryng.* 56 : 534-540.

LEYDEN, E., and JASTROWITZ, M., 1888, Beiträge zur Lehre von der Localisation im Gehirn. Leipzig, Thieme, p. 82.

LIDZ, T., 1939, A study of the effect of right frontal lobectomy on intelligence and temperament. *J. Neurol. & Psychiat.* 2 : 211-222.

LILLIE, R. D., ASHBURN, L. L., SEBRELL, W. H., DAFT, F. S., and LOWRY, J. V., 1942, Histogenesis and repair of the hepatic cirrhosis in rats produced on low protein diets and preventable with choline. *U.S. Public Health Rep.* 57 : 502-508.

LINDSAY, J. H., 1945, The significance of a positional nystagmus in oto-neurological diagnosis. *Laryngoscope* 55 : 527-551.

LIVINGSTONE, W. K., 1943, Pain mechanisms. New York, The Macmillan Company.

LOEB, J., 1902, Comparative physiology of the brain and comparative psychology. New York, G. P. Putnam Sons.

LYNN, J. G., LEVINE, K. N., and HEWSON, L. R., 1945, Psychologic tests for the clinical evaluation of late 'diffuse organic,' 'neurotic' and 'normal' reactions after closed head injury. *Proc. A. Research Nerv. & Ment. Dis.* 24 : 296-378.

McNALLY, W. J., 1947, The physiology of the vestibular mechanism in relation to vertigo. *Ann. Otol., Rhin. & Laryng.* 56 : 514-533.

MARBURG, O., 1924, Bemerkungen zu den pathologischen Veränderungen der Hirnrinde bei Psychosen. *Arb. neur. Inst. Wien* 26 : 245-251.

MARCHAND, L., 1928, Lésions de l'encéphale dans un cas de psychose périodique. *Bull. soc. clin. de méd. ment.* 16 : 176-179.

MARCUS, H., 1936, Etudes sur l'histopathologie de la démenca précoce. *Acta med. Scandinav.* 87 : 365-401.

MARIE, P., 1906, Revision de la question de l'aphasie: la troisième circonvolution frontale gauche ne joue aucun rôle spécial dans la fonction du language. *La sem. med., Paris* 26 : 241-247; see also pp. 343, 493-500, 563, 565-571, 574, 610.

MARMOR, J., and SAVITSKY, N. J., 1940, Electroencephalogram in cases of head injury. *Tr. Am. Neurol. A.* pp. 30-34.

MEAKINS, J. C., 1940, Hypoglycemia following encephalitis. *Ann. Int. Med.* 13 : 1830-1836.

MEDUNA, L. J., GERTZ, F. J., and URSE, V. G., 1942, Biochemical disturbances in mental disorders; anti-insulin effect of blood in cases of schizophrenia, *Arch. Neurol. & Psychiat.* 47 : 38-52.

METTLER, C. C., 1947, History of medicine. Philadelphia, The Blakiston Company.

METTLER, FRED A., 1942, Neuroanatomy. St. Louis, The C. V. Mosby Company.

METTLER, FRED A., 1943, Reticulocytosis following ablation of frontal cerebral cortex. *Arch. Surg.* 46 : 572-574.

METTLER, FRED A., 1944, Physiologic effects of bilateral simultaneous frontal lesions in the primate. *J. Comp. Neurol.* 81 : 105-136.

METTLER, FRED A., 1947, Extracortical connections of the primate frontal cerebral cortex. I. Thalamo-cortical connections. *J. Comp. Neurol.* 86 : 95-117.

METTER, FRED A., 1947a, Extracortical connections of the primate frontal cerebral cortex. II. Corticifugal connections, *J. Comp. Neurol.* 86 : 119-166.

METTLER, FRED A., 1948, The nonpyramidal motor projections from the frontal cerebral cortex. The frontal lobes, Res. Monogr. *A. Research Nerv. & Ment. Dis.* 27 : 162-200.

METTLER, FRED A., 1948a, Question in The frontal lobe. Res. Monogr. *A. Research Nerv. & Ment. Dis.* 27 : 607.

METTLER, FRED A., FINCH, G., GIRDEN, E. and CULLER, E. A., 1934, Acoustic value of the several components of the auditory pathway. *Brain* 57 : 475-483.

METTLER, FRED A., and METTLER, C. C., 1940, Labyrinthine disregard after removal of the caudate. *Proc. Soc. Exper. Biol. & Med.* 45 : 473-475.

METTLER, FRED A., and METTLER, C. C., 1942, The effects of striatal injury. *Brain* 65 : 242-255.

METTLER, FRED A., and ROWLAND, LEWIS P., 1948, Relation of the trephine opening (Freeman-Watts lobotomy point) to the underlying cerebrum. *Tr. Am. Neurol. As.* 73 meeting, 156-158.

METTLER, F., SPINDLER, J., METTLER, C. C., and COMBS, J. D., 1936, Disturbance in gastrointestinal function after localized ablations of cerebral cortex. *Arch. Surg.* 32 : 618-623.

METTLER, LEE H., 1904, A treatise on diseases of the nervous system. Chicago, Cleveland Press, see p. 747.

MEYER, F., 1934, Anatomisch-histologische Untersuchungen an schizophrenen. *Monatschr. f. Psychiat. u. Neurol.* 88 : 265-323.

MEYER, F., 1935, Anatomisch-histologische Untersuchungen an Manisch-Depressiven. *Monatschr. f. Psychiat. u. Neurol.* 91 : 137-159.

MILHORAT, A. T., SMALL, S. M., and DIETHELM, O., 1942, Leucocytosis during various emotional states. *Arch. Neurol. & Psychol.* 47 : 779-792.

MISIAK, H., 1947, Age and sex differences in critical flicker frequency. *J. Exper. Psychol.* 37 : 318-332.

MISKOLCZY, D., 1933, Über das anatomische Korrelat des schizophrenie. *Ztschr. f.d. ges. Neurol. u. Psychiat.* 147 : 509-554.

MISKOLCZY, 1937, Die örtliche Verteilung der Gehirnveränderungen bei der Schizophrenie. *Ztschr. f.d. ges. Neurol. u. Psychiat.* 158 : 203-208.

MIXTER, W. J., TILLOTSON, K. J., and WIES, D., 1941, Reports of partial frontal lobectomy and frontal lobotomy performed on three patients: one chronic epileptic and two cases of chronic agitated depression. *Psychosom. Med.* 3 : 26-37.

MONIZ, EGAS, 1936, Les premières tentatives opératoires dans le traitement de certaines psychoses. *Encéphale,* 31 (no. 2) : 1-29.

MORGAN, C. T., 1943, Physiological psychology, chapter X. New York, McGraw-Hill.

MORGAN, L. O., VONDERAHE, A. R., and MALONE, E. F., 1937, Pathological changes in the hypothalamus in diabetes millitus. A study of fifteen cases. *J. Nerv. & Ment. Dis.* 85 : 125-138.

MORISON, R. S., and BASSETT, D. L., 1945, Electrical activity of the thalamus and basal ganglia in decorticate cats. *J. Neurophysiol.* 8 : 309-314.

MOTT, F. W., 1919, Studies in the pathology of dementia praecox. *Proc. Roy. Soc. Med.* 13 (sect. of psychiat.) : 25-63.

MOUTIER, F., 1908, L'Aphasie de Broca. Paris, G. Steinheil, 774 pp.

MUNK, H., 1890, Ueber die Funktionen der Grosshirnrinde: gesammelte Mittheilungen mit Anmerkungen. Berlin, A. Hirschwald.

NAITO, I., 1924, Das Hirnrindenbild bei Schizophrenie. *Arb. neur. Inst. Wien.* 26 : 1-156.

NAÑAGAS, J. C., 1923, Anatomical studies on the motor cortex of Macacus rhesus. *J. Comp. Neurol.* 35 : 67-96.

NICHOLS, I. C., and HUNT, J. M., 1940, Case of partial bilateral frontal lobectomy: A psychopathological study. *Am. J. Psychiat.* 96 : 1063-1083.

NOBELE, 1835, Annal. de méd. belge, Février, Compte rendu, cited by H. Haeser, 1836, Fall einer bedeutenden Gehirnverletzung. Schmidt's Jahrbücher 9 : 321-322.

NOLTIE, H. R., 1938, The effect of pontine transection on the blood-sugar level of the decerebrated fasting cat. *Quart. J. Exper. Physiol.,* 28 : 99-114.

NYLÉN, C. O., 1939, The oto-neurological diagnosis of the brain. *Acta oto-laryng.,* Suppl. 33 : 5-151.

ORBISON, W. D., 1946, In D. Rapaport, 1946, Diagnostic psychological testing. vol. II, Chicago, Yearbook Publ.

OPPENHEIM, H., 1900, Diseases of the nervous system, translated by E. E. Mayer. Philadelphia, J. B. Lippincott, see p. 399.

PAPEZ, J. W., 1937, Proposed mechanism of emotion. *Arch. Neurol. & Psychiat.* 38 : 725-743.

PENFIELD, W., and CONE, W., 1926, Acute swelling of oligodendroglia. A specific type of neuroglial change. *Arch. Neurol. & Psychiat.* 16 : 131-153.

PENFIELD, W., and ERICKSON, T. C., 1941, Epilepsy and cerebral localization. Jasper, H. H.: Electroencephalography. Charles C Thomas, Springfield, Ill.

PENFIELD, W., and RASMUSSEN, T., 1947, Localization and arrest of speech. *Tr. Am. Neurol. As.* pp. 62-63, see discussion p. 64.

PENROSE, L. S., 1944, An economical method of presenting matrix intelligence tests. *Brit. J. M. Psychol.* 20 : 144-146.

PETERS, G., 1937, Zur Frage der pathologischen Anatomie der Schizophrenie. *Ztschr. f.d. ges. Neurol. u. Psychiat.* 160 : 361-380.

PETERS, JOHN P., and VAN SLYKE, DONALD D., 1946, Quantitative clinical chemistry, interpretations, vol. I, 2nd ed., Baltimore, Williams & Wilkins Co.

PETERSEN, F., 1939, Beobachtungen und Erfahrungen bei der Behandlung der Schizophrenie mit Cardiazol. *Allg. Ztschr. f. Psychiat.* 111 : 366-388.

PETERSEN, M. C., and BUCHSTEIN, H. F., 1947, Prefrontal lobotomy in chronic psychosis. *Am. J. Psychiat.* 104 : 426-430.

PEYTON, W. T., NORAN, H. N., and MILLER, E. W., 1948, Prefrontal lobectomy (excision of the anterior areas of the cerebrum). *Am. J. Psychiat.* 104 : 513-523.

POPPELREUTER, W., 1917, Die psychischen Schädigungen durch Kopfschuss. Band I. Leipzig, Voss.

PORTEUS, S. D., 1933, The maze test and mental differences. Vineland, N. J., Smith.

PORTEUS, S. D., 1942, Qualitative performance on the maze test. Vineland, New Jersey, Smith.

PORTEUS, S. D., and KEPNER, R. M., 1944, Mental changes after bilateral prefrontal lobotomy. *Genet. Psychol. Monogr.* 29 : 4-115.

PORTEUS, S. D., and PETERS, H., 1947, Maze test validation and psychosurgery. *Genet. Psychol. Monogr.* 36 : 3-86.

RAPAPORT, D., 1946, Diagnostic psychological testing, vol. II. Chicago, Yearbook Publ. Co.

RAVEN, J. G., 1941-1943, Standardization of progressive matrices. *Brit. J. M. Psychol.* 19 : 137-150.

REED, J. A., 1948, A study of gastric acids in prefrontal lobotomy. *Gastro-enterol.* 10 : 118-119.

RICHTER, C. P., and HINES, M., 1938, Increased spontaneous activity produced in monkey by brain lesions. *Brain* 61 : 1-16.

ROBERTI, C. E., 1931a, Contributo allo studeo del comportamento della nevroglia e degli elementi nervosi nelle sindromi mentali tossiche (amenza e demenza precoce iniziale). *Rassegna di studi psichiat.* 20 : 30-56.

ROBERTI, C. E., 1931b, Contributo allo studeo della microglia nei malati di mente (amenti e dementi prococi). *Riv. di pat. nerv.* 38 : 461-482.

ROBINSON, M. F., 1946, What price lobotomy? *J. Abnorm. & Social Psychol.* 41 : 421-436.

ROEDER-KUTSCH, T., 1939, Zur Frage der pathologischen Anatomie der schizophrenie. *Allg. Ztschr. f. Psychiat.* 112 : 63-74.

ROMANO, J., and COON, G. P., 1942, Physiologic and psychologic studies in spontaneous hypoglycemia, *Psychosom. Med.* 4 : 283-300.

ROTHMANN, E., 1934, Untersuchung eines Falles von umschriebener Hirnschadigung mit Stoerungen auf verschiedensten Leistungsgebieten. *Schweiz. Arch. f. Neurol. u. Psychiat.* 33 : 228-241.

ROWLAND, L. P., and METTLER, FRED A., 1948, Relation between the coronal suture and cerebrum. *J. Comp. Neurol.* 89 : 21-40.

RUBIN, E., 1921, Visuell wahrgenommene Figuren. Kopenhagen, Gyldendalski.

RUST, R. M., 1948, Some correlates of the movement response. *J. Personality.* In press.

RYLANDER, G., 1939, Personality changes after operations on the frontal lobes. *Acta psychiat. et neurol.*, suppl. 20 : 3-327.

RYLANDER, G., 1943, Mental changes after excision of cerebral tissue. *Acta psychiat. et neurol.*, suppl. 25 : 1-81.

SAKEL, M., 1935, Neue Behandlungsmethode der Schizophrenie. Vienna.

SCARFF, J. E., 1948, Unilateral prefrontal lobotomy with relief of ipsilateral, contralateral and bilateral pain. *J. Neurosurg.* 5 : 288-293. See also Koskoff in The Frontal Lobes. Res. Monogr. A. *Research Nerv. & Ment. Dis.* 27, 1948.

SCARFF, J. E., and RAHM, W. E., JR., 1941, The human electrocorticogram. *J. Neurophysiol.* 4 : 418-426.

SCIAMANNA, R., 1901, See abstract, Sur l'existence d'un centre moteur graphique. *Rev. neurol.* 9 : 1162. Sharp, H. C. and Baganz, C. N., 1940, A study of the problem of malnutrition in institutionalized psychotic patients. *Am. J. Psychiat.* 97 : 650-658.

SHARP, H. C. and BAGANZ, C. N., 1940, A study of the problem of malnutrition in institutionalized psychotic patients. *Am. J. Psychiat.* 97 : 650-658.

SHEEHAN, D., 1934, The effects of cortical stimulation on gastric movements in the monkey. *J. Physiol.* 83 : 177-184.

SIOLI, F., 1909, Histologische Befunde bei der Dementia praecox. *Allg. Ztschr. f. Psychiat.* 66 : 195-196.

SMITH, W. K., 1945, The functional significance of the rostral cingular cortex as revealed by its responses to electrical stimulation. *J. Neurophysiol.* 8 : 241-255.

SOLOMON, H. C., 1948, Prefrontal leukotomy, an evaluation. Veterans Admin. Techn. Bull., T. B. 10-46, May 21, p. 6.

SPEARMAN, C., 1927, The abilities of man. New York, The Macmillan Company.

SPIELMEYER, W., 1931, The problem of the anatomy of schizophrenia. A. Research Nerv. & Ment. Dis. vol. 10 (Schizophrenia). Baltimore, Williams and Wilkins.

STOOKEY, B., SCARFF, J. E., and TEITELBAUM, M. H., 1941, Frontal lobectomy in treatment of brain tumors. *Ann. Surg.* 113 : 161-169.

STRAUSS, I., and KESCHNER, M., 1935, Mental symptoms in cases of tumor of the frontal lobes. *Arch. Neurol. & Psychiat.* 33 : 986-1007.

STROM-OLSEN, R., LAST, S. L., BRODY, M. B., and KNIGHT, G. C., 1943, Results of prefrontal leucotomy in 30 cases of mental disorders. *J. Ment. Sc.* 89 : 165-181.

SWEET, W. H., KOTZIAS, G. C., SEED, J., and YAKOVLEV, P., 1948, Gastrointestinal hemorrhages, hyperglycemia, azotemia, hyperchloremia, and hypernatremia following lesions of the frontal lobe in man. In The Frontal Lobes. Res. Monogr. A. *Research Nerv. & Ment. Dis.* 27 : 795-822.

TEUBER, H., and BENDER, M., 1948, CFF in defective fields of vision. *Fed. Proc.* 7 : 123-124.

THOMPSON, J., 1941, The ability of children of different grade levels to generalize on sorting tests. *J. Psychol.* 11 : 119-126.

THURSTONE, L. L., 1938, Primary mental abilities. Psychometri. Monogr., No. 1.

THURSTONE, L. L., 1943, Factorial studies of perception. Chicago, University of Chicago Press.

THURSTONE, L. L., 1947, Multiple-factor analysis. Chicago, University of Chicago Press.

TIGGES, W., 1889, Das Gewicht des Gehirns und seiner Theile bei Geisteskranken. *Allg. Ztschr. f. Psychiat.* 45 : 97-223.

TYCHOWSKI, W. Z., and CROWELL, C., 1926, Pressure on the central nervous system in its relation to hyperglycemia: chronic piqure. *Arch. Int. Med.* 37 : 567.

VOGT, C., and VOGT, O., 1919, Allgemeinere Ergebnisse unserer Hirnforschung. *J. f. Psychol. u. Neurol.* Bd. 25, S. 277-462.

VOGT, C., and VOGT, O., 1922, Erkrankungen der Grosshirnrinde im Lichte der Topistik Pathoklise und Pathoarchitektonic. *J. f. Psychol. u. Neurol.* 28 : 1-171.

VON BONIN, G., 1944, Architecture of the precentral motor cortex and some adjacent areas, in The precentral motor cortex. *Univ. of Ill. Monogr. in Med. Sc.* 4 : 7-82.

VON BONIN, G., and BAILEY, P., 1947, The neocortex of Macaca mulatta. *Univ. of Ill. Monogr. in Med. Sc.*, vol. 5.

VONDERAHE, A. R., 1937, Central nervous system and sugar metabolism. Clinical, pathologic and theoretical considerations, with special reference to diabetes mellitus. *Arch. Int. Med.* 60 : 694-704.

VOTH, A. C., 1947, An experimental study of mental patients through the autokinetic phenomenon. *Am. J. Psychiat.* 103 : 793-805.

WADA, T., 1910, Beiträge zur pathologischen Anatomie einiger Psychosen. *Arb. neur. Inst. Wien* 18 : 313-345.

WALTER, F. K., 1919, Beiträge zur Histopathologie der endogenen verblödungen. *Ztschr. f.d. ges Neurol. u. psychiat.* 47 : 112-127.

WALTER, W. C., 1936, The location of cerebral tumors by electroencephalography. *Lancet* 2 : 305-308.

WALTER, W. G., and DOVEY, V. L., 1944, Electroencephalography in cases of subcortical tumor. *J. Neurol., Neurosurg. & Psychiat.* 7 : 57-65.

WARD, A. A. JR., 1948, The cingular gyrus; area 24. *J. Neurophysiol.* 11 : 13-23.

WATANABE, M., 1934, Beiträge zur Histopathologie des Gehirns von Dementia praecox. *Jap. J. M.Sc. VIII, Int. Med. Pediat. & Psychiat.* 3 : 97-107.

WATTS, J. W., and FULTON, J. F., 1934, Intussusception—studies on intestinal motility. *New England J. Med.* 210 : 883-896.

WECHSLER, D., 1944, Measurement of adult intelligence. Baltimore, Williams & Wilkins.

WEGROCKI, H. J., 1940, Generalizing ability in schizophrenia. *Arch. Psychol.* 36 (no. 254) : 76.

WEIGL, E., 1941, On the psychology of so-called processes of abstraction. *J. Abnorml. & Soc. Psychol.* 36 : 3-33.

WEIL, A., LIEBERT, E., and HEILBRUNN, G., 1938, Histopathologic changes in the brain in experimental hyperinsulinism. *Arch. Neurol. & Psychiat.* 39 : 467-481.

WEIL, A., and LIEBERT, E., 1940, Neuropathologic study of six cases of psychoses in which metrazol was used. *Arch. Neurol. & Psychiat.* 44 : 1031-1043.

WEISENBURG, T., and McBRIDE, K. E., 1935, Aphasia: A clinical and psychological study. New York, The Commonwealth Fund.

WELT, L., 1888, Ueber Charakterveränderungen des Menschen infolge von Läsionen des Stirnhirns. *Deutsches Arch. f. klin. Med. von Ziemssen* 42 : 339-390.

WILLIAMS, D., and GIBBS, F. A., 1939, Electroencephalography in clinical neurology. *Arch. Neurol. & Psychiat.* 41 : 519-534.

WILLIAMSON, R. T., 1896, On the symptomatology of gross lesions (tumors and abscesses) involving the praefrontal region of the brain. *Brain* 19 : 346-365.

WOLF, A., KABAT, E. A., and NEWMAN, W., 1943, Histochemical studies on tissue enzymes. III. A study of the distribution of acid phosphatases with special reference to the nervous system. *Am. J. Path.* 19 : 423-439.

WOODWORTH, R. S., 1938, Experimental psychology. New York, Holt.

WOOLLEY, E. J. S., 1936, Glycosuria and acetonuria in subarachnoid haemorrhage. A report of four cases. *Lancet* 1 : 894-896.

YEAGER, C. L., and LUSE, S., 1945, Electroencephalographic localization and differentiation of lesions of frontal lobes: pathological confirmation. *Arch. Neurol. & Psychiat.* 54 : 197-201.

ZEAMAN, JEAN, 1947, Effects of shock therapy on performance on the word association test. Unpublished Master's essay, Columbia University.

ZIMMERMANN, R., 1915, Beitrag zur Histologie der Dementia praecox. *Ztschr. f.d. ges. Neurol. u. Psychiat.* 30 : 354-378.

ZINGERLE, H., 1910, Zur pathologischen Anatomie des Dementia praecox. *Monatschr. f. Psychiat.* 27 : 285-321.

# INDEX

515